Series in Laboratory Medicine
Leo P. Cawley, M.D., Series Editor

Serum Protein Abnormalities

Diagnostic and Clinical Aspects

Serum Protein Abnormalities
Diagnostic and Clinical Aspects

Edited by

Stephan E. Ritzmann, M.D.

Clinical Professor of Medicine, University of
California, Irvine, California College of Medicine,
Irvine, California; Director, Consultation Laboratories,
Behring Diagnostics, Somerville, New Jersey
Formerly, Professor of Medicine and Pathology and
Director, Division of Experimental Immunology,
Department of Medicine, The University of Texas
Medical Branch at Galveston, Galveston, Texas

Jerry C. Daniels, M.D., Ph.D.

Assistant Professor of Internal Medicine and Chief,
Section of Clinical Immunology, Department of
Medicine, The University of Texas Medical Branch
at Galveston, Galveston, Texas
Formerly, Research Fellow, Department of
Medicine, Harvard Medical School and Robert
Breck Brigham Hospital, Boston, Massachusetts

Little, Brown and Company   Boston

Contributing Authors

Gerald A. Beathard, M.D., Ph.D., F.A.C.P.
Associate Professor, Departments of Internal Medicine and Pathology,
The University of Texas Medical Branch at Galveston, Galveston, Texas

Ludwig H. Bonacker, Ph.D.
Director, Diagnostics Research and Development, Behring Diagnostics,
American Hoechst Corporation, Somerville, New Jersey

Jerry C. Daniels, M.D., Ph.D.
Assistant Professor of Internal Medicine and Chief, Section of Clinical
Immunology, Department of Medicine, The University of Texas Medical Branch
at Galveston, Galveston, Texas; Formerly, Research Fellow, Department of
Medicine, Harvard Medical School and Robert Breck Brigham Hospital, Boston,
Massachusetts

Craig L. Fischer, M.D.
Head, Department of Pathology, and Director, Clinical Laboratories,
Eisenhower Medical Center, Palm Desert, California

Charles W. Gill, M.S.
Research Associate, Department of Immunology, Eisenhower Medical Center,
Palm Desert, California

Richard C. Hevey, Ph.D.
Research Associate, Behring Diagnostics, American Hoechst Corporation,
Somerville, New Jersey

Harumi Kuno-Sakai, M.D., D.M.Sc.
Research Scientist, Section of Clinical Immunology,
Department of Medicine, The University of Texas Medical Branch at Galveston,
Galveston, Texas

Monica Lawrence, M.T. (A.S.C.P.), S.B.B.
Supervisor, Immunodiagnostics Laboratory, Division of Experimental Immunology,
Department of Medicine, The University of Texas Medical Branch at Galveston,
Galveston, Texas

William C. Levin, M.D.

President, The University of Texas Medical Branch at Galveston, and Professor, Department of Internal Medicine, the University of Texas Medical Branch at Galveston, Galveston, Texas

Robert M. Nakamura, M.D.

Department of Molecular Immunology, Scripps Clinic and Research Foundation; Head, Department of Pathology, The Hospital of Scripps Clinic, La Jolla, California; Adjunct Professor of Pathology, University of California, San Diego, School of Medicine, La Jolla, California

Stephan E. Ritzmann, M.D.

Clinical Professor of Medicine, University of California, Irvine, California College of Medicine, Irvine, California; Director, Consultation Laboratories, Behring Diagnostics, Somerville, New Jersey; Formerly, Professor of Medicine and Pathology and Director, Division of Experimental Immunology, Department of Medicine, The University of Texas Medical Branch at Galveston, Galveston, Texas

Ernest S. Tucker, III, M.D.

Associate Clinical Professor of Pathology and Pediatrics, University of California, San Diego School of Medicine, La Jolla, California; Director of Laboratories, Immunodiagnostics, Inc., San Diego, California

Robert E. Wolf, M.D., Ph.D.

Research Associate, Dallas Veterans Administration Hospital, and Assistant Professor of Medicine, The University of Texas Health Science Center at Dallas Southwestern Medical School, Dallas, Texas

Preface

The history of many classic disciplines has shown periods of extraordinary ferment accompanied by logarithmic increases in verifiable knowledge. A decade ago it became evident that proteinology and immunology, encompassing such diverse disciplines as biochemistry, cell physiology, physics, genetics, and anthropology, were, and still are, in such a logarithmic phase. Immunology has become an established discipline in its own right; it has provided insight into the biological roles of proteins, such as the immunoglobulins, and has produced the modern diagnostic tools that aid in the detection and characterization of numerous proteins and their clinical effects. Many of the major advances of the past ten years are presently in clinical use for the benefit of our professional "raison d'être"–the patient; many more are potentially applicable and clinically relevant.

This book provides the personnel involved in health care delivery with a distillation and integration of current information on serum proteins and their counterparts in other biological fluids and on the related clinical and immunological aspects in a practical and selective, rather than an encyclopedic, fashion. The book is supplemented profusely with illustrations.

Foremost among the potential audience of this book is the clinician, but a broader audience–medical students, house officers, and practicing physicians–will find a spectrum of useful information and presentations. It is hoped that the book will prove useful as well for clinical pathologists, medical technologists, and other laboratory personnel. However, the intended emphasis is on the relationship between human disease, pathophysiology, and immunobiology as they relate to diagnosis, therapy, and prevention. Illustrated case reports are utilized to create condensed, albeit idealized, views of the protein functions with associated clinical disorders. We sincerely hope that the busy professional charged with the responsibility for patient care will find this book a useful addition to his armamentarium and a reliable companion in times of need.

S. E. R.
J. C. D.

Acknowledgments

Acknowledgments are due the Departments of Medicine and Pathology of The University of Texas Medical Branch at Galveston, which supported Stephan E. Ritzmann, and the Robert Breck Brigham Hospital of Harvard Medical School, Boston, which supported Jerry C. Daniels during the preparation of this book.

Acknowledgments are also due the contributing authors for their cooperation and for sharing their expertise with their colleagues in the medical community; to our editorial secretary, Mrs. Sandra Scales, for her dedicated, resourceful, and diligent supervision of the laborious tasks of manuscript preparation, collation, proofreading, and revision; to Mr. Edmund Stephenson for his unique insight and perception in providing medical illustrations as a uniform texture of presentation and for the countless hours he invested in bridging the gap of communication between authors and readers through his illustrations; to Mrs. Betty Herr Hallinger for her excellent indexing of the book; and finally to Little, Brown and Company for providing useful editorial assistance in order to unify diverse chapter presentations.

Contents

II Serum Protein Abnormalities

Introduction

Stephan E. Ritzmann and Jerry C. Daniels

Berzelius first used the term *protein* in 1838. In the words of Berzelius, "Protein (from Greek—*proteios*—of the first rank) is that important component of living matter without which life would not be possible." Initially, it was assumed that there was only one protein in all living matter, including plants and animals. With the advancement of analytical methodology, however, more and more different proteins have been recognized. The term *serum protein* now refers to a large, heterogeneous assortment of individual proteins. More than 100 serum proteins have been identified, but, at present, the functions of only about 40 of these have been elucidated (see Appendix).

Clinically useful techniques for the determination of the total serum protein concentration were introduced by modifying Kjeldahl's assays for nitrogen [1, 2]. The systematic study of serum proteins was facilitated by Howe's precipitation technique and its modifications [3], which utilizes sodium sulfate to salt out several protein fractions. By employing various concentrations of sodium sulfate, three fractions were identified: albumin, euglobulin (i.e., globulin precipitable with distilled water [4]), and pseudoglobulins [5]. The two globulins identified by this technique are now of historical interest only, but occasionally these terms still arise in clinical discussions and in the literature (e.g., the euglobulin lysis test or euglobulin test [6]). The now obsolete albumin-globulin (A/G) ratio is also based upon this precipitation technique.

With the introduction of the moving-boundary, or "free" electrophoresis, device by Tiselius [7], the serum proteins could be fractionated on the basis of their electrical charge at a particular pH. This technique allowed the delineation of four major protein groups, namely, albumin, α-globulin, β-globulin, and γ-globulin. The pseudoglobulin fraction that had been identified by the Howe precipitation technique was found by moving-boundary electrophoresis to be composed of about 85 percent α-globulin and 15 percent γ-globulin. The euglobulin that had been precipitated by the Howe technique was found to be composed of less α-globulin but more β- and γ-globulins. The subsequent use of zone electrophoretic methods (e.g., paper [8, 9] and cellulose-acetate [10, 11] electrophoresis) has resulted in even further distinctions among the serum protein fractions. These methods enabled the subdivision into α_1-

Table 1. Methodology of Serum Protein Analysis

Technique	Author(s)	Year	Reference	Sensitivity (per 100 ml)	Fractions, Terms
Total serum protein determination (TSP)					
Modified Kjeldahl method	Cullen and Van Slyke	1920	[1]	0.1 gm	1 Fraction: TSP
	Kabat and Mayer	1961	[2]	0.1 gm	
Biuret method	Kingsley	1939	[21]	0.1 gm	
	Kingsley and Getchell	1957	[22]	0.1 gm	
Refractometry	Reiss	1902	[23]	0.1 gm	
	Naumann	1964	[24]	0.1 gm	
Salting-out techniques					
Sodium sulfate precipitation	Howe	1921	[3]	0.1 gm	2 Fractions: albumin and globulin (TSP minus albumin)
Methanol precipitation	Pillemer and Hutchinson	1945	[25]	0.1 gm	
Analytical ultracentrifugation (UC)	Svedberg and Pederson	1940	[12]	0.1 gm	3 Fractions: 4.5S, 7S, and 19S components
Protein electrophoresis (PE)					
Free boundary electrophoresis	Tiselius	1937	[7]	0.1 gm	4 Fractions: albumin, α-, β-, and γ-globulins
Filter-paper electrophoresis	König	1937	[8]	0.1 gm	5 Fractions: albumin, α_1-, α_2-, β-, γ-globulins
	Durrum	1958	[9]	0.1 gm	
Cellulose-acetate electrophoresis	Kohn	1957	[10]	0.1 gm	5 Fractions: albumin, α_1-, α_2-, β-, γ-globulins

Method	Author	Year	Ref.	Sensitivity	Application
Qualitative immunoelectrophoresis (IEP)	Grabar and Williams	1953	[13]	10 mg	Demonstration of more than 30 fractions
	Scheidegger	1955	[26]	10 mg	Demonstration of more than 30 fractions
Quantitative immunoelectrophoresis	Ressler	1960	[27]	3 mg	Quantitation of more than 20 protein fractions
	Clark and Freeman	1968	[28]	3 mg	Quantitation of more than 30 serum protein fractions
Countercurrent electrophoresis (cross-electrophoresis, CEP)	Gocke and Howe	1970	[20]	–	Quantitative and semi-quantitative detection of proteins
	Pesendorfer et al.	1970	[19]	–	Quantitative and semi-quantitative detection of numerous proteins
Radial immunodiffusion (RID)	Fahey and McKelvey	1965	[14]	2 mg	Quantitation of more than 25 fractions
	Mancini et al.	1965	[15]	2 mg	Quantitation of more than 25 fractions
Electroimmunodiffusion (EID)	Laurell	1966	[16]	0.5 mg	Quantitation of more than 30 fractions
	Hartley et al.	1966	[17]	0.5 mg	Quantitation of more than 30 fractions
Radioimmunoassays (RIA)	Berson and Yalow	1964	[18]	1 pg	Numerous proteins (e.g., serum proteins, hormones, peptides)

and α_2-globulins, thereby increasing the number of recognized major fractions to five (albumin, α_1-globulin, α_2-globulin, β-globulin, and γ-globulin).

Using the techniques of analytical ultracentrifugation [12], serum proteins can be categorized, primarily on the basis of their molecular weight, into 4.5S, 7S, and 19S components. The γ-globulin fraction, which is defined as such by its electrophoretic characteristics, can be fractionated ultracentrifugally into 7S and 19S components.

More recently, protein separation techniques, such as immunoelectrophoresis [13], have been developed that utilize antigen-antibody precipitation reactions to further separate and categorize the serum proteins. Using this approach, more than 35 serum proteins can be demonstrated. Quantitative immunodiffusion techniques, such as radial immunodiffusion [14, 15] and electroimmunodiffusion [16, 17], have truly revolutionized the entire field of protein quantitation by virtue of their specificity, sensitivity, and practicality. Radioimmunoassay techniques [18] have extended the element of sensitivity to the picogram range, thus enabling the replacement of tedious bioassay tests for numerous hormones and other biologically active substances. The recently introduced cross-electrophoresis technique [19, 20] provides a practical approach for the detection and semiquantitative determination of certain proteins, including α_1-fetoprotein, hepatitis-B antigen, and others.

A perplexing and confusing system of nomenclature for the serum proteins has evolved as a consequence of the different separation methods employed. Each new method of separation has resulted in additional fractions and the renaming of previously described protein groups (for example, the 19S γ-globulin that is determined by ultracentrifugation is identical with immunoglobulin M as determined by immunoelectrophoresis; the β_1C-globulin that is identified by immunoelectrophoresis is analogous to the third component of complement, or C3, which is defined by its specific biological activity). Table 1 summarizes the evolution of clinically applicable techniques for the analysis of serum proteins. The subsequent chapters will consider the presently available techniques and their applications in the clinical laboratory and in clinical medicine.

A brief review of some of the fundamentals of protein chemistry may be of value. Proteins are large macromolecules composed of covalently linked amino acids. Each amino acid has a carboxyl group (COOH) at one end of the molecule and an amino group (NH$_2$) at the other end. The amino-carboxyl covalent bond, the peptide bond, is a structural feature that is characteristic of proteins and polypeptides. The term *peptide* is often used for molecules consisting of a relatively short sequence of amino acids, which are too small in size to be considered a protein.

Depending upon the electron distributions resulting from covalent bonding, amino acids may be either polar or nonpolar at a given pH. The electrical charge characteristics of these protein building blocks are further altered by the ionic bonding of structural subgroups. Thus, depending upon the pH of its medium, a given amino acid may be electri-

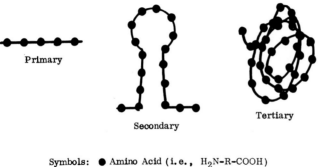

Primary

Secondary

Tertiary

Symbols: ● Amino Acid (i.e., $H_2N-R-COOH$)

– Peptide Bond (i.e., $R-C\overset{O}{\underset{NH-R}{}}$)

Figure 1
Basic levels of protein structure.

cally neutral, positively charged (cationic), or negatively charged (anionic); in other words, it may be either acidic or basic in nature depending upon the pH. The sequential arrangement of amino acids forms the *primary structure* of a protein. This amino-acid chain is folded within a two-dimensional plane by steric effects and other influences to form the *secondary structure,* which, when further twisted and convoluted in three-dimensional space by ionic attractions, van der Waals' forces, and hydrogen bonding, forms the protein's *tertiary structure.* The resulting molecule will, at this point, have electrical charge, again depending upon pH, and will exhibit a patchy distribution of charge densities that depends upon the summation of the contributory effects of its constituent structural units (Fig. 1). Polypeptide subunits may be coupled together to form a so-called *quaternary structure,* which represents the biologically active form of the protein.

The functional importance of the complex characteristics of protein molecular size, shape, and electrical properties cannot be overemphasized. It is the structural underpinning that dictates the behavior of the molecule in solution, in interactions with other molecules and ions, and in diffusion through various substances—in short, in virtually all of its biologically and biochemically important functions. One of the important functional parameters in protein chemistry is the isoelectric point (pI) of the molecule, which is defined as that pH at which the protein will not migrate within an electrical field; it is the point of equilibrium between the net electrical charge of the molecule and the prevailing electrical charge of the solution.

Proteins perform numerous vital functions throughout the body. They provide structural frameworks (e.g., collagen); they serve as bioactive and regulatory molecules (e.g., enzymes, hormones, and immunoglobulins); and they act as reservoirs for intrinsic chemical components or extrinsic transported substances (e.g., albumin).

For extensive discussions of protein chemistry, the reader is referred to the following sources:

White, A., Handler, P., and Smith, E. L. *Principles of Biochemistry* (5th ed.). New York: McGraw-Hill, 1973.

McGilvery, R. W. *Biochemistry: A Functional Approach.* Philadelphia: Saunders, 1970.

Mahler, H. R., and Cordes, E. H. *Basic Biological Chemistry.* New York: Harper & Row, 1968.

References

1. Cullen, G. E., and Van Slyke, D. D. Determination of the fibrin, globulin and albumin nitrogen of blood plasma. *J. Biol. Chem.* 41:587, 1920.
2. Kabat, E. A., and Mayer, M. *Experimental Immunochemistry.* Springfield, Ill.: Thomas, 1961. Pp. 476–483.
3. Howe, P. E. Use of sodium sulfate as a globulin precipitant in determination of proteins in blood. *J. Biol. Chem.* 49:93, 1921.
4. Schultze, H. E., and Heremans, J. F. *Molecular Biology of Human Proteins,* Vol. 1. Amsterdam: Elsevier, 1966.
5. Haurowitz, F. *Chemistry and Biology of Proteins.* New York: Academic, 1950.
6. Ritzmann, S. E., Wolf, R. E., Lawrence, M. C., Hart, J. S., and Levin, W. C. Sia euglobulin test—A re-evaluation. *J. Lab. Clin. Med.* 73:698, 1969.
7. Tiselius, A. A new apparatus for electrophoretic analysis of colloidal mixtures. *Trans. Faraday Soc.* 33:524, 1937.
8. König, P. Employment of Electrophoresis in Chemical Experiments with Small Quantities. *Acts and Works of the 3rd Congress of South American Chemists,* Rio de Janeiro, 1937. Vol. 2, p. 334.
9. Durrum, E. L. Paper Electrophoresis. In R. J. Block, E. L. Durrum, and G. Zweig (Eds.), *Paper Chromatography and Paper Electrophoresis,* Part II (2nd ed.). New York: Academic, 1958. Pp. 489–674.
10. Kohn, J. A cellulose acetate supporting medium for zone electrophoresis. *Clin. Chim. Acta* 2:297, 1957.
11. Sunderman, F. W. Micro-Kjeldahl Procedure for Determination of Serum Protein Nitrogen. In F. W. Sunderman and F. W. Sunderman, Jr. (Eds.), *Serum Proteins and the Dysproteinemias.* Philadelphia: Lippincott, 1964. Pp. 46–49.
12. Svedberg, T., and Pederson, K. O. *The Ultracentrifuge.* Oxford: Clarendon, 1940.
13. Grabar, P., and Williams, C. A. Méthode permettant l'étude conjugée des propriétés électrophorétiques immunochimiques d'un mélange de protéines. Application du sérum sanguin. *Biochim. Biophys. Acta* 10: 193, 1953.
14. Fahey, J. L., and McKelvey, E. M. Quantitative determination of serum immunoglobulins in antibody-agar plates. *J. Immunol.* 94:84, 1965.
15. Mancini, G., Carbonara, A. O., and Heremans, J. F. Immunochemical quantitation of antigens by single radial immunodiffusion. *Immunochemistry* 2:235, 1965.

16. Laurell, C. B.   Quantitative estimation of proteins by electrophoresis in agarose gel containing antibodies. *Anal. Biochem.* 15:45, 1966.
17. Hartley, T. F., Merrill, D. A., and Claman, H. N.   Quantitation of immunoglobulins in cerebrospinal fluid. *Arch. Neurol.* 15:472, 1966.
18. Berson, S. A., and Yalow, R. S.   Immunoassay of Protein Hormones. In G. Pincus et al. (Eds.), *The Hormones: Physiology, Chemistry and Applications,* Vol. 4. New York: Academic, 1964. P. 557.
19. Pesendorfer, F., Krassnitzky, O., and Wewalka, F.   Immunoelektrophoretischer Nachweis von "Hepatitits-Associated-Antigen" (Au/SH-Antigen). *Klin. Wochenschr.* 48:58, 1970.
20. Gocke, D. J., and Howe, C.   Rapid detection of Australia antigen by counter immunoelectrophoresis. *J. Immunol.* 104:1031, 1970.
21. Kingsley, G. R.   The determination of serum total protein, albumin and globulin by the biuret reaction. *J. Biol. Chem.* 131:197, 1939.
22. Kingsley, G. R., and Getchell, G.   The determination of microgram quantities of protein in biological fluid. *J. Biol. Chem.* 225:545, 1957.
23. Reiss, E.   Der Brechungskoeffizient des Blutserums als Indikator für den Eiweissgehalt. Inaugural Dissertation, Strassbourg, 1902.
24. Naumann, H. N.   Determination of Total Serum Proteins by Refractometry. In F. W. Sunderman and F. W. Sunderman, Jr. (Eds.), *Serum Proteins and the Dysproteinemias.* Philadelphia: Lippincott, 1964. Pp. 86–101.
25. Pillemer, L., and Hutchinson, M. C.   The determination of the albumin and globulin contents of human serum by methanol precipitation. *J. Biol. Chem.* 158:299, 1945.
26. Scheidegger, J. J.   Une microméthode de l'immunoélectrophorèse. *Int. Arch. Allergy Appl. Immunol.* 7:103, 1955.
27. Ressler, N.   Two-dimensional electrophoresis of serum protein antigens in an antibody containing buffer. *Clin. Chim. Acta* 5:795, 1960.
28. Clarke, M. H. G., and Freeman, T.   Quantitative immunoelectrophoresis of human serum proteins. *Clin. Sci.* 35:403, 1968.

Serum Protein Analysis: Methodology and Interpretation

I

Serum Protein Electrophoresis and Total Serum Proteins

Stephan E. Ritzmann and Jerry C. Daniels

Protein electrophoresis (from Greek *elektron,* electrical, plus *pherein,* to carry) is based on the movement of charged colloidal particles in an electrical field toward an electrode of opposite charge (Fig. 1-1). The rate of migration of proteins depends on the balance between the "driving" and "breaking" forces, which are brought about by such factors as viscosity of the medium and the net charge on the protein in the electrical field. The migration rate also depends on the structure and state of dissociation of acidic or basic groups of the protein molecule, as well as the pH and ionic strength of the solvents employed.

Moving boundary, or *"free," electrophoresis* was introduced by Tiselius in 1937 [1]; it employed an entirely fluid electrophoresis medium for the classification of proteins. *Zone electrophoresis* is a practical modification of the original Tiselius technique that permits satisfactory separation of the various protein components on an inert solid carrier medium, such as cellulose acetate. The amount of protein in each separate component can be quantitated by a number of methods, including the degree of dye absorption. Filter paper was introduced as a stabilizing medium by König [2], and this technique was subsequently adapted for use in clinical laboratories [3–6]. Cellulose acetate medium was introduced later by Kohn [7], and zone electrophoresis using cellulose acetate as the carrier medium is now used in most clinical laboratories.

Methodology

Among the various methodological approaches [6, 8–10] to cellulose acetate electrophoresis, microzone electrophoresis* has proved satisfactory. It requires only small samples (0.25 μ1), and a routine electrophoretic analysis of a set of eight samples can be completed within a few hours.

* Beckman Instruments, Inc., Fullerton, Calif. 92634.

Figure 1-1

Serum protein electrophoresis. *Top:* Separation of proteins in the electrical field. *Center:* Segregation of serum proteins into five distinct fractions. *Bottom:* Electrophoresis diagram of serum proteins and relative concentrations of albumin, α_1-, α_2-, β-, and γ-globulins. (Reproduced by permission. From Ritzmann, S. E., and Daniels, J. C. In G. J. Race (Ed.), *Tice's Practice of Medicine,* Vol. 2. New York: Harper & Row, 1974.)

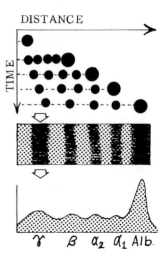

EQUIPMENT

Electrophoresis chambers are available commercially with the necessary accessories (Fig. 1-2). Any appropriate power supply is suitable, such as a Duostat (Beckman). The electrophoresed proteins are coagulated in a ventilated oven at 100°C, and the separation patterns are then scanned photometrically by scanning devices such as that shown in Figure 1-3.

PROCEDURE

The necessary reagents and cellulose acetate membranes are available from the manufacturer. The reservoirs of the microzone cell and a tray are filled with barbital buffer, pH 8.6, ionic strength 0.075 (i.e., B-2 buffer) (Fig. 1-4). The cellulose acetate membrane is wetted in the tray and is then placed on the bridge of the microzone cell; after the bridge has been attached to the cell, the membrane is allowed to equilibrate with the buffer. The serum samples (0.25 μl) are applied to the membrane with an applicator. After application of the samples (eight at most), the power supply is switched on and adjusted to a constant voltage (250 v) for 10 to 20 minutes of electrophoresis. After completion of the electrophoretic separation, the power supply is turned off, and the membrane is then removed from the bridge and submerged in the fixative-dye solution. Subsequently, the membrane is washed, alcohol-fixed, cleared, and baked.

The technique for *urine protein electrophoresis* is identical to that for serum protein electrophoresis except for the sample preparation. Usually, urine samples are concentrated 20 to 200 times prior to electrophoresis. This step, however, is time-consuming. In general, it may suffice to apply the urine sample three times to the membrane prior to electrophoresis; this technique effectively results in threefold concentration.

Figure 1-2
Microzone electrophoresis cell. (Courtesy of Beckman Instruments, Inc., Fullerton, Calif.)

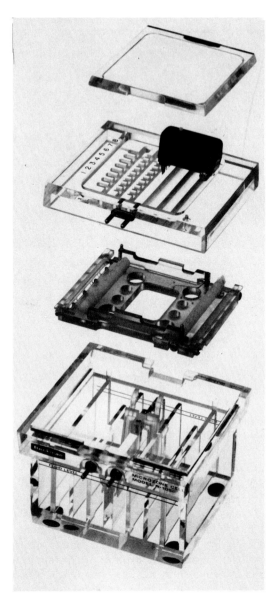

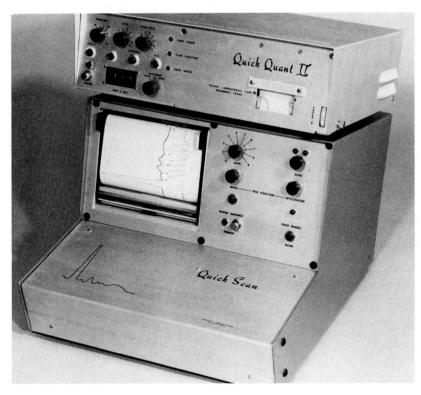

Figure 1-3
Densitometer: Basic unit (Quick Scan) and computer printout (Quick Quant). (Courtesy of Helena Laboratories, Beaumont, Tex.)

SOURCES OF ERROR

Sample preparation is important. Hemolyzed specimens should be avoided since they cause distorted patterns (e.g., hemoglobin bound by haptoglobin results in abnormal α_2-globulin fractions). The tubes containing blood or serum should be capped to prevent desiccation of the sample. Serum samples must be distinguished from plasma specimens, since fibrinogen in the latter may yield misleading electrophoretic peaks (see p. 22, Fig. 1-17). Reagents must be checked for their expiration dates and proper pH, and their reutilization should be limited (e.g., buffer should be used no more than five times, stain solution no more than 12 runs, and alcohol rinse and clearing solutions for no more than two runs per day). Equipment maintenance is imperative, and attention should be given particularly to the applicator (e.g., applicator ribbons that are not in parallel position may lead to "bowing" of the protein peaks on the membranes). Other technical errors include careless handling of the membranes, inappropriate sample application, and excessive electrophoresis.

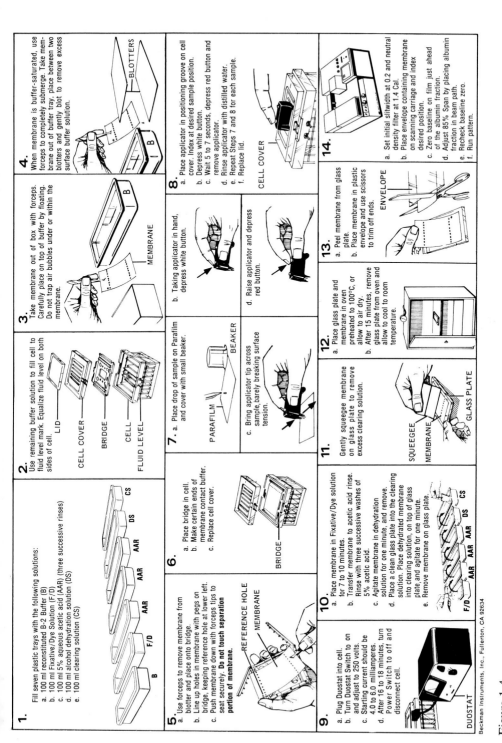

1.
Fill seven plastic trays with the following solutions:
a. 100 ml reconstituted B-2 Buffer (B)
b. 100 ml Fixative/Dye Solution (F/D)
c. 100 ml 5% aqueous acetic acid (AAR) (three successive rinses)
d. 100 ml alcohol dehydration solution (DS)
e. 100 ml clearing solution (CS)

CS DS AAR AAR AAR F/D B

2.
Use remaining buffer solution to fill cell to fluid level mark. Equalize fluid level on both sides of cell.

CELL COVER
LID
BRIDGE
CELL
FLUID LEVEL

3.
Take membrane out of box with forceps. Carefully place on top of buffer by floating. Do not trap air bubbles under or within the membrane.

MEMBRANE
B

4.
When membrane is buffer-saturated, use forceps to completely submerge. Take membrane out of buffer tray, place between two blotters and gently blot to remove excess surface buffer solution.

BLOTTERS
B

5.
a. Use forceps to remove membrane from blotter and place onto bridge.
b. Line up holes in membrane with pegs on bridge, keeping reference hole at lower left.
c. Push membrane down with forceps tips to seat securely. **Do not touch separation portion of membrane.**

REFERENCE HOLE
MEMBRANE

6.
a. Place bridge in cell.
b. Make certain ends of membrane contact buffer.
c. Replace cell cover.

BRIDGE

7.
a. Place drop of sample on Parafilm and cover with small beaker.

PARAFILM
BEAKER

b. Bring applicator tip across sample, barely breaking surface tension.

8.
a. Place applicator in positioning groove on cell cover. Index at desired sample position.
b. Depress white button.
c. Wait 5 to 7 seconds, depress red button and remove applicator.
d. Rinse applicator with distilled water.
e. Repeat Steps 7 and 8 for each sample.
f. Replace lid.

b. Taking applicator in hand, depress white button.

d. Raise applicator and depress red button.

CELL COVER

9.
a. Plug Duostat into cell.
b. Turn Duostat Switch to on and adjust to 250 volts. Starting current should be 4.0 to 6.0 milliamperes.
d. After 16 to 18 minutes, turn Power Switch to off and disconnect cell.

DUOSTAT

10.
a. Place membrane in Fixative/Dye solution for 7 to 10 minutes.
b. Transfer membrane to acetic acid rinse. Rinse with three successive washes of 5% acetic acid.
c. Agitate membrane in dehydration solution for one minute, and remove.
d. Place a clean glass plate into the clearing solution. Place dehydrated membrane into clearing solution, on top of glass plate, and agitate for one minute.
e. Remove membrane on glass plate.

11.
Gently squeegee membrane on glass plate to remove excess clearing solution.

SQUEEGEE
MEMBRANE
GLASS PLATE

12.
a. Place glass plate and membrane in oven preheated to 100°C, or allow to air dry.
b. After 15 minutes, remove glass plate from oven and allow to cool to room temperature.

13.
a. Peel membrane from glass plate.
b. Place membrane in plastic envelope and use scissors to trim off ends.

ENVELOPE

14.
a. Set initial slitwidth at 0.2 and neutral density filter at 1.4 Cal.
b. Place envelope containing membrane on scanning carriage and index at desired position.
c. Zero baseline on film just ahead of the albumin fraction.
d. Adjust 85% Span by placing albumin fraction in beam path.
e. Recheck baseline zero.
f. Run pattern.

Beckman Instruments, Inc., Fullerton, CA 92634

Figure 1-4
Microzone electrophoresis procedure. (Courtesy of Beckman Instruments, Inc., Fullerton, Calif.)

ANALYSIS OF RESULTS

The direct photometric scanning of the stained membranes yields a pattern based on the electrophoretic mobility and concentrations of the major protein fractions. The area under the curves corresponding to each protein fraction is proportional to the quantity of stained proteins present in that fraction.

The type of scanning equipment will be dictated by the volume of serum protein electrophoresis work. Analysis of small volumes (i.e., 10 to 15 samples per day) requires a scanning densitometer, such as the Analytrol (Beckman) or the Quick Scan*, which converts the protein separation patterns on the cellulose acetate membrane into scan patterns (Fig. 1-5). These instruments provide an optical density pattern of the electrophoretically separated protein fractions, and, below the pattern, the integrator readout is printed. By counting the number of spaces crossed by the integrator pen, one can determine the percent of each fraction in relation to that of the whole pattern. The area under each peak is determined by dividing the value of each area by the total value, thus giving the relative concentration, i.e., the percent of each fraction.

Analysis of large volumes (i.e., more than 50 electrophoresis samples per day) may be handled by automatic analysis employing high-speed scanning and quantitating devices (see Fig. 1-3). This computer system provides a printout of both the percent and, by entering the total serum protein (TSP) values, the gm per 100 ml values.

Manual quantitation, however, may be required in cases of certain abnormal electrophoretic patterns, such as M proteins, β-γ-globulin bridging, or low α_1-globulin values.

Normal Values

Normally, serum proteins are separated into five fractions, designated as *albumin* and α_1-, α_2-, β-, and γ-*globulins* (Fig. 1-6). Since interlaboratory variations are inevitable, each laboratory must establish its own normal values, using standardized techniques. Normal adult serum protein electrophoretic (SPE) values in our laboratories are shown in Table 1-1 [9, 10]. During infancy, the γ-globulin levels undergo a considerable increase (Table 1-2).

Determination of Total Serum Proteins (TSP)

The determination of the TSP values is a prerequisite for calculating the absolute values of the electrophoretic serum protein fractions. Measurement of total serum proteins may be accomplished by several techniques [11], including chemical methods, such as Kjeldahl [12] and biuret [13, 14] analyses, and physical means, such as refractometry [15]. The TS meter† has found wide application. It is a Goldberg refractometer that yields accurate, rapid, and reproducible results while requiring only

---

* Helena Laboratories, Beaumont, Tex. 77704.
† American Optical Instrument Co., Buffalo, N.Y. 14215.

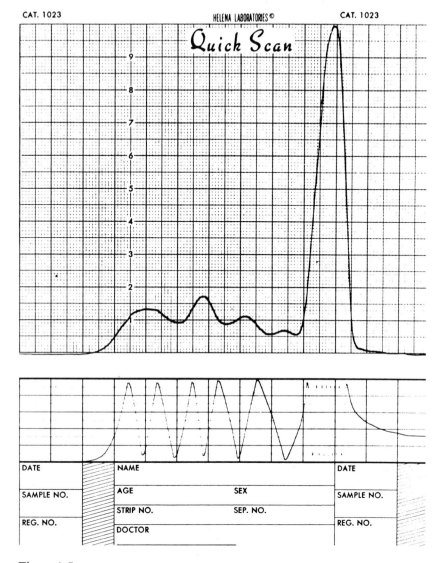

Figure 1-5
Normal serum protein electrophoresis pattern (*top*). The vertical lines separate the protein fractions, allowing their quantitation by the integrator scale (*bottom*).

Figure 1-6
Normal serum protein electrophoresis
pattern. From right to left: albumin,
α_1-, α_2-, β-, and γ-globulin fractions.

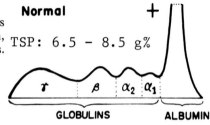

Normal

TSP: 6.5 – 8.5 g%

GLOBULINS   ALBUMIN

Table 1-1.   Normal Adult Concentration of Fractions by Serum Protein
Electrophoresis

Fraction	Percent of Total	Mean Value (gm/100 ml)	±2 SD Range (gm/100 ml)
Albumin	45–70	4.2	3.2–5.2
α_1-Globulin	2–5	0.2	0.1–0.3
α_2-Globulin	8–14	0.8	0.6–1.0
β-Globulin	10–15	0.9	0.7–1.1
γ-Globulin	11–22	1.2	0.8–1.6
Total serum proteins		7.3	6.3–8.3

Reproduced by permission. From Ritzmann, S. E., Daniels, J. C., Alami, S. Y., and
Lawrence, M. C.   In G. J. Race (Ed.), *Laboratory Medicine*. New York: Harper
& Row, 1975.

Table 1-2.   Microzone Serum Protein Electrophoresis: Serum γ-Globulin
Concentrations in Children

Age	Mean Value (gm/100 ml)	± 2 SD Range (gm/100 ml)
1 wk.	0.75	0.5–1.0
1–3 mo.	0.35	0.2–0.5
3–6 mo.	0.4	0.2–0.6
6–12 mo.	0.5	0.3–0.7
12–18 mo.	0.7	0.5–0.9
18–24 mo.	0.8	0.5–1.1
Over 2 yr.	Rapid increase to normal adult values	

Reproduced by permission. From Ritzmann, S. E., Daniels, J. C., Alami, S. Y.,
and Lawrence, M. C.   In G. J. Race (Ed.), *Laboratory Medicine*. New York:
Harper & Row, 1975.

small amounts of sample. Although the actual measurement is that of the refractive index, conversion tables are supplied for the assay of total solids, percentage composition (gm per 100 ml), and specific gravity for urine and serum protein concentrations (Fig. 1-7). It requires only a single drop of fluid sample. Determination of TSP is precise and reproducible (less than ± 2.5 percent deviation) within a wide range of TSP values (at least within ± 50 percent of normal, i.e., between 3.5 and 11.0 gm per 100 ml). Samples with TSP values above 11.0 gm per 100 ml may require dilution before assay, and those with TSP values below 3.5 gm per 100 ml may require assay by chemical means (e.g., microbiuret analysis).

Normal TSP values in our laboratories at the University of Texas Medical Branch, Galveston, Texas, range from 6.3 to 8.3 gm per 100 ml (± 2 SD) with a mean value of 7.3 gm per 100 ml.

Hyperproteinemia [9, 16] may be defined in terms of TSP values of more than 9.0 gm per 100 ml. Hyperproteinemia is almost exclusively due to hypergammaglobulinemia of either the polyclonal or the monoclonal variety. The highest TSP levels (which rarely exceed 20.0 gm per 100 ml) are found in patients with monoclonal gammopathy, and significantly increased levels (rarely higher than 14.0 gm per 100 ml) may be found in patients with polyclonal gammopathy.

Pseudohyperproteinemia due to sample desiccation (e.g., from serum storage in unstoppered test tubes at 4°C) can usually be recognized by the essentially normal relative concentrations of the albumin and globulin fractions on electrophoresis. Spuriously high TSP levels (usually between 8.0 and 9.0 gm per 100 ml) may be encountered in sera obtained from patients with hypovolemic shock or after prolonged application of tourniquets.

Hypoproteinemia [9] is usually caused by hypoalbuminemia, either alone (e.g., in liver diseases) or in combination with hypogammaglobulinemia (e.g., in nephrotic syndrome) or by an absolute decrease of all electrophoretic fractions. Hypoproteinemia associated with an essentially normal relative concentration of the electrophoretically separated serum protein fractions suggests "bulk loss" of proteins, i.e., the loss of proteins regardless of their molecular weight, such as that which occurs in patients with protein-losing gastroenteropathies or skin lesions (thermal burns or extensive eczema).

Application and Interpretation

The full value of an electrophoretic report can be obtained only by correlation of the quantitative values with both the configuration of the serum electrophoretic pattern (with TSP values) and the clinical findings [8, 9, 11, 17–19]. The application of electrophoretic analysis of serum proteins has led to the recognition of certain abnormal patterns that are pathognomonic for distinct disorders, while other, less specific patterns have proved useful as aids in the diagnosis and prognosis of certain diseases. It has contributed to the recognition of deficiency states,

Figure 1-7
TS meter. *A*. Application of serum to TS meter. *B*. Conversion grid to convert refractive index to grams per 100 ml protein. (Courtesy of American Optical Instrument Co., Buffalo, N.Y.)

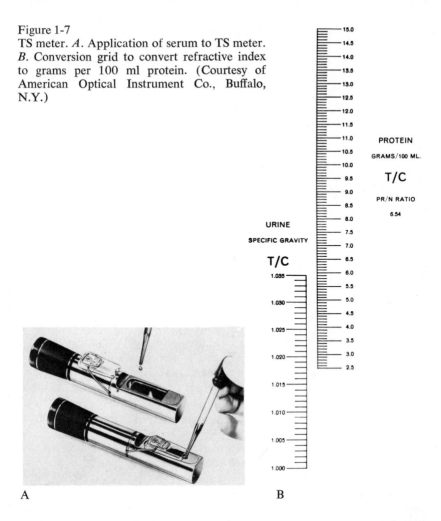

A

B

such as agammaglobulinemia and analbuminemia, as well as overproduction states, including hyperalpha-2-globulinemia and the hypergammaglobulinemias (Fig. 1-8).

It must be recognized that minor quantitative deviations (less than ±25 percent of normal means) of the electrophoretic fractions are often overinterpreted. As a rule of thumb, the normal adult α_1-globulin value may be considered to be 0.3 gm per 100 ml, and the α_2-, β-, and γ-globulin values represent increments of 0.3 gm per 100 ml of this value, i.e., 0.6, 0.9, and 1.2 gm per 100 gm, respectively; the remainder of the total protein is accounted for by albumin.

The interpreter of serum protein electrophoresis (SPE) patterns should master the subconscious process of "pattern reading," i.e., the visual recognition of certain recurrent constellations of changes on the SPE or subtle asymmetries of possible significance, rather than merely

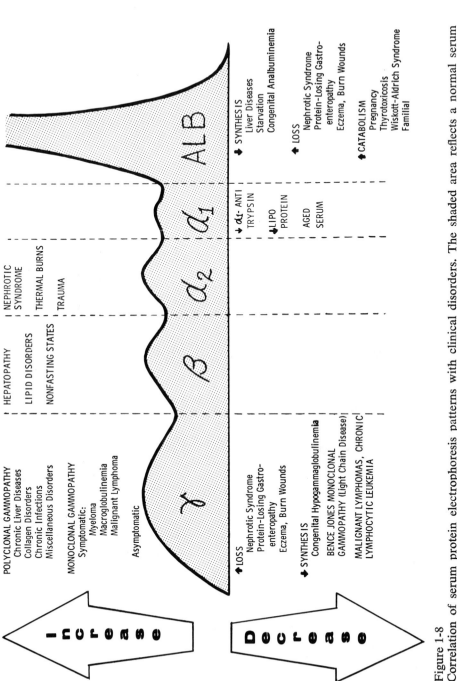

Figure 1-8

Correlation of serum protein electrophoresis patterns with clinical disorders. The shaded area reflects a normal serum protein electrophoresis pattern. Five major fractions are separated (*from right to left*): albumin, α_1-, α_2-, β-, and γ-globulins. (Reproduced by permission. From Ritzmann, S. E., Daniels, J. C., Alami, S. Y., and Lawrence, M. C. In G. J. Race (Ed.), *Laboratory Medicine*. New York: Harper & Row, 1975.)

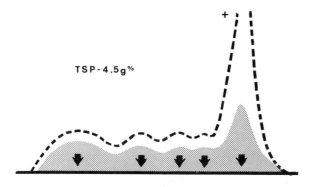

TSP-4.5g%

Figure 1-9
Pattern of hypoproteinemia associated with decrease of all serum protein fractions suggests "bulk loss" of serum proteins regardless of their molecular weight (e.g., protein-losing gastroenteropathies). (Reproduced by permission. From Ritzmann, S. E., and Daniels, J. C. In G. J. Race (Ed.), *Tice's Practice of Medicine,* Vol. 2. New York: Harper & Row, 1974.)

comparing observed numerical values with a table of "normals" for each electrophoretic fraction. A simplistic description, such as "slight decrease of albumin" or "split β-globulin fraction," without further interpretation, should be avoided.

HYPOPROTEINEMIA DUE TO "BULK LOSS" OF PROTEINS
Hypoproteinemia associated with essentially normal relative concentrations of the serum protein fractions suggests "bulk loss" of proteins (Fig. 1-9).

ALBUMIN ABNORMALITIES
Hypoalbuminemia of varying degrees is the most frequently encountered serum protein abnormality (Fig. 1-10) (see also Chap. 13). It is a nonspecific finding, and it may be due to: (1) loss of albumin from the kidney (nephrotic syndrome), the gastrointestinal tract (protein-losing gastroenteropathies), the skin (thermal burns or eczematous lesions), or into serous cavities (e.g., ascites with frequent tapping); (2) decreased synthesis of albumin by the liver (various liver diseases or congenital analbuminemia); (3) increased catabolism of albumin; or (4) various combinations of these factors.

In the case of hypoproteinemia and a decrease of all globulin fractions, an underlying disorder resulting in protein-losing gastroenteropathy must be excluded. Considerable degrees of hypoalbuminemia (i.e., albumin levels of less than 2.0 gm per 100 ml) may be accompanied by impaired oncotic pressure (e.g., edema) or transport functions (e.g., hypocalcemia). A naturally occurring hyperalbuminemia has not been observed. Spurious hyperalbuminemia, however, must be ruled out insofar as it may be caused by clinical dehydration or laboratory desiccation.

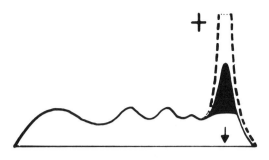

Figure 1-10
Hypoalbuminemia. Normal albumin fraction is indicated by the dotted line. Hypoalbuminemia is the most frequently encountered serum protein abnormality. Congenital analbuminemia or a double albumin peak (bisalbuminemia) may be encountered rarely. There is no naturally occurring hyperalbuminemia. (Reproduced by permission. From Ritzmann, S. E., and Daniels, J. C. In G. J. Race (Ed.), *Tice's Practice of Medicine,* Vol. 2. New York: Harper & Row, 1974.)

α_1-GLOBULIN FRACTION

DECREASED α_1-GLOBULIN FRACTION

The main portion (about 90 percent) of the α_1-globulin fraction consists of α_1-antitrypsin (see Chap. 15). Significant decreases of this fraction (i.e., levels of 0.1 gm per 100 ml or less; see Fig. 1-11A) are encountered in patients with congenital α_1-antitrypsin deficiency (often associated with juvenile emphysema), cases of hypo-alphalipoproteinemia, and in most aged samples that have been refrigerated for prolonged times. Compared with the SPE fractions other than albumin, the α_1-globulin fraction is somewhat unique in that a diminution suggests the possibility of a single specific protein deficiency, i.e., of α_1-antitrypsin, a diagnostic clue which is precluded by the multiplicity of individual proteins comprising the other globulin fractions.

INCREASED α_1-GLOBULIN FRACTION

Besides inhibiting the functions of several proteases (such as trypsin or plasmin), α_1-antitrypsin acts as an acute-phase protein (see Chap. 18).

Due to increases of α_1-antitrypsin in many inflammatory conditions, the α_1-globulin fractions may sometimes be increased excessively (e.g., as high as 0.8 gm per 100 ml; see Fig. 1-11B). Such an acute-phase increase of α_1-antitrypsin may temporarily obscure an underlying heterozygous α_1-antitrypsin deficiency.

α_2-GLOBULIN FRACTION

The α_2-globulin fraction is of some diagnostic and prognostic value. For practical purposes, however, only an increase of the α_2-globulin fraction needs to be considered.

1. Slight to moderate degrees of hyperalpha-2-globulinemia may be

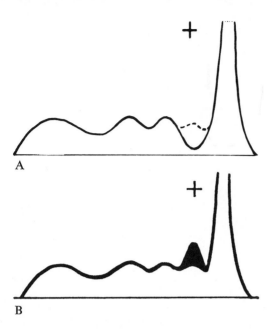

Figure 1-11

A. Hypoalpha-1-globulinemia pattern. Normal α_1-globulin fraction is indicated by the dotted line. A significant degree of hypoalpha-1-globulinemia may indicate α_1-antitrypsin deficiency, hypoalpha-1-lipidemia, or aged serum samples. (Reproduced by permission. From Ritzmann, S. E., and Daniels, J. C. In G. J. Race (Ed.), *Tice's Practice of Medicine,* Vol. 2. New York: Harper & Row, 1974.)

B. Hyperalpha-1-globulinemia pattern. Normal α_1-globulin fraction is indicated by the unshaded area. A significant degree of hyperalpha-1-globulinemia may indicate an acute-phase response of α_1-antitrypsin to inflammatory conditions.

encountered in chronic infections (e.g., pulmonary tuberculosis) or malignancies (e.g., Hodgkin's disease). The increase is due to elevated levels of certain glycoproteins and haptoglobin (see Chap. 18).

2. Considerable degrees of hyperalpha-2-globulinemia are typically seen in two conditions: nephrotic syndrome and thermal burns. Both disorders are also associated with hypoalbuminemia (Fig. 1-12). Rarely, significant increases of α_2-globulin are seen in certain lipid disorders [17] and neoplasms [17, 20, 21] (see Chap. 19).

Nephrotic syndrome is characterized by the renal excretion of low molecular weight proteins with the retention of certain high molecular weight proteins. This leads to hypoalbuminemia, hypogammaglobulinemia, and increases of lipoproteins and α_2M-globulin. The α_2M-globulin is an antiprotease similar to α_1-antitrypsin in its action, neutralizing proteolytic enzymes such as trypsin, plasmin (fibrinolysin), and kallikrein.

A similar SPE pattern is seen in patients with thermal burns during

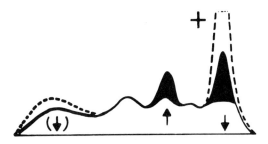

Figure 1-12
Hypoalbuminemia–hyperalpha-2-globulinemia pattern. This combination is typically associated with nephrotic syndrome. The γ-globulin fraction is often decreased. Similarly, patients with acute thermal burns may exhibit this pattern during the recovery stages. (Reproduced by permission. From Ritzmann, S. E., and Daniels, J. C. In G. J. Race (Ed.), *Tice's Practice of Medicine*, Vol. 2. New York: Harper & Row, 1974.)

the recovery stages. The significant and long-lasting increase of the α_2-globulin fraction in these patients, however, is not due to an increase of α_2M-globulin as in nephrotic syndrome, but due to increased levels of haptoglobin, another α_2-globulin. Haptoglobin (Hp) is the hemoglobin-binding protein. Hemoglobin (Hb) released from erythrocytes is taken up by Hp and the Hb-Hp complexes are removed by the reticuloendothelial system (RES), especially the Kupffer cells in the liver. This mechanism results in conservation of the body's iron stores.

β-GLOBULIN FRACTION
The diagnostic significance of the β-globulin fraction is limited to a few conditions. The β-globulin fraction may be increased in a variety of diseases, including liver and lipid disorders (primary or secondary hyperlipoproteinemias), as well as in sera from nonfasting subjects. The only β-globulin aberration of definite diagnostic significance is that of the presence of M protein (see p. 21).

γ-GLOBULIN FRACTION
The γ-globulin fraction contains most of the antibodies, or *immunoglobulins* (see Chaps. 3 and 19), and increases or decreases of this fraction reflect immunoglobulin aberrations. The electrophoretic migration ranges and relative concentrations of the five known classes—IgG, IgA, IgM, IgD, and IgE—are indicated in Figure 1-13. It is evident that routine SPE allows neither the precise quantitation of the total or individual serum immunoglobulins (although IgG may compose up to 90 percent of the γ-globulin fraction) nor the determination of the different immunoglobulin classes that may be altered in the various disorders of humoral immunity. The various immunoglobulin classes contain specific antibodies, which, in their entirety, provide humoral immunity.

Immunoglobulin abnormalities can be classified as either hypogamma-

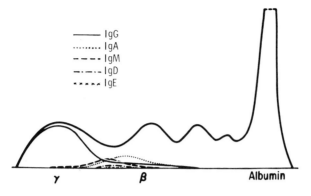

——— IgG
········· IgA
– – –· IgM
—·—·– IgD
· · · · · IgE

γ   β   Albumin

Figure 1-13
Normal serum protein electrophoresis pattern indicating migration ranges
and relative concentrations of IgG, IgA, IgM, IgD, and IgE. (Modified from
Fahey, J. L. *J.A.M.A.* 194:71, 1975.)

globulinemia or hypergammaglobulinemia. The latter can be either polyclonal gammopathy or monoclonal gammopathy (see also Chap. 19).

Hypo- OR AGAMMAGLOBULINEMIA

The SPE pattern of hypo- or agammaglobulinemia is depicted in Figure
1-14. General agreement has not been reached regarding the quantitative definitions of hypo- and agammaglobulinemias; however, adult γ-
globulin values of 10 percent of normal or less (i.e., not more than 0.1
gm per 100 ml) qualify generally for a diagnosis of agammaglobulinemia, and levels between 10 and 50 percent of normal (i.e., between 0.1
and 0.7 gm per 100 ml) fulfill the criteria for a diagnosis of hypogammaglobulinemia. Since the initial description of agammaglobulinemia by
Löffler in 1951 (see Chap. 19), a large number of patients with a wide
variety of immune deficiencies have been described.

Serum protein electrophoresis is an essential technique for the detection of such immunoglobulin deficiencies. In general, hypo- or agammaglobulinemias result from (1) defective synthesis, (2) excessive loss,
(3) increased catabolism of immunoglobulins, or (4) a combination of
these factors. Specifically, hypogammaglobulinemia *in children* may be
encountered after the first few months of life on a transient basis; rarely
is it encountered on a permanent basis (as in, e.g., Bruton's sex-linked
agammaglobulinemia). Hypogammaglobulinemia *in adults* may be due
to a variety of causes, including late manifestations of genetically determined decreased γ-globulin production (i.e., late onset, common variable type of "primary" hypogammaglobulinemia); certain malignant
lymphomas (e.g., chronic lymphocytic leukemia or lymphosarcoma);
loss of immunoglobulins (e.g., from burn sites, the gastrointestinal tract
in protein-losing gastroenteropathies, or the kidneys in nephrotic syndrome—see Figure 1-12); (in autoimmunologically caused nephrotic syndrome [e.g., systemic lupus erythematosus] a polyclonal gammopathy

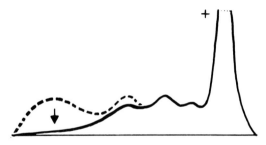

Figure 1-14
Agammaglobulinemia pattern. Normal γ-globulin fraction is indicated by the dotted line. (Reproduced by permission. From Ritzmann, S. E., and Daniels, J. C. In G. J. Race (Ed.), *Tice's Practice of Medicine,* Vol. 2. New York: Harper & Row, 1974.)

may be encountered instead of the customary hypogammaglobulinemia); and malignant plasma-cell disorders (i.e., monoclonal gammopathies, including Bence Jones monoclonal gammopathy or light-chain disease). In contrast to the nephrotic syndrome, protein loss from sites other than the kidneys (e.g., thermal burns or protein-losing gastroenteropathies) is nonselective, i.e., all serum proteins may be decreased, regardless of their molecular weights. All adult patients with hypogammaglobulinemia should be examined for the presence of Bence Jones proteins (see Chaps. 19 and 20). The detection of hypo- or agammaglobulinemia necessitates further studies to delineate the nature of the abnormality, including immunoelectrophoresis and quantitation of the various immunoglobulins by, for example, radial immunodiffusion.

Hypergammaglobulinemia
Polyclonal gammopathy. The SPE pattern in polyclonal gammopathy is characterized by a broad, diffuse increase of the γ-globulin fraction (Fig. 1-15). Usually, all three major immunoglobulins are increased, with variable relative concentrations. *PG is the second most frequent electrophoretic serum protein abnormality after hypoalbuminemia.* There is some prognostic value provided by PG. Clinical improvement of hepatitis, for instance, is associated with a decrease of the polyclonally increased γ-globulin fraction. PG is not a primary disease entity but is an expression of an underlying disease. It may accompany a wide range of clinical disorders, including (1) chronic liver diseases (Laennec's cirrhosis, infectious hepatitis, chronic active hepatitis [lupoid hepatitis], or biliary cirrhosis), (2) collagen disorders (rheumatoid arthritis, Sjögren's syndrome, Felty's syndrome, or lupus erythematosus), (3) chronic infections (tuberculosis, syphilis, deep fungus diseases, lymphogranuloma venereum, osteomyelitis, or chronic bronchitis with bronchiectasis), and (4) miscellaneous disorders (e.g., metastatic carcinoma, recovery stages of thermal burns, cystic fibrosis).
  Monoclonal Gammopathy. In monoclonal gammopathy (MG), one

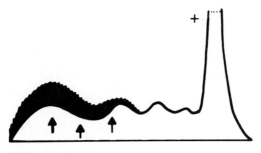

Figure 1-15
Polyclonal gammopathy pattern. In polyclonal gammopathy, the major serum immunoglobulins are usually increased to a varying extent, resulting in increased γ-globulin and often also β-globulin fractions (*solid area*). (Reproduced by permission. From Ritzmann, S. E., and Daniels, J. C. In G. J. Race (Ed.), *Tice's Practice of Medicine,* Vol. 2. New York: Harper & Row, 1974.)

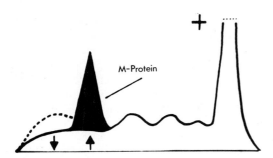

Figure 1-16
Monoclonal gammopathy pattern. In monoclonal gammopathy, one segment of one immunoglobulin class is greatly increased. The position of such an M protein (*solid area*) may be anywhere within the normal distribution range of serum immunoglobulins, i.e., between the γ- and α_2-globulin fractions. Often, the uninvolved immunoglobulin classes ("background γ-globulins") are decreased. (Reproduced by permission. From Ritzmann, S. E., and Daniels, J. C. In G. J. Race (Ed.), *Tice's Practice of Medicine,* Vol. 2. New York: Harper & Row, 1974.)

clone of the plasma cell proliferates, producing one homogeneous immunoglobulin in excessive amounts. The remainder of the plasma cell lines and their "normal" immunoglobulin products tend to be decreased. On electrophoresis of serum or urine samples, MG is characterized by the presence of an M protein (Fig. 1-16). A spike occurs in the SPE pattern, which is found most frequently in the γ-globulin region, less frequently in the γ-β regions, rarely in the β-α_2 positions, and, in a few instances, even in the α_1-globulin fraction (Table 1-3) [17]. The frequent association of these spikes with myeloma, macroglobulinemia, and, rarely, malignant lymphoma-like disorders led to the use of the term *M protein* (see Chap. 19). M protein in this sense should not be confused with the M protein of group A–hemolytic streptococci or the 19S "M" component obtained on ultracentrifugation of normal human serum that contains IgM.

Careful inspection of the SPE separation patterns on the membranes and on the resulting diagrams is essential for the recognition of M proteins. Small M fractions may easily be missed, especially when they are hidden in the main γ- or β-globulin fractions or when they are present in the "valleys" between the normal fractions. Such subtle clues on SPE patterns cannot be dismissed as insignificant. Often the uninvolved "residual" background immunoglobulins are decreased (see Fig. 1-16). In instances when the occurrence of Bence Jones proteins is the only abnormality (i.e., in light-chain disease), no discernible M protein may be present in serum, but it may be seen in the urine due to the small size of the overproduced entity. The SPE patterns in such cases may simply reflect hypogammaglobulinemia. In such instances, immunoelectrophoretic analyses and immunological tests for Bence Jones proteins are indicated.

The frequency with which MG occurs has undoubtedly been underestimated in the past. At the University of Texas Medical Branch, at least two new cases of MG are being diagnosed per week, which represents a frequency exceeding that of chronic lymphocytic leukemia, systemic lupus erythematosus, and Hodgkin's disease combined.

Table 1-3. Electrophoretic Mobility of 463 M Proteins

Immunoglobulin Category	Electrophoretic Mobility						
	γ_3	γ_2	γ_1	β_2	β_1	α_3	α_2
IgG	86	92	29	4	1	0	0
IgA	0	3	21	51	42	11	0
IgM	11	50	24	5	1	0	0
Bence Jones proteins	3	11	2	4	8	2	2
Total	100	156	76	64	52	13	2

Reproduced by permission. From Ritzmann, S. E., and Levin, W. C. In H. Dettelbach and S. E. Ritzmann (Eds.), *Lab Synopsis,* Vol. 2 (2nd ed.). Somerville, N.J.: Behring Diagnostics, 1969. P. 21.

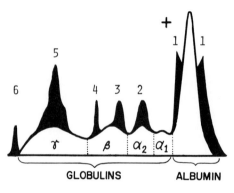

Figure 1-17

Pseudo-M proteins. The following must be considered in the differential diagnosis of M-protein disorders: (*1*) *Bisalbuminemia* or double albuminemia. The "abnormal" albumin fraction is positioned either anodically or cathodically from the "normal" albumin fraction. (*2*) *Hyperalpha-2-globulinemia,* associated with nephrotic syndrome, thermal burns, hyperlipidemia, etc. (*3*) *Hyperbetaglobulinemia* due to hemoglobin ("hemolyzed" serum); hypertransferrinemia associated with iron deficiency, pregnancy, or oral contraception; hyperlipidemia, especially in a nonfasting sample; unique proteins associated with malignant melanoma; etc. (*4*) *Peak near point of application* due to lipoprotein deposits (especially in nonfasting samples), fibrinogen (plasma), bacterial contamination, or desiccated specimens. (*5*) *Hypergammaglobulinemia* due to γ-globulin immune complexes, especially in sera with excessively high rheumatoid-factor activity. (*6*) *Postgamma peaks* due to hyperlysozymemia often associated with renal insufficiency or myelomonocytic leukemia. (Reproduced by permission. From Ritzmann, S. E., Daniels, J. C., Alami, S. Y., and Lawrence, M. C. In G. J. Race (Ed.), *Laboratory Medicine.* New York: Harper & Row, 1975.)

Pseudomonoclonal Gammopathies and Pseudo-M Proteins. M proteins may be mimicked by conditions other than MG. In the differential diagnosis of M-protein abnormalities, the conditions associated with pseudo-M proteins that are illustrated in Figure 1-17 must be considered. In almost all instances of doubt, immunoelectrophoretic analysis with the use of appropriate antisera permits the immunological characterization of "true" M proteins and distinguishes them from pseudo-M proteins.

Indications and Diagnostic Approach to Serum Protein Abnormalities

Serum protein electrophoresis, together with the determination of the total serum proteins, should be considered a routine procedure to be performed on patients admitted to the hospital and on those seen in the physician's office. As a result of the often decisive contribution made by SPE analysis, the clinical care of patients is improved.

Most assays for TSP and serum protein electrophoresis will be normal.

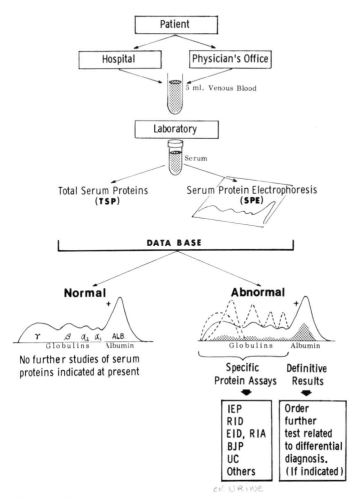

Figure 1-18
Diagnostic approach to serum protein abnormalities. (Reproduced by permission. From Ritzmann, S. E., and Daniels, J. C. In G. J. Race (Ed.), *Tice's Practice of Medicine*, Vol. 2. New York: Harper & Row, 1974.)

Protein abnormalities detected by SPE may, in general, either need no further protein studies (e.g., in cases of hypoalbuminemia and polyclonal gammopathy) or need additional evaluations by various adjunct techniques. For example, such techniques include:

1. Immunoelectrophoresis in the diagnosis of MG.
2. Quantitative immunodiffusion (i.e., radial immunodiffusion, electroimmunodiffusion, and radioimmunoassay) in the evaluation of protein deficiencies, including hypoceruloplasminemia, decreased complement levels, and hypogammaglobulinemia.

3. Analytical ultracentrifugation for the assay of immune complex disorders; assays for thermoproteins, including cryoglobulins, for the diagnosis of hyperviscosity syndrome and cryopathies; the determination of Bence Jones proteins; and other assays.

These various approaches, which are dictated by the individual abnormalities detected or suggested by SPE, constitute a functional approach to the numerous facets of serum protein abnormalities (Fig. 1-18).

References

1. Tiselius, A. A new approach for electrophoretic analysis of colloidal mixtures. *Trans. Faraday Soc.* 33:524, 1937.
2. König, P. Employment of Electrophoresis in Chemical Experiments with Small Quantities. *Acts and Works of the 3rd Congress of South American Chemists,* Rio de Janeiro, 1937. Vol. 2, p. 334.
3. Cremer, H., and Tiselius, A. Elektrophorese von Eiweiss in Filtrierpapier. *Biochem. Z.* 320:273, 1950.
4. Durrum, E. L. A Microelectrophoretic and microionophoretic technique. *J. Am. Chem. Soc.* 72:2943, 1950.
5. Sunderman, F. W., Jr. Recent Advances in Clinical Interpretation of Electrophoretic Fractionations of the Serum Proteins. In F. W. Sunderman and F. W. Sunderman, Jr. (Eds.), *Serum Proteins and the Dysproteinemias.* Philadelphia: Lippincott, 1964. Pp. 323–395.
6. Williams, F. G., Jr. Electrophoresis of Serum Proteins. B. Microzone Electrophoresis of Serum Proteins. In F. W. Sunderman and F. W. Sunderman, Jr. (Eds.), *Serum Proteins and the Dysproteinemias.* Philadelphia: Lippincott, 1964. Pp. 125–130.
7. Kohn, J. A cellulose acetate supporting medium for zone electrophoresis. *Clin. Chim. Acta* 2:297, 1957.
8. Cawley, L. P. *Electrophoresis and Immunoelectrophoresis.* Boston: Little, Brown, 1969.
9. Ritzmann, S. E., Alami, S., Van Fossan, D. D., and McKay, G. Electrophoresis, Immunoelectrophoresis, Quantitative Immunodiffusion (Radial Immunodiffusion, Electroimmunodiffusion) and Thermoproteins. In G. J. Race (Ed.), *Laboratory Medicine.* New York: Harper & Row, 1973. Pp. 1–56.
10. Ritzmann, S. E., Vyvial, T. M., Lawrence, M. C., and Daniels, J. C. Serum Protein Electrophoresis (SPE). In J. B. Fuller (Ed.), *ASCP Workshop Manual, Selected Topics in Clinical Chemistry* (4th ed.). Chicago: American Society of Clinical Pathologists' Commission on Continuing Education, 1973. Pp. 7–31.
11. Schultze, H. E., and Heremans, J. F. *Molecular Biology of Human Proteins,* Vol. 1. New York: Elsevier, 1966.
12. Sunderman, F. W. B. Micro-Kjeldahl Procedure for Determination of Serum Protein Nitrogen. In F. W. Sunderman and F. W. Sunderman, Jr. (Eds.), *Serum Proteins and the Dysproteinemias.* Philadelphia: Lippincott, 1964. Pp. 46–49.
13. Kingsley, G. R. The direct biuret method for determination of serum proteins as applied to photoelectric and visual colorimetry. *J. Lab. Clin. Med.* 27:840, 1942.

14. De La Huerga, J., Smetters, G. W., and Sherrick, J. C. Colorimetric Determination of Serum Proteins: The Biuret Reaction. In F. W. Sunderman and F. W. Sunderman, Jr. (Eds.), *Serum Proteins and the Dysproteinemias.* Philadelphia: Lippincott, 1964. Pp. 52–65.
15. Naumann, H. N. Determination of Total Serum Proteins by Refractometry. In F. W. Sunderman and F. W. Sunderman, Jr. (Eds.), *Serum Proteins and the Dysproteinemias.* Philadelphia: Lippincott, 1964. Pp. 86–107.
16. Hart, J. S., Lawrence, M. C., Ritzmann, S. E., and Levin, W. C. Hyperproteinemia. Correlation of elevated total serum protein values and their responsible globulin fractions with various polyclonal and monoclonal gammopathies. A study of 173 sera. *Tex. Rep. Biol. Med.* 23:445, 1965.
17. Ritzmann, S. E., and Levin, W. C. Polyclonal and Monoclonal Gammopathies. In H. Dettelbach and S. E. Ritzmann (Eds.), *Lab Synopsis,* Vol. 2 (2nd ed.). Somerville, N.J.: Behring Diagnostics, 1969. Pp. 9–54.
18. Royal Australian College of General Practitioners. Plasma Proteins in General Practice. *Annals of General Practice,* Sydney, Australia, 1971.
19. McKelvey, E. M. Studies of the serum proteins. VI. Advances in clinical interpretation of electrophoretic fractionations. *Am. J. Clin. Pathol.* 42:1, 1964.
20. McPhedran, P., Finch, S. C., Nemerson, Y. R., and Barnes, M. G. Alpha-2 globulin "spike" in renal carcinoma. *Ann. Intern. Med.* 76:439, 1972.
21. Vermillion, S. Renal carcinoma and alpha-2 globulin. *Ann. Intern. Med.* 77:324, 1972.

Qualitative Immunoelectrophoresis   **2**

Stephan E. Ritzmann and Monica Lawrence

Immunoelectrophoresis (IEP) was introduced by Grabar and Williams in 1953 [1, 2], and a practical microtechnique was reported subsequently by Scheidegger [3]. Much of our knowledge in the areas of proteinology and immunology is derived from the application of IEP as a research and diagnostic tool [4–13]. IEP is a two-step procedure in which proteins are characterized by both their electrophoretic and immunological properties. The proteins are separated by electrophoresis, and, subsequently, they are allowed to react with corresponding antibodies, which results in the formation of precipitin lines reflecting individual proteins (Figs. 2-1 and 2-2). With the use of polyvalent or specific antisera, more than 50 individual human serum proteins can be demonstrated, even if present in trace amounts (i.e., 5 to 10 mg per 100 ml) (see Fig. 2-2). In the clinical laboratory, IEP allows the diagnosis of serum protein deficiencies (e.g., homozygous α_1-antitrypsin deficiency); detection of clinically important "abnormal" proteins (e.g., α_1-fetoprotein); characterization of immunoglobulin abnormalities, including deficiencies (e.g., selective IgA deficiency) and overproduction states (i.e., polyclonal and monoclonal gammopathies and their distinction from pseudomonoclonal gammopathies); the study of phenotypes of certain proteins (e.g., Gc groups); and the recognition of certain types of immune complexes.

Methodology

IEP kits are commercially available that provide ready-to-use agar or agarose plates or rehydratable agarose films (Fig. 2-3) [14]. In general, agar or agarose is the most suitable medium for IEP. Other carrier media, such as cellulose acetate, yield satisfactory results under controlled laboratory conditions, but they are inferior to agar or agarose under the demanding "field conditions" of the clinical laboratory. Electrophoresis chambers (Fig. 2-4) and other accessories are also available on a commercial basis.

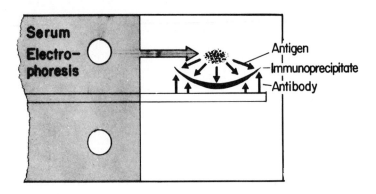

Figure 2-1
Immunodiffusion events in IEP. During the storage period after electrophoresis and the application of antiserum, diffusion of both the antigens (e.g., serum proteins) and antibodies (contained in antiserum) occurs, which results in an antigen-antibody reaction and the formation of visible precipitin lines. These precipitin lines reflect individual proteins. (Reproduced by permission. From Ritzmann, S. E., Daniels, J. C., Alami, S. Y., and Lawrence, M. C. In G. J. Race (Ed.), *Laboratory Medicine*. New York: Harper & Row, 1975.)

The IEP method using rehydratable agarose films (e.g., Immunotec*) is a practical approach to IEP in the clinical laboratory. The following reagents are required. (1) *Buffers:* Barbital buffer, pH 8.2, ionic strength 0.04, is most commonly used for IEP. (2) *Rehydratable agarose films:* These commercially prepared films can be easily readied for use in the laboratory (see Fig. 2-3A). Rehydration is achieved in distilled water and, subsequently, in barbital buffer for a total period of one hour. The procedural steps are as follows (Fig. 2-3B):

1. *Sample application:* Approximately 4 μl of the antigen solution (serum, urine, or cerebrospinal fluid) is placed in the wells with a micropipet or microliter syringe.
2. *Electrophoresis:* Electrophoresis is performed at 3 v per centimeter (i.e., 90 v per agarose plate) for approximately 55 minutes.
3. *Antisera Application:* The antibody troughs are then filled with 80 to 100 μl of antiserum. The choice of antisera and their pattern of application depends upon the specific problem under investigation. For instance, for the routine IEP screening of immunoglobulin abnormalities, the pattern shown in Table 2-1 usually suffices. On the other hand, a complete IEP analysis for serum protein abnormalities, including immunoglobulin aberrations, may require a pattern such as that shown in Table 2-2. In this approach, two agarose films are used for the systematic screening of two serum samples (see Chap. 19). A routine application of one additional serum sample that has been diluted, say, 1:3, is advocated in order to avoid antigen excess (see Fig. 2-5 and p. 34).

* Behring Diagnostics, Somerville, N.J. 08876.

Figure 2-2

Correlation of serum protein electrophoretic pattern with serum immunoelectrophoretic pattern. (Reproduced by permission. From Ritzmann, S. E., et al. *Lab Notes #3: Serum Proteins.* Somerville, N.J.: Behring Diagnostics, 1973.)

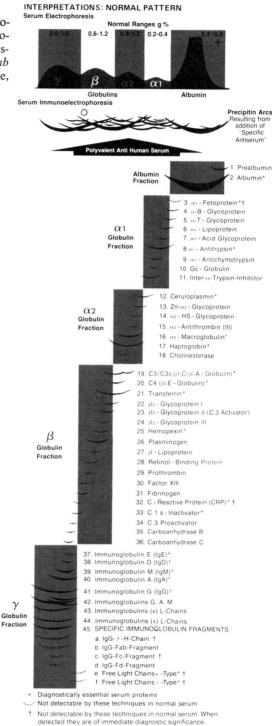

INTERPRETATIONS: NORMAL PATTERN
Serum Electrophoresis

Normal Ranges g %

0.8-1.5   0.8-1.2   0.8-1.2   0.2-0.4   3.2-5.0

γ   β   α2   α1   Albumin

Globulins

Serum Immunoelectrophoresis

Precipitin Arcs
Resulting from
addition of
"Specific
Antiserum"

Polyvalent Anti Human Serum

Albumin Fraction
1. Prealbumin
2. Albumin*

α1 Globulin Fraction
3. α₁ - Fetoprotein*†
4. α₁B - Glycoprotein
5. α₁T - Glycoprotein
6. α₁ - Lipoprotein
7. α₁ - Acid Glycoprotein
8. α₁ - Antitrypsin*
9. α₁ - Antichymotrypsin
10. Gc - Globulin
11. Inter-α-Trypsin-Inhibitor

α2 Globulin Fraction
12. Ceruloplasmin*
13. Zn-α₂ - Glycoprotein
14. α₂ - HS - Glycoprotein
15. α₂ - Antithrombin (III)
16. α₂ - Macroglobulin*
17. Haptoglobin*
18. Cholinesterase

β Globulin Fraction
19. C3/C3c (β₁C/β₁A - Globulin)*
20. C4 (β₁E - Globulin)*
21. Transferrin*
22. β₂ - Glycoprotein I
23. β₂ - Glycoprotein II (C 3 Activator)
24. β₂ - Glycoprotein III
25. Hemopexin*
26. Plasminogen
27. β - Lipoprotein
28. Retinol - Binding Protein
29. Prothrombin
30. Factor XIII
31. Fibrinogen
32. C - Reactive Protein (CRP)* †
33. C 1 s - Inactivator*
34. C 3 Proactivator
35. Carboanhydrase B
36. Carboanhydrase C

γ Globulin Fraction
37. Immunoglobulin E (IgE)*
38. Immunoglobulin D (IgD)*
39. Immunoglobulin M (IgM)*
40. Immunoglobulin A (IgA)*
41. Immunoglobulin G (IgG)*
42. Immunoglobulins G, A, M
43. Immunoglobulins (κ) L-Chains
44. Immunoglobulins (λ) L-Chains
45. SPECIFIC IMMUNOGLOBULIN FRAGMENTS:
   a. IgG- γ -H-Chain †
   b. IgG-Fab-Fragment
   c. IgG-Fc-Fragment †
   d. IgG-Fd-Fragment
   e. Free Light Chains κ -Type* †
   f. Free Light Chains λ -Type* †

* Diagnostically essential serum proteins
···· Not detectable by these techniques in normal serum
† Not detectable by these techniques in normal serum. When detected they are of immediate diagnostic significance.

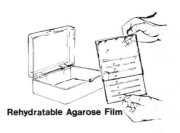

Rehydratable Agarose Film

1. Rehydration 2. Buffer 3. Lift out 4. Blot

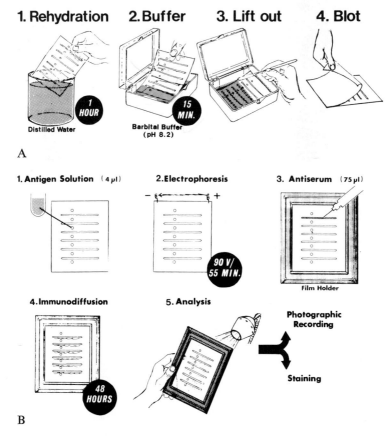

1 HOUR

Distilled Water

15 MIN.

Barbital Buffer
(pH 8.2)

A

1. Antigen Solution (4 μl)

2. Electrophoresis

− +

90 V/ 55 MIN.

3. Antiserum (75 μl)

Film Holder

4. Immunodiffusion

5. Analysis

48 HOURS

Photographic
Recording

Staining

B

Figure 2-3
Immunoelectrophoresis: *A*. Preparation. *B*. Procedure. (Reproduced by permission. From Ritzmann, S. E., Daniels, J. C., Alami, S. Y., and Lawrence, M. C. In G. J. Race (Ed.), *Laboratory Medicine*. New York: Harper & Row, 1975.)

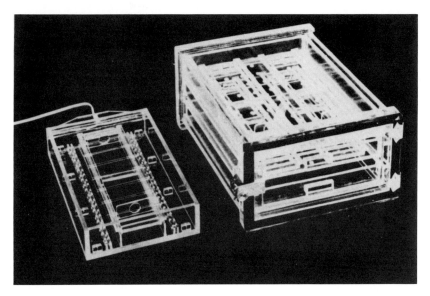

Figure 2-4
IEP equipment. Electrophoresis cell (*left*) and chamber (*right*). (Reproduced by permission. From Ritzmann, S. E., Daniels, J. C., Alami, S. Y., and Lawrence, M. C. In G. J. Race (Ed.), *Laboratory Medicine*. New York: Harper & Row, 1975.)

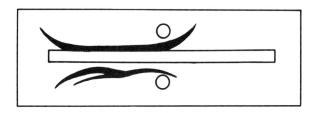

Figure 2-5
IEP pattern resulting from antigen excess (*top*). The same serum sample diluted 1:3 (*bottom*) reveals the characteristic abnormality of IgG monoclonal gammopathy. (Reproduced by permission. From Ritzmann, S. E., Daniels, J. C., Alami, S. Y., and Lawrence, M. C. In G. J. Race (Ed.), *Laboratory Medicine*. New York: Harper & Row, 1975.)

Table 2-1. Antigen (Serum)-Antiserum Combinations for Routine IEP Screening (Sequence from Top to Bottom of Rehydratable Agarose Film or Comparable Slide)

Well or Trough	Antigen-Antiserum Combinations
Antigen well #1	Normal control serum—undiluted
Antibody trough #1	Anti-IgG antiserum (H- and L-chain specific)—undiluted
Antigen well #2	Serum—patient #1—undiluted
Antibody trough #2	Anti-IgA antiserum (α-chain specific)—undiluted
Antigen well #3	Normal control serum—undiluted
Antibody trough #3	Anti-IgM-antiserum (μ-chain specific)—undiluted
Antigen well #4	Serum—patient #1—undiluted
Antibody trough #4	Anti-human serum antiserum (polyvalent antiserum)—undiluted
Antigen well #5	Normal control serum—undiluted
Antibody trough #5	No antiserum applied here (may be used for quality control)
Antigen well #6	Normal control serum—1:3 dilution
Antibody trough #6	Anti-IgG antiserum (γ H-chain specific)—undiluted
Antigen well #7	Serum—patient #1—1:3 dilution

Polyvalent antihuman sera (i.e., antisera containing antibodies against most serum proteins), anti-immunoglobulin sera (i.e., antisera containing antibodies against the major immunoglobulins IgG, IgA, and IgM), or antisera specific for individual proteins may be employed. Such specific antisera include those which react only with individual proteins, such as albumin, α_1-antitrypsin, α_2-macroglobulin, haptoglobin, transferrin, or complement C4 (β_1E-globulin); with specific protein moieties such as complement C3c (β_1A-globulin); with the immunoglobulins IgG, IgA, IgM, IgD, and IgE; with immunoglobulin types (e.g., anti-κ or λ type immunoglobulins); or with immunoglobulin fragments (e.g., anti-free κ or λ light chains) (see Fig. 2-2). Monospecific antisera to the various immunoglobulin classes contain antibody activity against the heavy chains of these immunoglobulins; such heavy-chain specific antisera (i.e., anti-γ, α, μ, δ, and ϵ chain antisera for IgG, IgA, IgM, IgD, and IgE, respectively) are also a prerequisite for the precise immunochemical quantitation of these immunoglobulins by radial immunodiffusion or electroimmunodiffusion. Antisera that are directed against the whole immunoglobulin molecule (e.g., anti-IgG-H+L-chain specific antisera) react with both the light and heavy chains, and therefore cross-react with the other immunoglobulin classes via their L-chain determinants. The latter antisera are useful for the sceening of Bence Jones proteins (see Chaps. 5 and 20). A wide variety of antisera is available on a commercial basis (see Fig. 2-2).

4. *Immunodiffusion:* After application of the antisera in the above

Table 2-2. Antigen (Serum)-Antiserum Combinations for Complete IEP Analysis (Sequence from Top to Bottom of Rehydratable Agarose Film)

Well or Trough	Antigen-Antiserum Combinations
Agarose Film #1	
Antigen well #1	Normal control serum—undiluted
Antibody trough #1	Anti-human serum antiserum (polyvalent antiserum)—undiluted
Antigen well #2	Serum—patient #1—undiluted
Antibody trough #2	Anti-immunoglobulin antiserum (anti-IgG, IgA, IgM)—undiluted
Antigen well #3	Normal control serum—undiluted
Antibody trough #3	Anti-IgG antiserum (H- and L-chain specific)—undiluted
Antigen well #4	Serum—patient #1—undiluted
Antibody trough #4	Anti-IgG antiserum (γ H-chain specific)—undiluted
Antigen well #5	Normal control serum—undiluted
Antibody trough #5	Anti-IgA antiserum (α H-chain specific)—undiluted
Antigen well #6	Serum—patient #1—undiluted
Antibody trough #6	Anti-IgM antiserum (μ H-chain specific)—undiluted
Antigen well #7	Normal control serum—undiluted
Agarose Film #2	
Antigen well #1	Normal control serum—undiluted
Antibody trough #1	Anti-IgD antiserum (δ H-chain specific)—undiluted
Antigen well #2	Serum—patient #1—undiluted
Antibody trough #2	Anti-IgE antiserum (ϵ H-chain specific)—undiluted
Antigen well #3	Normal control serum—undiluted
Antibody trough #3	Anti-immunoglobulin κ-type antiserum
Antigen well #4	Serum—patient #1—undiluted
Antibody trough #4	Anti-immunoglobulin λ-type antiserum
Antigen well #5	Normal control serum—undiluted
Antibody trough #5	No antiserum (may be used for quality control)
Antigen well #6	Serum—patient #1—1:3 serum dilution
Antibody trough #6	Anti-IgG antiserum (γ H-chain specific)
Antigen well #7	Normal control serum—1:3 serum dilution (to prevent antigen excess)

IEP method, the agarose plates are placed in a moisture chamber at room temperature for the diffusion of antigens and antibodies and the development of the characteristic precipitin arcs. The optimal diffusion time is between 24 and 48 hours. For routine analysis, the examination of unstained precipitin patterns is usually sufficient. Photographic records of unstained or stained patterns may also be obtained.

Sources of Error

Errors may be caused by impurities or imperfections in the agarose gel, desiccation of agarose films, improper rehydration procedure, use of aged or unreliable antisera, faulty techniques in applying the antigen or antibody solutions, insufficient electrical contact, improper voltage control, excessively long or short periods of electrophoretic separation, unsuitable buffers, and unfavorable antigen-antibody ratios (Fig 2-5).

The IEP analysis of sera from patients with either high protein concentrations (e.g., M proteins) or low protein concentrations (e.g., hypoalbuminemia, hypogammaglobulinemia, or α_1-antitrypsin deficiency) frequently requires considerable adjustment of the antigen concentrations regardless of the source and quality of the antiserum. Antigen excess may be encountered when the concentration of one protein (e.g., IgG) is greatly increased, resulting in the migration of this protein close to or into the antibody trough. Such a degree of antigen excess may result in misinterpretation of the IEP patterns. For this reason, a routine application of a diluted serum sample (e.g., 1:3 dilution) to be assayed for IgG abnormalities may have to be considered (see Table 2-2). Similar dilutions may be necessary for the analysis of other immunoglobulin patterns if antigen excess exists. It is important to realize that under routine service conditions, the antigen-antibody ratios vary between extremely low concentrations (e.g., 50 mg of IgG per 100 ml) and excessively high levels (e.g., 5000 mg of IgG per 100 ml), i.e., a 100-fold variation of concentrations. For these reasons, three important technical aspects of the IEP procedure in the clinical laboratory need to be emphasized:

1. The use of cellulose acetate instead of agar or agarose is not recommended. Although, under ideal laboratory conditions, satisfactory IEP patterns can be obtained with cellulose acetate, under the "field conditions" of the clinical laboratory, an unacceptably high percentage of serum protein abnormalities will be missed if it is used as the medium for IEP analysis. In particular, M proteins in low concentrations often escape detection.
2. The use of polyvalent antihuman antiserum as the only antiserum, without the additional use of antisera against specific proteins (e.g., anti-IgG antisera), is not advisable. Such a practice often does not allow the recognition of less conspicuous abnormalities, such as M proteins present in low concentrations.
3. The use of rabbit antisera is preferable to the use of horse antisera for the screening of serum protein abnormalities. The former yield

satisfactory precipitin arcs over a wider range of antigen-antibody ratios.

Indications for Immunoelectrophoresis

IEP analysis is indicated in most instances of suspected protein abnormalities. More specifically, IEP is the method of choice for the diagnosis and characterization of monoclonal gammopathies, including IgG, IgA, IgM, IgD, and IgE monoclonal gammopathies (MG) as well as light- and heavy-chain diseases (Figs. 2-6 and 2-7; see also Chap. 19). Both serum and urine specimens are used. IEP analysis is indicated in all instances of cryoglobulinemia and pyroglobulinemia, since a high percentage of these immunoglobulin abnormalities is associated with MG. IEP assays aid in the detection of the occurrence of "new" proteins (e.g., α_1-fetoproteins; see Chap. 21, Fig. 21-1), and the recognition and characterization of antibody deficiency syndromes (e.g., sex-linked agammaglobulinemia, selective IgA deficiency, or secondary immunoglobulin deficiencies associated with chronic lymphocytic leukemia). The presence of serum immune complexes can often be suspected (see Chap. 9).

Application and Interpretation

The shape of the precipitin lines may serve as a guide to the cathodic (negative) and anodic (positive) poles of the IEP pattern, i.e., albumin migrates toward the anode and displays symmetric precipitin lines, whereas IgG migrates toward the cathode and shows asymmetric arcs (see Fig. 2-2). Bromphenol-blue markers appear at the anode.

In general, *decreased* serum protein concentrations are reflected by weaker and shortened precipitin lines that are situated more distant from the antibody trough than their counterpart in the control serum (see Figs. 2-6 and 2-7). Significantly decreased immunoglobulins may reveal two parallel precipitin arcs. This phenomenon of two separate, parallel lines reflects the two light-chain types of these immunoglobulins, e.g., κ and λ types of IgG (Fig. 2-8).

Increased concentrations of serum proteins are reflected by thick and elongated precipitin arcs that are located closer to the antibody trough. In polyclonal gammopathies (PG), the increase of the major immunoglobulins is reflected by long heavy IgG, IgA, and IgM arcs near the antibody trough (see Figs. 2-6 and 2-7). IEP is, at best, a semiquantitative technique. In general, increases or decreases of proteins can only be detected with some degree of certainty if a ±50 percent deviation from normal values has occurred.

IMMUNOGLOBULIN ABNORMALITIES

TERMINOLOGY AND BACKGROUND
Inasmuch as the appropriate IEP analysis of immunoglobulin abnormalities requires a certain degree of background information, a brief

Immunoelectrophoresis

Normal

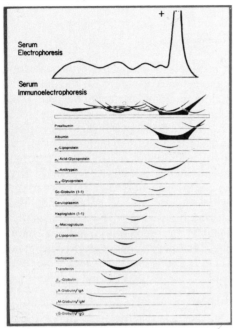

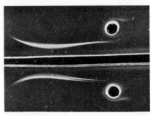

Ig G
Decreased

Control

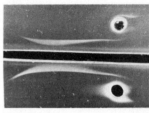

Ig G
Increased

A

Figure 2-6

A. IEP patterns of individual serum proteins (*left*), hypogammaglobulinemia (*right, top*), and increased IgG in association with polyclonal gammopathy (*right, bottom*). The top pattern in each panel indicates a normal precipitin line.

B. Abnormal IEP patterns (*bottom*) and normal patterns (*top*) of monoclonal gammopathies. (IgE myeloma serum kindly supplied by Dr. O. R.
McIntyre, University of New Hampshire, Hanover, N.H. Reproduced by
permission. From Ritzmann, S. E., and Daniels, J. C. In G. J. Race (Ed.),
Tice's Practice of Medicine, Vol. 2. New York: Harper & Row, 1974.)

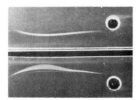

Ig G
Monoclonal
Gammopathy

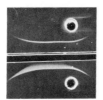

Ig A
Monoclonal
Gammopathy

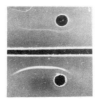

Ig M
Monoclonal
Gammopathy

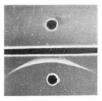

Ig D
Monoclonal
Gammopathy

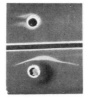

Ig E
Monoclonal
Gammopathy

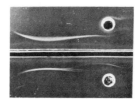

Bence Jones
Monoclonal
Gammopathy

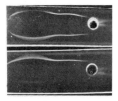

Ig G (κ)
Monoclonal
Gammopathy

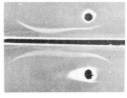

Immune
Complexes

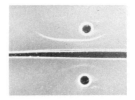

Isolated
Ig A
Deficiency

B

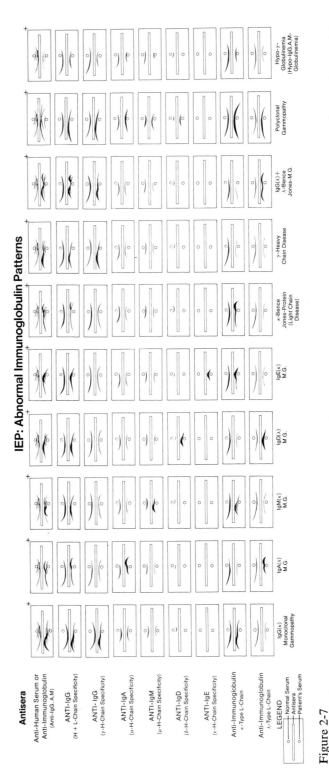

IEP: Abnormal Immunoglobulin Patterns

Antisera

Anti-Human Serum or
Anti-Immunoglobulin
(Anti-IgG, A,M)

ANTI-IgG
(H + L-Chain Specificity)

ANTI-IgG
(γ-H-Chain Specificity)

ANTI-IgA
(α-H-Chain Specificity)

ANTI-IgM
(μ-H-Chain Specificity)

ANTI-IgD
(δ-H-Chain Specificity)

ANTI-IgE
(ε-H-Chain Specificity)

Anti-Immunoglobulin
κ-Type L-Chain

Anti-Immunoglobulin
λ-Type L-Chain

LEGEND
○ — Normal Serum
⊢⊣ — Antisera
⊢—⊣ — Patient's Serum

Column labels (left to right):
IgG(κ)
Monoclonal
Gammopathy

IgA(λ)
M.G.

IgM(κ)
M.G.

IgD(λ)
M.G.

IgE(κ)
M.G.

κ-Bence
Jones-Protein
(Light Chain
Disease)

γ-Heavy
Chain Disease

IgG(λ) +
λ-Bence
Jones-M.G.

Polyclonal
Gammopathy

Hypo-γ-
Globulinemia
(Hypo-IgG,A,M-
Globulinemia)

Figure 2-7

Abnormal IEP patterns associated with monoclonal gammopathies. For comparison, the IEP patterns of polyclonal gammopathies and hypogammaglobulinemia are depicted at right. (Reproduced by permission. From Ritzmann, S. E., et al. *Lab Notes #3: Serum Proteins.* Somerville, N.J.: Behring Diagnostics, 1973.)

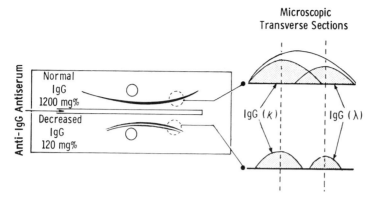

Microscopic
Transverse Sections

Figure 2-8
Normal and decreased IgG precipitin lines and their κ and λ light-chain type constituents. *Left:* Sera with normal IgG concentration (*top;* 1200 mg per 100 ml) and from patient with hypogammaglobulinemia (*bottom;* 120 mg per 100 ml). Antiserum to IgG (heavy- and light-chain specific) is contained in antibody trough. Note the shortened and split IgG precipitin arc that is situated farther away from the antibody trough than the normal IgG in the top pattern. *Right:* Cross sections through the precipitin arcs of normal IgG (*top*) and decreased IgG (*bottom*). In the former, the two light-chain constituents of IgG, i.e., IgG(κ) and IgG(λ), which are normally present in a ratio of 2:1, overlap each other, resulting in one solid precipitin line. The decreased IgG concentration in the lower pattern results in non-fusion of two light-chain types of IgG, thereby yielding two individual precipitin lines.

summary of the essential aspects of immunoglobulins is presented (see also Chaps. 1, 19, and 20).

The basic structure of the five known classes of immunoglobulins—IgG, IgA, IgM, IgD, and IgE—includes two pairs of polypeptide chains that are linked by disulfide and hydrogen bonds. Two of these chains, each with a molecular weight of approximately 25,000, are light (L) chains; these are linked to two heavy (H) chains, each with a molecular weight of approximately 50,000. The L chains are common to all immunoglobulins and may be of either κ or λ type. In normal human serum, the κ type immunoglobulins predominate over the λ type in an approximate ratio of 2:1. The H chains are unique for each class of immunoglobulins. They are termed γ, α, μ, δ, and ϵ *chains* for IgG, IgA, IgM, IgD, and IgE, respectively. In normal adult serum, there are four known subclasses of IgG (IgG$_1$, IgG$_2$, IgG$_3$, and IgG$_4$) and two subclasses of IgA (IgA$_1$ and IgA$_2$). The high molecular-weight IgM is a pentamer with an approximate molecular weight of 900,000. Cleavage of this molecule by mercaptans results in the formation of five monomeric subunits. In addition to the 7S serum IgA, there exists secretory IgA in the mucosal secretions. It is composed of two IgA subunits that are linked by S (secretory) and J (joining) pieces (see Chap. 19).

Normally, a single plasma cell produces the H and L chains in a synchronous fashion that results in the assembly and secretion of a complete immunoglobulin molecule. The normal serum immunoglobulin mixture of classes, subclasses, and types represents the sum of the immunoglobulin products of a multitude of plasma cell clones. The serum immunoglobulin levels are age-dependent; this fact needs to be considered when assaying these proteins in the pediatric age group. In patients with hypo- or agammaglobulinemia, there is usually a significant deficiency of all components of the immunoglobulin system. In selective IgA deficiency, however, only the IgA class is absent. In patients with PG, there is usually an increase, to various proportions, of all immunoglobulin classes, subclasses, and types, which generally preserves the normal ratios of these subclasses and types. In MG, however, one plasma cell clone proliferates out of proportion, resulting in the production and accumulation of either a homogeneous "complete" immunoglobulin molecular species of only one class, subclass, and type, such as $IgG_2(\kappa)$, or it produces excess amounts of "incomplete" immunoglobulin molecules, i.e., either L chains (κ or λ) or H chains (γ, α, μ, δ, and ϵ). These free monoclonal L or H chains are the result of an asynchronous synthesis of the H and L chains by these abnormal plasma cells. The free monoclonal L chains are identical with Bence Jones proteins.

The term *paraprotein* was introduced by Apitz in 1940 [15] to denote such "foreign" proteins in the blood, urine, or tissues produced by myeloma cells. Gutman in 1948 [16] coined the term *M proteins* for the discrete proteins demonstrated by electrophoresis in sera of patients suffering from myeloma. In 1957, Riva [17] applied this term to those narrow bands on electrophoresis patterns that were also found in association with macroglobulinemia. The term *monoclonal gammopathies* was introduced by Waldenström in 1961 and 1962 [18, 19] as a more comprehensive label for such abnormal immunoglobulins and their associated clinical conditions. Osserman uses the designation *plasma cell dyscrasias* [20, 21] and Engle and Wallis, *paraimmunoglobulinopathies* [11] for the same disorders.

The technical approach to IEP analysis of the immunoglobulin abnormalities consists of a stepwise sequence that requires special consideration (see Fig. 2-7 and Tables 2-1 and 2-2):

Step 1. Use of polyvalent antiserum to human serum. Such an antiserum provides general information as to the serum protein content and the presence or absence of major proteins or unusual patterns, such as fusion of albumin and IgA (see Fig. 2-10). The use of these antisera, however, often does not allow a reliable evaluation of immunoglobulin and other protein abnormalities; thus, these antisera are useful mainly in conjunction with the use of specific antisera.

Step 2. Use of polyvalent antisera to the major immunoglobulins IgG, IgA, and IgM and specific antisera to the individual immunoglobulin classes IgG, IgA, IgM, IgD and IgE. The use of these antisera is essential for a complete and systematic IEP analysis. Polyvalent antiimmunoglobulin antisera are directed to the major immunoglobulins

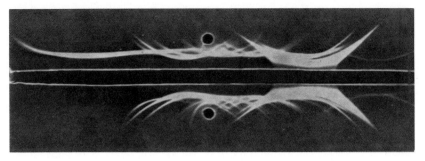

Figure 2-9
Agammaglobulinemia reflected by the absence of IgG, IgA, and IgM precipitin
arcs (*bottom*). Normal serum IEP pattern (*top*). *Antibody trough:* polyvalent
antihuman antiserum.

IgG, IgA, and IgM, and they not only allow the detection and characterization of deficiencies of these immunoglobulins but also the recognition
of most MGs of IgG, IgA, and IgM and of Bence Jones proteins. Rare
forms, such as IgD and IgE MGs, require the use of such specific antisera to the individual immunoglobulin classes. Specific antisera against
IgG, IgA, IgM, IgD, and IgE either are reactive with the entire immunoglobulin molecule (i.e., both the H and L chains) or are monospecific
and reactive with the H chains or the Fc fragments of the respective immunoglobulin class. The former cross-react with the L chains of all immunoglobulins and are able to detect free L chains (either polyclonal,
i.e., both κ and λ L chains, or monoclonal, i.e., either κ or λ L chains),
thus allowing screening for Bence Jones proteins. The latter antisera do
not cross-react with other immunoglobulin classes (e.g., H-chain specific anti-IgG antiserum reacts only with the IgG class), and therefore
are useful for immunochemical quantitation of immunoglobulins. Both
of these categories of antisera are useful for a systematic and complete
IEP analysis of monoclonal gammopathies.

Step 3. Anti-κ and anti-λ immunoglobulin antisera. These antisera
are essential for the typing of the immunoglobulins, the estimation of
κ/λ ratios, and the establishment of the monoclonal nature of M proteins.

HYPOGAMMAGLOBULINEMIAS
Depending upon the type of the antibody deficiency syndrome (see Figs.
2-6 and 2-7 and Chap. 19), several patterns may be encountered. All
major immunoglobulin classes may be virtually absent (Fig. 2-9), or
they may be moderately to considerably decreased. Only one or two of
the immunoglobulin classes may be deficient (e.g., as in isolated IgA deficiency; see Figs. 2-6 and 2-7), or an imbalance between the various
immunoglobulin classes may occur (e.g., decreased IgG and IgA but increased IgM may be found [22]). For verification and precise quantitation of such antibody deficiency patterns, immunochemical quantitation

of the immunoglobulins—including IgD and IgE, secretory IgA, and, occasionally, IgG subclasses—is often required.

POLYCLONAL GAMMOPATHIES

In general, the finding of a PG on serum protein electrophoresis is no indication for IEP analysis (see Figs. 2-6 and 2-7). The expected IEP finding in such sera is an increase of the major immunoglobulins IgG, IgA, and IgM. In doubtful cases with a questionably homogeneous γ-globulin fraction, the employment of IEP analysis will usually resolve such a diagnostic dilemma. For instance, patients with chronic active hepatitis frequently demonstrate a considerably increased γ-globulin fraction that is more compact than the usual form found in PG [23, 24]; it is usually due to an excessive, selective increase of the IgG class of both κ and λ types [25]. Such a pattern has been referred to as *oligoclonal gammopathy* (see Chaps. 1 and 19).

MONOCLONAL GAMMOPATHIES

IEP allows the diagnosis of MGs and their differential diagnosis into the various immunochemical categories (see also Chaps. 1 and 19). The immunoglobulin abnormalities of the MGs are accompanied by characteristic IEP patterns [2, 4, 6–8, 10–14, 24, 26–34] (see also Figs. 2-6 and 2-7). M protein on serum protein electrophoresis (SPE) results in localized antigen excess and in an abnormal bending (i.e., arc) of the corresponding precipitin lines on IEP. The arc on IEP corresponds to the identical electrophoretic position of the M protein on SPE (see Table 2-3). Occasionally, "fusion" of the M protein (especially IgA and IgM) with albumin or other anodically migrating proteins occurs [6] (Fig. 2-10). The MGs described to date include those due to an overproduction of IgG, IgA, IgM, IgD, and IgE as well as of free L chains and H chains. Occasionally, two different M proteins (biclonal gammopathy) or, rarely, three M proteins (triclonal gammopathy) are observed.

The series of monoclonal and biclonal gammopathies at the University of Texas Medical Branch at Galveston, Texas (compiled since 1962) may be representative of the relative frequency of the various categories of MG encountered in adult patients in a large referral institution (see Table 2-4). Additionally, there are the following rare monoclonal gammopathies:

1. Triclonal gammopathies
2. IgE MG (5 known cases)
3. Heavy-chain diseases, including γ H-chain disease (35 known cases), α H-chain disease (more than 60 known cases), and μ H-chain disease (10 known cases)
4. Low molecular weight IgM MG
5. Half-molecule MG
6. Deleted H and L chain diseases

Table 2-3.   Characteristic IEP Precipitin-Line Patterns of Immunoglobulin Abnormalities of Monoclonal Gammopathies[a]

1. IgG MG   a. Abnormal arc with:

           1. polyvalent antihuman serum;
           2. anti-immunoglobulin (G, A, M) serum;
           3. anti-IgG (H- + L-chain specific) serum; and
              with arcs in identical position as IgG arc):
           4. anti-IgG (γH-chain specific) serum[b] and abnormal arc
           5. either anti-immunoglobulin (κ type) serum;
           6. or anti-immunoglobulin (λ type) serum.
           FINAL DIAGNOSIS: Either IgG (κ) MG or IgG (λ) MG.

      b. Abnormal arc with 1, 2, 3, and 4 and two abnormal arcs with (one arc in identical position as IgG arc):
           5. either anti-immunoglobulin (κ type) serum;
           6. or anti-immunoglobulin (λ type) serum.
           FINAL DIAGNOSIS: Either IgG (κ) and BJP (κ) MG or IgG (λ) and BJP (λ) MG.

      c. Abnormal arc with 1, 2, 3, and 4 but no abnormal arc with either 5 or 6.
           PROBABLE DIAGNOSIS: γ heavy-chain disease. Confirmatory tests consist of serum fractionation by Sephadex G-200; molecular weight should be approximately 50,000).[c]

2. IgA MG   a. Abnormal arc with:

           1. polyvalent antihuman serum;
           2. anti-immunoglobulin (G, A, M) serum;
           3. anti-IgG (H- + L-chain specific) serum; and
           4. anti-IgA (α H-chain specific) serum and abnormal arc with (in identical position as IgA arc):
           5. either anti-immunoglobulin (κ type) serum;
           6. or anti-immunoglobulin (λ type) serum.
           FINAL DIAGNOSIS: Either IgA (κ) MG or IgA (λ) MG.

      b. Abnormal arc with 1, 2, 3, 4 and two abnormal arcs with (one arc in identical position as IgA arc):
           5. either anti-immunoglobulin (κ type) serum;
           6. or anti-immunoglobulin (λ type) serum.
           FINAL DIAGNOSIS: Either IgA (κ) and BJP (κ) MG, or IgA (λ) and BJP (λ) MG.

      c. Abnormal arc with 1, 2, 3, 4 but no abnormal arc with either 5 or 6.
           PROBABLE DIAGNOSIS: α heavy-chain disease.

[a] This IEP approach to the diagnosis of MG also allows the recognition of biclonal gammopathies, i.e., the presence of 2 different M proteins (e.g., lgG (κ) *and* IgA (λ) BG; IgG (κ) and IgG (λ) BG; BJP (κ) and BJP (λ) BG; etc.), or triclonal gammopathies (e.g., IgG (κ), IgA (κ) and IgM (λ) triclonal gammopathies).
[b] It is also advisable to use a dilution (e.g., 1:3) of the MG serum, in order to avoid antigen excess which may obscure the abnormal arc.
[c] Confirmation can also be obtained by the use of antisera to IgG Fc-fragments which will result in an abnormal precipitin arc. Serum with γ H-chain disease, however, does not show an abnormal precipitin arc with antisera specific for IgG Fab- and Fd-fragments.

43

Table 2-3 (*Continued*)

3. IgM MG   a. Abnormal arc with:
    1. polyvalent antihuman serum;
    2. anti-immunoglobulin (G, A, M) serum;
    3. anti-IgG (H- + L-chain specific serum; and
    4. Anti-IgM (μ H-chain specific) serum and abnormal arc with (in identical position as IgM arc):[d]
    5. either anti-immunoglobulin (κ type) serum;
    6. or anti-immunoglobulin (λ type) serum.
    FINAL DIAGNOSIS: Either IgM (κ) MG or IgM (λ) MG.

    b. Abnormal arc with 1, 2, 3, 4 and two abnormal arcs with (one arc corresponding with IgM arc):[d]
    5. either anti-immunoglobulin (κ type) serum;
    6. or anti-immunoglobulin (λ type) serum.
    FINAL DIAGNOSIS: Either IgM (κ) and BJP (κ) MG or IgM (λ) and BJP (λ) MG.

    c. Abnormal arc with 1, 2, 3, 4 but no abnormal arc with either 5 or 6.[d]
    PROBABLE DIAGNOSIS: μ heavy-chain disease.

4. IgD MG   a. Abnormal arc with:
    1. polyvalent antihuman serum;
    2. anti-immunoglobulin (G, A, M) serum;
    3. anti-IgG (H- + L-chain specific) serum; and
    4. anti-IgD (δ H-chain specific) serum and abnormal arc with (in identical position as IgD arc):
    5. either anti-immunoglobulin (κ type) serum;
    6. or anti-immunoglobulin (λ type) serum.
    FINAL DIAGNOSIS: Either IgD (κ) MG or IgD (λ) MG.

    b. Abnormal arc with 1, 2, 3, 4 and two abnormal arcs with (one arc corresponding with IgD arc):
    5. either anti-immunoglobulin (κ type) serum;
    6. or anti-immunoglobulin (λ type) serum.
    FINAL DIAGNOSIS: Either IgD (κ) and BJP (κ) MG or IgD (λ) and BJP (λ) MG.

    c. Abnormal arc with 1, 2, 3, 4 but no abnormal arc with either 5 or 6.
    PROBABLE DIAGNOSIS: δ heavy-chain disease (not reported yet).

5. IgE MG   a. Abnormal arc with:
    1. polyvalent antihuman serum;
    2. anti-immunoglobulin (G, A, M) serum;
    3. anti-IgG (H- + L-chain specific serum); and
    4. anti-IgE (ϵ H-chain specific) serum and abnormal arc with (in identical position as IgE arc):

---

[d] Sometimes, L-chain typing of the IgM MG is not possible. This is due to the fact that the IgG moves ahead of the IgM, toward the antibody trough, during immunodiffusion and neutralizes the antiserum before it can reach and react with IgM. Under these conditions, 6-mercaptoethanol (6 ME) may be used[e] to depolymerize the IgM molecules resulting in smaller IgM units. These subunits diffuse towards the antibody trough at least as fast as the IgG molecules, and react with the anti-κ or anti-λ sera.

Table 2-3 (*Continued*)

     5. either anti-immunoglobulin (κ type) serum;

     6. or anti-immunoglobulin (λ type) serum.

     FINAL DIAGNOSIS: Either IgE (κ) MG or IgE (λ) MG.

  b. Abnormal arc with 1, 2, 3, 4 and two abnormal arcs with (one arc corresponding with IgE arc):

     5. either anti-immunoglobulin (κ type) serum;

     6. or anti-immunoglobulin (λ type) serum.

     FINAL DIAGNOSIS: Either IgE (κ) and BJP (κ) MG or IgE (λ) and BJP (λ) MG.

  c. Abnormal arc with 1, 2, 3, 4 but no abnormal arc with either 5 or 6.

     PROBABLE DIAGNOSIS: ϵ heavy-chain disease (not reported yet).

6. Bence Jones MG (light-chain disease): [f]

  a. Abnormal arc with:

     1. polyvalent antihuman serum;

     2. anti-immunoglobulin (G, A, M) serum);

     3. anti-IgG (H- + L-chain specific serum); and

     4. either anti-immunoglobulin (κ type) serum;

     5. or anti-immunoglobulin (λ type) serum;

     but no abnormal arc with:

     6. anti-IgG (γ H-chain specific) serum;

     7. anti-IgA (α H-chain specific) serum;

     8. anti-IgM (μ H-chain specific) serum;

     9. anti-IgD (δ H-chain specific) serum;

    10. anti-IgE (ϵ H-chain specific) serum.

     FINAL DIAGNOSIS: Either Bence Jones Protein (κ) MG or Bence Jones Protein (λ) MG (i.e., κ or λ light-chain disease).

Other Immunoglobulin Abnormalities:

  1. Polyclonal gammopathy: All immunoglobulins increased. Normal but increased precipitin lines with all antisera (except IgD and IgE which may not be visible).

  2. Hypo-γ-globulinemia: All immunoglobulins decreased. Normal but decreased precipitin lines with all antisera (except IgD and IgE which will not be visible).

  3. Isolated IgA deficiency:

    IEP detects the isolated absence of IgA (i.e., all precipitin lines essentially normal but line with anti-IgA antiserum is absent). This defect is found in about 1 of 700 Americans. Half of them are healthy, the others suffer from autoimmune diseases, frequent infections, etc.

---

[e] See Dettelbach, H., and Ritzmann, S. E. (Eds.), *Lab Synopsis,* Vol. 2 (2nd ed.). Somerville, N.J.: Behring Diagnostics, 1969. Pp. 21, 27.

[f] Confirmation can be obtained by the use of antisera to *free* kappa or *free* lambda light chains.

Note: BJP = Bence Jones proteins; MG = monoclonal gammopathy; BG = biclonal gammopathy.

Reproduced by permission. From Ritzmann, S. E., et al. *Lab Notes #3: Serum Proteins.* Somerville, N.J.: Behring Diagnostics, 1973.

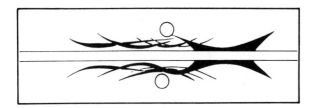

Figure 2-10
IEP pattern for albumin-IgA fusion. *Top:* normal serum precipitin pattern developed with antihuman serum. *Bottom:* serum from a patient with IgA-myeloma. The continuous precipitin line indicates complex formation between IgA and albumin. (Reproduced by permission. From Dettelbach, H., and Ritzmann, S. E. (Eds.). *Lab Synopsis,* Vol. 2 (2nd ed.). Somerville, N.J.: Behring Diagnostics, 1969.)

Table 2-4. Cases of Monoclonal and Biclonal Gammopathy[a]

Immunoglobulin Categories	Number	Total Number	Percent
1. IgG-MG	364	443	62.7
IgG-MG + BJP	79		
2. IgA-MG	77	105	14.9
IgA-MG + BJP	28		
3. IgM-MG	87	97	13.7
IgM-MG + BJP	10		
4. BJP-MG	57	57	8.1
5. IgD-MG	1	2	0.3
IgD-MG + BJP	1		
6. IgG + IgM-BG	1	2	0.3
IgG (λ) + BJP (κ)-BG	1		
Total	706	706	100.0

[a] Diagnosed at the University of Texas Medical Branch between 1962 and 1974.
Note: The recent application of sensitive and specific assays for free L chains in serum and urine has resulted in an incidence of Bence Jones proteins which is more than twice that shown above. MG = monoclonal gammopathy, BG = biclonal gammopathy, BJP = Bence Jones protein.

In summary, more than 95 percent of all MGs consist of (1) IgG with or without Bence Jones proteins, (2) IgA with or without Bence Jones proteins, (3) IgM with or without Bence Jones proteins, and (4) Bence Jones MG (i.e., L-chain disease).

IMMUNE COMPLEXES
"Milky" or clear spots on unstained agar or agarose IEP slides are frequently seen with sera containing M proteins. This finding is due to the focal accumulation of M proteins following electrophoresis, and their po-

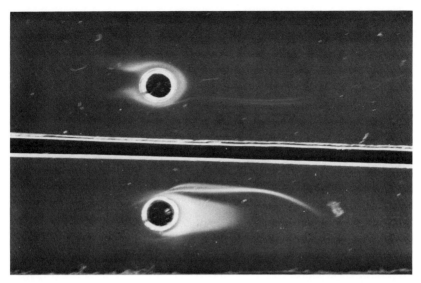

Figure 2-11
Normal IgM precipitin line (*top*). "Milky" area (*bottom*) reflects IgM monoclonal gammopathy in serum from patient with macroglobulinemia (Waldenström). Antibody trough contains antiserum to IgM. (Reproduced by permission. From Ritzmann, S. E., Daniels, J. C., Alami, S. Y., and Lawrence, M. C.
In G. J. Race (Ed.), *Laboratory Medicine*. New York: Harper & Row,
1975.)

sitions usually correspond to those found on cellulose acetate electrophoresis.

Another phenomenon is that of "milky" trailing precipitates on unstained IEP films that originate from the point of application and may
spread either cathodically or anodically (Fig. 2-11). This nonspecific
pattern is often encountered with viscous sera, such as in cases of IgM
monoclonal gammopathy.

Immune complexes, such as rheumatoid factors or lupus erythematosus factors, often produce nonspecific precipitation in the agar or
agarose during electrophoresis (Fig. 2-12; see also Chap. 9). Such a
pattern suggests the presence of serum immune complexes, and confirmatory assays are required.

ADDITIONAL APPLICATIONS
IEP can be applied to the examination of body fluids other than serum,
including cerebrospinal fluid, urine, colostrum and others (Fig. 2-13).
Concentration of the specimens prior to IEP analysis may be required
(e.g., an Amicon B-15* concentration device may be used, which al-

* Amicon Corporation, 21 Hartwell Avenue, Lexington, Mass. 02173.

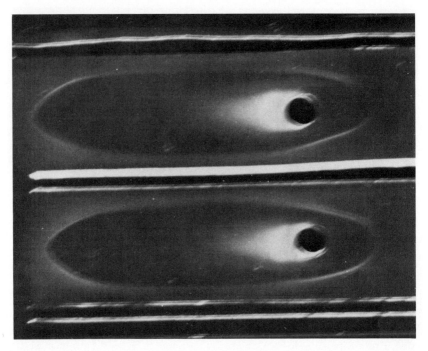

Figure 2-12
IEP pattern developed with anti-IgG antiserum demonstrating "trailing" from
the antigen well toward the cathode (*left*). This pattern reflects the presence of
circulating immune complexes. (Reproduced by permission. From Ritzmann,
S. E., Daniels, J. C., Alami, S. Y., and Lawrence, M. C. In G. J. Race (Ed.),
Laboratory Medicine. New York: Harper & Row, 1975.)

lows a 10- to 100-fold concentration, resulting in the retention of immunoglobulins and their derivatives).

Examining unconcentrated urine specimens by IEP with polyvalent
antiserum to human serum allows the recognition of several individual
proteins and the evaluation of the analog of the selectivity index of renal
function (Fig. 2-14) [35]. The determination of proteins with sequentially higher molecular weights—e.g., the series (1) α_1-antitrypsin, MW
45,000, (2) albumin, MW 65,000, (3) transferrin, MW 90,000,
(4) IgG, MW 150,000, (5) C4, MW 230,000, and (6) α_2-macroglobu-
lin, MW 820,000—can be easily monitored. The inverse relationship between the molecular size of a protein and its quantitative urinary excretion in health and disease [35–37] may thus be quickly estimated.

IEP can be used for the identification of individual proteins, even in a
mixture. Unknown antigens can be identified immunoelectrophoretically
by various criteria [2, 4, 6, 14], namely:

1. Different electrophoretic mobility and relative positions of the precipitin lines aid in the identification of certain proteins, such as the various Gc types (Fig. 2-15).

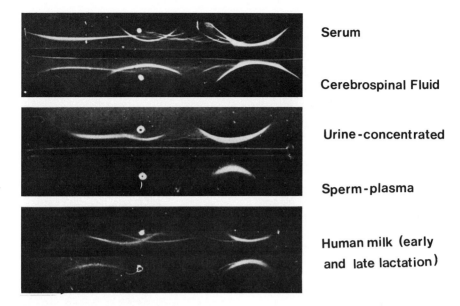

Figure 2-13
IEP analysis of various body fluids: serum, cerebrospinal fluid, urine, sperm fluid, and breast milk (early lactation and late lactation colostrum; the colostrum contains large amounts of secretory IgA).

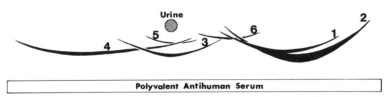

Figure 2-14
Analog of urinary selectivity index: IEP pattern of urinary proteins with increasing molecular weights (see text). (Reproduced by permission. From Ritzmann, S. E., Daniels, J. C., Alami, S. Y., and Lawrence, M. C. In G. J. Race (Ed.), *Laboratory Medicine.* New York: Harper & Row, 1975.)

2. The use of specific antisera in conjunction with polyvalent antihuman serum demonstrates individual serum proteins, such as transferrin (Fig. 2-16).
3. The employment of purified antigens allows the identification of the corresponding precipitin arcs within the precipitin patterns of human serum proteins, such as α_1-antitrypsin (Fig. 2-17).
4. Specific staining reactions allow the detection of certain proteins with specific biological properties, such as haptoglobin, hemopexin (peroxidase reactions), lipoproteins (oil red O), or cholinesterase (indoxyl acetate).
5. The "interrupted trough" technique [4] may be employed for the

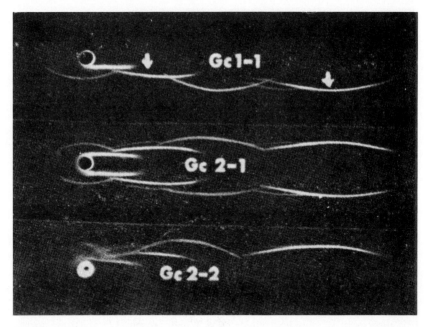

Figure 2-15
Gc 1-1 globulin precipitin line (*top*); Gc 2-1 globulin precipitin line (*center*);
Gc 2-2 globulin precipitin line (*bottom*). The α_2M-globulin precipitin arc
(*left arrow*) and α_1-lipoprotein precipitin arc (*right arrow*) serve as marker
lines. (Reproduced by permission. From Dettelbach, H., and Ritzmann, S. E.
(Eds.). *Lab Synopsis,* Vol. 2 (2nd ed.). Somerville, N.J.: Behring Diagnostics, 1969).

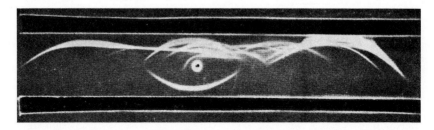

Figure 2-16
Identification of transferrin precipitin arc by use of antiserum specific to
transferrin. *Top trough:* antiserum to human serum. *Bottom trough:* antiserum to transferrin. *Antigen well:* human serum. (Reproduced by permission. From Dettelbach, H., and Ritzmann, S. E. (Eds.). *Lab Synopsis,* Vol. 2
(2nd ed.). Somerville, N.J.: Behring Diagnostics, 1969.)

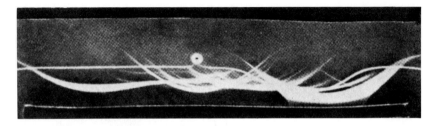

Figure 2-17
Identification of the α_1-antitrypsin. The α_1-antitrypsin precipitin line remains straight in the area devoid of α_1-antitrypsin (*left*), but fuses with its identical counterpart (*right*), thus positively identifying this protein. *Top trough:* α_1-antitrypsin. *Bottom trough:* antiserum to human serum. *Antigen well:* human serum. (Reproduced by permission. From Dettelbach, H., and Ritzmann, S. E. (Eds.), *Lab Synopsis,* Vol. 2 (2nd ed.). Somerville, N.J.: Behring Diagnostics, 1969.)

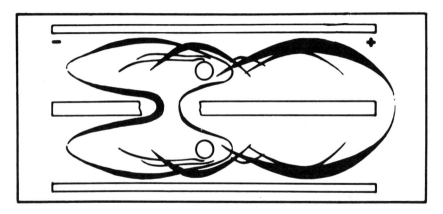

Figure 2-18
Identity of two IgG precipitin arcs as shown by the interrupted trough technique. Top and bottom troughs contain antiserum to human serum. Interrupted trough contains antiserum to IgG. Precipitin line, which is fused through the interrupted trough, indicates identity of antigens in top and bottom sections. (Reproduced by permission. From Dettelbach, H., and Ritzmann, S. E. (Eds.). *Lab Synopsis,* Vol. 2 (2nd ed.). Somerville, N.J.: Behring Diagnostics, 1969.)

identification of individual proteins or their derivatives, such as "abnormal" immunoglobulins and their cleavage products, fibrinogen-split products, and so on (Fig. 2-18).

6. The use of isotope-labeled antigens or antibodies aids in the detection of proteins in biological fluids, i.e., radioimmunoelectrophoresis.

References

1. Grabar, P., and Williams, L. A., Jr.   Méthode permettant l'étude conjugée des propriétés électrophoretiques et immunochemiques d'un mélange de proteines. Application au sérum sanguin. *Biochim. Biophys. Acta* 10:193, 1953.

2. Grabar, P., and Burtin, P.   *Immunoelectrophoretic Analysis. Application to Human Biological Fluids.* Amsterdam: Elsevier, 1964.

3. Scheidegger, J. J.   Une microméthode de l'immunoélectrophorèse. *Int. Arch. Allergy Appl. Immunol.* 7:103, 1955.

4. Osserman, E. F.   A modified technique of immunoelectrophoresis facilitating the identification of specific precipitin arcs. *J. Immunol.* 84:93, 1960.

5. Ouchterlony, O.   *Handbook of Immunodiffusion and Immunoelectrophoresis.* Ann Arbor, Mich.: Ann Arbor Sciences Publ., 1968.

6. Heremans, J. F.   *Les globulines sériques du système gamma. Leur nature et leur pathologie.* Brussels: Arscia, and Paris: Masson, 1960.

7. Korngold, L.   Plasma Proteins: Methods of Study and Changes in Disease. In M. Stefanini (Ed.), *Progress in Clinical Pathology,* Vol. 1. New York: Grune & Stratton, 1966. Pp. 340–397.

8. Terry, W. D., and Fahey, J. L.   Principles of Immunoelectrophoresis and Application to the Evaluation of Serum Gamma Globulins. In F. W. Sunderman and F. W. Sunderman, Jr. (Eds.), *Serum Proteins and the Dysproteinemias.* Philadelphia: Lippincott, 1964. Pp. 182–193.

9. Smith, J. B.   Alpha-fetoprotein: Occurrence in certain malignant disease and review of clinical applications. *Med. Clin. North Am.* 54:797, 1970.

10. Levin, W. C., and Ritzmann, S. E.   The Immunoglobulins. In C. E. Mengel, E. Frei, III, and R. Nachman (Eds.), *Hematology: Principles and Practice.* Chicago: Year Book, 1972. Pp. 544–567.

11. Engle, R. L., and Wallis, L. A.   *Immunoglobulinopathies. Immunoglobulins, Immune Deficiency Syndromes, Multiple Myeloma, and Related Disorders.* (American Lecture Series.) Springfield, Ill.: Thomas, 1969.

12. Cawley, L. P.   *Electrophoresis and Immunoelectrophoresis.* Boston: Little, Brown, 1969.

13. Osserman, E. F., Takatsuki, K., and Talal, N.   The Pathogenesis of "Amyloidosis." In P. A. Miescher (Ed.), *Multiple Myeloma.* Seminars in Hematology. New York: Grune & Stratton, 1964. Pp. 1–86.

14. Ritzmann, S. E., Daniels, J. C., Alami, S. Y., and Lawrence, M. C.   Characterization and Separation of Proteins: Qualitative and Quantitative Assays. In G. J. Race (Ed.), *Laboratory Medicine.* New York: Harper & Row, 1975.

15. Apitz, K.   Die Paraproteinosen. Über die Störung des Eiweissstoffwechsels bei Plasmozytom. *Virchow's Arch. Pathol. Anat.* 305:631, 1940.

16. Gutman, A. B.   The plasma proteins in disease. *Adv. Chem.* 4:155, 1948.

17. Riva, G. *Das Serumeiweissbild.* Bern: Huber, 1957.
18. Waldenström, J. Studies on conditions associated with disturbed gamma globulin formation (gammopathies). *Harvey Lect.* 56:211, 1961.
19. Waldenström, J. Monoclonal and polyclonal gammopathies and the biological system of gamma globulins. *Prog. Allergy* 6:320, 1962.
20. Osserman, E. F., and Fahey, J. L. Plasma cell dyscrasias: Current clinical and biochemical concepts. Combined staff clinic. *Am. J. Med.* 44: 256, 1968.
21. Osserman, E. F., and Takatsuki, K. Considerations regarding the pathogenesis of the plasmacytic dyscrasias. *Ser. Haematol.* 4:28, 1965.
22. Janeway, C. A., Rosen, F. S., Merler, E., and Alper, C. A. *The Gamma Globulins.* Boston: Little, Brown, 1967.
23. Demeulenaere, L., and Wieme, R. J. Special electrophoretic anomalies in the serum of liver patients: A report of 1145 cases. *Am. J. Dig. Dis.* 6:661, 1961.
24. Kyle, R. A., Bieger, R. C., and Gleich, G. J. Diagnosis of syndromes associated with hyperglobulinemia. *Med. Clin. North Am.* 54:917, 1970.
25. Osserman, E. F., and Takatsuki, K. The plasma proteins in liver disease. *Med. Clin. North Am.* 47:679, 1963.
26. Bachmann, R. The diagnostic significance of serum concentration of pathological proteins (M-components). *Acta Med. Scand.* 178:801, 1965.
27. Ritzmann, S. E., Daniels, J. C., and Levin, W. C. Paralymphomatous Disease: The Syndrome of Macroglobulinemia. In *Leukemia-Lymphoma.* (A collection of papers presented at the 14th Annual Clinical Conference on Cancer, 1969, at the University of Texas M. D. Anderson Hospital and Tumor Institute, Houston.) Chicago: Year Book, 1970. Pp. 169–222.
28. Pruzanski, W., and Ogryzlo, M. A. The changing pattern of diseases associated with M components. *Med. Clin. North Am.* 56:371, 1972.
29. Lee, B. J., Pinsky, C., and Miller, D. G. The management of plasma cell neoplasms. *Med. Clin. North Am.* 55:703, 1971.
30. Ritzmann, S. E., Daniels, J. C., Lawrence, M. C., Beathard, G. A., and Levin, W. C. Monoclonal gammopathies—Present status. *Tex. Med.* 68:91, 1972.
31. Zawadzki, Z. A., and Edwards, G. A. Nonmyelomatous Monoclonal Immunoglobulinemia. In R. Schwartz (Ed.), *Progress in Clinical Immunology,* Vol. 1. New York: Grune & Stratton, 1972. Pp. 105–156.
32. Ritzmann, S. E., and Levin, W. C. Polyclonal and Monoclonal Gammopathies. In H. Dettelbach and S. E. Ritzmann (Eds.), *Lab Synopsis,* Vol. 2 (2nd ed.). Somerville, N.J.: Behring Diagnostics, 1969. Pp. 9–54.
33. Waldenström, J. *Diagnosis and Treatment of Multiple Myeloma.* New York: Grune & Stratton, 1970.
34. Snapper, I., and Kahn, A. *Myelomatosis. Fundamentals and Clinical Features.* Baltimore: University Park Press, 1971.
35. Cameron, J. S., and White, R. H. R. Selectivity of proteinuria in children with the nephrotic syndrome. *Lancet* 1:463, 1965.
36. Hardwicke, J., Cameron, J. S., Harrison, J. F., Hulme, B., and Soothill, J. F. Proteinuria, Studied by Clearances of Individual Macromolecules. In Y. Manuel (Ed.), *Proteins in Normal and Pathological Urine.* Basel: Karger, 1970. Pp. 111–152.
37. Braun, W. E., and Merrill, J. P. Urine Protein Selectivity in Human Renal Allografts. In Y. Manuel (Ed.), *Proteins in Normal and Pathological Urine.* Basel: Karger, 1970. Pp. 281–291.

Quantitative Immunoelectrophoresis 3

Stephan E. Ritzmann and Robert M. Nakamura

Two-Dimensional Immunoelectrophoresis

The principle of quantitative two-dimensional immunoelectrophoresis (IEP) is similar to that of single-directional electroimmunodiffusion [1] (see Chap. 4). It is a combination of single agarose-gel electrophoresis and subsequent electroimmunodiffusion. Serial dilutions of known amounts of antigens (e.g., IgG or C1-esterase inhibitor) are placed in wells. The applied electrical field forces the antigens into the antibody-containing agarose gel, and, in the face of temporary antigen excess, the antigen-antibody complexes partly redissolve and continue to move forward. When optimal antigen-antibody ratios are reached, rocket-like precipitin areas form at the completion of the electrophoretic run. In electroimmunodiffusion employing one specific antiserum, one antigen can be quantitated on one plate at a time, whereas two-dimensional IEP, which uses a polyvalent antiserum, allows the quantitation of numerous individual proteins simultaneously (Fig. 3-1).

The technique of two-dimensional IEP, which was first described in 1960 [2], subsequently modified [1], and developed into a quantitative procedure by Clarke and Freeman [3], now lends itself to semi-automated, routine clinical procedures [4].

METHODOLOGY

The first step (or dimension) of two-dimensional IEP consists of the electrophoretic separation of a protein mixture (e.g., serum) in agarose gel. The second step (or dimension) of this procedure takes place during electrophoresis in an agarose gel that contains oligospecific or poly-specific antiserum. The latter step results in rocket-like immunoprecipitates that allow quantitation of the respective proteins.

Versey et al. [4] have recently described a technique that appears both practical and economical for routine use. In this procedure a prepoured plate containing a strip of agarose is filled with agarose that contains antiserum (e.g., anti-whole human serum). Electrophoresis is carried out while the plate is in an inverted position for about one hour. The

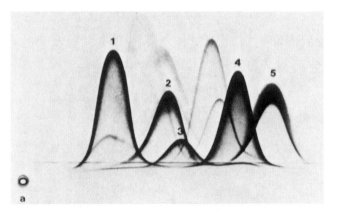

Figure 3-1
Two-dimensional immunoelectrophoresis. Application well (*a*) of the first dimension was filled with human serum. The agar gel of the second dimension contained an oligospecific antiserum. The numbered precipitates represent the following proteins: (*1*) transferrin, (*2*) α_2-macroglobulin, (*3*) ceruloplasmin, (*4*) α_1-antitrypsin, and (*5*) acid α_1-glycoprotein. (Reproduced by permission. From Becker, W. *Methods of Qualitative and Quantitative Immunoelectrophoresis*. Somerville, N.J.: Behring Diagnostics, 1973.)

power supply allows the delivery of current at right angles by means of a time switch. During the second step, the antigens are carried into the antiserum region by electrophoresis. After completion, the plate is stained, and the concentration of the individual proteins is determined by comparison with standards, such as albumin or transferrin [4] or standardized human serum* [5]. This is achieved either by measuring the peak areas by planimetry or by the single-area measurement technique (i.e., measuring the area in square millimeters by multiplying the length of half of the base-line of each peak by its height) [4].

APPLICATION
Two-dimensional IEP lends itself to the quantitation of numerous proteins in biological fluids (e.g., serum, urine, or cerebrospinal fluid). This technique may eventually compete with radial immunodiffusion and electroimmunodiffusion, especially in clinical laboratories with large volumes of quantitative assays.

SOURCES OF ERROR
The sources of error include those listed for electroimmunodiffusion (see Chap. 4, p. 76). Additional sources of error include alterations of electrophoretic mobility of protein fractions as a result of specimen storage (e.g., α_1-lipoprotein and C factors) and the presence of genetic variants (e.g., α_1-antitrypsin and haptoglobin) [5]. Technical sources of errors [6]

* Behring Diagnostics, Somerville, N.J. 08876.

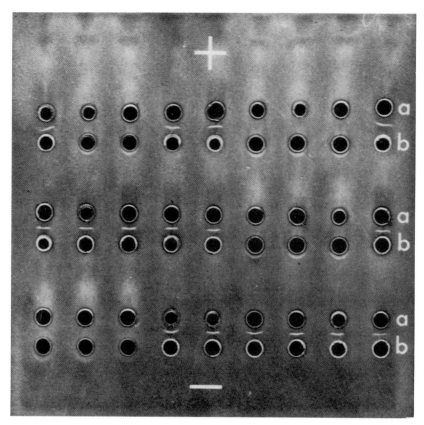

Figure 3-2
Countercurrent electrophoresis. Application wells *a:* anti-HAA serum raised
in rabbits. Application wells *b:* HAA-positive and HAA-negative human sera.
(Reproduced by permission. From Becker, W. *Methods of Qualitative and
Quantitative Immunoelectrophoresis.* Somerville, N.J.: Behring Diagnostics,
1973.)

include those resulting from excessive condensation during electrophoresis, double contoured peaks (tunnel phenomena) due to excessive temperature differences between the upper and lower gel surfaces, absent or distorted precipitates due to faulty electrical contact, inadequate antisera, and so on.

Cross-Immunoelectrophoresis

Various terms are used for this technique, including *cross-electrophoresis
(CEP)* [7], *counter-immunoelectrophoresis (CIEP)* [8, 9, 10], *cross-immunoelectrophoresis, crossover-electrophoresis* [11], *electroosmodiffusion (EOD)* [12], and *countercurrent electrophoresis* [6]. We prefer to

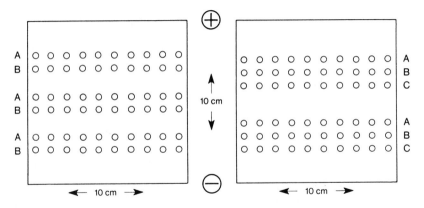

Figure 3-3
Countercurrent electrophoresis. (*A*) Wells for antiserum. (*B*) Wells for test samples. (*C*) Wells for HAA-positive sera. The well pattern in this plan enables sera to be tested simultaneously for HAA and anti-HAA. (Reproduced by permission. From Becker, W. *Methods of Qualitative and Quantitative Immunoelectrophoresis.* Somerville, N.J.: Behring Diagnostics, 1973.)

use *cross-immunoelectrophoresis* (*CIEP*). CIEP depends on the formation of visible immune complexes when anodically migrating antigens meet cathodically migrating antibodies during electrophoresis. For instance, precipitin lines are formed when such antibodies meet the hepatitis-associated antigens (HB-Ag), which possess α-globulin hepatitis antigens (Fig. 3-2).

METHODOLOGY
Appropriate antigens and antisera are applied to wells in the agar or agarose plates, and electrophoresis is then performed. Staining enhances the visibility of the precipitin lines [6].

SOURCES OF ERROR
These are identical with those described previously for two-dimensional IEP.

APPLICATION
Cross-immunoelectrophoresis is a suitable method for qualitative and semiqualitative assays of those proteins that possess an electrophoretic mobility which differs clearly from that of the corresponding antibodies. Such proteins include fibrinogen split products D and E [6], α_1-fetoprotein [13], IgE [10], and hepatitis-associated antigens (HB-Ag) [8, 9, 11, 12, 14], as well as antibodies against HB-Ag (Fig. 3-3).

References

1. Laurell, C. B. Antigen-antibody crossed electrophoresis. *Anal. Biochem.* 10:358, 1965.

2. Ressler, N.   Two-dimensional electrophoresis of serum protein antigens in an antibody-containing buffer. *Clin. Chim. Acta* 5:795, 1960.

3. Clarke, M. H. G., and Freeman, T.   Quantitative immunoelectrophoresis of human serum proteins. *Clin. Sci.* 35:403, 1968.

4. Versey, J. M. B., Slater, L., and Hobbs, J. R.   Semi-automated two-dimensional immunoelectrophoresis. *J. Immunol. Methods* 3:63, 1973.

5. Arvan, D. A., and Shaw, L. M.   2-Directional immunoelectrophoresis technique and applications in the clinical laboratory. *Separation Sci.* 8: 123, 1973.

6. Becker, W.   *Methods of Qualitative and Quantitative Immunoelectrophoresis.* Somerville, N.J.: Behring Diagnostics, 1973.

7. Nakamura, S.   *Cross Electrophoresis: Its Principles and Applications.* New York: Elsevier, 1966.

8. Gocke, D. J., and Howe, C.   Rapid detection of Australia antigen by counterimmunoelectrophoresis. *J. Immunol.* 104:1031, 1970.

9. Wallis, C., and Malnick, J. L.   Enhanced detection of Australia antigen in serum hepatitis patients by discontinuous counter-immunoelectrophoresis. *Appl. Microbiol.* 21:867, 1971.

10. Beng, C-G., Chan, G-L, Simons, M. J., and Lan, K-S.   Semi-quantitation of serum IgE by counter-immunoelectrophoresis. *Int. Arch. Allergy Appl. Immunol.* 45:352, 1973.

11. White, G. B. B., Lasheen, R. M., and Turner, G. L.   Rapid detection of Australia antigen by cross-over electrophoresis. *Lancet* 2:368, 1970.

12. Yap, E. H., Ee, T. I., and Simons, M. J.   Detection of Australia antigen by electroosmodiffusion (EOD). *Southeast Asian J. Trop. Med. Public Health* 2:486, 1971.

13. Kohn, J.   Method for the detection and identification of α-fetoprotein in serum. *J. Clin. Pathol.* 23:733, 1970.

14. Pesendorfer, F., Krassnitzky, O., and Wewalka, F.   Immunoelektrophoretischer Nachweis von "Hepatitis-Associated Antigen" (Au/SH-Antigen). *Klin. Wochenschr.* 48:58, 1970.

Quantitative Immunochemical Procedures

4

Stephan E. Ritzmann, Craig L. Fischer,
and Robert M. Nakamura

Quantitative knowledge of serum protein concentrations is essential for the diagnosis and management of numerous clinical conditions. Although standard serum protein electrophoresis (SPE) is a helpful tool, this procedure is limited as a quantitative method to a few proteins, such as albumin and most M proteins. It is now possible to accurately quantitate serum proteins by immunochemical techniques, specifically, by the techniques of single radial immunodiffusion (RID) and electroimmunodiffusion (EID), which permit the quantitation of more than 50 individual serum proteins. These techniques employ the use of specific antisera, and they are sensitive, rapid, reliable, and practical for routine quantitative protein studies (with the exception of M-protein studies) [1]. A wide selection of specific antisera (more than 50) is presently available commercially. The selection of appropriate antisera is critical for accurate and reproducible results [2–4]. Such antisera must be potent and specific; i.e., it must be devoid of antibody activity directed to other serum proteins or to certain moieties present in related proteins, such as the light chains common to all immunoglobulins. Further, such monospecific antisera should possess antibody activity that is constant from one batch to another.

Radial Immunodiffusion (RID)

The principle of RID is based upon the fact that any specific antigen (e.g., serum protein) will form a precipitin complex with its specific antiserum at a constant ratio of antigen to antibody. An antigen, when applied to a well in an agar substrate containing specific antiserum, will diffuse radially through the agar until the optimal ratio of antigen to antibody is achieved (Fig. 4-1). The diameters of the resulting precipitin rings are logarithmically related to the antigen concentration (i.e., the area of the precipitin ring varies directly as a function of the square of

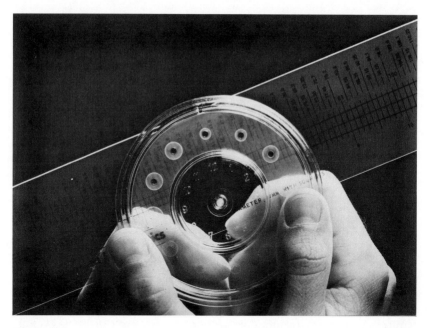

Figure 4-1
RID. The increasing diameters of the precipitin rings reflect increasingly larger protein concentrations. (Courtesy of Behring Diagnostics, Somerville, N.J.)

the diameter), whereas the area enclosed by the precipitin ring is linearly related to this parameter [4a, 4b]. Quantitation of the proteins is achieved by comparing the diameter produced by the serum protein in a patient's serum with the diameter of the precipitin rings produced by standard, commercially available serum solutions with known protein concentrations (Fig. 4-2).

There are basically two approaches to the RID procedure [5]: the *Mancini-Heremans technique* [6], which is based upon the analysis of results after the endpoint of immunodiffusion has occurred, and the *Fahey-McKelvey technique* [7], which is designed for early readout of results. Each of these approaches has its advantages as well as its disadvantages. For instance, early readout may be misleading if the concentration ranges of the test samples are highly abnormal; the endpoint methods may provide more accurate results at the expense of time. Within a certain range of antigen-antibody ratios, the concentration-diameter relation is linear in the endpoint approach. The shorter the diffusion time before reading the results, the more curvilinear the standard curve will be.

METHODOLOGY

EQUIPMENT AND SUPPLIES

RID immunodiffusion plates are available commercially. They allow the quantitation of numerous serum proteins, both in clinical and research

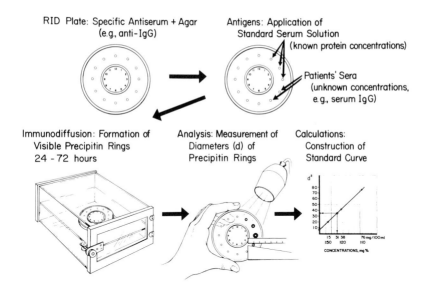

RID Plate: Specific Antiserum + Agar
(e.g., anti-IgG)

Antigens: Application of
Standard Serum Solution
(known protein concentrations)

Patients' Sera
(unknown concentrations,
e.g., serum IgG)

Immunodiffusion: Formation of
Visible Precipitin Rings
24 - 72 hours

Analysis: Measurement of
Diameters (d) of
Precipitin Rings

Calculations:
Construction of
Standard Curve

Figure 4-2
RID procedure. (Reproduced by permission. From Ritzmann, S. E., Daniels, J. C., Alami, S. Y., and Lawrence, M. C. In G. J. Race (Ed.), *Laboratory Medicine*. New York: Harper & Row, 1975.)

laboratories. The plates are used according to the manufacturer's directions, and quantitation and the results are calculated accordingly [8, 9]. A diagrammatic presentation of the RID approach is depicted in Figure 4-2. RID plates may also be prepared in individual laboratories [8, 9].

A standard serum solution with known protein concentrations is necessary for the construction of a standard curve from which the protein concentration of a patient's serum sample may be obtained (see Fig. 4-2). Such reference sera are provided with some manufacturer's kits for the construction of these standard curves; they are of a concentration range that covers the usual levels of such proteins.

PROCEDURE

After preparing the RID plates for use, reference serum dilutions of known concentrations are applied to the plate. Subsequently, the patient's serum is applied, usually in three different dilutions. Undiluted sera, however, may be added to the "low concentration" plates. The amounts of serum to be applied to each well vary among 2 μl, 5 μl, and 20 μl, depending upon the nature of the plate and the specific protein under assay. The plate is then stored in a horizontal position at room temperature. (If the lid of the RID plate is airtight, no immunodiffusion chamber is necessary.) The antigens are allowed to diffuse for varying periods of time depending upon the RID method, i.e., early readout method (approximately 6 to 20 hours) or the endpoint method (approximately 24 to 72 hours, depending upon the concentration and the type of protein under assay).

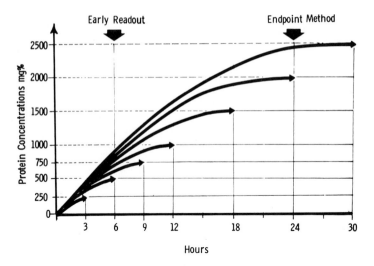

Figure 4-3
Relationship between protein concentration (mg per 100 ml) and the time (hours) required for complete reaction (i.e., endpoint) of all free proteins. For a given protein (e.g., IgG), the higher its concentration, the more the endpoint is protracted in time, and vice versa. Consequently, early readout (i.e., within 6 hours) can be promoted by assaying diluted samples with lowered protein concentrations.

ANALYSIS

After an appropriate incubation time, the diameters of the precipitin rings (see Figs. 4-1 and 4-2) are measured to the nearest 0.1 mm. In the case of Partigen Plates,* a standard curve is constructed by plotting the diameters squared (d^2 in square millimeters) of the precipitin rings produced by three standard protein concentrations against their respective concentrations on linear graph paper (Fig. 4-2 [ordinate: d^2; abscissa: $mg\%$]). The protein concentration in the patient's serum is calculated by squaring the diameter of the precipitin ring produced by the patient's serum, obtaining the corresponding concentration for d^2 from the standard curve, and multiplying this concentration by the dilution factor to obtain the concentration in the undiluted serum.

In the endpoint method (Mancini's technique [6]), the protein to be assayed is allowed to diffuse until all free protein molecules have reacted with the antiserum and no further extension of the precipitin ring occurs (Fig. 4-3). The various proteins are characterized by different diffusion times at which the endpoint is reached (e.g., the endpoint for IgG with normal adult serum concentration is approximately 24 hours, but for IgM with normal concentrations, it is approximately 50 hours). This difference of diffusion characteristics depends upon the protein concentration as well as the molecular weight (160,000 for IgG versus 900,000

* Behring Diagnostics, Somerville, N.J. 08876.

Figure 4-4
Distorted RID pattern due to nicked agar well. (Reprinted with permission from American Society for Medical Technology, *American Journal of Medical Technology*, Vol. 36, No. 10, p. 461, © 1970.)

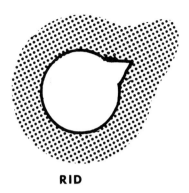

RID

for IgM). As a consequence, certain modified proteins yield concentration values that are either too high (e.g., low molecular weight IgM) or too low (e.g., secretory IgA or immune complexes) when compared with their respective "normal" counterparts.

In the early readout method (Fahey's technique [7]), the protein under assay is allowed to diffuse only for a limited time (e.g., 4 to 6 hours or 20 hours) before the diameter of the precipitin ring is determined (Fig. 4-3).

The endpoint method is the most accurate RID assay, but this is at the expense of prolonged diffusion time. With the early readout method, the advantage of rapid results is somewhat offset by the lesser degree of accuracy [10]. Some commercially available RID plates (e.g., Behring Partigen Plates) now offer a flexible approach in that they allow, with appropriate modification of sample preparation, either early readout after a few hours or endpoint readout. The latter approach provides high sensitivity (at least 0.02 mg per milliliter), good accuracy, and good reproducibility (better than ±6 percent).

Large-volume RID assays lend themselves to automated calculation of the results [8] using a computer program (e.g., the Olivetti program* for Partigen Plates).

SOURCES OF ERROR
Possible sources of error include the spilling of antigen outside the well; analysis of the standard serum solutions and patient's sera after different incubation periods; omission of standard serum solution from a plate; results obtained in the region of antigen or antibody excess; and unequal volumes of the solutions delivered to the wells. Also, during sample application, a cut in the agar may occur, resulting in distorted precipitin rings (Fig. 4-4). Protein complexes (e.g., haptoglobin-hemoglobin complexes or albumin-IgA complexes) or polymeric forms of IgM or IgA lead to an underestimation of the two concentrations, whereas low molecular weight moieties (e.g., 7S IgM) result in an overestimation of the true levels. Occasionally, IgM polymers or cryoglobulins do not diffuse

* Olivetti Corp. of America, 500 Park Avenue, New York, N.Y. 10022

into the agar or agarose of RID plates, thereby yielding spuriously low or even absent levels (see Chap. 19).

NORMAL VALUES

The approximate normal values (90th percentile ranges) of 25 serum proteins in adults, assayed by RID, are shown in Table 4-1 except for IgE, which requires radioimmunoassay (RIA) for precise quantitation.

The serum levels of the five immunoglobulin classes are age-dependent (Figs. 4-5 to 4-7), and their values must be expressed in age-related terms (e.g., an IgG value of 600 mg per 100 ml or 70 IU per milliliter is normal in a 9-month-old infant but decreased in adults).

APPLICATION AND INTERPRETATION

RID can be applied to the quantitation of proteins in serum and other body fluids. It allows quantitation of most proteins for which specific antisera are available, which at present total more than 40. This technique has been adapted for the use of capillary or venous blood obtained by a finger-prick [11]. Special low-concentration RID plates are available commercially for the assay of immunoglobulins in cerebrospinal fluid as well as for the screening of cord blood for increased levels of IgM that may indicate intrauterine infections [12]. RID represents a simple and reliable method for the screening and monitoring of most serum protein abnormalities, but monoclonal gammopathies represent a notable exception (see Chap. 19).

LIMITATION OF RID: M PROTEIN ASSAYS

Immunoelectrophoresis is the method of choice for the verification and differential diagnosis of M proteins, whereas serum protein electrophoresis (SPE) is the most satisfactory technique for their quantitation [13] (see Chaps. 1 and 19). Quantitation of M proteins by RID is unreliable and often misleading, since the results generally do not correlate with the true M-protein concentrations [13–15].

RID assays of IgG M proteins usually lead to spuriously high values of such immunoglobulins [13]. For instance, an IgG M-protein concentration of 3.2 gm per 100 ml by SPE may yield 5.1 gm per 100 ml by RID (Fig. 4-8). M proteins of the IgA and IgM classes likewise yield results that are either too high or too low in comparison to those obtained by SPE. It should be noted, however, that in a given patient, the monitoring of M protein by RID will yield the same percentage of deviation from the results obtained by SPE; thus, such proteins will be *consistently* overestimated or underestimated.

In RID, the M proteins often lead to a steeper slope of the standard curve, as if the antibody concentration had been decreased (Fig. 4-9). The discrepancy between SPE and RID data is probably due to an IgG subclass predominance in the IgG M-protein. In RID plates, there exists an imbalance between the IgG subclass of the M protein and the corresponding antibody activity to the normal IgG subclasses. Normal serum contains a mixture of IgG subclasses—IgG_1, IgG_2, IgG_3, and IgG_4—

Table 4-1.   Radial Immunodiffusion Assays and Normal Values

RID Plates	Normal Serum Protein Concentrations (healthy adults)	
	Concentration	IU/ml[a]
Prealbumin	10–40 mg/100 gm	
Albumin	3500–5500 mg/100 gm	
α_1-Fetoprotein	absent	
α_1-Acid glycoprotein	55–140 mg/100 gm	
α_1-Antitrypsin	200–400 mg/100 gm	
Gc-Globulin	30–55 mg/100 gm	
Ceruloplasmin	10–40 mg/100 gm	
α_2-HS-Glycoprotein	40–85 mg/100 gm	
Antithrombin (III)	17–30 mg/100 gm	
α_2-Macroglobulin	150–400 mg/100 gm	
Haptoglobin	50–220 mg/100 gm	
C3c (β_1C/A-globulin)	80–140 mg/100 gm	
C4 (β_1E-globulin)	20–50 mg/100 gm	
Transferrin	200–400 mg/100 gm	
β_2-Glycoprotein I	15–30 mg/100 gm	
Hemopexin	70–130 mg/100 gm	
Plasminogen	20–40 mg/100 gm	
β-Lipoprotein	78–122% normal	
Fibrinogen (plasma)	200–450 mg/100 gm	
C-reactive protein (CRP)	absent	
Immunoglobulin D (IgD)	0–40 mg/100 gm	0–280
Immunoglobulin M (IgM)	70–210 mg/100 gm	80–240
Immunoglobulin A (IgA)	70–350 mg/100 gm	45–210
Immunoglobulin G (IgG)	700–1700 mg/100 gm.	80–200
Immunoglobulin E (IgE); RIA	10–1000 ng/ml	5–500

[a] Recently, a World Health Organization Committee has recommended that concentrations of IgG, IgA, IgM, IgD, and IgE in human serum should be quantitated by assays against an international reference preparation and be expressed in International Units (IU per ml) (Anderson, S. G., et al. *Clin. Chim. Acta* 36:276, 1972; WHO Expert Committee on Biological Standardization. *WHO Tech. Rep. Ser.* 463: 62, 1971). Geometric mean values of estimates of concentrations of IgG, IgA, and IgM in IU per ml (with 95 percent confidence limits) were obtained from a total of 982 selected male blood donors, aged 20–29 years, from 11 countries. The concentrations of serum immunoglobulins were quantitated by RID using the WHO standard 67/97 (Rowe, D. S. *Lancet* 2:1232, 1972). The normal values for IgG, IgA, IgM, IgD, and IgE obtained in our laboratories are shown above.

Reproduced by permission. From Ritzmann, S. E., Daniels, J. C., Alami, S. Y., and Lawrence, M. C. In G. J. Race (Ed.), *Laboratory Medicine*. New York: Harper & Row, 1975.

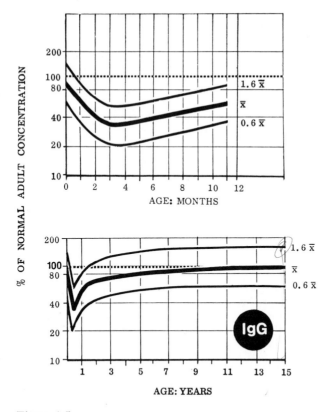

Figure 4-5
Serum concentrations of IgG. The immunoglobulin concentrations are shown during the first 12 months of life (*top panels*) and during the first 15 years of life (*bottom panels*). The concentrations are given in percent of normal adult levels (normal means and normal ranges). Normal absolute mean adult levels are: IgG, 1200 mg per 100 ml (140 IU/ml); IgA, 200 mg per 100 ml (125 IU/ml); IgM, 140 mg per 100 ml (160 IU/ml). IgG concentrations decrease rapidly after birth from the maternal level in umbilical cord serum to a low level at 3 to 4 months of age, indicating little synthesis during this period. (Reproduced by permission. From Ritzmann, S. E., et al. *Lab Notes #3: Serum Proteins.* Somerville, N.J.: Behring Diagnostics, 1973.)

that are present in a ratio of approximately 70, 25, 5, and 3 percent, respectively [16, 17]. In contrast, monoclonal IgG consists exclusively of one IgG subclass (e.g., IgG_3). On regular RID plates, such an M protein will only utilize that portion of the antibody activity which is directed to the IgG_3 subclass moiety, thus resulting in a larger precipitin ring and spuriously high concentrations.

Electroimmunodiffusion Technique (EID)

Electroimmunodiffusion is a method for quantitating antigens that combines the speed of electrophoresis with the specificity and sensitivity of

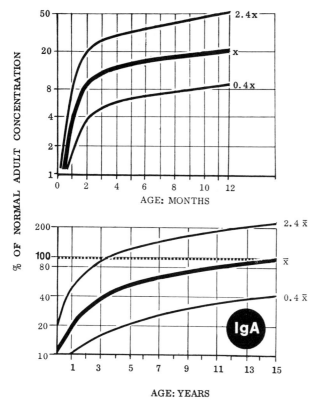

Figure 4-6
Serum concentrations of IgA during the first 12 months of life (*top*) and during the first 15 years of life (*bottom*). IgA concentrations are given in percent of normal adult levels (normal means and ranges). Normal absolute mean adult levels are approximately 210 mg per 100 ml (70–350 mg per 100 ml). Serum IgA increases slowly during infancy and childhood. IgM is detectable in trace amounts at birth, increases rapidly, and continues to rise for the first year. IgD and IgE levels also gradually rise to normal adult levels at 16 years of age (3 mg per 100 ml or 25 IU/ml and 0.03 mg per 100 ml or 150 IU/ml, respectively). Maximum serum immunoglobulin concentrations are attained in the third decade. IgM concentrations decrease significantly by the sixth decade, and IgG decreases significantly from the third to the sixth decade. Changes in serum IgA after maturity are small and not significant. (Reproduced by permission. From Ritzmann, S. E., et al. *Lab Notes #3: Serum Proteins.* Somerville, N.J.: Behring Diagnostics, 1973.)

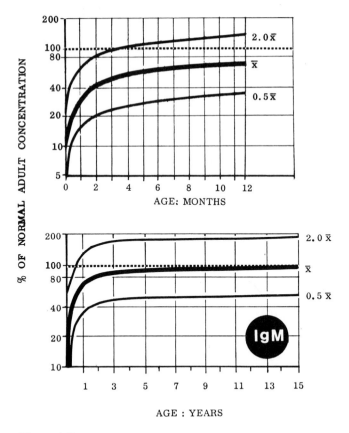

Figure 4-7
Serum concentrations of IgM during the first 12 months of life (*top*) and during the first 15 years of life (*bottom*). IgM concentrations are given in percent of normal adult levels (normal means and ranges). Normal absolute mean adult levels are approximately 140 mg per 100 ml (70–210 mg per 100 ml). (Reproduced by permission. From Ritzmann, S. E., et al. *Lab Notes #3: Serum Proteins.* Somerville, N.J.: Behring Diagnostics, 1973.)

immunodiffusion. In the EID procedure, the antigens move through an antibody-containing matrix within an electrical field, resulting in rocket-shaped precipitin patterns (Fig. 4-10). The lengths of the "rockets" are proportional to the concentration of the antigen [17a]. EID is also referred to as *quantitative immunoelectrophoresis* in antiserum containing agarose gel.

EID can be used to assay quantitatively all proteins possessing an electrophoretic mobility that differs from that of the antibodies incorporated into the agarose gel (see Table 4-2). The mobility of human immunoglobulins can be modified by carbamylation, which results in their anodic migration [18, 19].

EID is rapid (about 2 to 3 hours), sensitive (detecting at least 0.01 mg per milliliter), reproducible (less than 5 percent coefficient of variation)

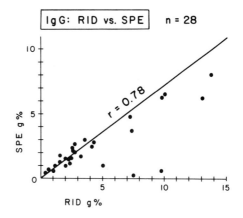

Figure 4-8
Comparison of SPE versus RID of 28 M proteins of the IgG class. An overestimation of IgG resulted to an unpredictable degree by RID.

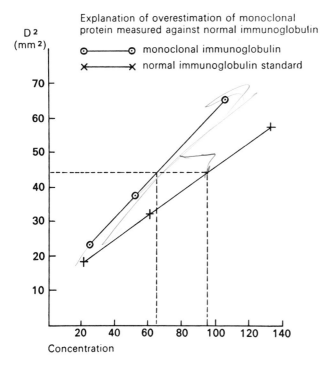

Figure 4-9
RID assays of monoclonal IgG (i.e., M proteins) usually result in overestimation of these immunoglobulins. RID assays of comparable amounts of "normal" immunoglobulins (e.g., IgG proteins from pooled normal serum) and "abnormal" M proteins (e.g., IgG proteins from myeloma patients) result in different slopes. The M-protein concentration in patients with IgG monoclonal gammopathy will usually be spuriously high. Similarly, misleading results may be obtained with protein polymers (e.g., IgA polymers), which lead to spuriously low concentrations. (Reproduced by permission. From Becker, W. *Methods of Qualitative and Quantitative Immunoelectrophoresis.* Somerville, N.J.: Behring Diagnostics, 1973.)

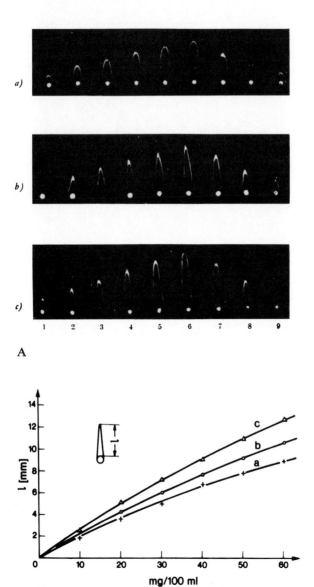

Figure 4-10
EID patterns and standard curves for the assay of hemopexin, C3c (β_1A-globulin), and α_1-acid glycoprotein. *A*. Quantitative determination of (*a*) hemopexin, (*b*) C3c (β_1A-globulin), and (*c*) α_1-acid glycoprotein by EID. *1–6:* Increasing concentrations of purified proteins (10, 20, 30, 40, 50, and 60 mg/100 ml); *7–9:* increasing serum dilutions. *B*. Standard curves for determination of (*a*) hemopexin, (*b*) C3c (β_1A-globulin), and (*c*) α_1-acid glycoprotein by EID. The length of the immunoprecipitin peaks is plotted against the concentrations of the purified proteins. (Reproduced by permission. From Ritzmann, S. E., Daniels, J. C., Alami, S. Y., and Lawrence, M. C. In G. J. Race (Ed.), *Laboratory Medicine*. New York: Harper & Row, 1975.)

Table 4-2. Electroimmunodiffusion of 19 Serum Proteins using Cellulose Acetate as the Carrier Medium

Serum Protein	Anti-serum Dilution	Buffers	Dilutions of Antigens (test sera)				Electrophoresis Time (minutes)	Milli-amperes
Prealbumin	1:40	Phosphate	1:2	1:4	1:8	1:16	25	3
Albumin	1:20	Phosphate	1:64	1:128	1:256	1:512	10	6
α_1-Acid glycoprotein	1:40	Phosphate	1:2	1:4	1:8	1:16	20	3
α_1-Antitrypsin	1:12	Phosphate	1:8	1:16	1:32	1:64	15	6
α_1-Antichymotrypsin	1:40	Barbital	1:2	1:4	1:8	1:16	15	3
Inter-α-trypsin inhibitor	1:40	Barbital	1:1	1:2	1:4	1:8	15	3
Ceruloplasmin	1:40	Phosphate	1:2	1:4	1:8	1:16	12	6
α_2-Macroglobulin	1:40	Barbital	1:8	1:16	1:32	1:64	20	3
Haptoglobin	1:12	Barbital	1:4	1:8	1:16	1:32	15	3
C3c (β_1A-globulin)	1:40	Barbital	1:16	1:32	1:64	1:128	30	3
C4 (β_1E-globulin)	1:40	Barbital	1:2	1:4	1:8	1:16	35	3
Transferrin	1:40	Phosphate	1:32	1:64	1:128	1:256	45	6
Hemopexin	1:40	Phosphate	1:4	1:8	1:16	1:32	25	6
C-reactive protein	1:40	Barbital	1:1	1:2	1:4	1:8	25	6
C1s-Inactivator	1:40	Barbital	1:1	1:2	1:4	1:8	20	3
IgG	1:20	Barbital	1:64	1:128	1:256	1:512	60	4
IgA	1:20	Barbital	1:16	1:32	1:64	1:128	35	4
IgM	1:20	Barbital	1:8	1:16	1:32	1:64	60	5
IgD	1:12	Barbital	1:1	1:2	1:4	1:8	45	6

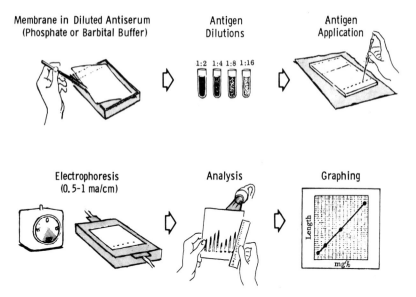

Figure 4-11
EID procedure.

[20], and economical. It is suitable for large-volume protein quantitation in the clinical laboratory.

METHODOLOGY

Several support media (e.g., agarose or cellulose acetate) can be utilized for EID. Agarose EID plates for the assay of IgG, IgA, IgM, and albumin are commercially available.* Cellulose acetate membranes [20a] provide an economical and convenient approach to EID [21]. Cellulose acetate EID is applicable to more than 20 serum proteins (Table 4-2). The technique of cellulose acetate EID is depicted in Figure 4-11.

EQUIPMENT AND SUPPLIES

The equipment includes an electrophoresis chamber (e.g., the Hyland Immunokit†), a current-stabilized power supply to maintain a current of 6 ma at a voltage of 100 to 200 v, a plastic template for use as a guide to sample application, and a magnetic stirrer.

The following supplies are required (see Table 4-2): barbital buffer (ionic strength 0.075; pH 8.6) or phosphate buffer (ionic strength 0.15; pH 7.4), cellulose acetate membranes with Mylar‡ backing, specific antisera to the proteins to be assayed (the antiserum dilutions are prepared using either a 1:4 dilution of barbital buffer or a 1:8 dilution of

* LKB Instruments, Inc., Rockville, Md. 20850; ICL Scientific, Fountain Valley, Calif. 92708.
† Hyland, Div. of Travenol Labs., Inc., Costa Mesa, Calif. 92626.
‡ Helena Laboratories, 1530 Lindberg Drive, Beaumont, Texas 77704.

phosphate buffer; such diluted antisera may be stored at 4°C for several weeks), reference samples (normal pooled serum that has been stored at −70°C produces satisfactory results), and staining dye (e.g., Ponceau S).

PROCEDURE

The cellulose acetate membrane is soaked in the diluted antiserum for approximately 10 minutes. The membrane is then placed on a moist base and covered with the application template. Next, 0.2 μl samples of three dilutions of the antigen are applied through the holes in the template by means of a Hamilton #7001 syringe* [22].

The cell is prepared for electrophoresis by filling the chamber sponges with the appropriate undiluted buffer. The membrane is placed on the cell with the cellulose acetate side down. The cell is then covered and, after an equilibration period of one minute, electrophoresis is performed using a constant current of 3 to 6 ma depending upon the protein examined. Subsequently, the membrane is removed from the cell, washed in diluted buffer (the same used for antiserum dilutions) on a magnetic stirrer, stained, and air dried.

ANALYSIS OF RESULTS

The lengths of the precipitin areas are measured to the closest 0.1 mm. A standard curve is constructed as for RID (see p. 63). The concentration of protein is obtained by comparing the length of the test "rockets" to those used for the reference curve (see Figs. 4-10 and 4-11).

SOURCES OF ERROR

For cellulose acetate EID, possible sources of error include incorrect application of samples; either incorrect dilutions, incorrectly applied volumes, or splattering, which can result in secondary rockets; drying of the cellulose acetate membrane before electrophoresis; pH changes; poor contact between the sponges and the membrane, which may result in a wavy precipitin pattern (this may be corrected by placing a glass microscope slide over the membrane and the sponges); and the use of inappropriate standard serum (e.g., certain commercial reference samples possess electrophoretic migration rates that differ from those of fresh or frozen serum).

NORMAL VALUES

The normal concentrations for serum proteins determined by RID (see Table 4-1) also apply to EID. The correlation between results with RID and EID systems is excellent, especially for the more anodically migrating proteins [20].

APPLICATION AND INTERPRETATION

In general, the applications of EID for the quantitation of serum proteins are similar to those of RID. Large-volume assays of numerous proteins benefit from the economy and speed of this technique.

* Hamilton Co., Whittier, Calif. 90608.

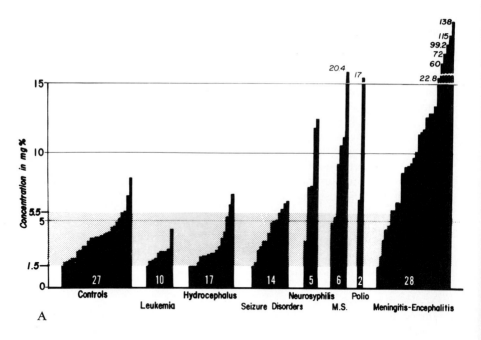

A

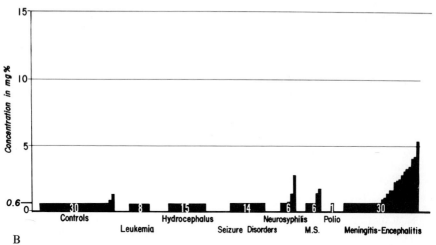

B

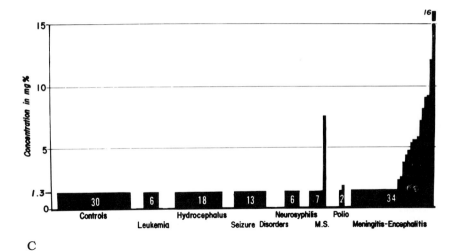

C

Figure 4-12
Results of EID immunoglobulin assays in CSF obtained from patients with a
variety of disorders. *A*. IgG in CSF: gray area represents 90th percentile
normal range (upper limits: 5.5 mg/100 ml). Significant increases of IgG
are seen in certain patients with multiple sclerosis (*M.S.*) and with meningitis, or encephalitis, or both. *B*. IgA in CSF: Normally, IgA is less than 0.6
mg/100 ml. In patients with meningitis, or encephalitis, or both, significant
increases of IgA may be encountered. *C*. IgM in CSF: Normally, IgM is not
detectable by EID. It is, however, greatly increased in certain patients with
meningitis, or encephalitis, or both.

Immunoglobulins in cerebrospinal fluid (CSF) can be scanned by electrophoresis [23, 24] and assayed more satisfactorily by immunochemical means, such as Ouchterlony double diffusion [25], immunoelectrophoresis [26, 27], radial immunodiffusion [24, 27, 28], radioimmunoassay [29], and electroimmunodiffusion [30–32]. EID appears to be the method of choice for the rapid quantitation of CSF albumin and immunoglobulins, allowing the measurement of the major immunoglobulins IgG, IgA, and IgM within 2 to 3 hours without prior concentration (Fig. 4-12). Normal CSF immunoglobulin concentrations (90th percentile ranges) as established in our laboratory (University of Texas Medical Branch, Galveston, Texas) are: IgG, undetectable to 5.5 mg per 100 ml; IgA, undetectable to 0.6 mg per 100 ml; and IgM, undetectable to 1.3 mg per 100 ml (see Fig. 4-12; see also references [33, 33a]).

Elevation of the immunoglobulins IgG, IgA, and IgM often occurs in numerous diseases that affect the blood-brain barrier, thus allowing an influx of serum immunoglobulins into the CSF. These disorders include meningitis and encephalitis. The quantitation of the total CSF proteins or CSF albumin simultaneously with that of IgG, IgA, and IgM in such patients allows the distinction between these intra– and extra–central nervous system (CNS) disorders.

Elevated IgG levels in CSF, which are often independent of elevations of the other immunoglobulins, occur in patients with active multiple sclerosis [26–28, 30, 34], and immunoglobulin fragments and free light chains are found frequently in the CSF of such patients [35]. Some of these light chains are of monoclonal nature [24] and IgG derivation [36]. Typically, in such patients the κ/λ ratios are altered.

Selectively increased CSF IgA levels are encountered in a variety of disorders, including diabetes mellitus complicated by retinitis proliferans (Fig. 4-13).

Selective increases of CSF IgM levels have been reported in conjunction with CNS-invading Burkitt's lymphoma, *Hemophilus influenzae* meningitis, and other disorders.

Decreased CSF IgG levels are encountered in patients with active CNS lupus erythematosus. It has been suggested that decreased IgG levels, rather than depressed C4 levels in the CSF, can aid in the differential diagnosis between CNS systemic lupus erythematosus and other causes for CNS symptoms, such as steroid-induced encephalopathy [25, 29].

The finding of abnormal CSF protein levels provides objective evidence of a disease process, but the precise clinical significance of these and other proteins, including IgD and IgE, remains to be established [37, 38].

LIMITATION OF EID
Quantitation of M proteins in patients with monoclonal gammopathy by EID leads to unreliable values, analogous to those obtained by RID (see p. 66). Each M protein has its own fixed electrophoretic mobility (e.g., the γ_1-globulin position), and the M protein will migrate only to

Figure 4-13
Selectively increased IgA concentration in CSF of a patient with diabetes mellitus complicated by retinitis proliferans, demonstrated by EID. Similarly, increased immunoglobulin concentrations can be demonstrated with this technique for IgA (as in poliomyelitis) and IgM (as in *Hemophilus influenzae* meningitis, etc.).

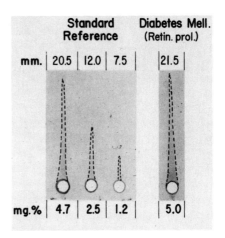

its characteristic electrophoretic position and not necessarily to the end of the precipitin rocket. Therefore, the true concentration of the M protein cannot be obtained (Fig. 4-14) unless it is performed by serum protein electrophoresis.

Automated Immunoprecipitation (AIP)

Antigen-antibody precipitin reactions have been utilized as quantitative assays for many years. The technique of Heidelberger and Kendall [39], which is based upon the assay of the nitrogen content of purified immunoprecipitates, possesses a high degree of reproducibility and sensitivity, but its disadvantage is its complexity and tediousness. A practical modification was provided in the technique of Schwick and others [40–42], which opened the era of immunochemical protein quantitation in the clinical laboratory. This approach utilizes the photometric determination of the degree of turbidity produced by antigen-antibody reactions (Fig. 4-15). The antigen and antibody constituents are allowed to react in highly diluted solutions. The resultant antigen-antibody complexes cause turbidity of the reaction mixture. The extinction at 436 to 450 nm can be used as a measure of the degree of turbidity and thus of the antigen concentration. This approach provides the basis for the automated immunoprecipitin reactions [43, 44].

If the quantity and potency of the specific antiserum is kept constant and the antigen concentration is varied, an optical density versus precipitin curve can be drawn (see Fig. 4-15). Antigen excess leads to soluble reaction products; therefore, only the ascending limb of the precipitin curve is used for the turbidimetric determination of proteins. Utilizing this portion of the standard curves, unknown antigen concentrations can be determined. Standard curves are established for the individual serum proteins to be assayed by mixing increasing amounts of purified antigens with constant amounts of antiserum. After a short reaction time (e.g., 30 minutes) at room temperature, the turbidity resulting from the anti-

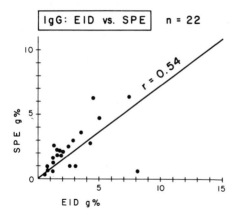

Figure 4-14
Comparison of results obtained by SPE and EID in the analysis of 22 M proteins of the IgG class. There is no correlation between these two techniques; only SPE yields accurate determinations.

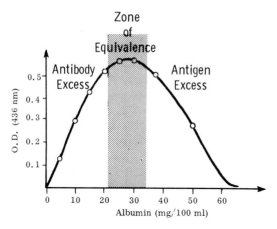

Figure 4-15
Standard curve for the photometric quantitation of serum albumin. Increasing amounts of antigen are added to a constant amount of antibody. At the equivalence zone, the precipitate is maximal and no unreacted antigen or antibody remains in solution. Soluble immune complexes occur on either side of the equivalence zone. *O.D.:* optical density. Modified from Becker, W., Rapp, W., Schwick, H. G., and Störiko, K. In E. Haaf (Ed.), *Lab Synopsis,* Vol. 1. Somerville, N.J.: Behring Diagnostics, 1969. Pp. 51–52.)

gen-antibody precipitin reaction is assayed spectrophotometrically at 436 to 450 nm. The test samples are prepared and assayed analogously, and the absolute protein concentrations are obtained from the standard curve after multiplication by the dilution factors.

Sources of error may be due to turbid or hemolyzed sera, the use of different antiserum batches for the standard curves, test cuvets with unsuitable transmittance characteristics, and temperature differences during the test procedures.

The automated immunoprecipitin (AIP) reaction follows the same principle as the described turbidity assay and is, therefore, liable to the same sources of error. In addition, AIP, at its present state of art, is subject to the capricious behavior of the electronic components. Its sensitivity varies from 2 μg per milliliter in CSF to approximately 250 μg per milliliter in serum [45, 46]. Newer technical approaches using a Technicon* instrument allow the processing of approximately 60 samples per hour, and the results may be obtained 20 minutes after sampling. The amounts of both the antiserum and serum used are in the microliter range. AIP undoubtedly will gradually assume its deserved place in the clinical laboratory when additional refinements of the instruments result in more compact units, improved reliability, and reduced cost factors.

References

1. Störiko, K.   Normal values for 23 different human plasma proteins determined by single radial immunodiffusion. *Blut* 16:3, 1968.
2. Reimer, C. B., Philipps, D. J., Maddison, S. E., and Shore, S. L.   Comparative evaluation of commercial precipitating antisera against human IgM and IgA. *J. Lab. Clin. Med.* 76:949, 1970.
3. Hosty, T. A., Hollenbeck, M., and Shane, S.   Intercomparison of results obtained with five commercial diffusion plates supplied for quantitation of immunoglobulins. *Clin. Chem.* 19:524, 1973.
4. Becker, W.   Determination of antisera titres using the single radial immunodiffusion method. *Immunochemistry* 6:539, 1969.
4a. Mancini, G., Vaerman, J. P., Carbonara, A. O., and Heremans, J. F. A Single Radial Immunodiffusion Method for the Immunological Quantitation of Proteins. In H. Peeters (Ed.), *Protides of the Biological Fluids,* Vol. 11. Amsterdam: Elsevier, 1964. Pp. 370–373.
4b. Vaerman, J. P., Lebacq-Verheyden, A. M., Scolari, L., and Heremans, J. F.   Further studies on single radial immunodiffusion. I. Direct proportionality between area of precipitate and reciprocal of antibody concentration. *Immunochemistry* 6:279, 1969.
5. Berne, B. H.   Differing methodology and equations used in quantitating immunoglobulins by radial immunodiffusion. A comparative evaluation of reported and commercial techniques. *Clin. Chem.* 20:61, 1974.
6. Mancini, G., Carbonara, A. O., and Heremans, J. F.   Immunochemical quantitation of antigens by single radial immunodiffusion. *Immunochemistry* 2:235, 1965.

* Technicon Instruments Corp., Tarrytown, N.Y. 10591.

7. Fahey, J. L., and McKelvey, E.   Quantitative determination of serum immunoglobulins in antibody-agar plates. *J. Immunol.* 94:84, 1965.
8. Ritzmann, S. E., Fischer, C. L., Mattingly, D. J., and Daniels, J. C. Quantitative Immunoassay—Radial Immunodiffusion (RID). In J. B. Fuller (Ed.), *ASCP Workshop Manual, Selected Topics in Clinical Chemistry* (4th ed.). Chicago: American Society of Clinical Pathologists' Commission on Continuing Education, 1973. Pp. 77–105.
9. Ritzmann, S. E., Alami, S. Y., Van Fossan, D. D., and McKay, G.   Electrophoresis, Immunoelectrophoresis, Quantitative Immunodiffusion and Thermoproteins. In G. J. Race (Ed.), *Laboratory Medicine*. New York: Harper & Row, 1973. Pp. 1–56.
10. Kalff, M. W.   Quantitative determination of serum immunoglobulin levels by single radial immunodiffusion. *Clin. Biochem.* 3:91, 1970.
11. Kassay, J. R., Muniz, F., Levin, W. C., and Ritzmann, S. E.   Quantitation of serum proteins on whole blood—Radial immunodiffusion technique applicable to capillary blood. *Aerosp. Med.* 41:26, 1970.
12. Alford, C. A., Jr.   Immunoglobulin determinations in the diagnosis of fetal infection. *Pediatr. Clin. North Am.* 18:99, 1971.
13. Daniels, J. C., Vyvial, T. M., Levin, W. C., and Ritzmann, S. E.   Methodologic differences in values for M-proteins in serum, as measured by three techniques. *Clin. Chem.* 21:243, 1975.
14. Kohler, P. F., and Farr, R. S.   Elevation of cord over maternal IgG immunoglobulin: Evidence for an active placental IgG transport. *Nature* 210:1070, 1966.
15. Hobbs, J. R., et al.   Six cases of gamma-D myelomatosis. *Lancet* 2:614, 1966.
16. Committee report.   *Bull. W.H.O.* 35:953, 1966.
17. Schur, P. H.   Human Gamma-G Subclasses. In R. S. Schwartz (Ed.), *Progress in Clinical Immunology,* Vol. 1. New York: Grune & Stratton, 1972. Pp. 71–104.
17a. Laurell, C. B.   Quantitative estimation of proteins by electrophoresis in agarose gel containing antibodies. *Anal. Biochem.* 15:45, 1966.
18. Weeke, B.   Carbamylated human immunoglobulins tested by electrophoresis in agarose and antibody-containing agarose. *Scand. J. Clin. Lab. Invest.* 21:351, 1968.
19. Weeke, B.   Quantitative estimation of human immunoglobulins following carbamylation by electrophoresis in antibody-containing agarose. *Scand. J. Clin. Lab. Invest.* 22:107, 1968.
20. Gill, C. W., Fischer, C. L., and Holleman, C. L.   Rapid method for protein quantitation by electroimmunodiffusion. *Clin. Chem.* 17:501, 1971.
20a. Kroll, J.   Quantitation of protein by electrophoresis in a cellulose acetate membrane impregnated with antiserum. *Scand. J. Clin. Lab. Invest.* 21:187, 1968.
21. Ritzmann, S. E., Fischer, C. L., Cobb, E. K., and Daniels, J. C.   Electroimmunodiffusion. In J. B. Fuller (Ed.), *ASCP Workshop Manual, Selected Topics in Clinical Chemistry* (4th ed.). Chicago: American Society of Clinical Pathologists' Commission on Continuing Education, 1973. Pp. 106–116.
22. Vyvial, T., Kiamar, M., and Ritzmann, S. E.   Cellulose acetate electroimmunodiffusion. *Am. J. Med. Technol.* In press.
23. Werner, M.   A combined procedure for protein estimation and electrophoresis of cerebrospinal fluids. *J. Lab. Clin. Med.* 74:166, 1969.
24. Zettervall, O., and Link, H.   Electrophoretic distribution of kappa and

lambda immunoglobulin light chain determinants in serum and cerebro-spinal fluid in multiple sclerosis. *Clin. Exp. Immunol.* 7:365, 1970.

25. Udeozo, I. O. K., Bezer, A. E., Osunkoya, B. O., Ngu, V. A., Luzzatto, L., and McFarlane, H. Cerebrospinal fluid immunoglobulins in Burkitt lymphoma. *J. Lab. Clin. Med.* 71:912, 1968.

26. Lamourezux, G., and Borduas, A. G. Immune studies in multiple sclerosis. *Clin. Exp. Immunol.* 1:363, 1966.

27. Gottesleben, A., and Bauer, H. J. Quantitative immunochemistry of cerebrospinal fluid proteins in inflammatory diseases of the nervous system. *Ger. Med. Mon.* 12:331, 1967.

28. Riddoch, D., and Thompson, R. A. Immunoglobulin levels in cerebrospinal fluid. *Br. Med. J.* 1:396, 1970.

29. Levin, A. S., Fudenberg, H. H., Petz, L. D., and Sharp, G. C. IgG levels in cerebrospinal fluid of patients with central nervous system manifestations of systemic lupus erythematosus. *Clin. Immunol. Immunopathol.* 1:1, 1972.

30. Hartley, T. F., Merrill, D. A., and Claman, H. N. Quantitation of immunoglobulins in cerebrospinal fluid. *Arch. Neurol.* 15:472. 1966.

31. Merrill, D. A., Hartley, T. F., and Claman, H. N. Electroimmunodiffusion (EID). A simple rapid method for quantitation of immunoglobulins in dilute biological fluids. *J. Lab. Clin. Med.* 69:151, 1967.

32. Schneck, S. A., and Claman, H. CSF immunoglobulins in multiple sclerosis and other neurologic diseases. Measurement by electroimmunodiffusion. *Arch. Neurol.* 20:132, 1969.

33. Bock, E. Quantitation of plasma proteins in cerebrospinal fluid. *Scand. J. Immunol.* 2[Suppl. 1]:111, 1973.

33a. Weeke, B., and Krasinikoff, P. A. The concentration of 21 serum proteins in normal children and adults. *Acta Med. Scand.* 192:149, 1972.

34. Nellhaus, G. Cerebrospinal fluid immunoglobulin G in childhood. *Arch. Neurol.* 24:441, 1971.

35. Koch, F., Becker, W., and Schwick, H. G. Fluid from patients with panencephalitis. *Ger. Med. Mon.* 15:149, 1970.

36. Link, H., and Zettervall, O. Multiple sclerosis. Disturbed kappa:lambda chain ratios of immunoglobulin G in cerebrospinal fluid. *Clin. Exp. Immunol.* 6:435, 1970.

37. CSF proteins in psychiatric disorders (Editorial). *Br. Med. J.* 1:582, 1970.

38. Kolar, O., Russell, D., and Hartlage, P. IgD and IgA in cerebrospinal fluid. *Lancet* 1:622, 1970.

39. Heidelberger, M., and Kendall, F. E. Quantitative studies on the precipitin reaction. The determination of small amounts of a specific polysaccharide. *J. Exp. Med.* 55:555, 1932.

40. Schultze, H. E., and Schwick, G. Quantitative Immunologische Bestimmung von Plasmaproteinen. *Clin. Chim. Acta* 4:15, 1959.

41. Schwick, G., and Störiko, K. Qualitative and Quantitative Determination of Plasma Proteins by Immunoprecipitation. In E. Haaf (Ed.), *Lab Synopsis*, Vol. 1. Somerville, N.J.: Behring Diagnostics, 1969. Pp. 1–79.

42. Becker, W., Rapp, W., Schwick, G., and Störiko, K. Methoden zur quantitativen Bestimmung von Plasmaproteinen durch Immunpräzipitation. *Z. Klin. Chem.* 6:113, 1968.

43. Larson, C., Gorman, J. M., and Becker, A. M. Automated Immunoprecipitin for Proteins in Body Fluids. Further Advances. In *AIP—Automated Immunoprecipitin Reactions; New Methods, Techniques and*

Evaluations. A collection of papers presented at the Colloquium on AIP, Technicon International Congress, New York, N.Y., 1972. Pp. 21–23.

44. Larson, C., Orenstein, P., and Ritchie, R. F. An Automated Method for Quantitation of Proteins in Body Fluids. In J. A. Preston and D. B. Troxel (Eds.), *Advances in Automated Analysis, Technicon International Congress, 1970,* Vol. 1. Miami: Thurman Associates, 1971. P. 101.

45. Riccomi, H., Masson, P. L., and Heremans, J. F. Evaluation of the Technicon Automated Specific Protein Analytical System. In *AIP—Automated Immunoprecipitin Reactions: New Methods, Techniques and Evaluations.* A collection of papers presented at the Colloquium on AIP, Technicon International Congress, New York, N.Y., 1972. Pp. 53–57.

46. Ritchie, R. F., Alper, C. A., Graves, J., Pearson, N., and Larson, C. Automated quantitation of proteins in serum and other biological fluids. *Am. J. Clin. Pathol.* 59:151, 1973.

Ouchterlony Double-Diffusion Technique

5

Stephan E. Ritzmann and Robert M. Nakamura

The Ouchterlony double-immunodiffusion method is a fundamental tool in most immunological areas [1–4]. The principle of the Ouchterlony double-immunodiffusion technique is based upon the simultaneous application of antigen and antibodies into separate wells of an agar or agarose layer, their subsequent immunodiffusion toward one another, and the development of precipitin lines resulting from the antigen-antibody interactions. The Ouchterlony double-diffusion reaction is a secondary antigen-antibody reaction that requires antigen and antibodies to form a precipitin line. Glass or plastic Petri dishes containing agar or agarose are used. The method is practical in the clinical laboratory for the detection of precipitin reactions in which the antigen molecular size is not excessively large (not more than 19S). A precipitin reaction may be seen within several hours after sample application and becomes optimal usually after 18 to 30 hours. The sensitivity of the Ouchterlony gel precipitation technique is in the range of 6.0 to 35.0 μg of antibody per milliliter of serum [5].

The Ouchterlony double-immunodiffusion technique is at best semiquantitative, and it lends itself primarily to qualitative tests for the presence and character of certain proteins. In particular, it detects immunological reactions of identity, partial identity, and nonidentity (Fig. 5-1). The sensitivity of the reaction is shown by the fact that a precipitin line may be uniformly obtained with concentrations of protein antigen of 50 μg per milliliter or less [5]. The double-immunodiffusion assays are subject to error if there are considerable excesses of antigen or antibody.

Methodology

Agar or agarose plates for double immunodiffusion can be readily prepared in the laboratory, and various cutting devices for antigen-antibody well patterns are commercially available. Such devices allow the preparation of either macro- or micropatterns ("rosettes"). Recently, rehy-

Figure 5-1
Three basic reaction patterns of Ouchterlony double immunodiffusion. *1.*
Pattern of immunological identity. The
antigens (*Aga, Aga*) in the lower wells
precipitate in a line of complete fusion,
reflecting the identity of the antigens.
2. Pattern of immunological partial
identity. The spur between the antibody (*Ab*) and the antigens [*Ag(a)*,
Ag(a)] indicates that the antigens in
the lower wells are related but not
identical. *3.* Pattern of immunological
nonidentity. The crossed precipitin
lines indicate that the antigens (*Aga,
Aga*) are unrelated.

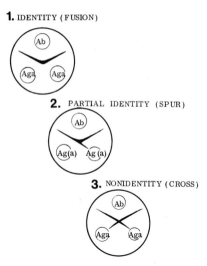

1. IDENTITY (FUSION)

2. PARTIAL IDENTITY (SPUR)

3. NONIDENTITY (CROSS)

dratable agarose films with precut rosettes* have become available that
require only rehydration prior to use (see Fig. 5-3).

Rehydratable agarose on 35-mm film strips with precut rosette patterns (MCI) is prepared, and the appropriate antigens and antisera are
added to the wells. After 24 hours of immunodiffusion at room temperature in a moisture chamber, the precipitin patterns are usually well visible.

Application and Interpretation

The Ouchterlony double-immunodiffusion technique lends itself to the
qualitative and semiquantitative assay of numerous proteins, including
Bence Jones proteins, secretory IgA, α_1-fetoprotein, myoglobin, and
C$\bar{1}$-INH. Additionally, under special circumstances, the technique may
be used to demonstrate the immunological identity, partial identity, or
nonidentity of proteins (see Figs. 5-1 to 5-3).

IMMUNOTEST FOR BENCE JONES PROTEINS (BJP)

Testing the urine and serum for Bence Jones proteins is an integral part
of the protein analysis in B-lymphocyte disorders, including monoclonal
gammopathies (see Chap. 19). Bence Jones proteins in urine may be
detected by the heat test [6–8] (see Chap. 20), electrophoresis, or immunochemical techniques (i.e., immunoelectrophoresis [see Chap. 2]
and double immunodiffusion) [9–13]. Whereas the former tests are rather
insensitive and often inconclusive, the latter immunochemical tests are
very sensitive and often allow the detection of trace amounts of Bence

---

* MCI, Biomedical Division of Marine Colloids, Inc., Rockland, Me. 04841.

Jones proteins in urine and serum. It should be noted that the Albustix* test may fail to detect urinary Bence Jones proteins, even if present in large amounts [14, 15]. Thus, the absence of proteinuria by routine urinalysis does not rule out the presence of Bence Jones proteins.

Immunoglobulins are composed of heavy and light polypeptide chains (see Chap. 19). Normally, light (L) and heavy (H) chains are produced in a synchronous fashion (i.e., in a ratio of 1:1) on the ribosomes within the endoplasmic reticulum (ER) of plasma cells (i.e., B-lymphocytes). Subsequently, these L and H chains are assembled into complete immunoglobulin molecules (e.g., IgG) which are secreted. In pathological conditions, L and H chains may be produced in an asynchronous fashion, in which case, either free L chains or free H chains will be produced.

Free monoclonal L chains (i.e., κ or λ chains) are identical with Bence Jones proteins, and their occurrence denotes the presence of monoclonal gammopathy. In certain renal diseases associated with nephron loss (e.g., systemic lupus erythematosus nephropathy), there occur free polyclonal L chains (i.e., κ and λ chains in an approximately normal 2:1 ratio) that must be distinguished from Bence Jones proteins. Free *monoclonal* L chains (i.e., BJP) are products of altered synthesis of immunoglobulins, whereas free *polyclonal* L chains are the result of altered catabolic pathways of immunoglobulins. The presence of BJP denotes the presence of a "malignant" disease [6, 11, 16–20] in distinct contrast to the "nonmalignant" nature of diseases associated with the production of polyclonal free L chains.

Free monoclonal or polyclonal L chains possess certain characteristics, including reversible heat precipitability (i.e., a positive *heat test*), an electrophoretic mobility within the immunoglobulin migration ranges (i.e., between the γ- and α_2-globulin positions, although most of them migrate to the γ- or β-globulin regions), and immunological cross-reactivity with all immunoglobulins. These characteristics provide the basis for the immunological detection of BJP. It must be noted, however, that the time-honored heat test is rather insensitive, requiring more than 1200 mg per day of urinary BJP. False-positive heat tests due to increased amounts of polyclonal free L chains occur, since this test does not distinguish between polyclonal and monoclonal free L chains and is usually not applicable to serum assays. The Albustix test may fail to detect urinary BJP, even if present in large amounts. Thus, the absence of proteinuria by routine urinalysis does not rule out the presence of BJP. Likewise, the *electrophoretic assay* for free L chains is insensitive. Furthermore, the detection of a band in the β- or γ-globulin areas on electrophoresis does not provide conclusive evidence for the presence of BJP. Myoglobin, lysozyme, free H-chain γ-globulin fragments, bacterial contamination, and so forth must be excluded as possible causes of such bands. Therefore, the immunological techniques for the detection of free L chains must be regarded as the assays of choice.

* Ames Company, Miles Laboratories, Elkhart, Ind. 46514.

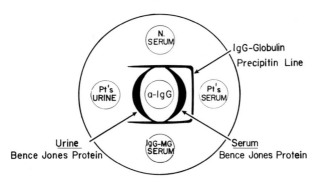

Figure 5-2
Ouchterlony double-diffusion technique for the detection of Bence Jones proteins (modified from Korngold [9]). *Top well:* Normal serum (normal control for IgG). *Bottom well:* IgG-myeloma serum (abnormal control for IgG). *Left well:* Patient's urine (concentration ranges 100:1 to 1:200). *Right well:* Patient's serum (concentration ranges 1:1 to 1:100). *Center well:* Antiserum to IgG containing antigenic determinants to both L-chain types κ and λ and γ H chains. Free L chains are indicated by the curved precipitin lines between center well, left well (urinary free L chains), and right well (serum free L chains). A negative test virtually rules out the existence of appreciable amounts of free L chains. A positive test, however, does not discriminate between free polyclonal and monoclonal L chains. Therefore, such positive samples are then reexamined with the aid of anti–free κ-chain antiserum and anti–free λ-chain antiserum on additional Ouchterlony plates. Polyclonal free L chains yield precipitin lines with both antisera, but monoclonal free L chains (BJP) react only with one antiserum, either the free anti-κ or the free λ-antiserum. (Reproduced by permission. From Ritzmann, S. E., Daniels, J. C., Alami, S. Y., and Lawrence, M. C. In G. J. Race (Ed.), *Laboratory Medicine.* New York: Harper & Row, 1975.)

Bence Jones proteins may be positively identified in serum or urine, even if present in small amounts, by immunoelectrophoresis (see Chap. 3) or Ouchterlony double diffusion (Figs. 5-2 and· 5-3). The Ouchterlony immunotest for BJP is a modification of Korngold's technique [9, 21]. After preparation of the rehydratable agarose, the serum or urine samples are applied to the antigen wells in various concentrations; the samples may require concentration or dilution ranging from 100:1 to 1:200. Polyvalent anti-IgG (H+L chain–specific) antiserum is added to the center well. After 24 hours, the plates are assayed for precipitin lines. Absence of precipitin lines reflects the absence of significant amounts of free L chains. The development of precipitin lines indicates the presence of free L chains. Since this screening test does not discriminate between polyclonal free L chains (κ and λ L chains) and monoclonal free light chains (κ or λ L chains, i.e., BJP), a specific immunotest* is then performed that utilizes antisera to free κ L chains and to free λ L chains (see Fig. 5-3). Occurrence of precipitin lines with *both* antisera

* Behring Diagnostics, Somerville, N.J. 08876.

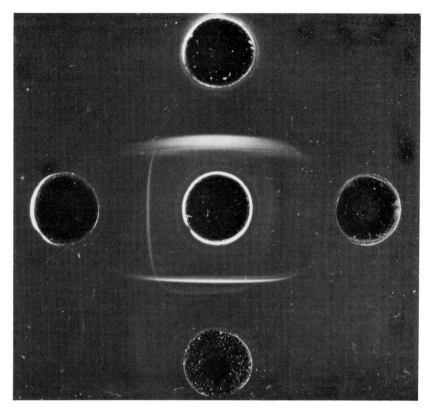

Figure 5-3
Positive Ouchterlony double-diffusion film (see text and Fig. 5-2). The center
well contains anti–free λ L-chain antiserum, which reveals the presence
of large amounts of free λ chains in a serum specimen (*left*); a parallel
immunotest with anti–free κ L-chain antisera revealed no precipitin line.
Such a reaction pattern is indicative of the presence of BJP(λ). The patient
was subsequently found to suffer from L-chain disease (i.e., myeloma associated with Bence Jones proteins as the only abnormal immunoglobulins).

indicates the presence of polyclonal light chains, but the presence of
appreciable amounts of *either* κ or λ L chains reflects the presence of
BJP.

False-positive tests may be obtained when testing sera from patients
with (1) IgA monoclonal gammopathy (one or more additional precipitin lines are found that are due to IgA polymers and are usually situated
peripherally to the IgG precipitin line), (2) γ H-chain disease (no reaction occurs with anti–L chain antisera), or (3) free polyclonal L chains
(e.g., κ and λ L chains in urine or serum from certain patients with lupus
erythematosus and tubular nephropathy). Such polyclonal free L chains
are *not* Bence Jones proteins. Confirmatory tests using anti–free L chain
antibodies are needed for this distinction.

False-negative tests may be encountered occasionally when using serum or urine specimens that have been stored for lengthy periods of time, when using antiserum with low antibody titers to light chains, or when dealing with antigen excess. Because of the last possibility, it is imperative to examine serum or urine specimens at different dilutions (e.g., up to 1:200) or, under special circumstances, concentrations (e.g., 10:1 to 100:1).

ASSAY FOR SECRETORY IgA

In this assay undiluted and 1:10 diluted saliva specimens are applied to the antigen wells; one sample is taken from a healthy control person and the other from the patient to be assayed. Anti-IgA antiserum is added to the center well. (Ideally, anti–secretory IgA antiserum should be applied, but, in the absence of such commercially available antisera, anti-IgA antiserum may be used since it cross-reacts sufficiently with the secretory IgA.) After 24 hours of immunodiffusion, the precipitin patterns are usually discernible between the undiluted and diluted saliva and the antiserum. This immunotest allows the detection of patients with secretory IgA deficiency.

The antibodies of the IgA class [22] belong to two separate systems [23, 24], namely, the IgA antibodies in the circulation (serum IgA) and those in the external secretions, such as saliva, gastric and intestinal juices, tears, urine, and colostrum (secretory IgA). Deficiency of such secretory IgA is usually associated with a general agammaglobulinemia, but it may also be associated with a selective serum IgA deficiency. The latter condition afflicts approximately one in 600 to 700 Americans [25–32]. Such subjects with isolated IgA deficiency either may be seemingly healthy or they may suffer from chronic otitis, bronchitis, colitis, or certain autoimmune phenomena [33–35].

ASSAY FOR α_1-FETOPROTEIN (AFP)

Alpha-fetoprotein (AFP) is produced by the fetal liver, and human fetal serum contains AFP in the α_1-globulin fraction. It is present in high concentrations during the early in utero period, but it decreases with maturation and is absent in normal adults (Fig. 5-4). If detectable in adult serum, it possesses clinical significance (see Chap. 21).

AFP is present in a high percentage of sera from African and Far Eastern patients with primary hepatoma and in approximately 50 percent of American patients with the disease. AFP may also be found occasionally in the sera of patients with teratocarcinoma, embryonal cell carcinoma, or infectious hepatitis [36]. The detection of AFP in serum is a useful screening test, and its monitoring may aid in the follow-up of these patients during treatment (see Fig. 21-1, Chap. 21).

The use of anti-AFP antiserum in the center wells of Ouchterlony double-diffusion plates and of the patient's serum in the outer wells allows the detection of AFP in most instances. Immunoelectrophoresis may also be used in detection of AFP.

Figure 5-4
Electrophoretic pattern of human fetal serum (*top*). Note the prominent fetal protein band (*dark area*) between albumin and α_1-globulin, representing α_1-fetoprotein. In the SPE pattern of maternal serum (*bottom*), AFP is absent.

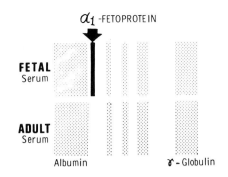

α_1-FETOPROTEIN

FETAL Serum

ADULT Serum

Albumin γ-Globulin

OTHER PROTEINS

C1s-INHIBITOR (C$\bar{1}$-INH)

This inhibitor of the first component of complement plays an essential role in maintaining the precarious balance between the activated and deactivated complement components (see Chap. 15). C$\bar{1}$-INH deficiency is often complicated by the characteristic manifestations of familial angioedema [37, 38]. The Ouchterlony assay technique and the use of anti-C$\bar{1}$-INH antiserum (Behring Diagnostics) allow a diagnostic approach to this disorder.

HEPATITIS-B ASSOCIATED ANTIGEN

Hepatitis-B associated antigen (HB-Ag) [39, 40] may be detected by various immunological techniques, which vary in their sensitivity. One such approach is the use of the Ouchterlony double-diffusion technique (see also Chap. 3, p. 58).

MYOGLOBIN

Myoglobin is frequently found in the urine following injuries [41, 42] or myocardial infarction [43]. Clinically, the detection of myoglobinuria should alert the physician to possible impending renal complications for which protective steps can be taken (e.g., vigorous hydration with diuretics or standby dialysis). The Ouchterlony immunotest with the use of specific anti-myoglobin antisera provides a sensitive, practical, economical approach.

IMMUNE COMPLEXES

Immune complexes in serum, joint fluid, and other biological fluids may be detected by the double gel-diffusion test (see Chap. 9). Agnello and co-workers [44] have demonstrated that the C1q component of complement will form a precipitin reaction with aggregated γ-globulin and immune complexes. The soluble immune complexes that are found in twofold to twentyfold antigen excess will react with C1q.

References

1. Ouchterlony, O. Diffusion-in-gel methods for immunological analysis. *Prog. Allergy* 5:1, 1958.
2. Ouchterlony, O. *Handbook of Immunodiffusion and Immunoelectrophoresis.* Ann Arbor, Mich.: Ann Arbor Science Publ., 1968.
3. Grabar, P., and Burtin, P. *Immunoelectrophoretic Analysis. Applications to Human Biological Fluids.* Amsterdam: Elsevier, 1964.
4. Weir, D. M., (Ed.). *Handbook of Experimental Immunology.* Oxford: Blackwell, 1967.
5. Kabat, E. A., and Mayer, M. M. *Immunochemistry* (2nd ed.). Springfield, Ill.: Thomas, 1961.
6. Snapper, I., and Kahn, A. I. Multiple myeloma. *Semin. Hematol.* 1:87, 1964.
7. Bence Jones, H. On a new substance occurring in the urine of a patient with mollities ossium. *Phil. Trans. London* 138:55, 1848.
8. Bernier, G. M., and Putnam, R. W. Polymerism, polymorphism and impurities in Bence Jones proteins. *Biochem. Biophys.* 86:295, 1964.
9. Korngold, L. Abnormal plasma components and their significance in disease. *Ann. N.Y. Acad. Sci.* 94:110, 1961.
10. Epstein, W. V., and Tan, M. Increase of L-chain proteins in the sera of patients with systemic lupus erythematosus and the synovial fluids of patients with peripheral rheumatoid arthritis. *Arthritis Rheum.* 9:713, 1966.
11. Osserman, E. F., Takatsuki, K., and Talal, N. The pathogenesis of "amyloidosis." *Semin. Hematol.* 1:3, 1964.
12. Tan, M., and Epstein, W. V. A direct immunologic assay of human sera for Bence Jones proteins (L-chains). *J. Lab. Clin. Med.* 66:344, 1965.
13. Heremans, J. F., and Heremans, M. Immunoelectrophoresis. *Acta Med. Scand. [Suppl.]* 367:27, 1961.
14. Clough, G., and Reah, T. G. A "protein error." *Lancet* 1:1248, 1964.
15. Huhnstock, K. Paraproteinurien mit negativem Ausfall des Albustix-Testes. *Klin. Wochenschr.* 40:1009, 1962.
16. McLaughlin, H., and Hobbs, J. R. Clinical Significance of Bence Jones Proteinuria. In H. Peeters (Ed.), *Proteins and Related Subjects. Protides of the Biological Fluids,* Vol. 20. Amsterdam: Elsevier, 1973. Pp. 251–254.
17. Damacco, F., and Waldenström, J. Serum and urine light chain levels in benign monoclonal gammopathies, multiple myeloma and Waldenström's macroglobulinemia. *Clin. Exp. Immunol.* 3:911, 1968.
18. Williams, R. C., Jr., Brunning, R. D., and Wollheim, F. A. Light chain disease. An abortive variant of multiple myeloma. *Ann. Intern. Med.* 65:471, 1966.
19. Pruzanski, W., and Ogryzlo, M. A. The changing pattern of diseases associated with M-components. *Med. Clin. North Am.* 56:371, 1972.
20. Hobbs, J. R. Immunocytoma o' mice an' man. *Br. Med. J.* 2:67, 1971.
21. Ritzmann, S. E., Alami, S. Y., Van Fossan, D. D., and MacKay, G. Electrophoresis, Immunoelectrophoresis, Quantitative Immunodiffusion and Thermoproteins. In G. J. Race (Ed.), *Laboratory Medicine.* New York: Harper & Row, 1973. Pp. 1–56.
22. Heremans, J. F. Gamma-1a-Globulin in Health and Disease. In S. E. Björkman (Ed.), *Gamma Globulins, Series Haematologica,* Vol. 4. Copenhagen: Munksgaard, 1965. Pp. 17–27.

23. Tomasi, T. B., Jr.   The gamma A globulins. First line of defense. *Hosp. Pract.* 2:26, 1967.
24. South, M. A., Cooper, M. D., Wollheim, F. A., and Good, R. A.   The IgA system. *Am. J. Med.* 44:168, 1968.
25. Ammann, A. J. and Hong, R.   Selective IgA deficiency. Presentation of 30 cases and a review of the literature. *Medicine* (Baltimore) 50:223, 1971.
26. Thompson, R. A., and Asquith, P.   Quantitation of exocrine IgA in human serum in health and disease. *Clin. Exp. Immunol.* 7:491, 1970.
27. Tomkin, G. H., Mawhinney, H., and Nevin, N. C.   Isolated absence of IgA with autosomal dominant inheritance. *Lancet* 2:124, 1971.
28. IgA-deficiency and coeliac disease (Editorial). *Lancet* 2:144, 1971.
29. Hobbs, J. R.   Immune imbalance in dysgammaglobulin type IV. *Lancet* 1:110, 1968.
30. Kaufman, H. S., and Hobbs, J. R.   Immunoglobulin deficiences in an atopic population. *Lancet* 2:1061, 1970.
31. Goldberg, L. S., Douglas, S. D., and Fudenberg, H. H.   Studies on salivary γA in agammaglobulinemia. *Clin. Exp. Immunol.* 4:579, 1969.
32. Good, R. A., and Choi, Y. S.   Relation of IgA and IgE to bodily defenses. *N. Engl. J. Med.* 284:552, 1971.
33. Heremans, J. F., and Crabbe, P. A.   IgA Deficiency: General Considerations and Relation to Human Diseases. In D. Bergsma and R. A. Good (Eds.), *Immunologic Deficiency Diseases in Man,* Vol. 4. (Birth Defects Original Article Series.) New York: The National Foundation for Birth Defects, 1968. Pp. 298–307.
34. Good, R. A., and Rodey, G. E.   IgA-deficiency, antigenic barrier and autoimmunity. *Cell. Immunol.* 1:147, 1970.
35. Case records of the Massachusetts General Hospital (case 1–1971). *N. Engl. J. Med.* 284:39, 1971.
36. Smith, J. B.   Alpha-fetoprotein: Occurrence in certain malignant diseases and review of clinical applications. *Med. Clin. North Am.* 54:797, 1970.
37. Dennehy, J. J.   Hereditary angioneurotic edema. Report of a large kindred with defect in C′1 esterase inhibitor and review of the literature. *Ann. Intern. Med.* 73:55, 1970.
38. Rosen, F. S., Alper, C. A., Pensky, J., Klemperer, M. R., and Donaldson, V. H.   Genetically determined heterogeneity of the C1 esterase inhibitor in patients with hereditary angioneurotic edema. *J. Clin. Invest.* 50:2143, 1971.
39. Blumberg, B.   Australia antigen. What it means to the hospital clinician. *Resident and Staff Physician,* Sept. 1972, pp. 66–84.
40. Sutnick, A. I., London, W. T., Millman, I., Coyne, V. E., and Blumberg, B. S.   Viral hepatitis. Revised concepts as a result of the study of Australia antigen. *Med. Clin. North Am.* 54:805, 1970.
41. Rowland, L. P., Fahn, S., Hirschberg, E., and Harter, D. H.   Myoglobinuria. *Arch. Neurol.* 10:537, 1964.
42. Kagen, L. J.   Immunofluorescent demonstration of myoglobin in the kidney. Case report and review of 43 cases of myoglobinemia and myoglobinuria identified immunologically. *Am. J. Med.* 48:649, 1970.
43. Adam, E. C., and Elliott, T. A.   Urinary myoglobin in myocardial infarction. *J.A.M.A.* 211:1013, 1970.
44. Agnello, V., Winchester, R. J., and Kunkel, H. G.   Precipitin reactions of the C1q component of complement with aggregated γ-globulin and immune complexes in gel diffusion. *Immunology* 19:909, 1970.

Radioimmunoassay

Harumi Kuno-Sakai, Robert M. Nakamura,
and Stephan E. Ritzmann

Radioimmunoassay (RIA) is a quantitative method that offers extreme sensitivity and specificity. It allows the quantitation of trace substances in biological fluids that cannot be assayed by other methods [1] (see Chaps. 11, 12). The principle of RIA (Fig. 6-1) [2, 3] is based upon the interactions of antibody with radiolabeled and unlabeled antigens. The extreme sensitivity (picogram range) of this technique is derived from the utilization of radiolabeled antigens and its specificity from that of specific antibodies. RIA requires three components: the unlabeled antigen (i.e., the substance to be assayed, such as IgE), a radiolabeled antigen (i.e., an antigen that is labeled with radioactive isotope, such as ^{125}I-IgE), and specific antibody (e.g., antibody against the substance to be assayed, such as anti-IgE antiserum).

The RIA procedure consists of five steps:

1. Mixing the three components (i.e., the unlabeled antigen, the radiolabeled antigen, and the specific antibody).
2. Incubation to allow completion of the antigen-antibody reaction.
3. Separation of the bound antigen (i.e., the unlabeled and the radiolabeled antigen bound to the antibody) from the free antigen (i.e., the unlabeled and the radiolabeled antigen not bound to the antibody).
4. Quantitation of the bound, radiolabeled antigen.
5. Calculation of the results.

Assuming that identical physicochemical properties exist for radiolabeled antigen (*Ag) and unlabeled antigen (Ag) and designating the ratio of bound *Ag to total *Ag as X, then the ratio of bound Ag to total Ag also becomes equal to X (see Fig. 6-1). This ratio, which can be determined by quantitating the bound radiolabeled antigen (*Ag) and the total radiolabeled antigen (total *Ag), decreases as the total concentration of antigen increases, if the concentrations of total *Ag and specific antibody are constant. An example is depicted in Figure 6-2.

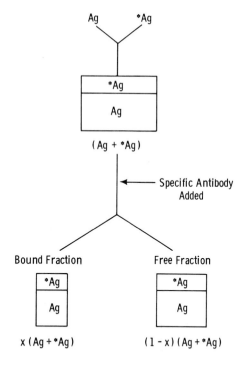

Figure 6-1
Principle of radioimmunoassay (RIA). *Ag:* Unlabeled antigen. **Ag:* Radiolabeled antigen. *X:* bound *Ag per total *Ag = bound Ag per total Ag.

Figure 6-3 depicts the dose-response curve (i.e., the standard curve) obtained from the three RIA standards illustrated in Figure 6-2. The amount of unlabeled antigen in a test sample is determined from such a standard curve. For example, if the amount of bound radiolabeled antigen is 2 (*ordinate*), the amount of unlabeled antigen will be 8 (*abscissa*).

Methodology

1. *Equipment and supplies.* A γ-counting system is used for the γ-emitting isotopes (e.g., ^{125}I), and a liquid scintillation counting system is used for β-emitting isotopes (e.g., ^{3}H). A wide range of RIA kits is commercially available [4].

2. *Technique.* The basic procedure (Fig. 6-4) consists of mixing the three main components (i.e., unlabeled antigen, radiolabeled antigen, and specific antibody), incubation, separation of free and bound antigens, radiation counting, and calculation of results.

3. *Analysis.* The amount of bound radiolabeled antigen in a test sample is compared with the standard curve, thereby obtaining the concentration of the antigen in the test sample.

4. *Sources of Error.* Errors may be caused by faulty sample preparation, such as the occurrence of hemolysis or fibrin clots, prolonged storage of samples or storage at inappropriate temperatures, and the presence of extraneous radioactivity (e.g., from diagnostic ^{125}I-uptake tests or contamination of the sample tube). Errors may also result from faulty

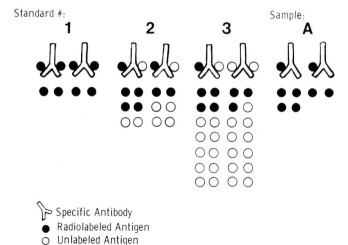

Standard #:

1   2   3   Sample: A

⋏ Specific Antibody
● Radiolabeled Antigen
○ Unlabeled Antigen

Figure 6-2
Principle of RIA. *Standard 1:* All antibody molecules are bound by the radiolabeled antigens in the absence of unlabeled antigen. *Standard 2:* Half of the antibody molecules are bound by the radiolabeled antigens in the presence of equal amounts of radiolabeled and unlabeled antigens. *Standard 3:* Only one-quarter of the antibody molecules are bound by radiolabeled antigens, because there are three times as many unlabeled antigens as radiolabeled antigens.

Figure 6-3
Standard curve obtained from the three RIA standards illustrated in Figure 6-2. (For explanation and details, see text.)

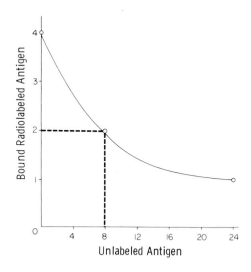

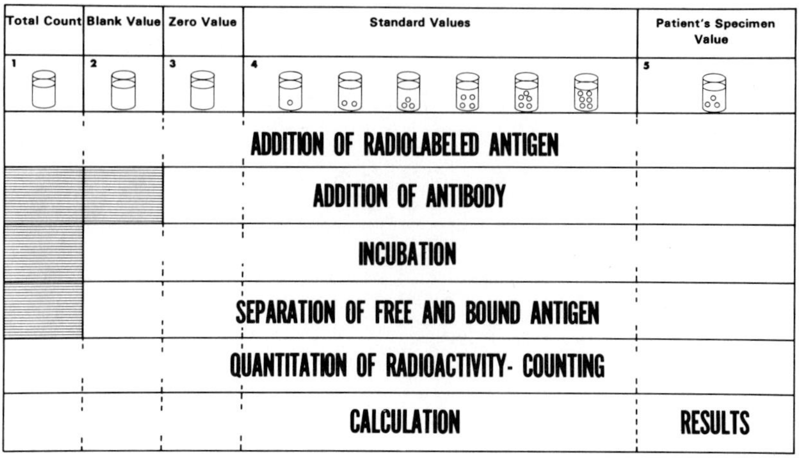

Total Count	Blank Value	Zero Value	Standard Values						Patient's Specimen Value
1	2	3	4						5
ADDITION OF RADIOLABELED ANTIGEN									
ADDITION OF ANTIBODY									
INCUBATION									
SEPARATION OF FREE AND BOUND ANTIGEN									
QUANTITATION OF RADIOACTIVITY- COUNTING									
CALCULATION									RESULTS

Figure 6-4
RIA procedure.

assay kits (i.e., degraded radiolabeled antigens, degraded standard antigens, or low antibody avidity) and faulty techniques (omitting reagents, careless dispensing of reagents, inadequate separation procedures, or extraneous radioactivity, for example from contaminated tubes or syringes).

Application and Interpretation

A large number of substances can be assayed by RIA, including the immunoglobulins IgG, IgA, IgM, IgD, and IgE; complement factors C3, C4, and $C\overline{1}$-INH; hormones; nonpeptide substances; and other larger and smaller molecular substances, including hepatitis-associated antigen (HB-Ag) and carcinoembryonic antigens (CEA) [1, 2, 4–7]. In general, any substance available in pure form to which specific antibodies can be produced is amenable to RIA. This includes low molecular weight substances that ordinarily are not antigenic (molecular weight of less than 1000) but which can be chemically conjugated as haptens to antigenic carrier proteins. Such an approach has led to the production of antibodies specific for steroid hormones, cardiac glycosides, morphine, and many other substances. Large hospitals with counting facilities for radiolabeled substances can perform RIA for the most important agents from a clinical standpoint (e.g., digoxin, digitoxin, renin, insulin, IgE, and HB-Ag). Small hospitals may have to rely upon neighboring large hospitals to perform these tests or upon dependable commercial laboratories.

RADIOIMMUNOLOGICAL TESTS FOR IgE
IgE possesses a molecular weight of 196,000 and a sedimentation coefficient of 8S [8, 9]. The IgE concentration in normal human serum is ex-

tremely low, approximately 1/40,000 that of IgG, and it is expressed in nanograms or international units per milliliter (see Chap. 4, p. 67; see also Fig. 6-7). RIA is therefore the method of choice for the quantitation of IgE. IgE contains reagenic antibodies, which are also known as anaphylactic, skin-sensitizing, atopic, allergic, or Prausnitz-Küstner antibodies. These are responsible for erythema or wheal skin reactions [10] and most anaphylactic reactions. The important role of IgE-mediated immune reactions requires specific diagnostic approaches. Prausnitz and Küstner [11, 12] first demonstrated that IgE-mediated allergy can be transferred passively by serum. However, this test, known as the Prausnitz-Küstner (PK) test, is dangerous and only of historical interest. Subsequently, skin tests were developed for testing IgE-mediated hypersensitivity. Such tests, however, are somewhat unreliable and are occasionally dangerous [13]. In vitro tests for IgE include RIA of total IgE and the radioallergosorbent techniques for specific IgE antibodies.

RIA for total IgE determines the total serum IgE by utilizing radiolabeled IgE and anti-IgE antibody. The radioallergosorbent test (RAST), which uses radiolabeled anti-IgE antibody and solid-phase antigen or allergen, allows the specific determination of specific IgE antibody to an antigen (e.g., penicillin or ragweed). It represents the in vitro analog of the in vivo skin test with specific antigens. When the inherent problems of sensitivity and complexity can be overcome, it may supplement or supplant the presently utilized in vivo skin tests.

Assays of total IgE

Two different RIA methods are available for assaying total IgE: double antibody radioimmunoassay and the radioimmunosorbent test (RIST).

The double antibody radioimmunoassay is the method that is most suitable for the determination of total serum IgE levels [14]. This method utilizes two kinds of antibodies; the first antibody is antibody that is directed against IgE and the second antibody is antibody 1, prepared in a different species 1, that is directed against the first antibody. Separation of bound IgE from free IgE can be performed by the collection of the precipitated complex of IgE-first antibody-second antibody. This procedure requires only minute quantities of purified IgE and specific antiserum against IgE, and it is exquisitely sensitive, being able to detect as little as 2 ng IgE per milliliter of serum.

The radioimmunosorbent test (RIST) [15] utilizes specific antibody to IgE which is coupled to Sephadex* particles. Therefore, the separation of bound IgE from free IgE can be performed easily by centrifugation. Problems exist with this method regarding reproducibility and sensitivity [14]. A RIST kit for total IgE levels is commercially available*. The procedure for the RIST is depicted in Figure 6-5.

There are several alternatives for the assay of IgE for laboratories that do not have access to γ- or β-radiation counters. The method of radioactive single radial diffusion (radio-radial immunodiffusion) described

* Pharmacia Laboratories, Inc., Piscataway, N.J. 08854.

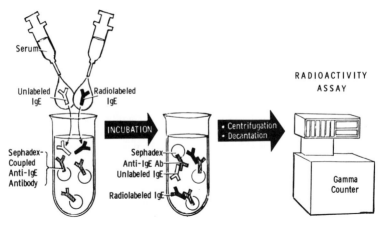

RADIOACTIVITY
ASSAY

Figure 6-5
Procedure for radioimmunosorbent test (RIST). (1) Radiolabeled IgE and serum sample containing unlabeled IgE are added to the suspension of Sephadex-coupled anti-IgE antibody; (2) during incubation, immune complexes of Sephadex-coupled antibody and IgE (unlabeled and radiolabeled) are formed; (3) these immune complexes are collected by centrifugation; and (4) the radioactivity of these immune complexes is assayed.

by Rowe [16] requires sheep anti-human IgE, ^{131}I-labeled rabbit γ-globulin containing antibody to the sheep immunoglobulin, and a reference preparation for IgE that is high in IgE content. Using this method, it is possible to detect IgE in concentrations as low as 40 ng per milliliter. A modification of this method was reported by Centifano and Kaufman [17] which employs fluorescein-labeled rabbit anti-sheep globulin.

Heiner and Rose [18] reported a Plexiglass micro-Ouchterlony technique. This method does not require radiolabeling. The lower limit of the detectable IgE concentration corresponds approximately with the upper limit of normal values. Therefore, this method is suitable for the assay of elevated levels of IgE.

RID plates for IgE quantitation are commercially available.*†

RADIOIMMUNOLOGICAL TEST FOR SPECIFIC IgE ANTIBODIES
(RADIOALLERGOSORBENT TEST; RAST)
The radioallergosorbent test [19] is an in vitro diagnostic test for IgE-mediated specific allergies. It quantitates the specific IgE antibodies to various antigens, such as pollens [20–22], certain drugs [23], animal dandruff [19, 24], house dust [19], and mites [20]. In vivo diagnostic tests for allergy (i.e., skin tests, passive transfer tests with the PK technique, and provocation tests) are potentially hazardous, somewhat unreliable, and, at the least, uncomfortable to the patient. In vitro tests, such

* Behring Diagnostics, Somerville, N.J. 08876.
† Hyland, Div. of Travenol Labs., Inc., Costa Mesa, Calif. 92626.

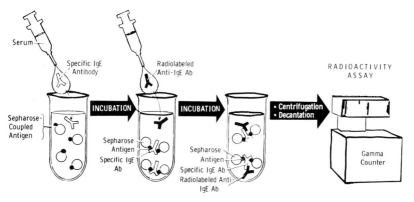

Figure 6-6

Procedure for radioallergosorbent test (RAST). (1) Serum containing specific IgE antibodies is added to the suspension of Sepharose-coupled antigen (e.g., ragweed, penicillin, etc.); (2) during the first incubation period, immune complexes of Sepharose-coupled antigen and specific IgE antibody are formed; (3) radiolabeled anti-IgE antibody is added; (4) during the second incubation period, immune complexes of Sepharose-coupled antigen-specific IgE antibody and radiolabeled anti-IgE antibodies are formed; (5) these immune complexes are collected by centrifugation; and (6) the radioactivity of the immune complexes is assayed.

as RAST, therefore provide a valuable addition to the diagnostic armamentarium.

The procedure for the RAST is depicted in Figure 6-6. RAST requires three components: the patient's serum containing specific IgE antibody, an antigen coupled to a solid matrix (e.g., Sepharose [Pharmacia Lab.] or filter paper disk), and the radiolabeled anti-IgE antibody. The RAST procedure consists of five steps: (1) incubation of the patient's serum with the antigen coupled to a solid matrix, (2) addition of the radiolabeled anti-IgE antibody followed by incubation, (3) washing out the unreacted radiolabeled anti-IgE antibody, (4) quantitation of the radioactivity of solid matrix, and (5) calculation of results.

Modifications of this basic method have been reported [25–29]. Significant correlations have been reported between RAST and various in vivo tests, such as the PK test [30], the provocation test [31], and the skin test [20, 32], as well as other in vitro tests (e.g., the chopped human lung test or CHLT [32]). The sensitivity of RAST is of the order of that of the outmoded PK test.

Sources of error include the lack of standardization of the antigens, since crude antigen extracts from different manufacturers or even from different lots from the same manufacturer vary greatly in their allergen concentrations. Currently, the allergen activity is assessed by skin tests using histamine as a standard [33], RIA of antigens [34], or RAST [35–41]. No diagnostic test kit for RAST is commercially available at this time.

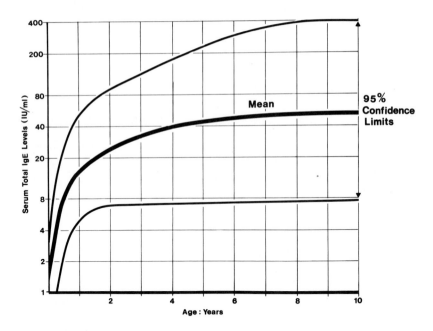

Figure 6-7
Age relationship of IgE serum levels. (Based on data from Foucard, T. *Acta Paediatr. Scand.* 63:129, 1974.)

CLINICAL IMPLICATIONS
Normal total serum IgE levels are age-dependent (Fig. 6-7). The mean IgE level of newborns is 3.2 ng per milliliter (1.6 IU per milliliter) [42, 43]. The level increases with age and reaches the adult level at about age 10 [43]. The mean IgE level of adults is approximately 140 to 300 ng per milliliter (70 to 150 IU per milliliter) [19, 44–48].

Decreased total IgE levels (Table 6-1) are seen in patients with certain primary and secondary forms of hypo- and agammaglobulinemia (i.e., antibody deficiency syndromes and dysgammaglobulinemias) [49]. It has been suggested that symptoms of IgE deficiency, either alone or in combination with IgA deficiency or ataxia-telangiectasia, may be related to the increased susceptibility to chronic sinopulmonary infections [50]. However, in patients with selective IgA deficiency there is a wide range of IgE levels, and a poor correlation exists between IgE levels and increased suspectibility to infections [51].

Increased total IgE levels (see Table 6-1) are characteristically found in patients with certain allergic disorders or parasitic infections. Two patients with idiopathic hyperimmunoglobulinemia-E had recurrent abscesses, growth retardation, coarse facies, chronic dermatitis, marked immediate hypersensitivity, eosinophilia, and depressed in vivo cellular immune reactions, but they were found to have normal serum levels of IgG, IgA, IgM, and IgD and intact antibody formation [52].

Table 6-1. IgE Levels in Various Disorders

Increased IgE Levels	Decreased IgE Levels

Atopic Diseases
  Bronchial asthma, extrinsic
  Hay fever
  Dermatitis
	Antibody deficiency syndromes
	
	Primary immune deficiencies:
	  Sex-linked agammaglobulinemia
	  Ataxia-telangiectasia

Parasitic infections
  Ascariasis
  Ankylostomiasis
  Visceral larva migrans
  Bilharziasis
  Trichinosis
  Capillariasis
	Combined IgA-IgE deficiency
	  Isolated IgE deficiency
	
	Secondary immune deficiencies:
	  Monoclonal gammopathies other
	  than IgE-myeloma (i.e., IgG,
	  IgA, IgM, and IgD monoclonal
	  gammopathies; L-chain and H-

Immune deficiency disorders
  Certain dysgammaglobulinemias
  Wiskott-Aldrich syndrome
  Hyperimmunoglobulinemia E
	chain diseases)

Monoclonal gammopathies IgE-myeloma	

In these disorders, the IgE increase is polyclonal in nature, whereas the IgE in patients with IgE myeloma is monoclonal. At least five patients with IgE monoclonal gammopathy have been described [53–55].

Increased levels of specific IgE antibodies have been reported in patients who are sensitive to ragweed [21, 22, 27, 30] or other pollens [20, 24], animal dandruff [19, 24], house dust [24], mites [20], penicillin [23], insulin [29], cod [32] or other fish [24], β-lactoglobulin and α-lactoalbumin [56], certain foods [26], snake venom [25], and others.

References

1. Radioimmunoassay (Special section). *Clin. Chem.* 19:145, 1973.
2. Berson, S. A., and Yalow, R. S. Radioimmunoassay: A Status Report. In R. A. Good and D. W. Fischer (Eds.), *Immunobiology.* Stamford, Conn.: Sinauer Associates, 1971. Pp. 287–293.
3. Ritzmann, S. E., Kuno-Sakai, H., Mattingly, D. F., and Daniels, J. C. Radioimmunoassays. In J. B. Fuller (Ed.), *ASCP Workshop Manual, Selected Topics in Clinical Chemistry* (3rd ed.). Chicago: American Society of Clinical Pathologists' Commission on Continuing Education, 1972. Pp. 207–233.
4. Kuno-Sakai, H., Mattingly, D. F., Gillum, R. L., Daniels, J. C., and Ritzmann, S. E. Radioimmunoassays (RIA). *ASCP Workshop Manual, Selected Topics in Clinical Chemistry* (4th ed.). Chicago: American Society of Clinical Pathologists' Commission on Continuing Education, 1973. Pp. 116–154.

5. Butler, V. P., Jr. Practical aspects of immunological assays. *Resident and Staff Physician*, Sept. 1972. Pp. 46–63.
6. Egan, M. L., Lautenschleger, J. T., Coligan, J. E., and Todd, C. W. Radioimmune assays of carcinoembryonic antigen. *Immunochemistry* 9:289, 1972.
7. A collaborative study of a test for carcinoembryonic antigen (CEA) in the sera of patients with carcinoma of the colon and rectum. *Can. Med. Assoc. J.* 107:25, 1972.
8. Bennich, H., and Johansson, S. G. O. Immunoglobulin E and immediate hypersensitivity. *Vox Sang.* 19:1, 1970.
9. Bennich, H., and Johansson, S. G. O. Studies on a New Class of Human Immunoglobulins. II. Chemical and Physical Properties. In J. Killander (Ed.), *Nobel Symposium 3, Gamma Globulins, Structure and Control of Biosynthesis.* Stockholm: Almqvist and Wiksell, 1967. P. 199.
10. Ishizaka, K., and Ishizaka, T. Human reagenic antibodies and immunoglobulin E. *J. Allergy* 42:330, 1968.
11. Prausnitz, C., and Küstner, H. Studien über die Uberempfindlichkeit. *Zentralbl. Bakteriol.* 86:160, 1921.
12. Sehon, A. H., and Gyenes, L. Antibodies in Atopic Patients and Antibodies Developed During Treatment. In M. Samter (Ed.), *Immunological Diseases* (2nd ed.). Boston: Little, Brown, 1971.
13. Vanarsdel, P. P., Jr. Identification of Causative Allergens in Allergic Diseases. In M. Samter (Ed.), *Immunological Diseases* (2nd ed.). Boston: Little, Brown, 1971.
14. Polmer, S. H., Waldmann, T. A., and Terry, W. D. A comparison of three radioimmunoassay techniques for the measurement of serum IgE. *J. Immunol.* 110:1253, 1973.
15. Wide, L. Radioimmunoassays employing immunosorbents. *Acta Endocrinol. [Suppl.]* (Kbh.) 142:207, 1970.
16. Rowe, D. S., and Wood, C. B. S. The measurement of serum immunoglobulin E levels in healthy adults and children and in children with allergic asthma. *Int. Arch. Allergy Appl. Immunol.* 39:1, 1970.
17. Centifano, Y. M., and Kaufman, H. E. A simplified method for measuring human IgE. *J. Immunol.* 107:608, 1971.
18. Heiner, D. C., and Rose, B. Elevated levels of IgE in conditions other than classical allergy. *J. Allergy* 45:30, 1970.
19. Johansson, S. G. O., Bennich, H. H., and Berg, T. The clinical significance of IgE. *Prog. Clin. Immunol.* 1:157, 1972.
20. Stenius, B., Wide, L., Seymour, W. M., Holford-Strevens, V., and Pepys, J. Clinical significance of specific IgE to common allergens. *Clin. Allergy* 1:37, 1971.
21. Lichtenstein, L. M., Ishizaka, K., Norman, P. S., Sobotka, A. K., and Hill, B. M. IgE antibody measurements in ragweed hay fever. *J. Clin. Invest.* 52:472, 1973.
22. Yunginger, J. W., and Gleich, G. J. Seasonal changes in IgE antibodies and their relationship to IgG antibodies during immunotherapy for ragweed hay fever. *J. Clin. Invest.* 52:1268, 1973.
23. Wide, L., and Lennart, J. Detection of penicillin allergy of the immediate type by radioimmunoassay of reagins (IgE) to penicilloyl conjugates. *Clin. Allergy* 1:171, 1971.
24. Aas, K., and Johansson, S. G. O. The radioallergosorbent test in the in vitro diagnosis of multiple reaginic allergy. *J. Allergy Clin. Immunol.* 48:134, 1971.
25. Kelly, J. F., and Patterson, R. Allergy to snake venom. The use of

radioimmunoassay for the detection of IgE antibodies against antigens not suitable for cutaneous tests. *Clin. Allergy* 3:385, 1973.

26. Galant, S. P., Bullock, J., and Frick, O. L.   An immunological approach to the diagnosis of food sensitivity. *Clin. Allergy* 3:363, 1973.

27. Zeiss, R. C., Pruzanski, J. J., Patterson, R., and Roberts, M.   A solid phase radioimmunoassay for quantitation of human reaginic antibody against ragweed antigen E. *J. Immunol.* 110:414, 1973.

28. Sarsfield, J. K., and Gowland, G.   A modified radioallergosorbent test for the in vitro detection of allergen antibodies. *Clin. Exp. Immunol.* 13:619, 1973.

29. Patterson, R., Mellies, C. J., and Roberts, M.   Immunologic reactions against insulin. *J. Immunol.* 110:1135, 1973.

30. Evans, R., Colonel, L., Reisman, R. E., Wypych, J. I., and Arbesman, C. E.   An immunologic evaluation of ragweed sensitive patients by newer techniques. *J. Allergy Clin. Immunol.* 49:285, 1972.

31. Berg, T., Bennich, H., and Johansson, S. G. O.   In vitro diagnosis of atopic allergy. *Int. Arch. Allergy Appl. Immunol.* 40:770, 1971.

32. Foucard, T., Aas, K., and Johansson, S. G. O.   Concentration of IgE antibodies, PK titers, and chopped lung titers in sera from children with hypersensitivity to cod. *J. Allergy Clin. Immunol.* 51:39, 1973.

33. Aas, K., and Belin, L.   Standardization of diagnostic work in allergy. *Int. Arch. Allergy Appl. Immunol.* 45:57, 1973.

34. Yunginger, J. W., and Gleich, G. J.   Measurement of ragweed antigen E by double antibody radioimmunoassay. *J. Allergy Clin. Immunol.* 50:326, 1972.

35. Foucard, T., Johansson, S. G. O., Bennich, H., and Berg, T.   In vitro estimation of allergens by a radioimmune antiglobulin technique using human IgE antibodies. *Int. Arch. Allergy Appl. Immunol.* 43:360, 1972.

36. Cesca, M.   Column chromatography of allergens and assessment of their activities by the paper disc radioallergosorbent method. *Int. Arch. Allergy Appl. Immunol.* 45:405, 1973.

37. Aronsson, T., and Wide, L.   The radioallergosorbent test used for characterization of allergenic extracts. *Int. Arch. Allergy Appl. Immunol.* 45:50, 1973.

38. Johansson, S. G. O., Bennich, H., and Foucard, T.   Quantitation of IgE antibodies and allergens by the radioallergosorbent test, RAST. *Int. Arch. Allergy Appl. Immunol.* 45:55, 1973.

39. Ceska, M., Eriksson, R., and Varga, J. M.   Radioimmunosorbent assay of allergens. *J. Allergy Clin. Immunol.* 49:1, 1972.

40. Varga, J. M., and Ceska, M.   Characterization of allergen extracts by gel isoelectrofocusing and radioimmunosorbent allergen assay. *J. Allergy Clin. Immunol.* 49:274, 1972.

41. Ceska, M., and Brandt, R.   Ultracentrifugation patterns of allergens in sucrose gradients and assessment of their activities by the paper disc radioallergosorbent method. *Int. Arch. Allergy Appl. Immunol.* 45:808, 1973.

42. Bulletin: Measurements of concentrations of human serum immunoglobulins. *J. Immunol.* 107:1798, 1971.

43. Foucard, T. A.   Follow-up study of children with asthmatoid bronchitis. *Acta Paediatr. Scand.* 63:129, 1974.

44. Gleich, G. J., Averbeck, A. K., and Swedlung, H. A.   Measurement of IgE in normal and allergic serum by radioimmunoassay. *J. Lab. Clin. Med.* 77:690, 1971.

45. Smith, H. J., Ozkaragoz, K., and Gocken, M.   A simplified radioim-

munoassay technique for measuring human IgE. *J. Allergy Clin. Immunol.* 50:193, 1972.

46. Bazaral, M., Orgel, H. A., and Hamburger, R. N. IgE levels in normal infants and mothers and an inheritance hypothesis. *J. Immunol.* 107:794, 1971.

47. Leonardy, J. G., and Peacock, L. B. An evaluation of quantitative serum immunoglobulin determinations in clinical practice. *Ann. Allergy* 30:378, 1972.

48. Warren, C. P. W., and Tse, K. S. Serum and sputum immunoglobulin E levels in respiratory disease in adults. *Can. Med. Assoc. J.* 110:425, 1974.

49. Hong, R., Ammann, A. J., Cain, W. A., and Good, R. A. Immunoglobulin E. *Am. J. Med. Sci.* 259:1, 1970.

50. Ammann, J. R., and Hong, R. Recurrent sinopulmonary infections, mental retardation and combined IgA and IgE deficiency. *J. Pediatr.* 77:802, 1970.

51. Stites, D. P., Ishizaka, K., and Fudenberg, H. H. Serum IgE concentrations in hypogammaglobulinemia and selective IgA deficiency. *Clin. Exp. Immunol.* 10:391, 1972.

52. Buckley, R. H., Wray, B. B., and Belmaker, E. Z. Extreme hyperimmunoglobulinemia E and undue susceptibility to infection. *Pediatrics* 49:59, 1972.

53. Johansson, S. G. O., and Bennich, H. Immunological studies of an atypical (myeloma) immunoglobulin. *Immunology* 13:381, 1967.

54. Ogawa, M., Kochwa, S., Smith, C., Ishizaka, K., and McIntyre, O. R. Clinical aspects of IgE myeloma. *N. Engl. J. Med.* 281:1217, 1969.

55. Fishkin, B. G., Orloff, N., Scaduto, L. E., Brouchi, D. T., and Spiegelberg, H. L. IgE multiple myeloma. A report of the third case. *Blood* 39:361, 1972.

56. Freier, S., and Berger, H. Disodium cromoglycate in gastrointestinal protein intolerance. *Lancet* 1:913, 1973.

Analytical Ultracentrifugation

Stephan E. Ritzmann and Robert M. Nakamura

Ultracentrifugation was introduced by Svedberg in 1924 [1], and it has subsequently been applied to the study of normal [2, 3] and abnormal [4] human sera. Ultracentrifugation involves the application of high centrifugal forces to effect the separation or redistribution of solutes and solvents. Ultracentrifugation methods may be either preparative or analytical. The former is mainly a quantitative method in which the contents of the tubes are analyzed after centrifugation, and the latter is chiefly a qualitative method in which the protein distribution is observed during the ultracentrifugal run.

Several major ultracentrifugation methods are used to exploit the differences in size, shape, mass, or density of molecules or particles in a solution [5]. These include methods involving moving-boundary, moving-zone, isodensity, or sedimentation equilibria.

The moving-boundary method is the most frequently used ultracentrifugation technique; it is identical in practice with pelleting or conventional analytical ultracentrifugation. The solute (e.g., serum protein) originally is distributed uniformly throughout the sample tube (t_0 in Fig. 7-1). During ultracentrifugation, transport of the solute occurs within the solvent. Depending upon the relative densities of solute and solvent, the direction of the transport may be to the bottom of the tube (sedimentation) or to the top of the tube (flotation). Most ultracentrifugation assays are concerned with the sedimentation method, such as the differential sedimentation of proteins with different molecular weights (e.g., the separation of 7S IgG from 19S IgM). The flotation method is most useful for the separation of serum lipoproteins. As centrifugation and transport proceed, boundaries develop between adjacent plateaus (tubes t_1 and t_2 in Fig. 7-1). After completion of the centrifugation run, pelleting of the solute results (tube t_∞ in Fig. 7-1). Since differences in the indices of refraction occur between the boundaries, an ingeniously designed optical transmission system employing Schlieren optics allows the translation of the boundaries into curve patterns according to Figure 7-1.

The Svedberg (S) or sedimentation coefficient provides a common unit of measure for the behavior of proteins in the centrifugal field. Nu-

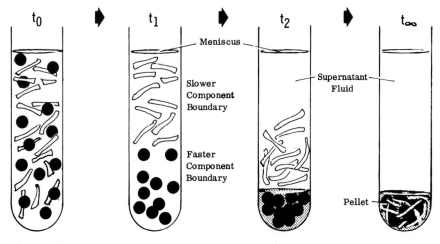

Figure 7-1
Moving-boundary ultracentrifugation. Circles represent protein particles that
are faster (i.e., larger or more symmetrical) but less dense than the protein
particles marked as rods. t_0 = initial loading; t_1, t_2 = two successive time
periods during ultracentrifugation; t_∞ = equilibrium. (Modified from Trautman, R., and Cowan, K. M. In C. A. Williams and M. W. Chase (Eds.),
*Methods in Immunology and Immunochemistry, Physical and Chemical
Methods,* Vol. 2. New York: Academic, 1968, Pp. 81–118.)

merous factors influence the sedimentation rates, including the molecular size, shape, and mass; the centrifugal force; the density of the solution; the specific volume; the temperature; and so on. The S coefficient
is computed from an observed, terminal velocity that is divided by the
strength of the centrifugal field. The practical S unit is equal to 10^{-13} second. S values are usually converted to standard conditions of infinite dilution in water at 20°C and are denoted as $S_{20,w}^{0}$ constants.

Methodology

1. *Equipment.* The most frequently used analytical ultracentrifuge is
the Spinco Model E.* This instrument allows the sedimentation of serum
proteins in a gravitational field generated by 60,000 or more revolutions
per minute of the rotor. Complete separation of the three major serum
protein fractions (4.5S, 7S, and 19S) is achieved within two hours. Several types of rotors and cells are available.

2. *Technique.* Approximately 0.2 ml of serum is diluted 1:5 with
0.9 percent NaCl or with appropriate buffers. Approximately 0.8 ml of
the serum dilution is inserted into the analytical cell, which is then placed
in the rotor. During the run, photographic recordings are obtained at
various intervals.

* Beckman Instruments, Fullerton, Calif. 92634.

3. *Analysis*. The complete separation sequence of the serum proteins can be monitored visually and photographically (see Fig. 7-2). From the photographic record, the quantity of the various fractions and their sedimentation characteristics can be derived. The S coefficients are determined by measuring the distances between a boundary in the sample cell and the axis of rotation at a given time, taking into account the magnification of the camera lens and other factors [6–10].

In normal human serum, there are three major components demonstrable by ultracentrifugation (see Fig. 7-2*A*): (1) *4.5S component,* which is also termed the *A component* because of its albumin content (it is quantitatively the major serum protein fraction); (2) *7S component,* also termed the *G component* because of its globulin content, including IgG, IgA, and IgD; and (3) *19S component,* which is also termed the *M component* because it contains the macroglobulins IgM and α_2M. (M component in this context should not be confused with the M proteins associated with monoclonal gammopathies or the M protein of certain β-hemolytic streptococci.) The 19S fraction is quantitatively a minor fraction.

NORMAL CONCENTRATIONS OF 4.5S, 7S, AND 19S COMPONENTS
The absolute concentrations of these fractions can be determined by planimetry of enlarged photographic prints and correlation with the percentage values of total serum protein levels. In 40 healthy adults, the following normal ranges (grams per 100 ml $\pm$ 2 SD) have been found in our laboratories:

4.5S Components	5.4–6.9
7S Components	0.6–1.2
19S Components	0.12–0.44

The ultracentrifugally determined normal values appear to remain constant, at least throughout the age groups between 30 and 70 years [11].

The mode of reporting S values varies greatly in the literature, which leads to difficulties in comparing the values obtained in various laboratories. They may be expressed as:

1. S_{20} coefficients, i.e., S values obtained at 20°C;
2. $S_{20, w}$ coefficients, i.e., S values obtained at 20°C but corrected for water as diluent;
3. $S_{20, w}^{0/0}$ coefficients, i.e., rates obtained at 20°C, corrected for water as diluent, and based on certain protein concentrations (indicated in superscript); or
4. $S_{20, w}^{0}$ constants, i.e., S values obtained at 20°C, corrected for water as diluent, and either calculated or extrapolated to zero protein concentration. In this expression, the fact that S rates depend partly upon the protein concentration is taken into consideration; the lower the

Figure 7-2

Synopsis of normal and abnormal serum and urine ultracentrifugal patterns. All serum samples have been ultracentrifuged in 1:5 dilutions with buffered phosphate solution at 60,000 rpm and 20°C for 120 minutes. The urine sample was analyzed undiluted.

A. Normal serum protein pattern. Pictures were taken sequentially at 12, 20, 30, 60, 90 and 120 minutes. The separation of the three main components proceeds from left to right: 19S M-component, containing mainly α_2-macroglobulin and IgM; 7S G-component, containing IgG, IgA, and IgD; and 4.5S A-component, containing mainly albumin.

B. Synopsis of normal and various abnormal ultracentrifugal serum and urine protein patterns. (*1*) Normal serum protein pattern depicting the 19S component (*left pattern, right peak*) and the 4.5S and 7S components (*right pattern, left two peaks*) (*2*) Agammaglobulinemia. The 19S component is usually discernible due to its normal α_2M-globulin contents; the 7S component is absent. (*3*) Polyclonal gammopathy. Both the 19S and 7S component are increased as a reflection of increased concentrations of IgM; and IgG, IgA (and IgD). (*4*) IgG monoclonal gammopathy. The 19S component is decreased but the 7S component is increased. (*5*) IgA monoclonal gammopathy. This form of MG is variously characterized by a selective increase of 7S; or the additional occurrence of 1, 2, 3, 4 or, rarely, 5 intermediate fractions reflecting dimers (9S), trimers (11S), tetramers (13S), pentamers (15S), or hexamers (17S) of IgA. Although the 7S or the 9S component or both are usually the principle fractions, any one of the other fractions may be predominant. (*6*) IgM monoclonal gammopathy. The 19S component is increased and peaked in appearance, and is usually accompanied by additional, larger macromolecular components of approximately 22S, 26S and 32S. (*7*) Light-chain disease (Bence Jones monoclonal gammopathy) in urine. A 3.6S component is visible in urine corresponding to a dimeric moiety of free light chains. The serum in this patient resembled that of marked hypogamma-globulinemia with reduced 7S and 19S components. (*8*) Nephrotic syndrome. The electrophoretic hyperalpha-2-globulinemia due to increased α_2M-globulin that is characteristic for nephrotic syndrome, is reflected by an increased 19S component (in contrast to IgM MG, there are no higher molecular components). The electrophoretic hypogammaglobulinemia and hypoalbuminemia are demonstrated on ultracentrifugation, by decreased 7S and 4.5S components.

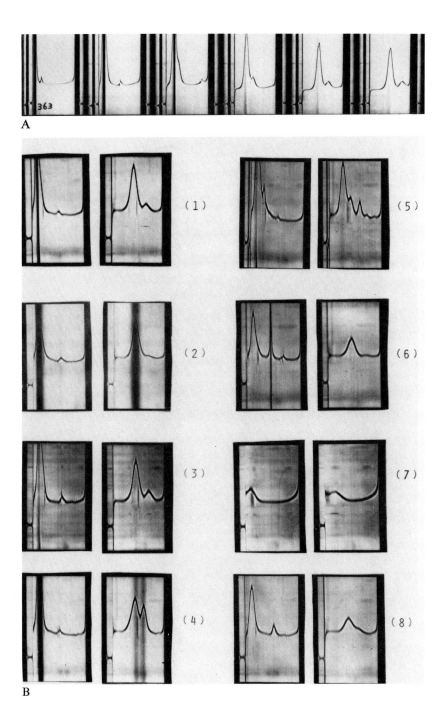

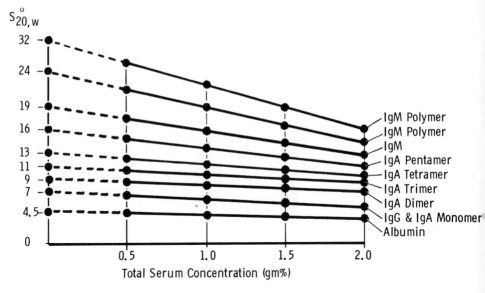

Figure 7-3
Diagrammatic presentation of the relationship between M-protein concentrations (*abscissa*) and the $S_{20,\,w}^{0/0}$ coefficients and the $S_{20,\,w}^{0}$ constants obtained by extrapolation to zero protein concentration (- - - -).

protein concentration, the higher the sedimentation rate (see Fig. 7-3).

SEDIMENTATION COEFFICIENTS OF M PROTEINS

S values calculated from the extrapolation of data obtained from a single ultracentrifugation run may be misleading, since the dependence of the S value upon protein concentration may result in slopes that differ from one M protein to another, even within the same immunoglobulin class. This significant degree of dependence of the S coefficients upon protein concentrations is influenced by several factors [8], including the molecular weight of the protein, viscosity of the solution, complex formation, the density of the solution, and others [10, 12]. The precise evaluation of $S_{20,\,w}^{0}$ constants of M proteins requires the ultracentrifugation of serum at various dilutions, or, preferably, at several dilutions of the purified proteins, with subsequent extrapolation to zero protein concentrations (Fig. 7-3).

Application and Interpretation

During recent years, newer techniques have relegated analytical ultracentrifugation to an adjunct role for the deciphering of difficult clinical problems rather than routine use. Its most useful application is in the differential diagnosis of monoclonal gammopathies (MG) and certain immune complex disorders.

MONOCLONAL GAMMOPATHIES

The characteristic ultracentrifugation patterns found in MG are depicted in Figures 7-2 and 7-4. The ultracentrifugal sedimentation patterns of the various MGs reveal the following patterns:

1. *IgG MG* [8, 13–15]: Slightly to considerably increased and peaked 7S components but decreased 19S components.

2. *IgA MG* [8, 14–17]: Slightly to considerably increased and peaked 7S components that are usually accompanied by the presence of one or more peaked intermediate components (9S dimer, 11S trimer, 13S tetramer, 15S pentamer, or 17S hexamer) and often decreased 19S components.

3. *IgM MG* [8, 14–16, 18, 19]: Slightly to considerably increased and peaked 19S components that are usually associated with the presence of one or more macromolecular peaked components (22S to 24S or 32S) and often decreased 7S components. The $S_{20, w}^0$ constants for the monoclonal IgM components are approximately 19S [8, 15], yet the reported S values in the literature are extremely diverse, ranging from 12S to more than 22S [8]. This is mainly due to calculation rather than actual determination of the S constants at infinite serum protein concentration. In certain patients with IgM MG, the 7S component may be increased due to low molecular weight 7S monoclonal IgM [20].

In the nephrotic syndrome (see Fig. 7-2), there is usually an increased 19S component without the presence of additional higher molecular weight fractions. The increase of the 19S component in this disorder is due to the selective increase of α_2-macroglobulin [21].

4. *IgD MG* [13, 22]: Slightly to considerably increased 7S component but decreased 19S fraction.

5. *IgE MG* [23]: Increased 8S component.

6. *Light-chain disease* [8, 15]: Decreased 7S and 19S components. Occasionally, a skewing "shoulder" configuration of 4.5S component occurs toward the low molecular weight side due to Bence Jones proteins (3.2S to 3.8S) that partially overlap the 4.5S component. Samples from urine often show a single component.

7. *Heavy-chain disease* (γ, α, *or* μ *chains*) [24–29]: Serum patterns often characterized by decreased 7S and 19S components. Urine contains low molecular weight components (3S to 4S).

8. *Low molecular weight IgM MG* [20, 30]: Increased 7S component but decreased 19S fraction.

HYPO- OR AGAMMAGLOBULINEMIA

The various forms of immunoglobulin deficiencies (see Chap. 19) are associated with a variety of ultracentrifugal patterns, depending upon the immunoglobulin classes affected. The classic agammaglobulinemia with deficiency of IgG, IgA, and IgM is reflected in ultracentrifugation studies by a deficiency of both 7S and 19S components (see Fig. 7-2).

POLYCLONAL GAMMOPATHIES

In sera from patients with polyclonal gammopathies (PG), there is usually an increase of both 7S and 19S components (see Fig. 7-2). The in-

Figure 7-4

Ultracentrifugal patterns of monoclonal gammopathies. *A.* Abnormal ultracentrifugal patterns of sera containing M proteins correlated with immunoelectric patterns. (Reproduced by permission. From Levin, W. C., and Ritzmann, S. E. In C. E. Mengel, E. Frei, III, and R. Nachman (Eds.), *Hematology: Principles and Practice.* Chicago: Year Book, 1972. Pp. 544–567.)

B. Ultracentrifugal sedimentation patterns of three variants of each of the three main monoclonal gammopathy categories: (*a*) IgG MG. *Top:* Slightly increased 7S component. *Center:* Moderate increase of 7S component. *Bottom:* Greatly increased peaked 7S component. Decreased 19S component. (*b*) IgA MG. *Top:* Increased peaked 7S component as sole abnormality. *Center:* Slightly increased 7S component, presence of one large intermediate (11S) component. *Bottom:* Increased, peaked 7S component; presence of large 9S, moderate 11S, small 13S, and minute 15S components. Decreased 19S component. (*c*) IgM MG. *Top:* Increased 19S M_1 and small, heavier M_2 components. *Center:* Large, peaked 19S M_1 and heavier M_2 components. *Bottom:* Small M_1' (17.8 $S_{20,w}^0$ component), large 19S M_1, moderate M_2 (24–26S), and small M_3 (approximately 32S) components. Decreased 7S component. (Reproduced by permission. From Ritzmann, S. E., and Levin, W. C. In H. Dettelbach and S. E. Ritzmann (Eds.), *Lab Synopsis,* Vol. 2 (2nd ed.). Somerville, N.J.: Behring Diagnostics, 1969. Pp. 9–50.)

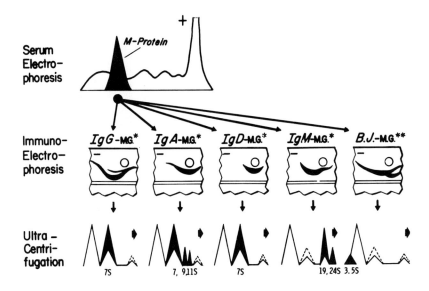

* Monoclonal Gammopathy
** Bence Jones Monoclonal Gammopathy

A

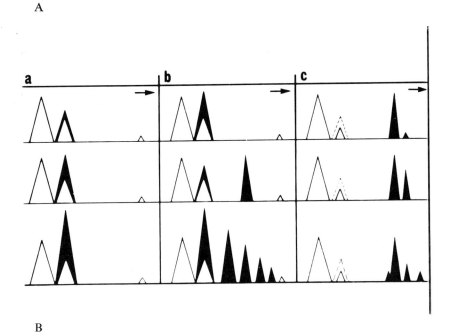

B

Figure 7-5
Top: Ultracentrifugal pattern of immune complexes of the macromolecular variety (greater than 19S) associated with IgM monoclonal gammopathy and high rheumatoid-factor activity. *Bottom:* After reduction with 0.1 molar 6-mercaptoethanol, the peak of macromolecular immune complexes have disappeared concomitantly with an increase of the 7S component (sedimentation from left to right).

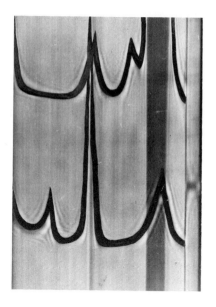

crease in the 7S component is due to an elevation of IgG mainly and of IgA partly, whereas the increase in the 19S component is due to elevated IgM levels. Such ultracentrifugation patterns are mostly encountered in patients with chronic liver diseases, collagen disorders, chronic infections, and others. The increase of both 7S and 19S components may be profound [31], or the 7S component may be almost exclusively increased, as, for example, in patients with active chronic hepatitis. In other patients, the 19S component may be preferentially elevated, such as in certain patients with liver cirrhosis [8], congenital syphilis [32], kala-azar [33], toxoplasmosis [34], leishmaniasis and trypanosomiasis [5], and others. This last pattern of a selective polyclonal increase of 19S IgM has been referred to as *symptomatic* or *secondary* macroglobulinemia [8, 33] in contrast to *primary, idiopathic,* or *essential* Waldenström's macroglobulinemia [4], which is associated with a monoclonal increase of 19S IgM (see Chap. 19).

IMMUNE-COMPLEX DISORDERS
The value of ultracentrifugation analysis of sera from patients with such disorders lies in its diagnostic and differential diagnostic potential (see also Chaps. 9 and 20).

MONOCLONAL GAMMOPATHIES
In a certain number of patients with IgM and IgA MG, the IgA or IgM M proteins do not sufficiently penetrate agar or agarose to allow a precise characterization of this protein by immunodiffusion assays (e.g., radial immunodiffusion or immunoelectrophoresis). Some of these immunoglobulins are associated with a high activity of monoclonal rheu-

Figure 7-6
Pattern of intermediate (7S to 19S) and macromolecular (greater than 19S) immune complexes in the serum of a patient with rheumatoid arthritis. *Top:* After treatment with 6 molar urea, the pattern of immune complexes has disappeared; 6-mercaptoethanol had no effect on these immune complexes. *Bottom:* Untreated serum showing peaks representing intermediate and macromolecular immune complexes (sedimentation from left to right).

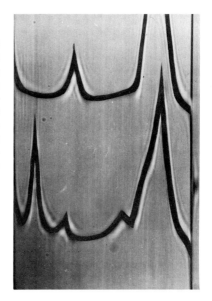

matoid factor, cryoglobulin properties, or both. Under such circumstances, the depolymerization of these proteins with mercaptans [35, 36] usually allows their immunoelectrophoretic analysis. Alternatively, ultracentrifugation assay of the untreated serum offers a direct diagnostic approach (Fig. 7-5).

POLYCLONAL GAMMOPATHIES
Problems in the differential diagnosis of IgM MG may arise if the increased 19S is accompanied by the occurrence of 22S to 24S components. Sera from patients with high rheumatoid factor activity often reveal such soluble 22S complexes [37, 38] (Fig. 7-6). Differential diagnostic difficulties also occur with IgA MG, especially those that exhibit intermediate IgA polymers (Figs. 7-2, 7-4). High rheumatoid factor activity that is associated with immune complexes intermediate between the 7S and 19S components [36, 39], macromolecular complexes (greater than 19S), or both are observed in patients with rheumatoid arthritis and nonthrombocytopenic purpura [36, 39, 40, 41], Felty's syndrome, and bizarre collagen or autoimmune disorders, some of which may be mistaken for chronic lymphocytic leukemia or Waldenström's macroglobulinemia [42–45] (see Fig. 7-6).

Both the intermediate and macromolecular immune complexes of this type can be dissociated to 7S moieties by treatment with 6 molar urea [36] or acid buffers [36, 46], but treatment with mercaptans has no significant effect. In distinct contrast, the intermediate IgA and macromolecular IgM components associated with IgA and IgM MG are usually not affected by 6 molar urea or acid buffers, but they are dissociated by mercaptans [17, 35, 36, 47, 48] (see Fig. 7-5).

References

1. Svedberg, T., and Rinde, H.   The ultracentrifuge, a new instrument for the determination of size and distribution of size particle in amicroscopic colloids. *J. Am. Chem. Soc.* 46:2677, 1924.
2. Von Mutzenbecher, P.   Untersuchung der bei Serumelektrodialyse auftretenden Eiweissfraktion mit der Ultrazentrifuge. *Biochem. Z.* 235:425, 1931.
3. Von Mutzenbecher, P.   Die Analyse des Serums mit der Ultrazentrifuge. *Biochem. Z.* 266:226, 1933.
4. Waldenström, J.   Incipient myelomatosis or essential hyperglobulinemia and fibrinogenopenia—a new syndrome? *Acta Med. Scand.* 117:216, 1944.
5. Trautman, R., and Cowan, K. M.   Preparative and Analytical Ultracentrifugation. In C. A. Williams and M. W. Chase (Eds.), *Methods in Immunology and Immunochemistry,* Vol. 2. New York: Academic, 1968. Pp. 81–118.
6. Resnik, R. A.   Ultracentrifugation of the Serum Proteins. In F. W. Sunderman and F. W. Sunderman, Jr. (Eds.), *Serum Proteins and the Dysproteinemias.* Philadelphia: Lippincott, 1964. Pp. 136–147.
7. Schachman, H. K.   *Ultracentrifugation in Biochemistry.* New York: Academic, 1959.
8. Jahnke, K., and Scholtan, W.   *Die Bluteiweisskörper in der Ultrazentrifuge, Sedimentation-Flotation.* Stuttgart: Thieme, 1960.
9. Svedberg, T., and Pedersen, K. O.   *The Ultracentrifuge.* Oxford: Clarendon, 1940.
10. Schultze, H. E., and Heremans, J. F.   *Molecular Biology of Human Proteins,* Vol. 1. New York: Elsevier, 1966.
11. Böttiger, L. E., Carlson, L. A., and Hedman, S.   Ultracentrifugal plasma protein pattern and age in healthy men. *Acta Med. Scand.* [*Suppl.*] 445: 93, 1966.
12. Laurell, H.   Präparative Verfahren and Sedimentations-Analytik. In C. Steffin (Ed.), *Methods of Immunohaematologic Research.* Bibliotheca Haematologica. Basel: Karger, 1963. P. 180.
13. Hanson, U. B., Laurell, C. B., and Bachmann, R.   Sedimentation constants of IgG and IgD myeloma proteins compared with those of normal IgG. *Acta Med. Scand.* [*Suppl.*] 445:89, 1966.
14. Laurell, A. H. F.   Sera from patients with myeloma, macroglobulinemia, and related conditions as studied by ultracentrifugation. *Acta Med. Scand.* 170 [Suppl. 367]:69, 1961.
15. Heremans, J.   Proteins in Myeloma and Macroglobulinaemia. In C. Steffin (Ed.), *Methods of Immunohaematologic Research.* Bibliotheca Haematologica. Basel: Karger, 1963. P. 139.
16. Fessel, W. J.   Clinical analysis of 142 cases with high molecular weight serum proteins. *Acta Med. Scand.* 173 [Suppl. 391]:1, 1962.
17. Levin, W. C., Ritzmann, S. E., Seuwen, J. P., and Nanninga, L.   Some properties of β_2A-myeloma proteins. *Clin. Chim. Acta* 10:12, 1964.
18. Imhof, J. W., Ballieux, R. E., and Mijinieff, P. F.   Ultracentrifuge investigation of the serum proteins in Waldenström's macroglobulinemia. *Clin. Chim. Acta* 5:801, 1960.
19. Ratcliff, P., Soothill, J. F., and Stanworth, D. R.   Physicochemical and immunological studies of pathological serum macroglobulinemias. *Clin. Chim. Acta* 8:91, 1963.

20. Busch, S. T., Sewedelund, H. A., and Gleich, G. J. Low molecular weight IgM in human sera. *J. Lab. Clin. Med.* 73:194, 1969.
21. Eriksen, N. Serum macroglobulin levels in relation to age, sex and disease. *J. Lab. Clin. Invest.* 51:521, 1958.
22. Rowe, D. S., and Fahey, J. L. A new class of human immunoglobulins. I. A unique myeloma protein. *J. Exp. Med.* 121:171, 1965.
23. Bennich, H., and Johansson, S. G. O. Immunoglobulin E and immediate hypersensitivity. *Vox Sang.* 19:1, 1970.
24. Franklin, E. C., Lowenstein, J., Bigelow, B., and Meltzer, M. Heavy chain disease—A new disorder of serum γ-globulins. Report of the first case. *Am. J. Med.* 37:332, 1964.
25. Osserman, E. F., and Takatsuki, K. Clinical and immunochemical studies of four cases of heavy (H γ_2) chain disease. *Am. J. Med.* 37: 351, 1964.
26. Ellman, L. L., and Block, K. J. Heavy-chain disease. Report of a seventh case. *N. Engl. J. Med.* 278:1195, 1968.
27. Zawadzki, Z. A., Baucdek, T. G., Ein, D., and Easton, J. M. Rheumatoid arthritis terminating in heavy chain disease. *Ann. Intern. Med.* 70: 335, 1969.
28. Seligmann, M., and Basch, A. The Clinical Significance of Pathological Immunoglobulins. *Proceedings of the Plenary Session Papers, XII Congress International Soc. Hematology,* New York, 1968. Pp. 21–31.
29. Seligman, M., and Rambaud, J. C. IgA abnormalities in abdominal lymphoma (α-chain disease). *Isr. J. Med. Sci.* 5:151, 1969.
30. Solomon, A., and Kunkel, H. J. A. "Monoclonal" type, low molecular weight protein related to γM-macroglobulins. *Am. J. Med.* 42:958, 1967.
31. Coleman, R. W., Osterlund, C. K., Dorfman, R. F., and Chaplin, H. A. Unique lymphoproliferative disorder associated with an IgM platelet agglutinin, diffuse hypergammaglobulinemia, amyloid deposition and excessive urinary excretion of IgG fragments. *Am. J. Med.* 45:607, 1968.
32. Oehme, J. Symptomatische Makroglobulinämie bei Lues Connata. *Klin. Wochenschr.* 36:869, 1958.
33. Waldenström, J. Abnormal proteins in myeloma. In W. Dock and I. Snapper (Eds.), *Advances in Internal Medicine,* Vol. 5. Chicago: Year Book, 1952. Pp. 398–440.
34. Cleve, H., and Schwick, G. Immuno-Elektrophoretische Serum-Analyse bei Makroglobulinämie Waldenström. *Z. Naturforsch.* [B] 112:375, 1957.
35. Ritzmann, S. E., Cobb, E. K., and Levin, W. C. Electrophoretic differentiation of myeloma and macroglobulinemia M-proteins. Effects of D,L-penicillamine and ephacridine lactate on M-proteins. *Tex. Rep. Biol. Med.* 25:273, 1967.
36. Kunkel, H. G., Müller-Eberhard, H. J., Fudenberg, H. H., and Tomasi, T. B. Gamma globulin complexes in rheumatoid arthritis and certain other conditions. *J. Clin. Invest.* 40:117, 1961.
37. Franklin, E. C., Holman, H. R., Müller-Eberhard, H. J., and Kunkel, H. G. An unusual protein component of high molecular weight in the serum of certain patients with rheumatoid arthritis. *J. Exp. Med.* 105: 425, 1957.
38. Franklin, E. C., and Kunkel, H. G. Immunologic differences between the 19S and 7S components of normal human γ-globulin. *J. Immunol.* 78:11, 1957.
39. Bloch, K. J., Buchanan, W. W., Wohl, M. J., and Bunim, J. J. Sjögren's syndrome. A clinical, pathological, and serological study of sixty-two cases. *Medicine* (Baltimore) 44:187, 1965.

40. Tomasi, T. B., Jr.   Human gamma globulin. *Blood* 25:382, 1965.
41. Bloch, K. J., Buchanan, W. W., Franklin, E. C., and Kunkel, H. G. Immunologic differences between the 19S and 7S components of normal human γ-globulin. *J. Immunol.* 78:11, 1957.
42. Wolf, R. E., Ritzmann, S. E., and Levin, W. C.   Rheumatoid factors and serum immune complexes. Differentiation of rheumatoid complex syndrome from rheumatoid factor clonal macroglobulinemia. In press.
43. Marmont, A., Chiappino, G., Damasio, E., and D'Amore, E.   Démonstration par microscopie en immunofluorescence des eléments cellulaires macroglobulinopoiétiques dans la maladie de Waldenström. *Schweiz. Med. Wochenschr.* 93:1445, 1963.
44. Ritzmann, S. E., Daniels, J. C., and Levin, W. C.   Paralymphomatous Disease—: The Syndrome of Macroglobulinemia. In *Leukemia-Lymphoma*. (A collection of papers presented at the 14th Annual Clinical Conference on Cancer, 1969, at the University of Texas M. D. Anderson Hospital and Tumor Institute, Houston.) Chicago: Year Book, 1970. Pp. 169–222.
45. Kritzmann, J., Kunkel, H. G., MacCarthy, J., and Mellors, R. C.   Studies of a Waldenström-type macroglobulin with rheumatoid factor properties. *J. Lab. Clin. Med.* 57:905, 1961.
46. Rees, E. D., and Resner, R.   Dissociation of a human serum macroglobulin in acid buffer. *Clin. Chim. Acta* 4:272, 1959.
47. Deutsch, H. F., and Morton, J. I.   Dissociation of human serum macroglobulins. *Science* 125:600, 1957.
48. Glenchur, H., Zinneman, H. H., and Briggs, D. R.   Macroglobulinemia: Report of two cases. *Ann. Intern. Med.* 48:1055, 1958.

Assays for Complement Activity   8

Ernest S. Tucker, III, and Robert M. Nakamura

Various methods for assaying the activity of the complement system have been described. The most useful are those that allow quantitation of individual components by means of a radial immunodiffusion (RID) technique based on the method of immunochemical determination that was originally described by Mancini et al. [1, 2]. For the determination of functional complement activity, a hemolytic assay utilizing a sheep red-blood cell system and rabbit antibody as the sensitizing hemolysin is recommended [3]. This total hemolytic assay affords a general screening test to determine the activity of the entire complement sequence and the presence of inhibitor activity. Although total hemolytic activity is best suited for screening for a complement abnormality, individual component determinations are more applicable for the precise definition of the defect.

By the use of selective measurements of complement components C3 and C4 along with the quantitation of C3 activator (properdin factor B), one can estimate the contribution of the classic antibody-mediated intrinsic pathway [4–6] and the alternate (properdin) extrinsic pathway [6–8, 12] for complement activation in a given disease process. These assays may be performed by a RID method.

Specialized assays for complement components and activities are available in certain laboratories. These include hemolytic titrations for specific complement components; measurements of the peptidase and esterase activity of components; biological tests such as phagocytosis, chemotaxis, and the generation of anaphylatoxin; and tests for inhibitor activity such as C1 esterase inhibitor [9].

Diagnostic Approach

The suggested approach to determining the complement abnormalities that are associated with various clinical disorders is as follows:

1. Measure the total hemolytic activity on fresh or fresh frozen ($-40°C$) serum. If it is low, proceed to step 2.

2. Determine the serum C3 level by RID. Proceed to step 3 if the value is abnormal.
3. Determine the serum C4 and C3 activator (properdin factor B; β_2-glycoprotein II) by RID to differentiate between intrinsic and extrinsic complement pathway activation. If these values are normal and the hemolytic activity is low, proceed to step 4.
4. Determine the levels of other complement components by either RID or hemolytic titrations on fresh serum or serum rapidly frozen and preserved at $-40°C$. (Consult with special reference laboratories for these assays.)

If the total hemolytic complement screening test reveals abnormal values, quantitation of C3, C4, and C3 activator usually will indicate the following: (1) *Low C3*—activation of either the classic pathway, the alternate (properdin) pathway, or both of complement sequence; (2) *Low C4*—classic antibody activation of complement in cases such as serum sickness or immune complex diseases [4, 5, 6]; (3) *Low C3 activator*—activation of the alternate pathway of complement [7, 8]. Both pathways of complement activation may be involved simultaneously [10] or the alternate pathway alone may be involved [11]. If the total hemolytic complement screening test reveals abnormal values, but the C3, C4, and C3 activator levels are found to be normal, the specific factor deficiency should be indicated by consulting special reference laboratories (step 4).

Methodology

ASSAY OF TOTAL SERUM HEMOLYTIC
COMPLEMENT (CH$_{50}$ UNITS) [3, 9]
1. Prepare veronal buffer (VB++) diluent from the following: 83.8 gm NaCl, 2.52 gm NaHCO$_3$, 3.0 gm Na 5,5-diethyl barbiturate, 4.6 gm 5,5-diethyl barbituric acid, 1.0 gm MgCl $\cdot$ 6H$_2$O, and 0.14 gm CaCl$_2$ (anhydrous) or 0.20 gm CaCl$_2$ $\cdot$ 2H$_2$O.
Dissolve the last three components in 500 ml of hot distilled water. Dissolve the other components in 500 to 1000 ml of distilled water, combine with the above solution and bring to a total volume of *2000 ml* with distilled water. This solution is five times isotonicity. Store at 1°C to 4°C, and label "stock solution." For use, dilute the stock solution by adding exactly four volumes of distilled water.
2. Collect the serum (either fresh or stored below $-40°C$).
3. Prepare or use commercially available* sensitized sheep (EA) erythrocytes and standardize the cell suspension to give an optical density (OD) of 0.680 at 541 nm (0.5 cm light path). An optical density of 0.680 is equivalent to 1×10^9 cells per milliliter. When sensitizing the cells, add an appropriate dilution of hemolysin to the washed erythrocytes and incubate for 30 minutes at 37°C.

* Cordis Laboratories, P.O. Box 428, Miami, Fla. 33137.

4. Prepare the protocol for complement titration. Place 0.5 ml EA in each test tube. Dilute the human serum 1 to 40 and add, to each tube, amounts increasing by increments of 0.1 ml. Prepare the appropriate controls. Add VB++ diluent as appropriate to each tube to a volume of 1.5 ml, and prepare the appropriate controls. Incubate the tubes with gentle shaking at 37°C for one hour, and add VB++ diluent to a final total volume of 5.0 ml. Centrifuge the tubes at 1800 rpm for 15 minutes, decant the supernatant, and read the optical density at 412 mμ.

The Y value is calculated as follows:

$$Y = \frac{\text{color corrected OD of tube}}{\text{OD 100\% lysis}}$$

Using logarithmic graph paper, plot the curve of Y versus the milliliters of serum (complement) for each tube. The CH_{50} is determined by:

$$CH_{50} = \frac{\text{original serum (C) dilution}}{\text{vol. of serum (C) at } Y = 0.5}$$

HEMOLYTIC ASSAYS FOR SPECIFIC COMPLEMENT COMPONENTS
These assays are based on the addition of a specific component to a reaction mixture containing all the other intermediates in the hemolytic sequence. Such intermediates are commercially available (Cordis Lab.) or can be prepared.

ASSAYS FOR C3 AND C4 COMPONENTS BY IMMUNODIFFUSION
For this method, see Chapter 4.

References

1. Mancini, G., Vaermann, J. P., Carbonara, A. O., and Heremans, J. F. Single Radial Diffusion Method for Immunological Quantitation of Proteins. In H. Peeters (Ed.), *Protides of Biological Fluids,* Vol. 11. Amsterdam: Elsevier, 1964. Pp. 370–373.
2. Mancini, G., Carbonara, A. O., and Heremans, J. F. Immunochemical quantitation of antigens by single radial immunodiffusion. *Immunochemistry* 2:235, 1965.
3. Rapp, H. J., and Borsos, T. *Molecular Basis of Complement Action.* New York: Appleton-Century-Crofts, 1970.
4. Müller-Eberhard, H. J. Chemistry and reaction mechanisms of the complement system. *Adv. Immunol.* 8:1, 1968.
5. Müller-Eberhard, H. J. Complement. *Annu. Rev. Biochem.* 38:389, 1969.
6. Ruddy, S., Gigli, I., and Austen, K. F. The complement system of man. *N. Engl. J. Med.* 287:489, 545, 591, 641, 1972.
7. Gotze, O., and Müller-Eberhard, H. J. The C3 activator system; an alternate pathway of complement activation. *J. Exp. Med.* 134 [Suppl.]: 90, 1971.

8. Lachmann, P. J., and Nicol, P. Reaction mechanism of the alternate pathway of complement activation. *Lancet* 1:465, 1973.
9. Tucker, E. S. The Role of Complement and Other Biochemical Mediators in Immunologic Disease. In R. M. Nakamura (Ed.), *Immunopathology: Clinical Laboratory Concepts and Methods.* Boston: Little, Brown, 1974.
10. Hunsicker, L. D., Ruddy, S., Carpenter, C. B., Schur, P. H., Merrill, J. P., Müller-Eberhard, H. J., and Austen, K. F. Metabolism of third component of complement (C3) in nephritis: Involvement of the classic and alternate (properdin) pathways for complement activation. *N. Engl. J. Med.* 287:835, 1972.
11. Johnston, R. B., Newman, S. L., and Struth, A. G. An abnormality of the alternate pathway of complement activation in sickle cell disease. *N. Engl. J. Med.* 288:803, 1973.
12. Perrin, L. H., Lambert, P. H., Nydegger, U. E., and Miescher, P. A. Quantitation of C3PA (properdin factor B) and other complement components in diseases associated with a low C3 level. *Clin. Immunol. Immunopathol.* 2:16, 1973.

Assays for Immune Complexes

9

Robert M. Nakamura and Ernest S. Tucker, III

The pathogenic role of antigen-antibody complexes in autoimmune disorders is unquestioned. Immune complexes play a significant role in the pathogenesis of vascular, glomerular, and joint lesions in a wide variety of diseases, including glomerulonephritis, periarteritis nodosa, systemic lupus erythematosus, and rheumatoid arthritis [1–4].

The presence of large quantities of immune complexes in serum and other biological fluids when accompanied by depression of serum complement is correlated with disease activity [1–4]. During the past several years, various laboratory tests for the detection of serum and joint fluid immune complexes have been developed [4–6]. The tests have been useful for diagnosis and therapeutic monitoring of the diseases. The methods for the detection of immune complexes may be classified as follows:

1. Routine clinical laboratory tests for screening suspected cases of immune-complex disease
2. Physicochemical methods
3. Immunochemical methods
4. Immunofluorescent methods (tissue biopsy material)

Methods and Application

ROUTINE CLINICAL LABORATORY TESTS
These tests are presumptive and may be of value if positive results are obtained. Other tests elaborated below should be performed if the patient has clinical evidence of immune-complex disease. The common laboratory tests are immunoelectrophoresis (IEP) (see Chap. 2) and tests for cryoglobulins (see Chaps. 19 and 20).

IMMUNOELECTROPHORESIS
Immune-complex diseases may be suggested when the serum immuno-electrophoresis (IEP) pattern shows a trailing effect from the antigen

Figure 9-1

Immunoelectrophoretic pattern of patient with serum immune complexes. The immunoelectrophoretic pattern was developed with specific anti-IgG antiserum. *Top well:* Normal patient's serum. *Lower well:* Serum from SLE patient with serum cryoglobulins and DNA-anti-DNA immune complexes. Note the IgG precipitin arcs and trailing phenomenon extending toward the cathode from the lower well.

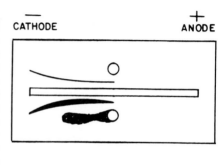

well—usually within the IgG area—toward the cathode. Such trailing is indicated by an opaque, diffuse, oblong area in the agar gel and is due to nonspecific precipitation of the immune complexes [7]. The dense area is connected with the antigen well, but it appears to narrow just to the anodic side of the antigen well (Fig. 9-1). Opacities that are confined closely to either the cathodic or anodic side of the antigen well indicate the possible presence of an abnormal immunoglobulin (monoclonal gammopathy). Such areas differentially do not show the constriction on the cathodic side of the antigen well (Fig. 9-2), and they are often present as well-circumscribed milky or clear areas or spots.

IEP patterns of certain sera may show arcs close to the antigen well, but they usually exhibit definite crescent-shaped precipitin arcs on the anodic side. This pattern is demonstrated better in agar than in agarose. The precipitate may be due to lipoproteins and euglobulins [8]. Although the IEP patterns described above are not diagnostic (since certain immune complexes do not present a cathodic trailing effect), they are extremely helpful. A positive result is one more piece of evidence to confirm suspected immune-complex disease. Conversely, an IEP pattern lacking such trailing effects does not rule out the possibility of the presence of immune complexes, especially if agarose is used instead of agar.

TESTS FOR CRYOGLOBULINS

The sera of patients with suspected immune-complex disease also should be tested for cryoglobulins (see Chap. 20). Many mixed cryoglobulins behave biologically as immune complexes, and they are capable of inducing tissue injury [9, 10].

PHYSICOCHEMICAL METHODS

The physicochemical methods for studying immune complexes are analytical ultracentrifugation [4, 11], preparative ultracentrifugation [12, 13], and column chromatography [13, 14].

ANALYTICAL ULTRACENTRIFUGATION

Analytical ultracentrifugation is the quantitative application of centrifugal force to a solution of particles, which causes molecules or particles

Figure 9-2
Immunoelectrophoretic pattern of
patient with monoclonal macroglobulinemia. Immunoelectrophoretic
pattern was developed with specific
anti-IgM antiserum. *Top well:* Normal serum. *Lower well:* Serum from
patient with monoclonal macroglobulinemia. Note the scooped
monoclonal type of IgM arc near
the lower well. The large, diffuse
protein precipitate adjacent to the
lower well differs from the trailing
effect with the constriction produced by certain serum immune
complexes, as seen in Figure 9-1.

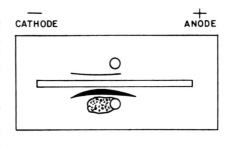

of varying size to sediment at different rates in a standard solution (see
Chap. 7). The sedimentation coefficient is calculated from the observed
velocity of sedimentation divided by the strength of the centrifugal force.
The various immunoglobulins, such as IgG and IgM, have different sedimentation rates. The IgG and IgM immunoglobulin sedimentation rates
are 7S and 19S, respectively. Immune complexes can be definitively detected in sera by analytical ultracentrifugation if they are present in significant amounts.

Immune complexes in virus antibody in the sera of minks with Aleutian mink disease have been demonstrated by this method [11]. Complexes of rheumatoid factor and γ-globulin can often be demonstrated by
analytical ultracentrifugation (see Chap. 7).

PREPARATIVE ULTRACENTRIFUGATION
A sucrose density gradient is frequently employed as a medium to separate molecules of different sizes by ultracentrifugation. The contents of
the sample tube are analyzed after the centrifugation cycle, and the heavier molecules or particles will migrate to the bottom of the tube. The
various particles are fractionated by punching a hole in the bottom of
the tube and collecting sequential fractions. With the use of known markers such as specific antibody or radiolabeled IgM, immune complexes
may be fractionated from a serum sample [12, 13].

COLUMN CHROMATOGRAPHY
Column chromatography by gel filtration is based on the separation of
molecules on the basis of size. Different gel columns, such as Sephadex
G-200 or agarose gel beads (Sepharose 2B or Sepharose 4B),* are used
to isolate immune complexes. The immune complexes, which may have
a molecular weight of more than 1,000,000, will be noted in the end volume or initial protein elution peak during column fractionation of the

* Pharmacia Laboratories, Inc., Piscataway, N.J. 08854.

Figure 9-3
Isolation of immune complexes by column chromatography. (For details, see text.)

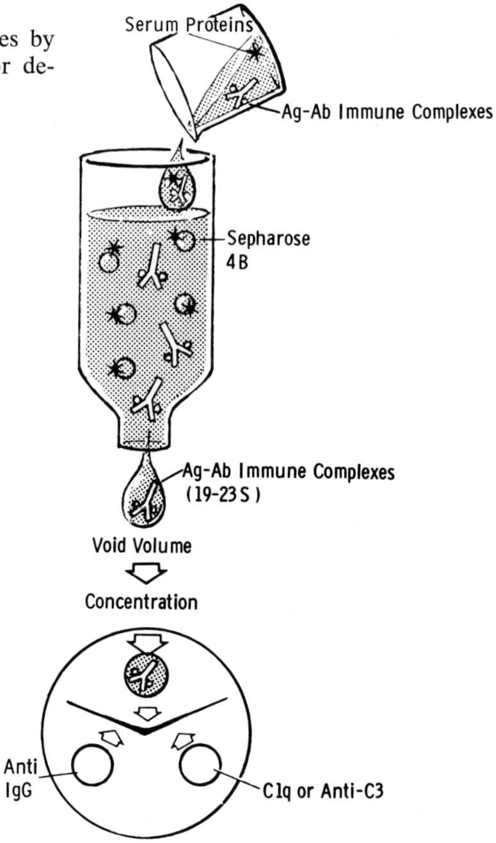

Serum Proteins

Ag-Ab Immune Complexes

Sepharose 4B

Ag-Ab Immune Complexes (19-23 S)

Void Volume

Concentration

Anti IgG

C1q or Anti-C3

protein [13, 14]. The eluate is then concentrated and the immune complexes are detected by double-diffusion gel reactions by reaction against the C1q component of complement and anti-IgG or anti-IgM antisera (Fig. 9-3). Soothill and Hendricks [14] have isolated circulating immune complexes from the sera of patients with malarial nephrosis on Sephadex G-200 and demonstrated that C3 was attached to high molecular weight complexes.

IMMUNOCHEMICAL REACTIONS
Biological reagents that can detect immune complexes by immunochemical reactions are the C1q component of complement [15–17] and monoclonal rheumatoid factor [16, 17]. The platelet aggregation test is also useful in the clinical laboratory in this respect [18, 19].

C1q REACTIONS
Recent studies have shown that certain circulating immune complexes in serum, synovial fluid, and other body fluids may be detected by reaction with C1q [15, 16] and monoclonal rheumatoid factor [17]. C1q is

Figure 9-4
C1q precipitation of serum immune complexes. Well *1:* C1q component of complement. Well *2:* Serum from patient with systemic lupus erythematosus during acute phase of disease. Well *3:* Serum of same patient with SLE during remission. A precipitin line is seen between wells 1 and 2 and demonstrates the presence of immune complexes in the serum placed in well 2. The sample placed in well 3 from the same patient showed no evidence of immune complexes.

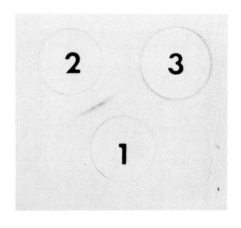

one of the 11 components of complement. It has a molecular weight of about 400,000 and is the first component of complement to attach to immunoglobulin in an antigen-antibody reaction [20]. It may be isolated from normal serum by precipitation with calf thymus deoxyribonucleic acid (DNA) [15] or by precipitation in the presence of a chelating agent such as ethyleneglycol bis(aminoethyl)tetraacetic acid at low ionic strength [21]. Agnello and co-workers [15] have described a gel diffusion method for demonstrating precipitin reactions of C1q with aggregated γ-globulin and immune complexes (Fig. 9-4). Optimal reactions are observed with 0.6 percent agarose in 0.01 molar EDTA at pH 7.2 and ionic strength 0.09. Precipitation with C1q usually occurs with γ-globulin aggregates greater than 19S and with other soluble immune complexes found in twofold to twentyfold antigen excess. Generally, C1q reacts with large γ-globulin molecules and immune complexes. A positive control that can be used in the clinical laboratory test is heat-aggregated γ-globulin, since this will give a precipitin line with C1q similar to that of immune complexes [15].

MONOCLONAL RHEUMATOID FACTOR
The classic rheumatoid factor (RF) that is found in sera of patients with rheumatoid arthritis is polyclonal in nature and has the ability to react with large aggregates of γ-globulin and large immune complexes [17]. Monoclonal rheumatoid factor is found in certain lymphoproliferative disorders as macroglobulinemia [9, 10]. The monoclonal RF can be isolated from the sera of such patients and can be used to detect the presence of immune complexes—which may be either small (less than 19S) or large (more than 19S)—using a gel precipitin reaction similar to the C1q precipitin test [16, 17]. The reactivity of monoclonal RF is enhanced in the cold. Both the C1q component of complement and polyclonal RF will react with and precipitate large complexes and large aggregates of γ-globulin in the joint fluid of patients with rheumatoid

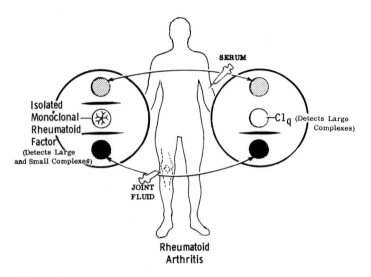

Figure 9-5
Immunodiffusion gel reactions of small and large immune complexes with C1q and monoclonal rheumatoid factor. Note that C1q does not demonstrate a precipitin reaction with serum containing small immune complexes, while the isolated monoclonal rheumatoid factor obtained from a patient with Waldenström's macroglobulinemia shows a precipitin reaction with both the large and small immune complexes found in the joint fluid and serum of the same rheumatoid arthritis patient.

arthritis but not with smaller complexes from their serum. In contrast, the immune complexes from both the joint fluid and sera of rheumatoid arthritis patients will show an in vitro precipitin reaction with monoclonal RF [17] (Fig. 9-5).

PLATELET AGGREGATION TEST
This test may be used to detect circulating immune complexes [18, 19]. A standardized suspension of washed, fresh human platelets is incubated overnight at 5° to 8°C with dilutions of the serum or joint fluid, which has previously been heat-inactivated at 56°C for 30 minutes (Fig. 9-6).

The aggregation patterns are read against dark background illumination, and a smooth white button or a dark even pattern on the bottom of the well indicates negative or positive reactions, respectively. The validity of this procedure in detecting immune complexes has been confirmed by ultracentrifugal sedimentation analysis [19].

IMMUNOFLUORESCENCE STUDY OF TISSUE BIOPSY MATERIAL
Glomerulonephritis is often noted in patients with immune complexes; it is the hallmark of classic immune-complex disease [4, 22–24] (see Chap. 17). Immune complexes play an important role in the pathogenesis of joint lesions in rheumatoid arthritis [5]. The immune complexes

Figure 9-6
Immune complexes detected by platelet aggregation test. (For details, see text.)

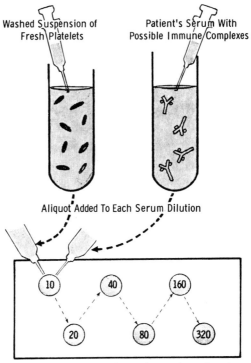

Washed Suspension of Fresh Platelets

Patient's Serum With Possible Immune Complexes

Aliquot Added To Each Serum Dilution

10   40   160

20   80   320

Incubate for one hour at room temperature, then incubate at 5-8°C and observe for agglutination titer.

in joint fluid obtained from rheumatoid arthritis patients are large (more than 19S), whereas the immune complexes found in the sera of such patients are often smaller in size [17]. The difference in the sizes of the immune complexes found in the joint fluid and serum in patients with rheumatoid arthritis may help explain the low incidence of glomerulonephritis in this group [5, 6, 17].

The glomerulonephritis of systemic lupus erythematosus, poststreptococcal glomerulonephritis, and other related diseases are most likely due to immune complexes [4, 22–24]. A diagnosis of immune-complex glomerulonephritis can be made by fluorescent antibody studies of kidney biopsy specimens. The demonstration of deposits of IgG or IgM along with deposits of C3 in similar areas and the distribution of an irregular "lumpy-bumpy" pattern along the epithelial side of the basement membrane provides strong evidence for the pathogenic role of immune complexes in kidney lesions [4, 22–24]. Figure 9-7 shows irregular deposits of IgG along the glomerular basement membrane in a kidney biopsy specimen. C3 was also noted to be deposited in a similar distribution to that of IgG. The nature of the antigen in immune-complex glomerulonephritis is unknown.

Immunofluorescence studies of biopsy specimens from the joint synovial tissues of patients with rheumatoid arthritis may demonstrate the

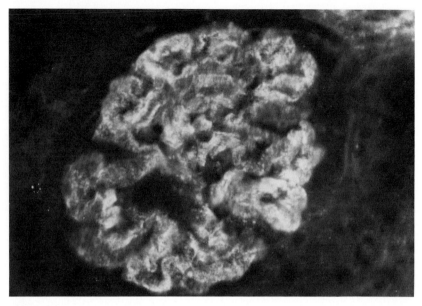

Figure 9-7
Immune-complex glomerulonephritis. By the direct fluorescent antibody test, there is evidence of localization of IgG in an irregular pattern along the basement membrane. A similar fluorescent staining pattern was seen when the section was reacted with fluorescein-labeled anti-C3. The patient showed a clinical picture of progressive glomerulonephritis. The nature of the antigen is not known. (Approx. ×400.)

presence of immune complexes [6]. Deposits of IgG, IgM, and C3 along the synovial epithelium may be found with the use of fluorescent-labeled antisera, and this observation is characteristic of cases of active rheumatoid arthritis [5, 6].

Vasculitis is also a hallmark lesion of immune-complex disease [4]. Patients with periarteritis nodosa and chronic Australia antigenemia have provided evidence that immune complexes of Australia antigen (hepatitis B) are probably involved in the pathogenesis of the vascular lesions. Biopsy specimens from patients with periarteritis and chronic Australia antigenemia showed localization of IgM, Australia antigen, and complement along the basement membrane of the arterial wall in the periarteritis lesion in fluorescent antibody studies [25].

Limitations

1. Immunoelectrophoresis is nonspecific, but the results are better if agar is used instead of agarose.
2. Ultracentrifugation analyses suffer from low sensitivity.
3. Column chromatography is not practical for routine use in most hospital clinical laboratories.

4. C1q is reactive with large complexes, which are usually pathogenic, but it is not reactive with smaller complexes.
5. Monoclonal rheumatoid factor is sensitive and will react with both large and small complexes. Many of the smaller complexes, however, may not be pathogenic.
6. The platelet aggregation test is very sensitive, but rigorous controls must be instituted since many other nonspecific factors can cause platelet aggregation.
7. Immunofluorescence provides an excellent method for demonstrating immune complexes having a pathogenic role, but this procedure requires tissue biopsy specimens.

References

1. Weigle, W. O.   Fate and Biological Action of Antigen-Antibody Complexes. In W. H. Taliaferro and J. H. Humphrey (Eds.), *Advances in Immunology*, Vol. 1. New York: Academic, 1961. P. 283.
2. Dixon, F. J.   The role of antigen-antibody complexes in disease. *Harvey Lect.* 58:21, 1963.
3. Cochrane, C. G., and Dixon, F. J.   Cell and Tissue Damage Through Antigen-Antibody Complexes. In P. Miescher and H. Müller-Eberhard (Eds.), *Textbook of Immunopathology*. New York: Grune & Stratton, 1969. P. 94.
4. Cochrane, C. G., and Koffler, D.   Immune Complexes in Experimental Disease and Man. In F. J. Dixon and H. G. Kunkel (Eds.), *Advances in Immunology*, Vol. 16. New York: Academic, 1973. P. 186.
5. Broder, I., Vrowitz, M. B., and Gordon, D. A.   Appraisal of rheumatoid arthritis as an immune complex disease. *Med. Clin. North Am.* 56:529, 1972.
6. Zvaifler, H. J.   The Immunopathology of Joint Inflammation in Rheumatoid Arthritis. In F. J. Dixon and H. G. Kunkel (Eds.), *Advances in Immunology*, Vol. 16. New York: Academic, 1973. P. 265.
7. Ritzmann, S. E., Daniels, J. C., Alami, S. Y., and Lawrence, M. C. Electrophoresis, Immunoelectrophoresis, Quantitative Immunodiffusion, and Thermoproteins. In G. J. Race (Ed.), *Laboratory Medicine*. New York: Harper & Row, 1975.
8. McKay, G. G.   Practical Application of Immunoelectrophoresis. In H. R. Dettelbach and S. E. Ritzmann (Eds.), *Lab Synopsis*, Vol. 2 (2nd ed.). Somerville, N.J.: Behring Diagnostics, 1969.
9. Barnett, E. V., Bluestone, R., Cracchiolo, A., Goldberg, L. S., Kantor, G. L., and McIntosh, R. M.   Cryoglobulinemia and disease. *Ann. Intern. Med.* 73:95, 1970.
10. Grey, H. M., and Kohler, P. F.   Cryoimmunoglobulins. *Semin. Hematol.* 10:87, 1973.
11. Porter, D., Dixon, F. J., and Larsen, A. E.   Metabolism and function of gamma globulin in Aleutian disease of mink. *J. Exp. Med.* 121:889, 1965.
12. Cochrane, C. G., and Hawkins, D.   Studies of circulating immune complexes.   III. Factors governing the ability of circulating complexes to localize in blood vessels. *J. Exp. Med.* 127:137, 1968.
13. Baumal, R., and Broder, I.   Studies into the occurrence of soluble antigen-antibody complexes in disease.   III. Rheumatoid arthritis and other human diseases. *Clin. Exp. Immunol.* 3:555, 1968.

14. Soothill, J. F., and Hendricks, R. G. Some immunological studies of the nephrotic syndrome of Nigerian children. *Lancet* 2:629, 1967.
15. Agnello, V., Winchester, R. J., and Kunkel, H. G. Precipitin reactions of the C1q component of complement with aggregated γ-globulin and immune complexes in gel diffusion. *Immunology* 19:909, 1970.
16. Agnello, V., Koffler, D., Eisenberg, J. W., Winchester, R. J., and Kunkel, H. G. C1q precipitins in the sera of patients with systemic lupus erythematosus and other hypocomplementemic states. Characterization of high and low molecular weight types. *J. Exp. Med.* 134 [Suppl.]:228, 1971.
17. Winchester, R. J., Kunkel, H. G., and Agnello, V. Occurrence of γ-globulin complexes in serum and joint fluid of rheumatoid arthritis patients. Use of monoclonal rheumatoid factor as reagents for their demonstration. *J. Exp. Med.* 134 [Suppl.]:286, 1971.
18. Penttinen, K., Vaheri, A., and Myelyla, G. Detection and characterization of immune complexes by the platelet aggregation test. I. Complexes formed *in vitro*. *Clin. Exp. Immunol.* 8:389, 1971.
19. Myelyla, G., Vaheri, A., and Penttinen, K. Detection and characterization of immune complexes by the platelet aggregation test. II. Circulating complexes. *Clin. Exp. Immunol.* 8:399, 1971.
20. Müller-Eberhard, H. J. Chemistry and Reaction Mechanisms of Complement. In F. J. Dixon and H. G. Kunkel (Eds.), *Advances in Immunology,* Vol. 8. New York: Academic, 1968. P. 2.
21. Yonemasu, K., and Stroud, R. M. C1q: Rapid purification method for the preparation of monospecific antisera and for biochemical studies. *J. Immunol.* 106:304, 1971.
22. McCluskey, R. T. The value of immunofluorescence in the study of human renal disease. *J. Exp. Med.* 134 [Suppl.]:242, 1971.
23. Churg, J., and Grishman, E. Ultrastructure of immune deposits in renal disease. *Ann. Intern. Med.* 76:479, 1972.
24. Roy, L. P., Fish, A. J., Michael, A. F., and Vernier, R. L. Etiologic Agents of Immune Deposit Disease. In R. S. Schwartz (Ed.), *Progress in Clinical Immunology,* Vol. 1. New York: Grune & Stratton, 1972. P. 1.
25. Gocke, D. J., Hsu, K., Morgan, C., Bombardieri, S., Lockshin, M., and Christian, C. L. Vasculitis in association with Australia antigen. *J. Exp. Med.* 134 [Suppl.]:330, 1971.

Fluorescent Antibody Assays 10

Robert M. Nakamura and Gerald A. Beathard

The fluorescent antibody method developed by Coons and co-workers in 1941 [1] has gained widespread applicability in the field of medicine. It has been used to identify and visualize antigens of many types, such as bacterial, viral, protozoal, and fungal antigens, as well as those of animal tissue origin. In recent years, it has been widely used for the localization of serum antibodies in tissue, a technique that is very important in the diagnosis and evaluation of a number of disease entities.

The immunofluorescence technique is based upon the successful conjugation of a specific antibody with a dye of high quantum yield, following exposure to light of short wavelength. The development of simple, efficient methods of conjugating the dye with the antibodies without denaturation, the methods for purification of the conjugates, improved methods for preparing materials to be studied, and the development of improved optical systems for the study of immunofluorescent materials have established this technique as a standard procedure in the clinical laboratory and have made it suitable for general clinical use. The fact that it combines the high level of specificity of immunological reactions with the sensitivity of fluorescence methods has made it invaluable to the field of medicine.

The technique depends upon the conjugation of a fluorochrome through a covalent bond to a specific antibody in such a way as not to alter its immunological reactivity. A fluorochrome is a substance that emits light following exposure to exciting radiation in the form of short wavelengths of light. The light emitted by the fluorochrome is of longer wavelength than the radiation to which it is exposed (Fig. 10-1); this light is called *fluorescence*. The isothiocyanate derivative of fluorescein, fluorescein isothiocyanate (FITC), and the sulfonic acid derivative of rhodamine, lissamine rhodamine B (RB 200), are the two fluorochromes most frequently used. FITC has a maximum absorption at 495 nm (see Fig. 10-1) and a maximum emission at 520 nm (green). RB 200 has a maximum absorption at 575 nm and two emission peaks, one at 595 nm (yellow) and the other at 710 nm (red) [2–4].

The green fluorescence of fluorescein offers several advantages over

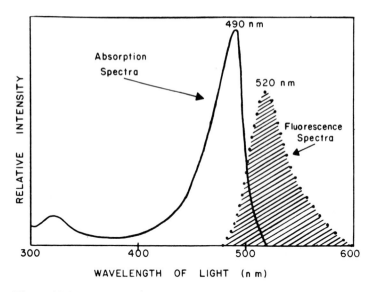

Figure 10-1
Comparison of light wavelengths absorbed and emitted by a fluorochrome.
(Absorption and fluorescence spectra of fluorescein at pH 7.1.)

the red fluorescence of rhodamine: the human eye is more sensitive to
the green color, and green autofluorescence is less common than red
autofluorescence, thus eliminating one source of error in the interpretation of fluorescent preparations.

General Methods for Use of Fluorescent Antibody

In practice, several immunofluorescence techniques may be used to detect the presence of unknown antigens in tissues or smears or the presence of unknown antibodies in the sera of patients suspected of having
certain diseases. The most commonly used methods are the direct, indirect, competitive inhibition, and complement-staining techniques [2,
3, 5].

DIRECT METHOD

With the direct technique, an unknown antigen is detected using an antibody of known specificity that is labeled with a fluorescent compound
(Fig. 10-2). The material suspected of containing the antigen is fixed to
a slide; then the fluorescent-labeled antibody (conjugate) is added in its
predetermined optimal dilution and allowed to react for a period of 30
minutes to 1 hour. The preparation is washed to remove the excess conjugate that has not been specifically bound to the antigen. The slide is
blotted and mounted with a coverslip using buffered glycerol. It is examined with a fluorescence microscope to detect the presence of the antigen
being studied.

Figure 10-2
Mechanism of direct immunofluorescence method. In this
technique, the antigen is localized through the use of an
antibody that has been conjugated with the fluorochrome.

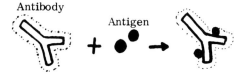

Figure 10-3
Mechanism of indirect im-
munofluorescence method.
In this method, two anti-
bodies are used. The pri-
mary antibody (step *1*) is
specific for the antigen but
is not conjugated with fluorochrome. The secondary
antibody (step *2*) is an
anti-immunoglobulin anti-
body that has been conju-
gated with the fluoro-
chrome so that it can be
localized using fluores-
cence microscopy. Note
the amplification that results through the use of
this technique.

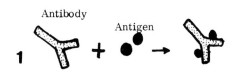

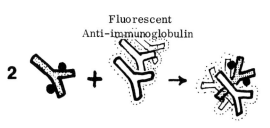

INDIRECT METHOD

This method is the one that is most widely used in the clinical laboratory.
It is utilized for the detection of either an unknown antigen in tissue sections or smears, or an unknown antibody in the serum of a patient. This
technique is based upon the principle that a specific antigen-antibody reaction can be visualized by the addition of a fluorescent-labeled antibody
directed against the immunoglobulin involved in the specific immune reaction (Fig. 10-3). This procedure involves a primary (specific) antibody and a secondary (nonspecific) antibody. Only the secondary antibody is labeled. The complex of the antigen plus antibody globulin
(primary antibody) plus labeled anti-immunoglobulin (secondary antibody) results in specific fluorescence, indicating the presence of the
antigen. The primary advantage of the indirect method lies in the fact
that a labeled anti-immunoglobulin preparation may be used to detect
a variety of different specific antigen-antibody reactions as long as the
antibody involved is from the species for which the anti-immunoglobulin
is specific. An additional advantage is the degree of amplification that
results from the fact that several molecules of the tagged secondary antibody react with each molecule of the untagged primary antibody.

The procedure used in this method involves "flooding" the tissue section or smear under study with the unlabeled primary antibody that is
specific for the antigen being tested. The antibody is allowed to react for

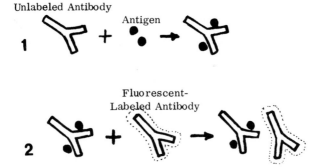

Unlabeled Antibody

Antigen

1

Fluorescent-
Labeled Antibody

2

Figure 10-4
Competitive inhibition method. In this technique, the antigen is first allowed to react with unconjugated antibody and then subsequently with the conjugated antibody. The principle of the technique is based on the tendency for the unlabeled antibody to saturate the antigen (step *1*), not leaving any reactive sites for the conjugated antibody to attach with in the subsequent reaction (step *2*).

30 minutes to 1 hour. The preparation is thoroughly washed to remove unbound antibody. The labeled secondary antibody is then applied and allowed to react for 30 minutes to 1 hour. Following this, the preparation is washed and mounted with a coverslip, using buffered glycerol. The preparation is examined for the presence of fluorescence, which indicates the presence of the antigen being studied.

COMPETITIVE INHIBITION METHOD
This method is primarily employed as a control for testing the specificity of antibodies used in the direct immunofluorescence technique. It has also been used to detect the presence of antibodies directed against certain microorganisms, such as *Toxoplasma gondii* in serum [6]. This procedure involves the use of two antibodies, both of which are specific for the antigen being studied. One antibody is labeled with the fluorescent compound; the other is not. The technique is based upon the principle that antigen, when treated with unlabeled specific antibody, becomes saturated so that it cannot bind the labeled specific antibody in a subsequent exposure. Such a sequence fails to result in fluorescence (Fig. 10-4). The technique is performed in a manner similar to that described for the indirect immunofluorescence technique. The optimal concentration of both the labeled and unlabeled antibody should be determined prior to performing the test.

COMPLEMENT-STAINING METHOD
This technique is quite similar to the indirect immunofluorescence technique except that the labeled antibody is directed against complement. Complement is added to the preparation in addition to the unlabeled primary antibody, which in this technique must be complement-binding. Guinea pig complement is frequently used for this purpose. The labeled

Figure 10-5
Anticomplement staining method. The antibody used in step *1* is a complement-fixing antibody that will attach to the antigen for which it is specific and bind complement in the process. The presence of complement can then be demonstrated as in step *2*, using a fluorochrome-tagged anticomplement antibody.

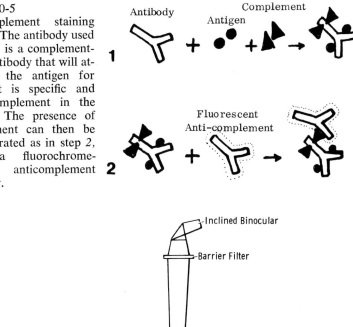

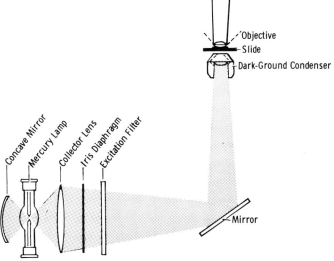

Figure 10-6
Instrumentation used in immunofluorescence microscopy.

secondary antibody is directed against the complement. The test is based on the principle that the antigen-antibody complex resulting from the interaction of the specific primary antibody with the antigen will bind complement to the complex (Fig. 10-5). When this is followed by the addition of labeled anticomplement globulin (species-specific), the presence of fluorescence in the preparation indicates the location of the antigen involved in this series of reactions.

Instrumentation

Factors that must be considered in the selection of appropriate equipment to be used for immunofluorescence studies include the light source, filters to select or eliminate certain light wavelengths, the microscope, the appropriate condenser, and microscope objectives [2, 3, 5, 7] (Fig. 10-6).

LIGHT SOURCE
For illumination, there are two widely used light sources. One is the mercury vapor lamp (Osram HBO 200*), which provides a steady, powerful source of ultraviolet light, and the other is a more recently developed halogen quartz lamp. The halogen quartz light source provides a higher intensity emission in the 400 to 500 nm range than does the mercury vapor lamp (Fig. 10-7). For this reason, it is preferred by many investigators for working with fluorescein isothiocyanate-labeled compounds, since the peak absorption of this material is approximately 495 nm.

FILTERS
Two types of filters are used in immunofluorescence microscopy: primary or excitor filters and secondary or barrier filters (see Fig. 10-6). The primary filter is placed between the light source and the condenser and allows the passage of light of the preferred wavelengths for excitation, blocking light of longer wavelengths. These filters are of two types: those designed to transmit ultraviolet and eliminate visible illumination (up to a wavelength of 410 nm) and those designed to transmit ultraviolet-blue light (up to a wavelength of 480 nm). The secondary filter is placed between the objective and the ocular and prevents the passage of light of shorter wavelengths, such as the excitation light. It also aids in providing a relatively black background and in protecting the observer's eyes from the ultraviolet light. The primary and secondary filters must be appropriately paired to provide a black background.

MICROSCOPE
There are a number of microscopes available that can be utilized for immunofluorescence work. These vary more in price than in the quality of the optics. The availability of service, mechanical simplicity, and the availability of appropriate accessories are the primary factors that dictate selection of the basic microscope.

* Gesellschaft, Berlin, West Germany (available through local microscope dealers in U.S.).

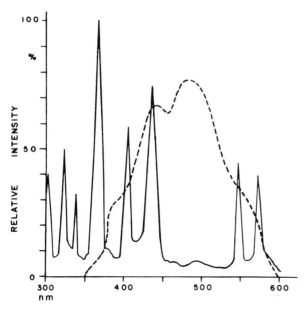

Figure 10-7
Light spectra emitted by an HBO-200 mercury vapor lamp (*solid line*) and a
halogen quartz lamp (*dotted line*).

CONDENSER

The choice of condensers to be used in fluorescence microscopy is of
considerable importance. The dark-field condenser is regarded as essential equipment. Its principal advantage is that it directs the primary illumination passed by the excitor filter away from the objective of the microscope so that, apart from light scattered by the object being viewed,
none is collected by the objective lens. This allows for the use of more
intense primary illumination. Dark-field condensers provide the additional advantage of rendering images of higher contrast than do bright-
field condensers. There are two types of dark-field condensers: oil immersion and dry. The oil immersion type is superior optically; however,
the dry dark-field condenser is easier to use for routine studies using low
to medium magnification.

Phase-contrast condensers and, more recently, phase-interference systems have been used in conjunction with fluorescence for special purposes.

MICROSCOPE OBJECTIVES

Microscope objectives that have nonfluorescent lenses must be obtained.
In general, the more highly corrected objectives tend to have more autofluorescence. Achromatic objectives are generally preferred to apochro-
matic objectives, because they have much less autofluorescence and are
quite suitable for the color ranges encountered in fluorescence microscopy.

INCIDENT-LIGHT IMMUNOFLUORESCENCE

Incident-light fluorescence microscopy or epifluorescence is a relatively new development in the field of microscopy. It is based upon the use of highly efficient interference mirrors designed to have a reflectance of 90 to 95 percent for the wavelengths of exciting light and 75 to 95 percent transmission for longer wavelengths. The light source and interference mirrors are arranged in such a way that the light is directed downward through the microscope tube and through the objective of the microscope to excite the fluorochrome in the preparation from above. In this way, the objective for the microscope also serves the same purpose as the condenser in transmission microscopy. The primary advantage of incident light fluorescence is the increased intensity of fluorescence that is obtained. This makes it especially suitable for the detection of fluorescence of very weak intensity, such as that resulting from cell-surface immunoglobulins and antigens in tumors or on lymphocytes [5].

Sources of Error

There are many potential sources of error in the various methods that have been described [2, 3, 5]. The chance of error can be considerably reduced or eliminated by the utilization of appropriate controls. The controls that are most frequently used are as follows:

1. Absorption of the labeled antiserum with the specific antigen against which it is directed, before staining the preparation. This should result in negative fluorescence.
2. Comparison of the fluorescence obtained with a known positive and a known negative slide of a similar or identical material.
3. The use of an unrelated labeled antiserum, such as labeled normal globulin, on both positive and negative controlled tissues. This will indicate whether the fluorescence noted is specific or not.
4. Inhibition or blocking of fluorescence by the prior application of unlabeled specific antibody. This should eliminate or significantly reduce the positive fluorescence.

Inherent difficulties in the standardization of procedures exist, since there is a wide variety of antigen substrates and antisera that are used in different procedures. There have been attempts by several international committees to formulate criteria for standard preparations of fluoresceinated antisera [8–14]. Standardization is very important since it is desirable for a laboratory to be able to reproduce its results with a relative degree of accuracy using different fluorescent antibody preparations [15].

Application of Immunofluorescence Methods

Immunofluorescence techniques have come to be widely used in clinical medicine for the localization and identification of antigens in a variety of different tissues and smears and for the identification of antibodies directed against a wide variety of substances. The application of an immunofluorescence technique in this manner provides the clinician with a test having a high degree of specificity, which is limited only by the immunological specificity of the antibody involved. The specificity of this reaction can be assured through the use of the control measures described above. In these tests, the direct immunofluorescence method has a sensitivity that is comparable to that of complement-fixation tests. It is somewhat less sensitive than tests such as hemagglutination and hemagglutination-inhibition [3]. The indirect fluorescent antibody method is about 5 to 10 times more sensitive than the direct method.

The application of various immunofluorescence methods can be considered under several categories.

MICROBIOLOGY
In the diagnostic area, the majority of human pathogens have been studied experimentally and, frequently, clinically as well. Almost all have been found to be suitable for identification by means of immunofluorescence. Using this technique, a tentative diagnosis may be given much sooner than by cultivation, and it can subsequently be confirmed through the isolation of the organism in the usual manner. It is important to note that this type of identification cannot replace the isolation of these organisms. Isolation continues to be essential to confirm the immunofluorescence information and for antibiotic sensitivity studies [16, 17].

DETECTION OF AUTOANTIBODIES
The field of medicine recognizes a family of diseases that is characterized by the presence of autoimmune phenomena, i.e., immunological reactions directed against the subject's own tissues. These diseases are diverse in their clinical presentation and severity. However, they all share one feature in common: the presence in the patient's serum of autoantibodies, i.e., antibodies capable of reacting with the individual's own tissue antigens. Clinical screening for the presence of autoantibodies by means of immunofluorescence, primarily by the indirect immunofluorescence method, has come to be a standard diagnostic test in most hospitals (Fig. 10-8). The autoantibodies considered to be important include antinuclear (Fig. 10-9), anti-mitochondrial, anti–smooth muscle, anti-thyroid, anti–thyroid epithelial cells, anti-parietal cells, anti-reticulum, anti–basement membranes, anti-skin, anti–skeletal muscle, and anti-colon antibodies [18–20].

IMMUNE-COMPLEX DISEASES
A variety of diseases encountered clinically have been shown to be caused by immunological mechanisms. One of the most frequent means by which these diseases occur is through a series of reactions initiated by the deposition of antigen-antibody complexes within the affected tissue structures. In this category, immunological renal disease has gained the widest attention, and immunofluorescence techniques, primarily the di-

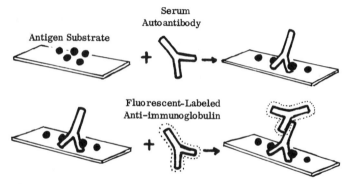

Figure 10-8
Immunofluorescence antibody method for detection of autoimmune antibody in serum. The general procedure used in demonstrating the presence of auto-antibody in the serum is shown. The antigen substrate on a slide is first treated with the patient's serum and subsequently with a fluorochrome-tagged anti-immunoglobulin antibody, which localizes the site of the reaction.

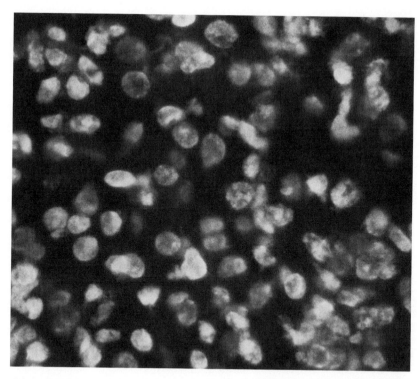

Figure 10-9
Antinuclear antibody demonstrated by immunofluorescence technique. (Approx. ×250.)

144

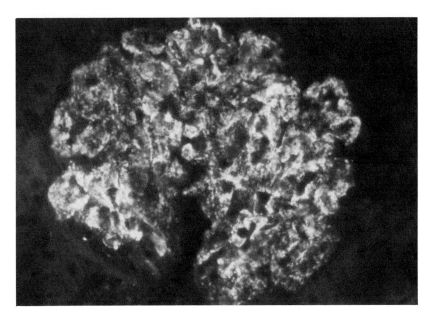

Figure 10-10
Deposition of the immunoglobulin in the glomerulus of a patient with membranous glomerulonephritis, demonstrated by immunofluorescence technique. (Approx. ×450.)

Figure 10-11
Surface immunoglobulins on a lymphocyte demonstrated by immunofluorescence technique. (Approx. ×450.)

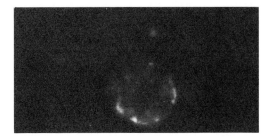

rect immunofluorescence method, have come to be used routinely as an aid in the diagnosis of such conditions (Fig. 10-10). It is now apparent that the immunofluorescence study of kidney biopsy material is a necessary, essential aspect of renal pathology [4].

Studies similar to those applied to kidney biopsy material may also be applied to a variety of other tissues, such as synovium, blood vessels, and lungs (see Chaps. 8 and 9).

MISCELLANEOUS APPLICATIONS
Immunofluorescence techniques may also be used for the detection of hormones, enzymes, organ-specific antigens, blood cell antigens, plasma

proteins, tumor-specific antigens, and, more recently, in the identification of lymphocytes (Fig. 10-11).

References

1. Coons, A. H., Creich, H. J., Jones, R. N., and Berliner, E. The demonstration of pneumococcal antigen in tissues by the use of fluorescent antibody. *J. Immunol.* 45:159, 1942.
2. Goldman, M. *Fluorescent Antibody Methods.* New York: Academic, 1968.
3. Kawamura, A. *Fluorescent Antibody Techniques and Their Application.* Baltimore: University Park Press, 1969.
4. McClusky, R. T. The value of immunofluorescence in the study of human renal disease. *J. Exp. Med.* 134:2425, 1971.
5. Nairn, R. C. *Fluorescent Protein Tracing* (3rd ed.). Baltimore: Williams & Wilkins, 1969.
6. Goldman, M. Staining toxoplasma gondii with fluorescein-labeled antibody. II. A new serological test for antibodies to toxoplasma based upon inhibition of specific staining. *J. Exp. Med.* 105:557, 1957.
7. Blundell, G. P. Fluorescent Antibody Techniques. In M. Stefanini (Ed.), *Progress in Clinical Pathology,* Vol. 3. New York: Grune & Stratton, 1970. P. 211.
8. Anderson, S. G., Addison, I. E., and Dixon, H. G. Antinuclear factor serum (homogeneous). An international collaborative study of the proposed research standard 66/233. *Ann. N.Y. Acad. Sci.* 177:337, 1971.
9. Barnett, E. V. Staining Activity of Conjugates in Relation to Their Antibody Content. In E. J. Holborow (Ed.), *Standardization of Immunofluorescence.* Oxford: Blackwell, 1970.
10. Beutner, E. H., Chorzelski, T. P., and Jordon, R. E. *Autosensitization in Pemphigus and Bullous Pemphigoid.* Springfield, Ill.: Thomas, 1970. P. 131.
11. Beutner, E. H., Holborow, E. J., and Johnson, G. D. Quantitative studies of immunofluorescence staining. I. Analysis of mixed immunofluorescence. *Immunology* 12:327, 1967.
12. Beutner, E. H., Sepulveda, M. R., and Barnett, E. V. Quantitative studies of immunofluorescent staining. II. Relationships of characteristics of unabsorbed anti-human IgG conjugates to their specific and non-specific staining properties in an indirect test for antinuclear factors. *Bull. W. H. O.* 39:587, 1968.
13. Chantler, S., and Haire, M. Evaluation of the immunological specificity of fluorescein-labeled anti-human IgM conjugates. *Immunology* 23:7, 1972.
14. Holborow, E. J., Brighton, W. D., Sander, G., and Taylor, C. E. D. Report of Subcommittee on Requirement for Specification of Anti-immunoglobulin Conjugates. In E. J. Holborow (Ed.), *Standardization of Immunofluorescence.* Oxford: Blackwell, 1970. P. 275.
15. Hebert, G. A., Pittman, B., and Cherry, W. B. The definition and application of evaluation techniques as a guide for the improvement of fluorescent antibody reagents. *Ann. N.Y. Acad. Sci.* 177:54, 1971.
16. Cherry, W. B., and Moody, M. D. Fluorescent antibody techniques in diagnostic bacteriology. *Bacteriol. Rev.* 29:222, 1965.
17. McEntegart, M. G. Immunological Tracing: Bacteria, Protozoa, Hel-

minths and Fungi. In R. C. Nairn (Ed.), *Fluorescent Protein Tracing.* Baltimore: Williams & Wilkins, 1969. P. 152.

18. Roitt, I. M.   Immunofluorescent Tests for Detection of Autoantibodies. In *Manual of Autoimmune Serology.* Geneva: World Health Organization, 1970.

19. Tan, E. M.   Relationship of nuclear staining patterns with precipitating antibodies in systemic lupus erythematosus. *J. Clin. Lab. Med.* 70:800, 1967.

20. Whittingham, S.   Serological Methods in Autoimmune Disease. In J. B. G. Kwapinski (Ed.), *Research in Immunochemistry and Immunobiology, I.* Baltimore: University Park Press, 1972. P. 173.

Immunoenzymatic Histochemical Assays 11

Robert M. Nakamura and Gerald A. Beathard

Since the first descriptions by Nakane and Pierce [1] and Avrameas and Uriel [2], immunoenzymatic techniques have been developed in which enzymes are used as antibody markers for both light and electron microscopy studies in a manner identical to that in which the fluorochrome is used in immunofluorescence studies. Enzymes such as peroxidase, alkaline phosphatase, acid phosphatase, glucose oxidase, tyrosinase, and lactic dehydrogenase have been used for light microscopy. Peroxidase and alkaline or acid phosphatase have been the primary enzymes used for electron microscopy [3]. These enzymes are coupled to antibody through a covalent bond in such a way that neither the antibody nor the enzyme is functionally altered. Whereas the antibody involved in the immunofluorescent reaction is localized by the fluorescence emitted by the fluorochrome, in the immunoenzymatic technique the antibody is localized by the deposition of a reaction product resulting from the catalytic effect of the enzyme [3–11]. In general, any technique that can be adapted to the immunofluorescence method can be adapted to the immunoenzymatic method. In addition, the technique is adaptable to ultrastructural studies.

Methodology

The immunoenzymatic techniques have been broadly classified into direct and indirect methods.

DIRECT METHOD

In the direct method, an antigen is detected using a specific antibody that has been tagged with the enzyme. A variant of this direct technique, which is very similar to the indirect immunofluorescence method, involves the use of untagged specific (primary) antibody directed against the antigen being studied and an anti-immunoglobulin (secondary) antibody that bears the enzyme tag. The procedure followed in this type of

Figure 11-1
Direct immunoenzymatic method. In step *1*, an antibody that has been conjugated with the enzyme is used to localize the presence of the antigen. In step *2*, the reaction is localized by treating it with the substrate specific for the enzyme involved.

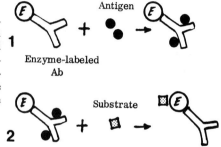

study is essentially the same as that followed in the immunofluorescence method. It differs in that once the antigen, which is fixed to a slide, is allowed to react with the enzyme-tagged antibody, it is treated with the specific substrate for the enzyme. This results in a reaction producing either a chromogenic or electron-dense deposit (Fig. 11-1). According to the terminology used in immunoenzyme staining, both of these techniques in which an enzyme is directly conjugated with an antibody are referred to as *direct methods*.

INDIRECT METHOD
Three types of indirect techniques have been described [3, 5]: the hybrid antibody method, the mixed antibody method, and the amplification antibody method. These are referred to as *indirect methods* because in each case an anti-enzyme antibody is used. In this sense, they are comparable to the indirect immunofluorescence method in which an anti-immunoglobulin antibody is used. They should not be confused with the type of direct immunoenzymatic method described above in which an enzyme-tagged anti-immunoglobulin is involved.

HYBRID ANTIBODY METHOD
The hybrid antibody method utilizes an antibody with double specificity that is prepared from purified preparations of anti-enzyme and anti-protein antibodies. These separate antibodies are first digested with pepsin, reduced, and then allowed to recombine. The hybrid antibody having the specific reactivity of both the parent immunoglobulins is then isolated using specific immunoabsorbent columns [12, 13]. The technique followed in this method allows the anti-protein portion of the hybrid antibody to react with the protein antigen being studied in the tissue or smear. The preparation is then treated with the enzyme against which the anti-enzyme moiety of the hybrid is directed. This results in the binding of the enzyme to the site of antigen localization. The substrate that is specific for the enzyme is added to the preparation and the reaction product is produced (Fig. 11-2).

MIXED ANTIBODY METHOD
This type of indirect immunoenzymatic technique utilizes two untagged antibodies: an anti-immunoglobulin and an anti-enzyme antibody. The technique as originally described [14] was used to detect the presence of

Figure 11-2
Hybrid antibody method. In step *1*, a hybrid antibody is produced having specificities for both the antigen being studied and the enzyme being utilized. This is allowed to react with both the enzyme and the antigen. In step *2*, the reaction sequence is then localized by use of the substrate specific for the enzyme, as in step *3*.

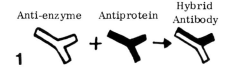

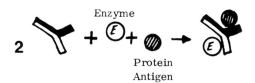

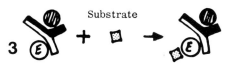

immunoglobulin in animal material. The anti-immunoglobulin antibody is allowed to react with the immunoglobulin in the animal tissue, and it is then treated with the anti-enzyme antibody derived from the same species as the tissue being studied. This technique is based upon the presumption that the species-specific anti-immunoglobulin reacts with the antigen using only one of its reactive sites, leaving the other available to react with the anti-enzyme antibody derived from the same animal species. Following the reaction of these two antibodies in sequence, the preparation is treated with enzyme. The reactive site is identified through the use of the substrate that is specific for that enzyme (Fig. 11-3).

A modification of this technique has been reported for use in identifying immunoglobulin deposition in kidney biopsy material from patients with glomerulonephritis [15]. This technique involves the use of a total of three antibodies: an anti-human immunoglobulin that is heavy-chain specific (antibody A), an anti-immunoglobulin antibody (antibody B), and an anti-enzyme antibody (antibody C). Antibody A and antibody C are derived from the same animal species (e.g., rabbit), and antibody B is specific for that species (anti-rabbit immunoglobulin). According to the technique of this method, antibody A is allowed to react with the tissue suspected of containing the antigen, and it is then treated with antibody B, which will attach to the first antibody, as well as antibody C with which the preparation is subsequently treated. Once the triple antibody complex is attached to the antigen in the tissue preparation, it can then be treated with the enzyme and, subsequently, with the substrate of the enzyme to produce a reaction product, thus allowing the localization of the antigen that initiated the total reaction (Fig. 11-4).

AMPLIFICATION ANTIBODY METHOD
The amplification antibody method is essentially a modified direct technique in which the sensitivity of the enzyme-labeled specific antibody is

Figure 11-3
Mixed antibody method (double antibody). In this method, an immunoglobulin antigen is localized through the use of untagged antibody and an anti-enzyme antibody. It is important to realize that the anti-enzyme antibody must have the same species-specificity as the immunoglobulin being detected. The anti-immunoglobulin antibody will then react with both the immunoglobulin antigen and the anti-enzyme antibody. Localization of the reaction sequence is then performed by treating the preparation with the enzyme and, subsequently, its specific substrates, as in steps 3 and 4.

Figure 11-4
Mixed antibody method (triple antibody). In this method, three antibodies are used in sequence. It is important to recognize that antibody A and antibody C must be derived from the same species. It is against the immunoglobulin of this species that antibody B is directed. The total reaction sequence is again localized using the enzyme against which antibody C is directed, followed by treatment with its substrate.

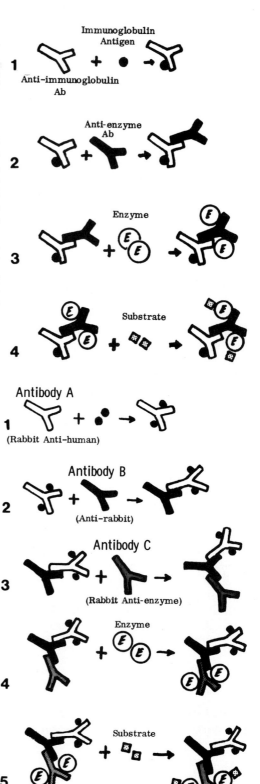

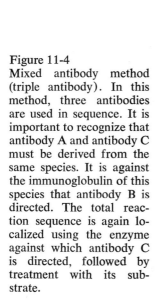

Figure 11-5
Amplification antibody method. This technique may be used to intensify the reaction in situations where only minimal reactivity is present. Step *1* of the method is identical with the direct immuno-enzymatic technique. The preparation, however, is subsequently treated with an anti-enzyme antibody and then free enzyme (step *2*), prior to treatment with the substrate for that enzyme to localize the site of the reaction (step *3*). The net result of this technique is amplification of the localized enzymatic reaction.

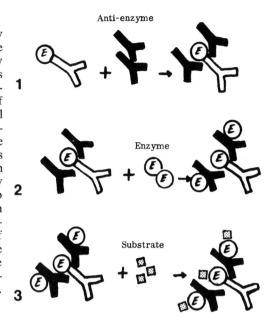

enhanced by the use of anti-enzyme antibody and additional free enzyme. The anti-enzyme antibody is allowed to react with the enzyme-tagged specific antibody, and the preparation is then treated with the free enzyme. This technique depends upon the assumption that the anti-enzyme antibody will react with the conjugated enzyme by using one of its reaction sites, leaving the other free to react with the free enzyme (Fig. 11-5). In this way, the specific immunological reaction that is initiated by the enzyme-labeled antibody is amplified through the binding of a greater amount of enzyme to the reaction site than would otherwise have been present. This feature makes this technique especially adaptable to situations in which the level of antibody binding is minimal.

Sensitivity

In a comparison between immunofluorescence techniques and immuno-enzymatic techniques using a variety of enzymes [4], the level of sensitivity of the enzymatic method was essentially the same or slightly better than the fluorescence method (see Chap. 10). In a comparison of staining patterns in glomerulonephritis, no difference was noted between the immunofluorescence and immunoenzymatic techniques [16].

Sources of Error

Immunoenzymatic techniques are subject to many of the same types of error that may be encountered in immunofluorescence methods. In addition, the histochemical enzyme reactions may not be specific in cases in which endogenous tissue enzymes may interfere with the assays [3, 5]. In studies in which immunoenzymatic techniques are used for the ultrastructural localization of antigen, the molecular size and its effect on penetration are an additional source of error.

CONTROLS

Essentially, the same controls that are used in immunofluorescence studies should be used for immunoenzyme studies [3]. These include:

1. Absorption of the enzyme-labeled antibody with its homologous antigen. This should remove the specific reactivity of the preparation so that subsequent staining does not occur.
2. Comparison of the appearance of a known positive preparation with similar material known to be negative.
3. Treating the preparation with an unrelated antibody coupled with the same enzyme, such as enzyme-labeled normal globulin. This process will indicate whether the reactivity that is seen is specific or not.
4. Inhibition or blocking of the reactivity by the prior application of unlabeled antibody. This should result, if the reaction is specific, in either elimination of, or a significant reduction in, reactivity.
5. Treating the preparation with the enzyme alone. If the enzyme alone binds to the preparation, the reactivity seen following treatment with the enzyme-labeled antibody may not be specific.

UNWANTED SPECIFIC REACTIVITY

Some tissues may contain the same enzyme that is being used as a label. In this instance, when the preparation is treated with the substrate for that enzyme, reactivity will occur at these locations. This can, if unrecognized, lead to confusion. Peroxidase, the most frequently used enzyme in immunoenzymatic studies, is contained in erythrocytes, leukocytes, and macrophages. When using these enzymes as labels, reactivity is to be expected in these sites following reactivity of the preparation with the substrate that is designed to produce the chromogenic reaction products [3].

PENETRATION OF ENZYME-ANTIBODY CONJUGATES

In electron microscope studies using the immunoenzymatic techniques, it is necessary for the conjugate to be able to penetrate the tissues. Enzyme-immunoglobulin conjugates are of such a size (e.g., peroxidase has a molecular weight of 40,000 and immunoglobulin a molecular weight of 90,000) that penetration of tissue is limited. This factor has to be taken into consideration in interpreting negative results. This problem has been partially solved through the use of Fab fragments of immunoglobulin rather than the entire immunoglobulin molecule in the preparation of conjugates. Even with this reduction in size, penetration continues to be a problem [8].

Advantages of Immunoenzymatic Methods

Immunoenzymatic methods have several advantages over immunofluorescence techniques. These advantages include:

1. The preparation can be examined and studied using an ordinary light microscope, obviating the necessity for expensive, special microscopic equipment.
2. Unlike immunofluorescent preparations, immunoenzyme preparations are permanent. This feature makes it possible to retain preparations for later comparison with other material of a similar nature or for later reference in the evaluation of material from patients being studied serially.
3. There are several principles involved in immunoenzymatic staining that make it especially adaptable to detecting multiple antigens within the same tissue preparation. Different enzymes having different substrates may produce reaction products of different colors. By using two different specific antibodies, each labeled with a different enzyme, two different antigens can be detected simultaneously. Since the immunoenzyme preparation is permanent, it is very easily adaptable to the additional application of radiolabeled antibody techniques to the same preparation, thus enabling the detection of additional antigens.
4. Ultrastructural studies may be performed using immunoenzymatic techniques since the reaction product of several of the enzyme substrates is electron-dense. Even though the molecular size of these conjugates presents a problem in relation to tissue preparation, the technique is superior to the immunoferritin technique, which, although it has been used for this purpose, is burdened to a greater extent by the much larger molecular size of the complex involved.

Disadvantages of Immunoenzymatic Methods

Even though the advantages of the immunoenzymatic technique are multiple and are amply sufficient to justify its inclusion in the armamentarium of both the researcher and the clinical pathologist, the technique does have several disadvantages.

1. Unlike the widespread availability of fluorescent conjugates, standardized preparations of enzyme-labeled antibodies are not readily available from commercial sources [17].
2. Enzyme-labeled preparations have not been the subject of the standardization procedures that have been utilized in connection with fluorescent reagents. Clinical laboratories, at this time, cannot obtain reproducible titers on the same individual materials using different reagents.

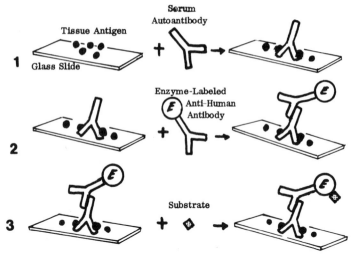

Figure 11-6
Enzyme-labeled antibody method for detection of autoimmune antibodies in serum. The procedure is shown that is followed in using the immunoenzymatic technique to demonstrate the attachment of autoantibodies in serum of patients with autoimmune disease to an antigen substrate on a glass slide.

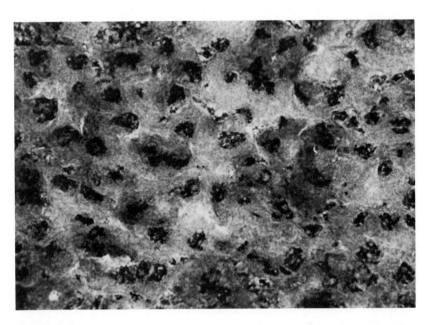

Figure 11-7
Antinuclear antibody demonstrated with the immunoenzymatic technique. (Approx. ×400.)

Applications

Immunoenzymatic methods are adaptable to any of the applications that have been developed for immunofluorescence techniques. The immuno-peroxidase technique has been the most widely developed and studied. It has been widely used for both light and electron microscopic localization of antigens and antibodies in a wide variety of situations.

MICROBIOLOGICAL

Immunoenzymatic techniques have not been widely utilized as of yet in the microbiological area. It has been shown, however, that it is possible to identify the presence of antibody directed toward *Treponema pallidum* performing this technique in the same manner as the fluorescent treponemal antibody (FTA) technique [18].

DETECTION OF AUTOANTIBODIES

The immunoperoxidase technique has become widely used in the detection of autoantibodies (Fig. 11-6), such as anti-nuclear antibody (Fig. 11-7) [18–20], anti-mitochondrial antibodies [18], anti–glomerular basement membrane antibody [16], anti–thyroid cytoplasmic antibody [18], anti–parietal cell antibody [21], anti–striated muscle antibodies, antibodies active against neurons [22], and antibodies present in both pemphigus and bullous pemphigoid [23].

IMMUNE-COMPLEX DISEASE

In the detection and study of tissues suspected of containing immune complexes, the immunoperoxidase technique has been found to be very useful [15, 16]. This approach has an added advantage in that the permanency of the preparation allows for the easy comparison of serial material from patients undergoing therapy for a disease, such as glomerulonephritis (Fig. 11-8).

MISCELLANEOUS

Since enzymes are proteins, they are antigenic. Using peroxidase as an antigen to immunize experimental animals, the morphology of cells that are capable of producing antibody following immunization has been studied [24–26]. This procedure is carried out by simply treating the tissue from the immunized animal with the free enzyme and then with its substrate to produce the electron-dense reaction products. Information gained from this technique has been important in identifying the morphology of cells capable of producing antibody and in determining the intracellular localization of the antibody that is produced. The immunoperoxidase technique has also been used in the detection of surface antigens on lymphocytes by electron microscopy [27], thus providing additional information in this very important area.

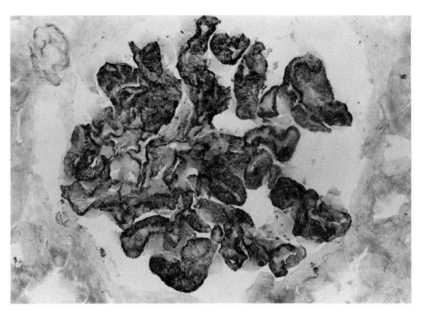

Figure 11-8
Demonstration of immunoglobulin deposition in the glomerulus from a patient with membranous glomerulonephritis using the immunoenzymatic technique. (Approx. ×450.)

References

1. Nakane, P. K., and Pierce, G. B.   Enzyme-labeled antibodies: Preparation and application for the localization of antigens. *J. Histochem. Cytochem.* 14:929, 1966.
2. Avrameas, S., and Uriel, J.   Méthode de marquage d'antigènes et d'anticorps avec des enzymes et son application en immunodiffusion. *C. R. Acad. Sci. [D]* (Paris) 262:2543, 1966.
3. Avrameas, S.   Immunoenzyme techniques: Enzymes as markers for the localization of antigens and antibodies. *Int. Rev. Cytol.* 27:349, 1970.
4. Avrameas, S.   Coupling of enzymes to proteins with glutaraldehyde. Use of the conjugates for the detection of antigens and antibodies. *Immunochemistry* 6:43, 1969.
5. Avrameas, S., and Bouteille, M.   Ultrastructural localization of antibody by antigen label with peroxidase. *Exp. Cell Res.* 53:166, 1968.
6. Avrameas, S., and Ternynck, T.   Biologically active water insoluble protein polymers.   I. Their use for isolation of antigens and antibodies. *J. Biol. Chem.* 242:1651, 1967.
7. Avrameas, S., and Ternynck, T.   The cross-linking of proteins with glutaraldehyde and its use for the preparation of immunoadsorbents. *Immunochemistry* 6:53, 1969.
8. Avrameas, S., and Ternynck, T.   Peroxidase labeled antibody and Fab conjugates with enhanced intracellular penetration. *Immunochemistry* 8:1175, 1971.
9. Nakane, P. K.   Simultaneous localization of multiple tissue antigens

utilizing peroxidase-labeled antibody method: A study on pituitary glands of the rat. *J. Histochem. Cytochem.* 16:557, 1968.

10. Nakane, P. K. Peroxidase-Labeled Antibody Method. In W. Montagna and R. E. Billingham (Eds.), *Advances in Biology of Skin,* Vol. 11. New York: Appleton-Century-Crofts, 1971. P. 283.

11. Nakane, P. K., and Pierce, G. B. Enzyme-labeled antibodies for the light and electron microscopic localization of tissue antigens. *J. Cell Biol.* 33:307, 1967.

12. Nisonoff, A., and Palmer, J. C. Hybridization of half molecules of rabbit gamma globulin. *Science* 143:376, 1964.

13. Nisonoff, A., and Rivers, M. M. Recombination of mixture of univalent antibody fragments of different specificity. *Arch. Biochem. Biophys.* 93:460, 1961.

14. Avrameas, S. Indirect immunoenzyme techniques for the intracellular detection of antigens. *Immunochemistry* 6:825, 1969.

15. Hoedemacker, P. J., Feenstra, K., Nijkenter, A., and Arends, A. Ultrastructural localization of heterologous nephrotoxic antibody in the glomerular basement membrane of the rat. *Lab. Invest.* 26:610, 1972.

16. Davey, F. R., and Busch, G. J. Immunohistochemistry of glomerulonephritis using horseradish peroxidase and fluorescein-labeled antibody: A comparison of two technics. *Am. J. Clin. Pathol.* 53:531, 1970.

17. Nakamura, R. M. Immunoenzyme Histochemical Methods. In R. M. Nakamura (Ed.), *Immunopathology: Clinical Laboratory Concepts and Methods.* Boston: Little, Brown, 1974.

18. Petts, V., and Roitt, I. M. Peroxidase conjugates for demonstration of tissue antibodies: Evaluation of technique. *Clin. Exp. Immunol.* 9:407, 1971.

19. Benson, M. D., and Cohen, A. S. Antinuclear antibodies in systemic lupus erythematosus. *Ann. Intern. Med.* 73:943, 1970.

20. Darling, J., Johnson, G. D., Webb, J. A., and Smith, M. E. Use of peroxidase conjugated antiglobulin as an alternative to immunofluorescence for the detection of antinuclear factor in serum. *J. Clin. Pathol.* 24:501, 1971.

21. Hoedemacker, P. J., and Ito, S. Ultrastructural localization of gastric parietal cell antigen with peroxidase-coupled antibody. *Lab. Invest.* 22:184, 1970.

22. Zeromski, J. Immunological findings in sensory carcinomatous neuropathy. Application of peroxidase labeled antibody. *Clin. Exp. Immunol.* 6:633, 1970.

23. Fukuyama, K., Douglas, S. D., Tuffanelli, D. L., and Epstein, W. L. Immunohistochemical method for localization of antibodies in cutaneous disease. *Am. J. Clin. Pathol.* 54:410, 1970.

24. Gudat, F. G., Harris, T. N., Harris, F., and Hunmeler, K. Studies on antibody-producing cells. I. Ultrastructure of 19S and 7S antibody-producing cells. *J. Exp. Med.* 132:448, 1970.

25. Leduc, E. H., Avrameas, S., and Bouteille, M. Ultrastructural localization of antibody in differentiating plasma cells. *J. Exp. Med.* 127:109, 1968.

26. Leduc, E. H., Scott, G. B., and Avrameas, S. Ultrastructural localization of intracellular immune globulins in plasma cells and lymphoblasts by enzyme-labeled antibodies. *J. Histochem. Cytochem.* 17:211, 1969.

27. Willingham, M. C., Spicer, S. S., and Graber, C. D. Immunocytologic labeling of calf and human lymphocyte surface antigens. *Lab. Invest.* 25:211, 1971.

Enzyme Immunoassays 12

Ludwig H. Bonacker and Richard C. Hevey

The detection and, particularly, the quantitative determination of biologically active components in plasma and other body fluids employ a variety of immunological methods [1–3]. Radioimmunoassay is currently the most sensitive method that is routinely used [4] (see Chap. 6). Although a radiolabeled component occupies a central position in the assay, the label need not be a radionuclide. Instead, radionuclides may be substituted with enzymes as markers, where the resulting catalytic indicator reaction allows the accumulation of the reaction product with time.

Enzyme conjugates are used for the localization of antigens and antibodies in histochemistry and histopathology [5] (see Chap. 11). More recently, the principle of immunoenzymatic histochemical assays, combined with the method of radioimmunoassays, has been applied to the determination of antigens and antibodies in solution [6–9]. Assays employing this combination are known as *enzyme-linked immunosorbent assays* (ELISA) [6], *enzyme immunoassays* [9, 10], and *solid-phase immunosorbent enzyme-linked assays* [11].

Methodology

"SANDWICH" TECHNIQUE

The assay requires the interaction of three types of molecules: (1) a specific antibody directed against the antigen to be assayed, which is coated to an insoluble carrier (e.g., cellulose or plastic tubes); (2) the antigen to be assayed; and (3) the enzyme-labeled antibody that is specific for the antigen. The antigen to be assayed is allowed to react with the immobilized specific antibody. The unreacted antigen is removed, and enzyme-labeled antibody directed against the antigen is then added. Following the reaction of the enzyme-labeled antibody, unreacted conjugate is separated from reacted conjugate by aspiration, and the remaining enzyme activity is measured spectrophotometrically on any accessible spectrophotometer. The enzyme activity is proportional to the amount of antigen in the sample (Fig. 12-1). Alternatively, as in the radioallergo-

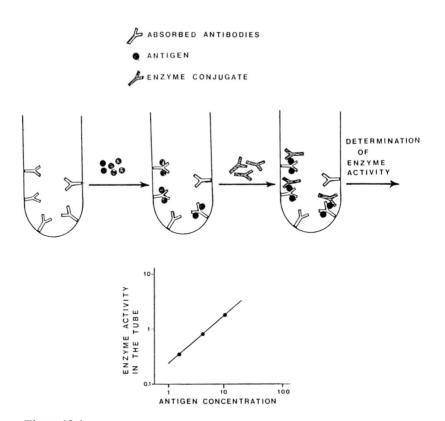

ABSORBED ANTIBODIES

ANTIGEN

ENZYME CONJUGATE

DETERMINATION
OF
ENZYME
ACTIVITY

Figure 12-1
Principle of the "sandwich" technique. A tube coated with antibodies is treated with the sample containing the antigen. Unreacted antigen is aspirated and enzyme-labeled antibody added. Unreacted conjugate is removed, and the remaining enzyme activity measured. The enzyme activity in the tube is proportional to the amount of antigen. A plot of log enzyme activity versus log antigen concentration gives a linear standard curve.

sorbent test (RAST) [12], an antigen may be adsorbed to a solid-phase carrier for the determination of its corresponding antibody. In this case, an enzyme-labeled, secondary antibody that is directed against the antibody to be determined is employed [7, 13, 14]. The "sandwich" technique has been applied in the determination of anti-DNA antibodies [11], α_1-fetoprotein [14], and rabbit IgG [8].

COMPETITIVE-BINDING ANALYSIS
Required for this assay are three components: (1) the insolubilized specific antibody (which may be adsorbed to polystyrene tubes) directed against the antigen to be determined, (2) the antigen to be assayed, and (3) the same antigen, which is enzyme-labeled.

The antigen to be assayed is incubated with a known amount of en-

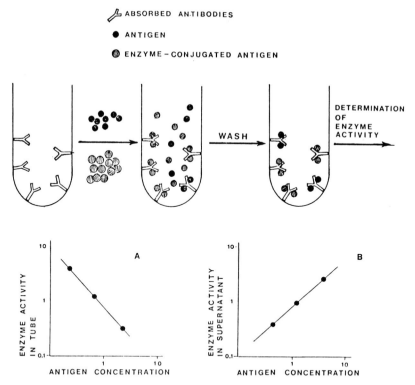

Figure 12-2
Principle of competitive-binding analysis. A tube coated with antibodies is incubated with the sample containing the antigen of unknown concentration and a known amount of enzyme-labeled antigen. After equilibration, unbound antigen is removed and the enzyme activity on the insoluble phase or in the supernatant is measured. The enzyme activity on the insoluble phase is inversely proportional to the antigen concentration in the sample (A). The enzyme activity in the supernatant is directly proportional to the antigen concentration in the sample (B). A plot of log enzyme activity versus log antigen concentration gives a linear standard curve.

zyme-labeled antigen. A competition is established between the antigen to be determined and a known amount of enzyme-labeled antigen for the binding sites of the insolubilized antibodies. After equilibration, the antigen that is bound to the insolubilized antibody is separated from the antigen in solution, and the enzymatic activity of the supernatant or of the insoluble phase is determined [6, 10, 13, 14]. The enzymatic activity in the insoluble phase is inversely proportional to the amount of antigen on the test sample, whereas the enzymatic activity in the supernatant is proportional to the amount of antigen (Fig. 12-2). Competitive-binding analysis has been used in the determination of insulin [9, 15] and human chorionic gonadotropin [10].

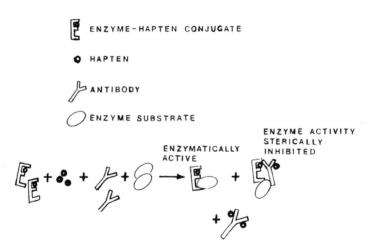

Figure 12-3

Principle of the homogeneous enzyme immunoassay. A hapten is covalently coupled near the active site of an enzyme. A competition for a defined amount of hapten-specific antibodies is established between the enzyme-labeled hapten and free hapten in the test sample. Unreacted enzyme-labeled hapten retains its enzymatic activity, but enzyme-labeled hapten that has reacted with antibodies is enzymatically inactive. Since the extent of neutralization of added antibodies is dependent on the hapten concentration in the sample, the amount of enzymatic activity remaining after reaction is proportional to the free hapten concentration.

HOMOGENEOUS ENZYME IMMUNOASSAY

A requirement of all radioimmunoassays and enzyme immunoassays is that the antigen which is bound to the antibody must be physically separated from the unreacted antigen. Immunoassay methods in which only one phase is used are known as *homogeneous immunoassays* [16–18], and these require no separation steps. In this homogeneous immunoassay system, an enzyme is coupled to a molecule (a hapten such as morphine, phenobarbital, or testosterone) in such a manner that the enzyme cannot catalyze the turnover of its substrate when the enzyme-labeled hapten is reacted with its corresponding antibody. The exact mechanism of the inhibition of the enzyme is not known, but it probably is caused by steric hindrance of the active site of the enzyme [17]. When the specimen is mixed with the antibody and enzyme-labeled hapten, free hapten molecules present in the specimen compete with the enzyme-labeled hapten for antibody binding sites. The higher the hapten concentration in the specimen, the greater is the neutralization of added antibodies. Since antibodies are consumed by free hapten, more enzyme conjugate remains unbound and enzymatically active. Therefore, the enzyme activity is proportional to the concentration of hapten in the specimen (Fig. 12-3). Opiates, barbiturates, and amphetamines can be determined by homogeneous enzyme immunoassay [16, 19].

Sources of Error

Uncertainties and possible sources of error in enzyme immunoassays may conceivably arise from variations of pH, temperature, and substrate concentration, which affect the enzyme activity. The extended use of unstable reagents or substrates could contribute significant errors in the enzymatic assay. It should also be considered that enzyme inhibitors which might be present in the samples and the inactivation of the enzyme during prolonged incubation may affect the results.

Advantages

Enzyme immunoassays have several advantages over other methods. They are simple, quantitative techniques with high sensitivity that do not require extensive training of laboratory personnel and that can be adapted to any laboratory that conducts routine enzymatic assays. Problems in the handling of radioisotopes are not encountered, and expensive equipment is not required.

Disadvantages

As with radioimmunoassays, the problems encountered are the need for highly specific antibodies and the relatively long incubation periods that are necessary to achieve the high sensitivity of the assay. With the exception of homogeneous enzyme immunoassays, which take only minutes to conduct, the time required to conduct enzyme immunoassays may range from 5 to 24 hours. Improvements in the procedures for the preparation of conjugates with high enzymatic and immunological activities are necessary in order to provide reagents for routine use.

Applications

There is no theoretical limit to the number or nature of biological compounds of interest—including proteins, hormones, and haptens—that can be determined by enzyme immunoassays. Enzyme-labeled proteins and haptens, which are the key constituents in the assay, can be prepared in various ways [10, 20, 21]. Bifunctional reagents, however, have been most frequently employed for the preparation of conjugates [22, 23, 24].

The enzyme that is chosen for conjugation should have a high specific activity and a facile procedure for its determination. A basic requirement is that enzymatic activity must be retained after conjugation. Horseradish peroxidase and alkaline phosphatase, while meeting these requirements, have the added advantage that they catalyze the turnover of achromatic substrates into chromatic products, and they have therefore been successfully used for conjugation [5, 7, 8, 9, 20, 25].

IMMUNOGLOBULIN G (IgG)

Enzyme immunoassays (EIA) were initially applied by Engvall and Perlmann [6–8] for the determination of rabbit IgG. Using glutaraldehyde as the coupling reagent for the conjugation of rabbit IgG to alkaline phosphatase, they demonstrated that the enzyme-linked immunosorbent assay (ELISA) was as sensitive and precise as the radioimmunosorbent test (RIST). By employing equilibrium competitive-binding analysis (see Fig. 12-2) with the antibody covalently bound to microcrystalline cellulose, an assay range of approximately 50 to 1000 ng per milliliter was obtained [6]. Modification of the above system by the use of polystyrene tubes simplified the assay procedure [7].

A sensitive method for the quantitative determination of antibodies that applies the principle of the radioallergosorbent test (RAST) has been reported [8]. When rabbit antisera against human serum albumin or the dinitrophenyl group (DNP) were tested, less than 1 ng per milliliter of specific antibodies could be detected. Typical standard curves that were obtained are shown in Figure 12-4.

An EIA employing glucose oxidase-conjugated anti-IgG has been utilized for the quantitative determination of human IgG [9].

IMMUNOGLOBULIN E (IgE)

A study of the quantitative determination of IgE by EIA has been conducted, and the results have been compared to those of the radioimmunosorbent test (RIST) for IgE. The EIA system consisted of IgE myeloma protein conjugated by glutaraldehyde to alkaline phosphatase and antibody-coated plastic tubes. In competitive protein-binding analysis, the IgE content in patients' sera and in standard preparations gave a rank-order correlation coefficient of 0.97 when compared to the RIST test [26].

α_1-FETOPROTEIN

Rat α_1-fetoprotein has been quantitatively determined by an EIA system in which both the competitive protein-binding procedure and the "sandwich" technique were employed [13]. The results of the EIA, when compared to electroimmunodiffusion (EID), were discrepant by 15 to 30 percent in the amount of rat α_1-fetoprotein determined [14].

An EIA for human α_1-fetoprotein has recently been reported [27]. The basic method of this assay consists of allowing α_1-fetoprotein to react with enzyme-labeled α_1-fetoprotein antibody in slight excess. After incubation, an immunosorbent of insolubilized α_1-fetoprotein is added to bind unreacted, excess conjugate. The enzymatic activity of the supernatant is proportional to the amount of antigen in the sample. The test gave reproducible results in the assay range of 0.7 to 15 ng per milliliter of α_1-fetoprotein. The coefficient of variation varied from 3 to 15 percent in the assay range. In testing sera of healthy adults, pregnant

Figure 12-4
Standard curves for determination of specific antibodies. *A.* Dilutions of standard anti-HSA serum, 5.2 mg/ml HSA antibodies. *B. Upper curve:* Dilutions of standard anti-DNP serum, 2.5 mg/ml DNP antibodies. *Lower curve:* Dilutions of an anti-DNP serum collected 13 days after one injection of 5 mg DNP-BGG. (Reproduced by permission. From Engvall, E., and Pearlmann, P. *J. Immunol.* 109: 133, © 1972 The Williams & Wilkins Co., Baltimore.)

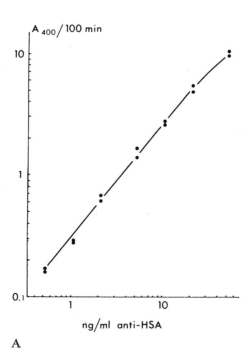

A

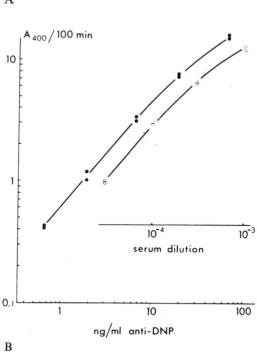

B

women, and adults with liver diseases by enzyme immunoassay and by radioimmunoassay, a correlation coefficient of 0.95 was obtained [27].

OTHER PROTEINS

EIA has also been applied to DNA-antibody determination in systemic lupus erythematosus [11] and to the quantitation of haptoglobin in human serum [28]. Another application has been the use of EIA for the determination of antibodies and antibody classes in hyperimmune sera obtained by the immunization of animals with antigens from microbiological organisms [25, 29, 30, 31].

DETERMINATION OF HORMONES AND HAPTENS

The application of EIA for the determination of hormones reflects the principles and procedures mentioned previously. Because of the relatively small size of hormone and hapten molecules, competitive protein-binding analysis has been exclusively utilized.

An immunosorbent assay for the determination of human chorionic gonadotropin (HCG) in urine has been reported [10]. The results of the competitive protein-binding assay for HCG that was conjugated to peroxidase had a sensitivity comparable to the hemagglutination-inhibition or complement-fixation tests.

In the insulin-anti-insulin system, variable sensitivity ranges for EIA have been reported. In one procedure, a sensitivity comparable to that of radioimmunoassay was obtained [15], while in another procedure, insulin could only be quantitated in a concentration range of 75 to 200 milliunits per milliliter [28].

An interesting new test system, homogeneous enzyme immunoassay (see Fig. 12-3), has been developed for the determination of haptens such as morphine [16–18]. In the test system for morphine, the hapten is chemically bound to lysozyme. Morphine concentrations in urine greater than 0.5 μg per milliliter could be quantitated [16, 18]. The sensitivity of the homogeneous enzyme immunoassay lies between the sensitivity range of radioimmunoassay and thin-layer chromatography for morphine, i.e., between 30 ng per milliliter and 1 μg per milliliter [19, 32].

References

1. Becker, W., Rapp, W., Schwick, H. G., and Störiko, K.   Quantitative determination of plasma proteins by immunoprecipitation. *Z. Klin. Chem.* 6:113, 1968.
2. Gill, T. J.   Methods for detecting antibody. *Immunochemistry* 7:997, 1970.
3. Schwick, H. G.   Immunological Methods in Clinical Chemistry. In O. Wieland (Ed.), *Sixth International Congress of Clinical Chemistry, Munich, 1966; Clinical Protein Chemistry,* Vol. 1. Basel: Karger, 1968. Pp. 93–105.

4. Skelly, D. S., Brown, L. P., and Besch, P. K. Radioimmunoassay. *Clin. Chem.* 19:146, 1973.
5. Avrameas, S. Immunoenzyme techniques: Enzymes as markers for the localization of antigens and antibodies. *Int. Rev. Cytol.* 27:349, 1970.
6. Engvall, E., and Perlmann, P. Enzyme-linked immunosorbent assay (ELISA). Quantitative assay of immunoglobulin G. *Immunochemistry* 8:871, 1971.
7. Engvall, E., Jonsson, K., and Perlmann, P. Enzyme-linked immunosorbent assay. II. Quantitative assay of protein antigen, immunoglobulin G, by means of enzyme-labelled antigen and antibody-coated tubes. *Biochim. Biophys. Acta* 251:427, 1971.
8. Engvall, E., and Perlmann, P. Enzyme-linked immunosorbent assay, ELISA. III. Quantitation of specific antibodies by enzyme-labeled anti-immunoglobulin in antigen-coated tubes. *J. Immunol.* 109:129, 1972.
9. Masseyeff, R., Maiolini, R., and Bouron, Y. A method of enzyme immunoassay. *Biomedicine* 19:314, 1973.
10. Van Weemen, B. K., and Schuurs, A. H. W. M. Immunoassay using antigen-enzyme conjugates. *F.E.B.S. Letters* 15:232, 1971.
11. Pesce, A. J., Mendoza, N., Boreisha, I., Gaizutis, M. A., and Pollak, V. E. Use of enzyme-linked antibodies to measure serum anti-DNA antibody in systemic lupus erythematosus. *Clin. Chem.* 20:353, 1974.
12. Johansson, S. G. O., Bennich, H. H., and Berg, T. The clinical significance of IgE. *Prog. Clin. Immunol.* 1:157, 1972.
13. Belanger, L., Sylvestre, C., and Dufour, D. Enzyme-linked immunoassay for alpha-fetoprotein by competitive and sandwich procedures. *Clin. Chim. Acta* 48:15, 1973.
14. Belanger, L., and Dufour, D. Le dosage immunoenzymologique de l'AFP. *Colloquium on Alpha Fetoprotein,* Nice, France, 1974.
15. Ishikawa, E. Enzyme immunoassay of insulin by fluorimetry of the insulin-glucoamylase complex. *J. Biochem.* (Tokyo) 73:1319, 1973.
16. Bastiani, R. J., Phillips, R. C., Schneider, R. S., and Ullman, E. F. Homogeneous immunochemical drug assays. *Am. J. Med. Technol.* 39:211, 1973.
17. Rubenstein, K. E., Schneider, R. S., and Ullman, E. F. Homogeneous enzyme immunoassay. A new immunochemical technique. *Biochem. Biophys. Res. Commun.* 47:846, 1972.
18. Schneider, R. S., Lindquist, P., Tong-in Wong, E., Rubenstein, K. E., and Ullman, E. F. Homogeneous enzyme immunoassay for opiates in urine. *Clin. Chem.* 19:821, 1973.
19. Mule, S. J., Bastos, M. L., and Jukofsky, D. Evaluation of immunoassay methods for detection, in urine, of drugs subject to abuse. *Clin. Chem.* 20:243, 1974.
20. Kawaoi, A., and Nakane, P. K. An improved method of conjugation of peroxidase with proteins. *Fed. Proc.* 32(3):3508, 1973.
21. Sternberger, L. A., Cuculis, J. J., Meyer, H. G., Lenz, D. E., and Kavanagh, W. G. Antibodies to organophosphorus haptens. Immunity to paraoxon poisoning. *Fed. Proc.* 33(3):2930, 1974.
22. Avrameas, S. Coupling of enzymes to proteins with glutaraldehyde. Use of the conjugates for the detection of antigens and antibodies. *Immunochemistry* 6:43, 1969.
23. Erlanger, B. F. Principles and methods for the preparation of drug protein conjugates for immunological studies. *Pharmacol. Rev.* 25:271, 1973.

24. Likhite, V., and Sehon, A. Protein-protein conjugation. In C. A. Williams and M. W. Chase (Eds.), *Methods in Immunology and Immunochemistry*. New York: Academic, 1967.
25. Herrmann, J. E., and Morse, S. A. Coupling of peroxidase to poliovirus antibody: Characteristics of the conjugates and their use in virus detection. *Infect. Immunity* 8:645, 1973.
26. Hoffman, D. R. Estimation of serum IgE by an enzyme-linked immunosorbent assay (ELISA). *J. Allergy Clin. Immunol.* 51:303, 1973.
27. Maiolini, R., Ferrua, B., and Masseyeff, R. Dosage enzymo-immunologique de l'alpha-foetoprotéine humaine. *Colloquium on Alpha Fetoprotein,* Nice, France, 1974.
28. Miedema, K., Boelhouwer, J., and Otten, J. W. Determinations of proteins and hormones in serum by an immunoassay using antigen-enzyme conjugates. *Clin. Chim. Acta* 40:187, 1972.
29. Carlsson, H. E., Lindberg, A. A., and Hammarstroem, S. Titration of antibodies to salmonella O antigens by enzyme-linked immunosorbent assay. *Infect. Immunity* 6:703, 1972.
30. Holmgren, J., and Svennerholm, A. M. Enzyme-linked immunosorbent assays for cholera serology. *Infect. Immunity* 7:759, 1973.
31. Saunders, G. C., and Wilder, M. E. Disease screening with enzyme-labeled antibodies. *J. Infect. Dis.* 129:362, 1974.
32. Walberg, C. B. Correlation of the "EMIT" urine barbiturate assay with a spectrophotometric serum barbiturate assay in suspected overdose. *Clin. Chem.* 20:305, 1974.

Serum Protein Abnormalities

Albumin Abnormalities 13

Gerald A. Beathard

Quantitative change in the level of serum albumin represents an important and frequently used indicator of the presence or progression of disease. For practical purposes, this is limited to varying degrees of hypoalbuminemia, since, with the exception of cases of acute dehydration, hyperalbuminemia does not occur [1, 2]. Serum albumin represents only a fraction of the total body pool of albumin. Its level at any given time depends upon the balance between the processes of synthesis, catabolism (i.e., endogenous degradation plus external loss), and distribution. Reductions in the body's total albumin pool, which are generally reflected by changes in serum albumin, can be produced by one or, in many instances, a combination of three separate mechanisms: reduced synthesis, excessive loss, or increased degradation. This chapter is concerned with a review of these processes and the examination of some of the more important clinical situations characterized by abnormalities in albumin metabolism.

Physiological Considerations

DISTRIBUTION OF ALBUMIN

Albumin is the major protein produced by the liver (see Appendix), and it represents more than half of the total protein present in serum. Only 30 to 40 percent of the body's total exchangeable albumin pool, however, is located in the intravascular compartment [1]. The remainder is extravascular and is found within the interstitial spaces (Fig. 13-1). The majority of the interstitial albumin in man is present in the muscles and skin. The liver, lung, heart, kidney, and spleen contain only minor portions. Although it constitutes only 6 percent of the total body weight, the skin contains 30 to 40 percent of the total extravascular albumin [3]. Lymph contains only 2 or 3 percent of the total interstitial albumin, and its concentration in different sites is quite variable [4, 5] (Table 13-1). Albumin is also found in small amounts in a variety of different body tissue fluids, such as sweat, tears, gastric juice, and bile [2].

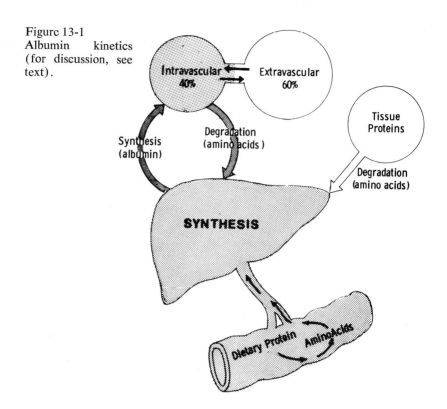

Figure 13-1
Albumin kinetics
(for discussion, see
text).

FUNCTIONS OF ALBUMIN

Albumin has two primary functions: the provision of colloidal osmotic pressure and the transport of long-chain fatty acids, bilirubin, hormones, calcium, metal anions, drugs, and vitamins. It also functions as an endogenous source of amino acids.

ONCOTIC FUNCTION

Although albumin accounts for only 50 to 60 percent of the total plasma protein, it contributes 80 percent of the colloid osmotic pressure because of its small molecular weight [6]. Even though hypoalbuminemia results in edema, a definite linear correlation between the incidence or degree of hypoproteinemic edema or serous effusions and the concentration of albumin in plasma does not exist. The presence or absence of edema in hypoalbuminemic states in large part depends upon sodium and water balance (see Fig. 13-4).

Albumin also plays a major role in regulating the size of the extravascular space. Albumin in the interstitial fluid competes with intravascular albumin in holding water that has been filtered into the extravascular area. This interstitial albumin may exert a greater osmotic effect than would be expected simply from a consideration of its concentration and the observed water content of the interstitium. Albumin may be excluded

Table 13-1. Lymph Albumin Concentrations

Source	Lymph/Plasma Ratio
Thoracic duct	0.51–0.87
Liver	0.90
Intestine	0.70 (average)
Muscle	0.20–0.30

Reproduced by permission. From Yoffey, J. M., and Courtice, M. C. *Lymphatics, Lymph and Lymphomyeloid Complex.* New York: Academic, 1970.

from much of the interstitial water space by substances such as hyaluronic acid, and it may actually be dissolved in only a fraction of it, thereby increasing its effective contribution to interstitial osmotic pressure [7].

TRANSPORT FUNCTION

The second major physiological function of albumin relates to its unusually strong affinity for a number of cations and other substances of considerable biological importance to the homeostasis of the individual [2, 6]. This affinity is the basis for its transport function. Of the substances bound to and transported by albumin, bilirubin and long-chain fatty acid anions are the most important. Their binding is so complete that less than $\frac{1}{5000}$ of their total remains free in the circulation [8]. Albumin plays an important role in fat metabolism, binding fatty acid anions released from adipose tissue and keeping them in a soluble form in the plasma [9]. The hyperlipemia occurring in patients with hypoalbuminemia demonstrates the importance of this function.

Hormones bound to albumin exist in a state of equilibrium that permits small quantities of free hormones to be available at all times [2]. Nearly all of the circulating esterol is bound to serum albumin [8]. Corticosteroids are bound primarily by a specific binding globulin; however, once this is saturated, albumin becomes the major means for transport [10]. Approximately 10 percent of thyroxine is bound to serum albumin [2, 11]. The relationship between serum albumin and the substances dependent upon it for transport is illustrated by the changes in serum levels of these substances that are seen in association with pathological states characterized by hypoalbuminemia. This is especially true for substances such as calcium. For this reason, the interpretation of a low serum calcium requires that the physician also know the serum albumin level [12] (see Fig. 13-5).

SOURCE OF ENDOGENOUS AMINO ACIDS

Albumin represents a good potential source for many essential amino acids. It has been considered to be a major reserve of amino acids, its rapid turnover providing for the recycling of these substances [13, 14]. The importance of this function has yet to be proved.

Table 13-2. Normal Albumin Levels

	Serum Levels (gm/100 ml)	Albumin Synthesis (mg/kg/day)	Total Exchangeable Pool (gm/kg)	Intravascular Pool (%)
Males	3.5–5.0	150–250	4.0–5.0	31–42
Females	3.5–5.0	150–180	3.5–4.5	31–42

NORMAL ALBUMIN LEVELS

The normal mean value for serum albumin is approximately 4.2 gm per 100 ml [1, 14], with a standard deviation of 0.35 gm per 100 ml and a range of 3.5 to 5.0 gm per 100 ml [1, 15] (Table 13-2). According to a study of normal Caucasians, the serum albumin level is 0.2 gm per 100 ml higher in males than in females between the ages of 20 and 50. This difference decreases after that time, becoming insignificant by age 70 [16, 17]. A slight decrease in albumin concentration has been reported with advancing age in patients of both sexes [18]. Racial differences in serum albumin levels have been reported [19, 20], with values in Caucasians being 0.33 gm per 100 ml higher than in Negroids. These differences may be due to socioeconomic rather than genetic factors [8].

The total exchangeable albumin pool for normal individuals ranges from 4.0 to 5.0 gm per kilogram of body weight for men and 3.5 to 4.5 gm per kilogram of body weight for women (see Table 13-2). The distribution of this pool in the body is such that 31 to 42 percent is intravascular and the remainder is extravascular. The existence of albumin in the intracellular fluid is doubtful. It has been identified within the cytoplasm of hepatic cells bound to cytoplasmic particles; however, this represents newly synthesized albumin [21]. Albumin taken up by cells of other organs is rapidly degraded [22].

BIOCHEMISTRY OF ALBUMIN

Albumin has a molecular weight of 65,000 daltons and contains 575 amino acids [1, 8]. Chemical groups on the surface of the molecule are such that two to five adaptable sites are presented that have a high affinity for large organic anions. These sites are critical for albumin's transport function [23]. Observations made after rupturing bonds within the albumin molecule indicate that it is a single peptide chain that is provided structure chiefly by the presence of 17 disulfide bonds [8]. Structurally, the single peptide chain is pictured as weaving through four connected globular segments of unequal size to form a molecule that has been determined to have an ellipsoid shape with major and minor axes of 140 and 40 A [8, 24].

Albumin is extremely soluble in water and has a negative charge of 19 at the normal pH of blood. This latter feature of albumin causes it to migrate rapidly toward the anode during serum protein electrophoresis (see Chap. 1) and is largely responsible for the Donnan effect of blood [25].

Causes of Heterogeneity. Heterogeneity, which results in alterations in electrophoretic mobility, has been frequently documented in studying preparations of human albumin under a variety of circumstances [26–29]. The causes for this have been ascribed to a variety of factors: impurities, polymerization, mixed disulfides, binding of anions, isomerization at pH 3 to 4, configurational variants, possible "molecular aging," and the occurrence of certain genetic variants [8].

Genetic variants of albumin. Albumin polymorphism was first described by Scheurlen [30], who found a double albumin peak on serum protein electrophoresis done on one of a series of patients with diabetes mellitus. This condition, referred to as *bisalbuminemia,* was found to be familial [31]. Since that time, 23 electrophoretically distinct variants of human albumin have been described in addition to the normal variety, which is referred to as *albumin A* [32].

An albumin variant appears to be inherited as a simple, autosomal, codominant trait, the locus for which is closely linked to that for the genes determining Gc protein variants [33]. The term *alloalbuminemia* has been recommended to designate the condition in which an individual exhibits any albumin variant other than albumin A [8]. Patients with alloalbuminemia who are heterozygotes have the condition referred to as *bisalbuminemia,* with a double albumin spike or band that is found on serum protein electrophoresis. Homozygotes show only a single albumin spike or band, and these are frequently overlooked because of a failure to take note of minor abnormalities in the single abnormal electrophoretic band [34]. The double band seen in heterozygous alloalbuminemia is not easily overlooked.

The molecular basis for the difference between an albumin variant and normal human albumin is presumably a single amino-acid residue substitution resulting from a single nucleotide change in the DNA codon [8]. Patients with alloalbuminemia of either the heterozygous or homozygous type have no significant associated clinical or biochemical abnormality other than the disorder of synthesis resulting in the variant serum protein [32].

ALBUMIN SYNTHESIS

Albumin synthesis takes place in the liver and amounts to approximately one-third of the total protein production of that organ [8]. The details of the protein-synthesizing mechanism that results in the production of albumin by the liver have not been completely elucidated; however, all available evidence indicates that albumin is produced by the hepatocyte, using free amino acids by the same general mechanism as the biosynthesis of proteins by other types of cells [8, 35, 36] (Fig. 13-2). Evidence obtained both in vivo and in vitro using labeled amino acids indicates that membrane-bound polysomes are the exclusive sites of serum albumin synthesis by the liver cell [37, 38]. This is in contrast to other proteins, such as ferritin, which are formed by free cytoplasmic polysomes [38].

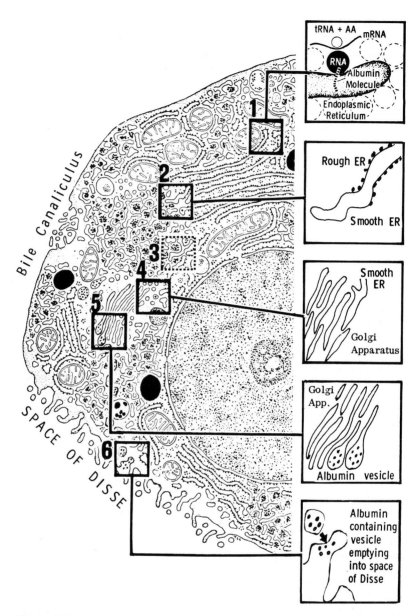

Figure 13-2
Albumin synthesis by hepatocyte. The sequential synthesis and secretion of albumin by the hepatocyte begins (*1*) with the formation of the polypeptide chain through the interaction of rRNA, mRNA, and tRNA. The albumin, once it is formed, passes into the cisternae of the smooth endoplasmic reticulum (*2* and *3*). The newly synthesized albumin ultimately arrives in the Golgi apparatus (*4*), from which small vesicles containing albumin develop (*5*). These vesicles then migrate to the cell surface, where they are discharged into Disse's spaces (*6*).

Studies using radioisotopically tagged leucine [39] have shown the appearance of albumin on membrane-bound polysomes within two minutes following intravenous injections. It then passes through the membrane system of the hepatocyte (see Fig. 13-2) and enters Disse's spaces. This space communicates freely with the hepatic sinusoid-containing portal blood which receives the newly synthesized protein [40, 41]. The processes leading to the synthesis of albumin and its transport to the point of release into the portal circulation require approximately 20 minutes [1, 39].

The equilibration of newly synthesized albumin with the total body pool is a process that can best be understood by a consideration of the equilibration kinetics of an intravenous injection of tagged albumin in man. A 90 percent intravascular equilibration occurs within 2 minutes [42]. Some intravascular areas apparently have slower rates of equilibration so that a total of 10 to 15 minutes is required for complete intravascular distribution to occur [2]. Loss of albumin from the intravascular compartment is a slow process. In most instances, less than 10 percent of the intravascular material is lost during the first two hours. This is true even in abnormal situations, such as heart failure with edema or cirrhosis with ascites [43, 44]. More than three-fourths of the injected protein equilibrates with the extravascular pool within 48 hours. Complete distribution equilibrium requires approximately one week [2].

The delivery of newly synthesized albumin into the circulation bypasses the lymph under normal conditions [40, 41], although lymph is important in the recirculation of albumin from extravascular areas to the plasma. In the cirrhotic patient, there is some transfer of newly synthesized albumin directly into the lymph [44].

RATES OF SYNTHESIS
The rate of albumin synthesis is constant in normal individuals at 150 to 250 mg per kilogram per day [45, 46]. This results in the production of 10 to 18 gm of albumin in a 70 kg man per day, or an average of approximately 14 gm.

Current evidence suggests that the albumin-synthesizing mechanism of the liver is not in constant use, but it usually is operating at about one-third of its potential capacity. This indicates the reserve capacity of the liver and suggests the operation of a control mechanism that prevents hyperalbuminemia [1, 39].

FACTORS AFFECTING ALBUMIN SYNTHESIS
The process of albumin synthesis can be significantly affected by a variety of factors, such as enzyme poisons, hormonal changes, energy imbalance, inadequate diet, disease, or environmental alterations [2]. Clinically, however, the primary factors (short of liver disease) are protein and amino acid nutrition, colloidal osmotic pressure, and the action of hormones [8].

Nutrition. With fasting or in the case of a grossly protein-deficient diet, there is a significant slowing of albumin synthesis, even with an adequate caloric intake [47, 48]. In patients with chronic malnutrition, e.g., in kwashiorkor, albumin synthesis is depressed to values that are less than half the normal rate [49]. In malnourished children, depressed albumin synthesis rates ranging from 100 to 148 mg per kilogram per day have been reported [48]. These studies have been confirmed in animal models, where fasting for 18 to 24 hours has been shown to cause a 30 to 40 percent reduction in albumin synthesis [13, 50].

Malnutrition affects the subcellular protein-synthesizing mechanism of the hepatocyte, resulting in a disaggregation of the polysome to a polysome with a lower ribosome content [13]. Reversion to the heavy type of polysome that is effective in albumin synthesis occurs rapidly in the whole animal after feeding protein [48] or after the feeding of an excessive amount of tryptophan [8]. Isoleucine has a similar but less efficient effect than tryptophan [51].

Clinically as well as experimentally, amino acid mixtures can be substituted for protein in supporting albumin synthesis. This effect depends, however, upon the quality as well as the quantity of the amino acids. Tryptophan-deficient mixtures lead to deficient albumin synthesis [52]. The role played by tryptophan is not clear, but it does not relate simply to the supply of this amino acid that is necessary for incorporation into albumin, since albumin contains less tryptophan than do most other proteins [8]. Current evidence suggests that trytophan plays a role in ribosome-mRNA-endoplasmic reticulum stability or complexing [1].

In the normal individual, albumin synthesis responds to the availability of amino acids provided by the portal blood following each protein-containing meal, which results in cyclic changes in the rate of albumin synthesis. This sensitivity to dietary amino acids appears to be specific for albumin, since the level of dietary protein affects the turnover of globulins only slightly [53].

Oncotic pressure. Since the concept that albumin synthesis in man might be related to changes in oncotic pressure first received attention [54], considerable in vivo and in vitro evidence has been accumulated to support the existence of such a relationship [55–58]. The exact mechanisms of this effect of oncotic pressure on albumin synthesis have been difficult to define, however. Studies investigating this relationship have shown that albumin synthesis actually reflects an inverse relationship not to plasma oncotic pressure, but to extravascular albumin levels [54, 56, 58]. This fact has suggested that the oncotic mechanism for the control of albumin synthesis is located at an extravascular site at or near the site of albumin synthesis [1, 59], a hypothesis which is supported by animal studies [54].

The relation between serum albumin levels and synthesis rates in man is somewhat variable. Anderson and Rossing [60] demonstrated a weakly inverse, nonlinear response of albumin synthesis in a normal individual made hyperalbuminemic by the infusion of albumin and hypoalbuminemic by plasmapheresis. A direct, linear relationship was seen between albumin catabolism and serum albumin levels. Thus, it appears that in man the rate of catabolism of albumin is much more sensitive to changes in albumin concentrations than is the rate of albumin synthesis.

In human disease, the effects of hypoalbuminemia on albumin synthesis are variable. High rates of synthesis have occasionally been observed in patients with hypoalbuminemia due to diseases such as nephrosis or cirrhosis [61, 62]; however, the absolute rate of synthesis is not consistently elevated in these diseases and it may even be decreased [61, 63, 64]. This variability is probably related to variability in the total and extravascular albumin pools.

In summary, changes in oncotic pressure can be shown to result in inverse changes in albumin synthesis, and these changes are related primarily to changes in the extravascular albumin concentration. Intravascular albumin levels do not always correlate with extravascular levels, so that albumin synthesis rates in patients who are hypoalbuminemic are somewhat variable. The infusion of albumin to raise the serum albumin level has a greater effect in increasing catabolism than it does in decreasing synthesis, and hypoalbuminemia is more effective in decreasing catabolism than in increasing synthesis [2].

Hormones. Several hormones have been shown to exert specific effects on albumin synthesis [2]. In experimental animals, albumin synthesis is decreased by the removal of the pituitary, adrenals, or thyroid gland, whereas anabolic hormones such as testosterone cause an increased synthesis rate [1].

Thyroid hormone has an important effect on the albumin-synthesizing mechanism of the liver. It stimulates rRNA synthesis, enhances the binding of rRNA to endoplasmic reticulum, and stimulates the synthesis of mRNA [1, 65, 66].

When thyroid is given in excessive doses of 0.4 to 1 gm per day, a rapid increase in albumin synthesis occurs. This is paralleled by an equivalent increase in albumin degradation, so that no overall change in the size of the albumin pool occurs [67] (Fig. 13-3). Similar changes have been noted in patients with spontaneous thyrotoxicosis [1, 68]. Because the increased rate of degradation is balanced against an increased synthesis rate, the long-range effects of thyrotoxicosis on albumin levels largely depend upon the continuance of good nutrition. Clinically, hypoalbuminemia is not usually seen [1].

In patients with myxedema, the reverse picture is seen: a low albumin synthesis rate and a decreased albumin degradation rate occur [16]. There is a shift in the normal distribution of albumin, however, so that the extravascular pool may contain as much as 80 percent of the exchangeable albumin [66, 68]. This contributes in part to the edematous appearance of these patients.

In normal animals [69] and man [70], corticosteroids cause an early increase in albumin degradation that is followed by a compensatory increase in the albumin synthesis rate. The net effect of increasing degradation and synthesis rates for albumin is little or no change in the size of the exchangeable albumin pool [1]. Corticosteroids do produce a change in the distribution of albumin, however, which results in a shift of extravascular albumin into the intravascular space. This decrease in extravascular albumin is reflected in the liver interstitial space and therefore could

Albumin Kinetics In Disease

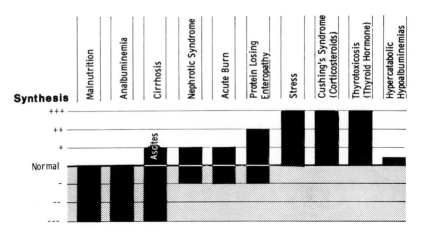

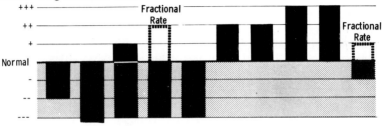

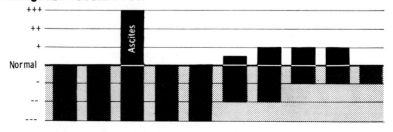

Figure 13-3

Albumin kinetics in disease: relationship between synthesis, absolute degradation rate, and exchangeable albumin pools in a variety of different disease situations. It should be noted that in many of these situations, one or more of these variables may range from negative to positive. This represents the variability that may be seen in different patients under varying circumstances.

contribute to the increase in albumin synthesis that results [59]. Studies of patients with Cushing's syndrome have shown that similar changes in albumin synthesis rates occur in this disease state [70] (see Fig. 13-3).

Studies concerning the mechanism by which corticosteroids affect albumin synthesis have indicated that cortisone stimulates the synthesis of liver RNA, including rRNA, tRNA, and mRNA [71]. In addition, there is evidence to suggest that cortisone promotes the binding of ribosomes to the endoplasmic reticulum to form the albumin-synthesizing mechanism of the hepatocyte [72].

Effect of liver damage on albumin synthesis. The serum albumin level seen clinically in the healthy individual represents the net effect of an interplay between nutrition, hormonal factors, and the effects of albumin distribution, as well as the minor contributory effects of the other factors that have been listed. Changes in any of these factors can cause changes in serum albumin; however, impaired hepatic function is the primary, single cause of pathologically depressed serum albumin levels [8]. The liver has a considerable reserve potential; only 10 to 25 percent of the hepatic cells are essential to provide a normal level of albumin synthesis. Since liver damage must be severe for serum albumin levels to be depressed [73], situations that affect all liver cells, such as toxins or disease processes associated with massive hepatic necrosis (hepatitis), are much more effective in producing hypoalbuminemia than are diseases, such as cirrhosis, which leave a number of hepatic cells unaffected [8].

In addition to these factors, there are a number of toxins that can affect the liver's ability to produce albumin. The most important toxin from the clinical viewpoint is alcohol, which has been shown to cause disruption of the endoplasmic reticulum of the hepatocyte of man [74] and to result in decreased albumin synthesis in perfused animal livers [75]. In addition, the secretion of albumin is highly sensitive to the membrane damage produced by such toxins as carbon tetrachloride [76]. Sublethal irradiation [77] also causes sufficient liver injury to impair albumin synthesis. The transport of newly synthesized albumin within the hepatocytes to its point of release from the cells is slowed by a reduced potassium level [78].

Miscellaneous factors affecting albumin synthesis. Albumin synthesis in the liver can also be affected by a number of other specific and nonspecific factors. Growth hormone, testosterone, and insulin have been shown to increase albumin synthesis to a degree [1, 79, 80]. Environmental factors also appear to play a role in the rate of albumin synthesis. In hot tropical climates, albumin levels are depressed, often in association with elevation of the γ-globulin fraction [81, 82]. It has been suggested that this decrease in albumin could be secondary to the elevated γ-globulin level [1]. When inhabitants of cold climate have moved to more tropical areas, their albumin levels fall, but increases in the rate of albumin synthesis during cold acclimation have not been documented [1]. Environmental factors such as altitude may cause changes in albumin metabolism. This has been reported in animals [83], but it has not been confirmed in man [84].

Stress of a variety of types may increase albumin synthesis (see Fig. 13-3). Fever, surgical procedures, and hemorrhage are ail followed by increases in albumin production in man [85–88]. The possibility that cortisone may play a key role in such changes associated with stress has been emphasized [2]. The stress resulting from extremely catastrophic events, which generally are associated with shock, has a different effect on albumin synthesis, resulting in a decreased rate. This is accompanied by an increase in acute-phase globulins, fibrinogen, and haptoglobin, and a decrease in other proteins such as lipoproteins, transferrin, and prealbumin. This contrasting effect may be due to liver damage accompanying these events [89].

ALBUMIN DEGRADATION

Even less is understood about albumin degradation than is known about albumin synthesis. This process must be considered from two viewpoints: the fractional degradation rate (the percentage of the total exchangeable albumin pool undergoing degradation each day) and the absolute degradation rate (the absolute amount lost, including both endogenous catabolism and external loss) [2]. The fractional albumin degradation rate may remain relatively constant in spite of large changes in the absolute degradation rate [62]. In hypoalbuminemia, the fractional albumin degradation rate may be normal or increased, while the absolute degradation rate is decreased [62, 90]. With albumin infusion, an increase in the fractional degradation rate occurs in association with an increase in the absolute degradation rate [91].

FACTORS AFFECTING RATES OF DEGRADATION

Normally, albumin degradation progresses at a constant rate in man [13], and, since albumin levels are rather constant [4], it follows that the albumin degradation rate should be equal to the synthesis rate for a given individual. Albumin degradation and albumin synthesis are independent processes, however, as indicated by the fact that with albumin infusion, there is a significant increase in albumin degradation with very little change in albumin synthesis [91].

The major hormones that affect albumin synthesis also affect the rate of degradation. With the administration of thyroid hormone or with spontaneous thyrotoxicosis, the albumin degradation rate rapidly increases as the rate of albumin synthesis increases, so that no overall change in the size of the albumin pool occurs, providing good nutrition is maintained [67] (see Fig. 13-3). With hypothyroidism, there are decreases in both the absolute and fractional degradational rate of albumin [68]. These are also accompanied by a shift in the normal distribution of albumin and a significant increase in the size of the extravascular pool [66, 68] (see Fig. 13-3). With corticosteroid administration or in Cushing's syndrome, there are significant increases in both the absolute and fractional degradation rates for albumin that are paralleled by an increase in the albumin synthesis rate (see Fig. 13-3). No change in the size of the total exchangeable albumin pool occurs [69, 70], even though the size of the intravascular pool increases at the expense of the extra-vascular pool [59].

In conditions associated with lowered serum albumin levels, such as malnutrition, nephrosis, or cirrhosis, the absolute albumin degradation rate is generally decreased [49, 61, 64, 92, 93]. The fall in the albumin degradation rate occurs after, and apparently in response to, a lowered albumin level, and it appears to be a compensatory mechanism repre-senting an attempt to conserve albumin [2].

In normal individuals, the albumin degradation rate is increased in a strongly positive, almost linear fashion following attempts to raise the serum albumin levels by albumin infusion. A negative change of lesser degree in the synthesis rate also occurs [60].

SITES OF ALBUMIN DEGRADATION

The primary sites for albumin degradation are not known [2]. There is evidence to indicate that albumin is metabolized by virtually every organ of the body, serving as a source of amino acids supplemental to those derived from plasma [94].

There is no evidence to indicate that a major portion of albumin ca-tabolism takes place in any specific organ. Normally, loss of albumin into the intestinal tract counts for approximately 6 percent of the total albumin catabolized daily [95, 96]. This albumin is broken down into amino acids within the gastrointestinal tract and reappears in the portal circulation, so it therefore is not lost to the body [8]. No significant level of albumin degradation has been identified in the liver using perfusion studies [2]. The kidney has been reported to account for less than 10 to 15 percent of the total daily albumin catabolism. In disease states such as nephrosis or protein-losing enteropathy, the level of albumin degrada-tion in the kidney or intestine may be considerably increased [97].

The metabolic breakdown of albumin occurs at locations that are in direct contact and capable of rapid equilibrium with the bloodstream [98]. Albumin is taken up into the cells involved with its metabolic breakdown where it is rapidly degraded by lysosomal enzymes [22], re-leasing amino acids that are in part utilized for the energy requirements of the cell and in part secreted into the pool of extracellular amino acids [8].

Pathological Considerations

HYPOALBUMINEMIA–GENERAL ASPECTS AND DEFINITIONS

Determination of serum albumin levels has long been used as a clinical guide to indicate the presence and, in some instances, the severity and progression of a variety of different diseases. In this regard, a definition of clinically significant hypoalbuminemia is an important consideration. Although values below 2.5 and 3.0 gm per 100 ml are considered sig-nificant from the viewpoint of potential or hypoalbuminemic edema, a serum level of 3.2 gm per 100 ml or less is sufficient to warrant a clinical evaluation. Serum albumin levels in the range of 1.5 to 1.8 gm per 100 ml or less are considered extreme.

The serum albumin concentration is the net result of three processes—synthesis, degradation, and distribution [8]—any of which can singly or in combination be altered in disease. In clinical medicine, hypoalbuminemia is generally not the result of a single mechanism. In alcoholic cirrhosis, for example, the liver disease, the toxic effects of alcohol intake, malnutrition, hormonal changes, and the volume disturbances associated with ascites all act together to produce the net effect reflected by the serum albumin level. Similar circumstances exist in other diseases.

CLINICAL CONSEQUENCES OF HYPOALBUMINEMIA

The clinical consequences of decreased serum albumin may be best examined by a consideration of each of the proposed functions of albumin: colloid osmotic pressure, transport function, and a possible endogenous source of amino acids.

COLLOID OSMOTIC PRESSURE

Albumin accounts for approximately 80 percent of the plasma colloid osmotic pressure [6]. The importance of this function is demonstrated by the frequency with which edema accompanies hypoalbuminemia. The presence of edema in the patient with a lowered serum albumin level represents the net result of the interaction of several mechanisms relating to two basic processes: alterations occurring at a local tissue level (Starling's forces) and alterations in the renal excretion of salt and water [99]. Starling's forces determine the distribution of fluid between the intravascular and the interstitial spaces. Under normal circumstances, intracapillary hydrostatic pressure and the interstitial osmotic pressure, which have a tendency to move fluid out of the intravascular compartment, are balanced by the interstitial fluid pressure and the osmotic pressure of the blood. With a fall in serum albumin, these forces become unbalanced. The net effect is loss of fluid from the intravascular space and the development of excessive interstitial fluid.

The loss of intravascular volume activates the receptors of the body's volume control system, of which an integral part is the system regulating sodium balance [100].

While the formation of edema in hypoalbuminemic conditions involves a dysequilibrium of Starling's forces at the tissue level, expansion of the extracellular fluid compartment depends ultimately on sodium and water retention by the kidney (Fig. 13-4). These mechanisms serve the physiological purpose of trying to preserve the volume of the intravascular compartment; however, the decrease in oncotic pressure within the capillaries as a consequence of the decreased plasma albumin content results in the constant translocation of fluid from the intravascular compartment into the interstitium. As a consequence, the intravascular compartment does not expand and stimuli for salt and water retention continue. The renal factors resulting in this retention (see Fig. 13-4) include a decrease in the glomerular filtration rate [101], increased aldosterone production [100], and a diminished natriuretic factor, or third

Figure 13-4

Renal factors resulting in sodium retention as a result of protein loss: the chain of events initiated by the loss of protein from the intravascular space. The net result is a retention of sodium and water by the kidneys, leading to the formation of edema (for details, see text). Note that the process can be altered at two points: by increased albumin synthesis by the liver to offset the effects of the lost protein, or by a decreased sodium and fluid intake to prevent accumulation of these substances that leads to edema formation.

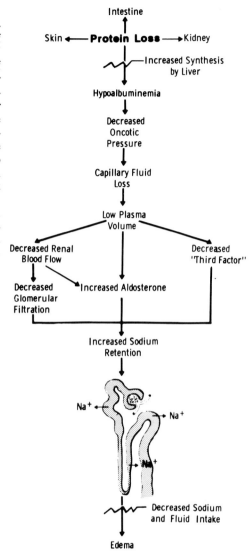

factor [100]. Knowledge of this pathophysiological relationship offers two possible means of controlling edema in the hypoalbuminemic patient: limiting sodium intake and increasing excretion of sodium and water through the use of diuretics. Variations in sodium and water intake and differences in the effectiveness of diuretics account for the fact that the degree of hypoalbuminemia does not correlate with the degree of edema present in individual patients.

TRANSPORT FUNCTION

Although albumin is considered to be very important in transporting a wide variety of substances (see p. 175), very few abnormalities can be attributed to a loss of this function in patients with hypoalbuminemia. This is perhaps best typified by the individual with congenital analbuminemia who shows no apparent effect from the loss of albumin transport function [32, 102]. Hyperlipemia is a frequent occurrence in patients with hypoalbuminemia and has been related to the function of albumin in the transport of fatty acids [9]. It has been postulated that the hyperlipemia that occurs in these patients may represent a risk factor in the development of arteriosclerotic vascular disease.

Perhaps the most important anomaly resulting from a loss of the transport function of albumin from the viewpoint of the clinician relates to its binding of calcium. Calcium exists in the circulation in three forms: ionized, albumin-bound, and complexed. Of these, the ionized fraction is the only form that is physiologically significant, but the protein-bound fraction represents the largest component. For this reason, when measuring total serum calcium levels, the albumin concentration must be taken into account (Fig. 13-5). Blood pH must also be taken into consideration to be completely accurate in relating these two values [12]. The best approach in patients with hypoalbumincmia would be to measure ionized calcium directly rather than total calcium.

SOURCE OF AMINO ACIDS
Even though albumin is listed as a potential endogenous source for amino acids, definite proof of this function is lacking and no problems are seen clinically that may be attributed to a loss of this function in patients that are hypoalbuminemic [13, 14].

CAUSES OF HYPOALBUMINEMIA
Decreased synthesis of albumin may be caused by malnutrition, liver disease, or congenital analbuminemia. Increased loss of albumin may occur through the kidney (nephrotic syndrome), the gastrointestinal tract (protein-losing enteropathies), or the skin (acute thermal burns or eczema). Increased degradation of albumin is found in idiopathic edema and miscellaneous disorders, such as familial idiopathic hypercatabolic hypoproteinemia and Wiskott-Aldrich syndrome.

DECREASED ALBUMIN SYNTHESIS
Malnutrition. As previously discussed, albumin synthesis rates are highly dependent upon the supply of amino acids derived from the diet. Even though severe protein malnutrition is not commonly seen in clinical medicine, inanition and anorexia undoubtedly contribute to the lowered albumin levels seen in many diseases [2]. In other instances, particularly in chronic renal failure, the dietary restrictions against protein contribute to the lowered serum albumin levels that are observed [103]. The malabsorption of protein in diseases such as sprue or celiac disease or following gastrointestinal surgery can result in hypoalbuminemia in spite of adequate or more than adequate dietary protein intake [104].

Observations made in protein-depleted infants and adults [47, 48] indicate that degradation rates for albumin are also decreased during peri-

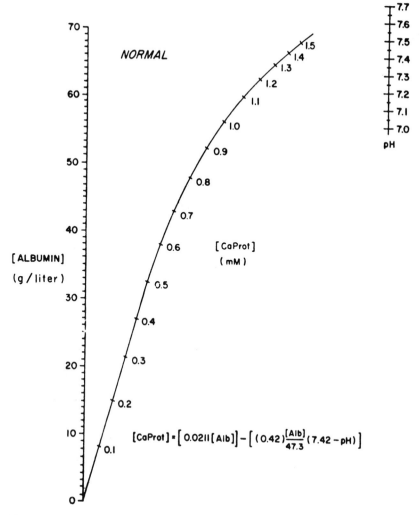

Figure 13-5

Nomogram relating protein-bound calcium to serum albumin concentration and pH. By connecting the albumin value to the pH values with a straight line, the normal protein-bound calcium value can be determined. At the bottom of the nomogram is the formula expressing this value. (Reproduced by permission. From Moore, E. W. *J. Clin. Invest.* 49:318, 1970.)

ods of decreased protein intake. The decrease, however, is of a lesser degree and occurs only after a short lag period, in contrast to the immediate change that occurs in the synthesis rate [105]. Serum albumin levels generally do not decrease for days or weeks, even in the face of severe protein restriction, because of shifts in albumin from the extravascular to the vascular space as the total exchangeable pool decreases. Ultimately, the total exchangeable albumin pool may decrease to one-third of normal [1] (see Fig. 13-3).

The end picture of protein depletion in man is seen in the disease *kwashiorkor*. This disease, though unusual in the United States, represents the most widespread and important dietary disease in the world today [106]. Kwashiorkor is seen primarily among young children in regions of the world where dietary animal protein has been replaced by other types of food. It generally develops soon after the child is weaned and is characterized clinically by retarded growth, alterations in skin and hair pigmentation, edema, dermatosis, gastrointestinal disorders, irritability, and apathy. It may ultimately be fatal. Albumin levels are typically low, often less than half of normal [107]. The presence and severity of the edema that is present in this disease correlates more closely with the total serum protein level than with albumin, however. An increase in serum γ-globulin accompanies the disease [107] and tends to offset the decreased oncotic effect of the hypoalbuminemia to a degree.

Cirrhosis. Liver disease, generally cirrhosis, is probably the most common condition associated with hypoalbuminemia [8]. This does not necessarily reflect a decrease in the actual rate of albumin synthesis in the liver, because, for this to occur, the liver damage must be so severe as to overcome the considerable reserve capacity of this organ [73]. In a study of 19 patients with alcohol-induced cirrhosis, each with depressed serum albumin, the albumin synthesis rates were elevated in 7, normal in 5, and depressed in 7 patients [62].

The hypoalbuminemia in these patients represents the end result of a combination of factors that may be present in varying degree: intrinsic liver disease [62], toxic effects of alcohol [74], abnormalities of albumin distribution, hormonal changes, and malnutrition [1] (see Table 13-3). Abnormalities in albumin distribution are especially important in cirrhotic patients with ascites, where as much albumin may be located in the ascitic fluid as in the plasma. In these patients, the total exchangeable albumin pool may actually be increased above normal [2] (see Fig. 13-3). With increased portal pressure, the pathway delivering newly synthesized albumin directly into the circulation is altered. A significant percentage of the newly synthesized albumin enters hepatic lymph, and a portion leaks across the capsule of the liver directly into the ascitic fluid [1, 2].

Since hypoalbuminemia in patients with cirrhosis represents the net effect of multiple factors, the serum albumin level in these patients is neither a good index of the synthesizing ability of the liver nor of the patient's overall prognosis [1, 2].

Congenital Analbuminemia. Analbuminemia, a rare condition char-

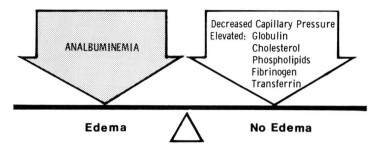

Figure 13-6
Pathophysiological characteristics of congenital analbuminemia with mild edema (for details, see text).

acterized by an almost complete absence of albumin from the serum, has been described in several patients [108, 109]. Consanguinity has been found in some of these cases. Genetic analysis indicates that the condition is most likely inherited as an autosomal recessive trait.

Examination of serum from homozygous patients using immunological techniques reveals the presence of small quantities of apparently normal albumin (in the range of 1.6 to 24 mg per 100 ml), although by routine electrophoresis it appears to be virtually absent [9]. This indicates that the defect is not complete. The serum albumin level of patients presumed to be heterozygotes appears to be normal [9].

In contrast to patients with acquired hypoalbuminemia, patients with congenital hypoalbuminemia are not clinically ill, and, in spite of the many functions ascribed to albumin, very few symptoms occur [32, 110]. Easy tiring, diarrhea, and anemia have been reported in addition to mild, generally episodic, edema. Cholesterol, phospholipid, fibrinogen, and transferrin levels are generally elevated [102]. These values return to normal following the restoration of serum albumin levels by infusion [109].

An increase in the elimination rate of intravenously injected Congo red and Evans blue dyes and a decreased blood calcium level are occasionally noted [9], suggesting a disorder of the transport function of albumin in these patients. No liver abnormalities have been detected in patients with this defect [110].

The effect of severely depressed serum albumin levels is not yet completely understood; when it is, it may explain the limited edema that is present in this disorder. It is thought to be related at least in part to a combination of compensatory factors (Fig. 13-6). Globulin levels are elevated to about 4.5 gm per 100 ml, which, in addition to the elevated cholesterol, phospholipid, fibrinogen, and transferrin levels, provide some increase in the colloid osmotic pressure of the serum. The blood pressure in these patients is generally reduced, being in the range of 90/65, which results in a decreased capillary pressure [102].

Congenital hypoalbuminemia is the result of a significar: decrease in the rate of albumin synthesis [108]. The fractional degradation rate for albumin in these patients is reduced 2 to 5 times [93] (see Fig. 13-3). Following the restoration of serum albumin levels to normal by the intravenous infusion of albumin, there is an increase in the degradation rate; however, normal levels are not achieved [1]. The exact metabolic defect that causes these derangements in albumin synthesis and degradation rates has yet to be defined [1].

EXOGENOUS LOSS OF ALBUMIN

There are a number of pathological states that can lead to hypoalbuminemia through the loss of albumin. When the loss is minimal, hypoalbuminemia does not occur, because of the ability of the liver to increase its synthesis rate and because of changes that occur in the distribution of albumin within the body. With a greater degree of loss, a point is reached at which compensatory mechanisms do not suffice, and hypoalbuminemia results. In these clinical conditions, just as in those diseases resulting in hypoalbuminemia due to decreased synthesis, several mechanisms often coexist that bring about the lowering of serum albumin (Table 13-3). In patients with burns, there is loss of albumin from the skin; however, alterations in distribution are often present as well. In patients with nephrosis or protein-losing enteropathies, increased catabolism of albumin is often present and is a factor, in addition to the external loss of albumin, in lowering serum levels.

Kidneys—nephrotic syndrome. The nephrotic syndrome has been classically defined as a clinical syndrome characterized by massive proteinuria, edema, hypoproteinemia, lipidemia, and lipiduria [111]. This clinical syndrome has a number of causes (Table 13-4), including glomerular diseases, metabolic diseases, collagen vascular diseases, and circulatory diseases. It may also be caused by toxins, such as mercurial diuretics and gold, or it may occur in congenital or familial form [111]. Seventy percent of the diseases causing the nephrotic syndrome in adults are intrinsic renal diseases. Glomerulonephritis, diabetes mellitus, lipoid nephrosis, and lupus nephritis lead the list.

All the diseases causing the nephrotic syndrome share one feature in common: a significant increase occurs in the permeability of the glomerular capillary filter. This increase in permeability is a functional one, which does not correlate with morphological alterations even at an ultrastructural level. The normal glomerular capillary structure allows some protein to pass, primarily albumin and other low molecular weight proteins. Normally, most of the filtered proteins are reabsorbed by the proximal tubules and only very small quantities appear in the urine [111]. This reabsorbed protein is apparently catabolized by the proximal tubules, and the products of this catabolism are added to the general body stores of peptides and amino acids [112]. In the nephrotic syndrome, the quantity of protein allowed to pass into the urine by the abnormal glomerular capillary filter is greatly increased. The reabsorptive capacity of the renal tubules becomes overburdened and proteinuria develops. In these cases, however, the amount of protein reabsorbed and catabolized by the tubules may be considerable.

Table 13-3. Pathogenic Factors Leading to Hypoalbuminemia in Various Pathological Conditions

Pathological Conditions	Pathogenic Factors

Liver disease	Decreased albumin synthesis
	  Intrinsic liver disease (if severe)
	  Toxic effects of alcohol (frequently present)
	  Malnutrition
	Abnormalities of albumin distribution (ascites)

Renal disease	Albumin loss (proteinuria) Increased degradation rate (fractional) Increased serum oncotic pressure (azotemia) Malnutrition (protein restriction) Shifts in distribution (edema)

Acute burns	Albumin loss
	  Transudation
	  Skin loss
	Shifts in distribution
	Inadequate recirculation of albumin (lymphatic blockade)
	Decreased synthesis (only in severe cases)
	  Liver damage (anoxia)
	  Associated with excessive production of γ-globulin and acute-phase reactants

Gastrointestinal disease	Albumin loss
	  Lymphatic abnormalities
	  Lymphatic obstruction
	  Mucosal disease
	Malabsorption
	Malnutrition

The relationship between the quantity of protein excreted in the urine and the occurrence of hypoalbuminemia is not clear-cut. Patients may be seen who excrete large quantities of protein each day with normal serum albumin levels, whereas other patients may be seen who excrete much smaller quantities with a definite hypoalbuminemia [112]. In some instances, this latter case relates to a decrease in urine protein secondary to decreased serum levels; in other cases it relates to differences in synthesis rates.

Clinically, the absolute albumin degradation rate is generally depressed, paralleling the decrease in the size of the body's albumin pool, while the fractional degradation rate may be significantly increased due primarily to increased degradation of albumin by the kidney [1] (see Fig. 13-3). The measured half-life of albumin in the nephrotic syndrome has been found in some patients to be reduced to 3 to 6 days [92].

The exchangeable albumin pool may be significantly reduced in patients with higher levels of albuminuria. In some instances, this reduction may be less than 15 percent of normal, and the absolute albumin

Table 13-4.   Causes of Nephrotic Syndrome

Lipoid nephrosis

Glomerulonephritis
   Idiopathic membranous
   Acute proliferative
   Rapidly progressive
   Chronic proliferative
   Focal

Metabolic diseases
   Diabetic glomerulosclerosis
   Amyloidosis
   Multiple myeloma

Hypersensitivity diseases involving multiple organ systems
   Systemic lupus erythematosus
   Periarteritis
   Henoch-Schönlein syndrome (anaphylactoid purpura)
   Goodpasture's syndrome

Circulatory diseases
   Renal vein thrombosis
   Constrictive pericarditis
   Congestive heart failure
   Tricuspid valvular insufficiency

Nephrotoxins
   Organic mercurial diuretics
   Inorganic mercury
   Bismuth
   Gold

Allergens and drugs
   Pollen
   Bee stings
   Poison oak and poison ivy
   Trimethadione and paramethadione

Diseases due to infection
   Cytomegalic inclusion disease
   Syphilis
   Malaria
   Subacute bacterial endocarditis

Heredofamilial causes

Miscellaneous causes
   Eclampsia
   Transplantation

turnover rate may exceed 50 percent of the intravascular pool each day [92]. An increased rate of synthesis is not uniformly seen [2]; in fact only one-third to one-half of nephrotic patients have albumin synthesis rates that are elevated above normal [2, 92, 113].

In summary, the changes occurring in the various parameters of albumin distribution and metabolism are somewhat variable from one patient to another. In general, however, the urinary loss of protein initiates a reduction in the size of the total exchangeable albumin pool. The absolute degradation rate of albumin decreases in conjunction with this decrease in pool size, but the fractional degradation rate for albumin is increased. Experimentally, there is an increased potential for synthesis in the liver [114]. Clinically, however, synthesis may be decreased, normal, or slightly increased (see Fig. 13-3). Synthesis is not, in general, sufficiently increased to compensate for the loss of protein and the increase in fractional degradation of albumin. Hypoalbuminemia is usually present, but in individual cases it may not correlate very well with the degree of proteinuria.

The hyperlipemia present in patients with nephrotic syndrome underscores the importance of the transport functions of albumin in lipid metabolism.

Case Report 1
A 42-year-old housewife was hospitalized for progressive swelling of the hands and feet. Physical examination revealed moderate hypertension, a slight pallor, periorbital edema, edema of both hands, and bilateral pitting pretibial edema. Urinalysis revealed proteinuria and a sediment containing double-reactile bodies ("maltese crosses") when examined by polarized light. Serum protein electrophoresis revealed hypoalbuminemia of 1.9 gm per 100 ml, an elevated α_2-globulin fraction, and a slight degree of hypogammaglobulinemia. The BUN and creatinine were normal and a creatinine clearance was normal. The serum calcium was decreased to 6.0 mg per 100 ml. Her serum cholesterol was 450 mg per 100 ml. Percutaneous renal biopsy revealed the presence of membranous glomerulonephritis. The patient received appropriate dietary management and steroids (Fig. 13-7).
Final Diagnosis: 1. Nephrotic syndrome, secondary to membranous glomerulonephritis. 2. Hypocalcemia, secondary to hypoalbuminemia. 3. Secondary hyperlipemia.

Skin—thermal burns. As in cirrhosis and nephrotic syndrome, the changes that occur in albumin metabolism in patients with severe thermal burns represent the complex interaction of a number of factors (see Table 13-3). Most important is the loss of albumin from and into the burned area. A considerable increase in capillary permeability occurring in association with the burn results in a significant loss of albumin from the intravascular space into the extravascular space. An amount of albumin equivalent to one plasma pool may be lost from the body, and an equivalent amount may be sequestered in the extravascular space during the first four days following a burn in patients with involvement of 50 percent or more of the body surface [115]. The intravascular pool is fur-

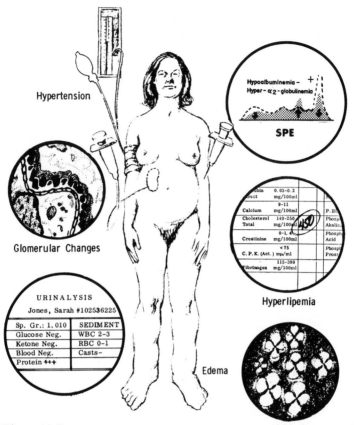

Figure 13-7
Clinical features of nephrotic syndrome (see Case Report 1). (Reproduced by permission. From Ritzmann, S. E., and Daniels, J. C. In G. J. Race (Ed.), *Tice's Practice of Medicine,* Vol. 2. New York: Harper & Row, 1974.)

ther compromised by the fact that lymphatics are unable to return extravascular albumin back to the plasma because they are overloaded by material derived from the burn area [116].

Another important concept in considering the changes in albumin that occur in burns is the fact that skin contains a major portion of the extravascular albumin. Loss of skin in the severely burned patient may result in the loss of a significant amount of the exchangeable albumin pool [1].

The effects on albumin metabolism of the stress that is associated with burn trauma are the same as those of other types of stress. In general, stress tends to increase the rate of synthesis. In severe burns, however, the patient's circulation may be compromised to the point that a degree of anoxia is imposed on the liver, thus decreasing its capacity for albumin synthesis. The polyclonal gammopathy that occurs following acute burns and the excessive production of acute-phase proteins during this period also act to decrease the rate of albumin synthesis [115, 117].

In summary, albumin metabolism in the patient with severe thermal burns may be characterized by either increased or decreased albumin synthesis and an accelerated rate of degradation. The total body albumin pool is reduced primarily at the expense of the intravascular compartment, while the extravascular albumin pool is expanded. These changes are superimposed on the albumin losses that occur secondarily to the loss of skin and the losses that occur from the surface of the burn area.

Case Report 2

A 32-year-old man sustained 38 percent total surface area (35 percent third degree) acute thermal burns when a gasoline heater exploded in his apartment. He was hospitalized on the plastic surgery service, and fluid and electrolyte therapy was instituted. Sulfamylon was applied locally to the burned areas. Shortly after admission, the patient spiked a temperature and *Pseudomonas aeruginosa* was cultured from his blood on multiple occasions. Within a week, the patient had become afebrile as a result of gentamicin therapy. Serum protein electrophoresis carried out shortly after admission revealed a significant degree of hypoalbuminemia with an elevated α_2-globulin fraction and a moderate degree of hypogammaglobulinemia. Split-thickness skin grafts were applied several weeks after admission. The patient was eventually discharged for further reconstructive surgery, with a contracture of the left arm that has persisted despite vigorous physical therapy (Fig. 13-8).

Diagnosis: Acute thermal injury.

Gastrointestinal tract. As previously mentioned, the gastrointestinal (GI) tract participates to some degree in the degradation of albumin in the normal individual. Enteric protein loss accounts for 2 to 15 percent, or an average of approximately 6 percent, of the overall degradation of albumin in the normal person. In some patients with hypoalbuminemia, the loss of albumin into the GI tract may be significantly increased, so that 25 percent [2] to 35 percent [96] of the albumin catabolism occurs in the GI tract. Studies in these patients have shown that from 2 to 60 percent of the intravascular pool may be cleared into the GI tract each day [96]. This loss of albumin is part of a "bulk" protein loss, which is not related to the molecular weight of the protein (see Chap. 1). This results in a decrease in total serum protein values, but essentially normal percentage values for serum protein fractions are found on electrophoresis. This feature may provide an important clue to the mechanism of this protein loss.

Excessive GI albumin loss, in association with the loss of other serum proteins, has been demonstrated in conjunction with a number of GI disorders of diverse causes [118] (Table 13-5). In many of these patients, GI symptoms are not present, and hypoproteinemia and edema may be the only clinical manifestations [113]. For this reason, protein-losing enteropathy should be suspected in all patients with unexplained hypoalbuminemia, especially when associated with "bulk" hypoproteinemia.

Protein-losing enteropathy may have several pathophysiological mechanisms (see Table 13-3) associated with a variety of diseases (see Table 13-5). It may be related to several types of lymphatic abnormalities: increased pressure, as in patients with constrictive pericarditis; lymphatic blockage due to tumors; or congenital abnormalities, as in primary in-

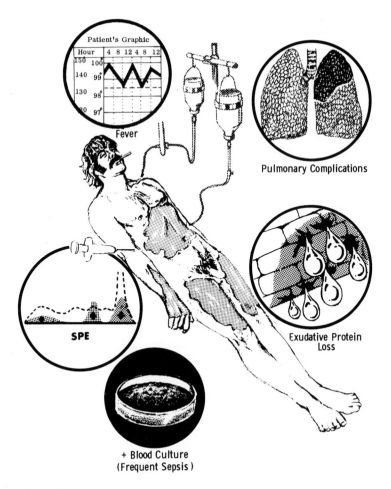

Patient's Graphic

Fever

Pulmonary Complications

SPE

Exudative Protein Loss

+ Blood Culture
(Frequent Sepsis)

Figure 13-8
Clinical features of acute thermal burn injury (see Case Report 2). (Modified from Ritzmann, S. E., and Daniels, J. C. In G. J. Race (Ed.), *Tice's Practice of Medicine,* Vol. 2. New York: Harper & Row, 1974.)

testinal lymphangiectasia. In other cases, it is secondary to mucosal disease with weeping or direct loss of serum into the intestine, such as in inflammatory bowel diseases or hypertrophic gastritis. In addition, there are several diseases associated with excessive loss of gastrointestinal albumin in which the mechanism of loss has not been defined [2, 96].

When albumin is lost into the GI tract, it is catabolized rapidly into its constituent amino acids, which are subsequently reabsorbed. These amino acids are transported to the liver by the portal circulation and are available for the resynthesis of albumin. Hypoalbuminemia develops when the rate of albumin degradation exceeds the liver's albumin-synthesizing capacity [118]. A factor probably more important than the limitation imposed by the synthesizing capacity of the liver is the in-

Table 13-5. Disorders Associated with Protein-Losing Enteropathy

Primary intestinal lymphangiectasia
Colonic lymphangiectasia
Congestive heart failure
   Constrictive pericarditis
   Tricuspid insufficiency
   Myocardiopathy
Regional enteritis
Ulcerative colitis
Hypertrophic gastritis (Ménétrier's syndrome)
Whipple's disease
Gastric carcinoma
Esophageal carcinoma
Colonic carcinoma
Gastric polyp
Tropical and nontropical sprue
Celiac disease
Lymphosarcoma of bowel
Nonspecific granulomatous disease of bowel
Acute gastrointestinal infections
   Shigella
   Salmonella
Chronic pancreatitis
Megacolon
Agammaglobulinemia
Nephrosis
Angioneurotic edema
Allergic gastroenteropathy
Acute transient protein-losing enteropathy

fluence of mucosal disease of the intestine on its absorptive capabilities. Malabsorption induced by these diseases may lead to a lowering of the albumin synthesis rate due to a lack of absorbed amino acids. In a study of patients with tropical sprue, no correlation could be found between the serum albumin level, intestinal losses, and the absolute albumin synthesis rate. However, the greater the degree of malabsorption, the lower the rate of albumin synthesis [104].

In chronic, debilitating inflammatory diseases of the GI tract, malnutrition, with its effects on albumin synthesis, may also play a role.

Albumin metabolism in patients with hypoalbuminemia due to protein-losing enteropathies is generally characterized by some degree of increase in albumin synthesis [1], as well as an increase in the fractional [96] and absolute [2] degradation rates (see Fig. 13-3). The presence of hypoalbuminemia and its severity when present is a reflection of an inability of the synthesis rate to keep pace with the degradation rate. The synthesis rate is determined by the intrinsic capacity of the liver, which is at times modified by an unavailability of amino acids due to malnutrition or malabsorption [2].

Congestive heart failure is frequently associated with some degree of hypoalbuminemia. In most instances, this decrease in the serum level is dilutional due to an increase in circulating plasma volume [1]. In some cases, however, significant GI protein loss may occur due to a considerably elevated venous pressure [118]. The increase in venous pressure results in partial obstruction to the entry of lymph into the central veins, an increase in lymphatic pressure, dilatation of lymphatic channels in the small intestine, and albumin leakage. Other serum proteins are also lost, and lymphocytopenia may occur, which is comparable to that seen in other disorders associated with the loss of lymph into the bowel [119, 120].

Protein-losing enteropathy associated with congestive heart failure is most frequently seen in conjunction with constrictive pericarditis. Cases have been reported, however, in patients with tricuspid insufficiency and in association with severe congestive heart failure related to cardiomyopathy, atrial septal defect, and congenital pulmonary stenosis [96]. The common denominator in all these cases is a significantly increased venous pressure.

Following cardiac compensation, a reversal of the GI protein loss, lymphocytopenia, and the abnormalities of intestinal lymphatics occurs [96, 119]. It should also be remembered that hypoalbuminemia in association with congestive heart failure may be due to renal losses (see Table 13-4).

Primary intestinal lymphangiectasia refers to a disorder in which there is gastrointestinal protein loss associated with dilatation of the mucosal and mesenteric lymphatics of the small intestine [121]. Changes of this same type, however, have been seen in association with other causes of protein-losing enteropathy. For this reason, it is necessary to demonstrate abnormalities of the intestinal lymphatics by intestinal biopsy and to rule out the presence of inflammatory disease of the intestine or any of the other well-defined causes of protein-losing enteropathy before the diagnosis of primary intestinal lymphangiectasia can be made.

Primary intestinal lymphangiectasia is but one component of a diffuse, congenital hypoplasia of the lymphatics [122–124]. In some patients, this abnormality of the lymphatics includes the regional absence of lymph nodes [124, 125]. Most cases are first recognized in children; however, in more severe cases, manifestations are present at birth or shortly thereafter [126], while in an occasional patient, the effects of the abnormality do not become apparent clinically until the second or third decade [122].

Clinically, peripheral edema is a prominent feature of the condition because of the lymphatic abnormalities that are present in the lower extremities as well as the hypoproteinemia that occurs secondarily to the intestinal loss [123, 124]. Other clinical features seen in this condition include severe hypoproteinemia, lymphocytopenia, hypocalcemia, reduced serum immunoglobulin levels, weight loss, and weakness [124, 127]. The intestinal component of this congenital abnormality of the lymphatics is characterized pathologically by significant dilatation of the lymphatics of the mucosa, submucosa, and serosa of the intestine [118].

Case Report 3

A 38-year-old shopkeeper in a small town had been troubled with recurrent but progressively more severe episodes of edema since adolescence. Earlier episodes had been confined to peripheral edema with a capricious course. The past ten years had seen three episodes of severe ascites for which the patient had required hospitalization, with resolution of symptoms on bed rest and infusion of salt-poor human serum albumin. The patient had also had a striking number of episodes of viral respiratory infections and viral gastroenteritis. The patient was known to be a very heavy "social" drinker, and, although no liver biopsy had been performed nor had jaundice ever been documented, he was assumed by his local physician to have some form of cirrhosis (either Laennec's or postnecrotic) dating to adolescence. About three years prior to admission, the patient had sustained an attack of thrush. The patient's deteriorating health eventually forced him to close his local shop. Upon the onset of severe anasarca, he was referred to a medical center for evaluation. No hepatomegaly was present, and liver function studies were normal. Serum protein electrophoresis revealed considerably diminished albumin with a considerable decrease of all other serum protein fractions. The total serum protein was diminished. The peripheral blood lymphocyte count was 550 per cubic millimeter. Anergy was found in response to all skin tests applied. The gastroenterology service performed a biopsy of the jejunum using a Rubin capsule, which revealed histopathological evidence of dilated lacteals compatible with lymphangiectasia and protein-losing gastroenteropathy (Fig. 13-9).

Final Diagnosis: Intestinal lymphangiectasia, complicated by lymphocytopenia and protein-losing gastroenteropathy.

Lymphangiectasia localized to the colon has been reported [128, 129]. These cases have been seen in adults and are characterized by diarrhea, hypoalbuminemia, and edema [128, 130]. Potassium loss has been considerable in some cases, resulting in hypokalemia and weakness. Pathologically, the abnormality is localized to the colon and is characterized by significant submucosal edema and dilatation of the colonic lymphatics [128]. Partial colectomy results in improvement or complete resolution of the symptoms of the disease [128].

Hypertrophic gastritis (Ménétrier's syndrome) is a disease characterized by considerable hypertrophy of the gastric mucosal folds, which is often associated with the presence of edema and ascites. The concentrations of plasma proteins in these patients are generally low. Hypoalbuminemia is often severe, especially in those cases with significant edema. The hypoproteinemia and hypoalbuminemia in these patients are related to the loss of protein into the stomach secondary to the mucosal abnormality that characterizes the disease [131].

Hypertrophic gastritis is a rare condition, which is difficult to distinguish from other causes of the apparent thickening of gastric mucosal folds. An accurate diagnosis can only be made on the basis of a full-thickness biopsy specimen from a wall of the stomach [131]. Histologically, prominent hypertrophy of the surface epithelium of the stomach is seen with hypertrophy and significant tortuosity of the glands. There is also an infiltration of moderate numbers of lymphocytes and plasma cells into the supporting stroma. The cause of the disease is not known. Clini-

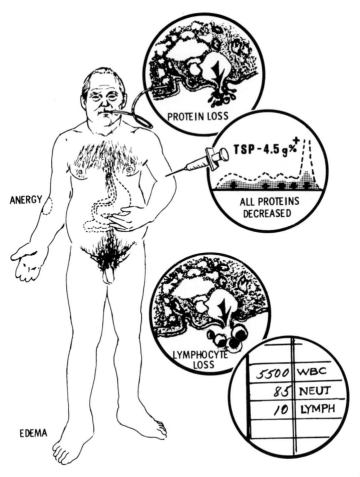

Figure 13-9
Clinical features of intestinal lymphangiectasia with protein-losing gastro-enteropathy (see Case Report 3). (Modified from Ritzmann, S. E., and Daniels, J. C. In G. J. Race (Ed.), *Tice's Practice of Medicine,* Vol. 2. New York: Harper & Row, 1974.)

cally, patients present with upper abdominal pain, weight loss, and edema. Normal or low gastric acid secretion is present [131].

Metabolic studies have indicated the passage of abnormally large quantities of albumin from the plasma across the gastric mucosa into the lumen of the stomach that is associated with an increase in the fractional degradation rate for albumin. These changes are present even in the absence of hypoalbuminemia. The absolute degradation rate is either within normal range or only slightly elevated [131].

The exact mechanism resulting in the loss of protein through the mucosa is unknown, but it does not appear to have an inflammatory basis [131]. Gastrectomy may be indicated because of the severity of the disease. Resolution of the sy1 ptoms follows this procedure [131].

In *chronic inflammatory diseases of the small intestine and colon*—such as regional enteritis and ulcerative colitis, acute inflammatory diseases such as shigellosis, or even diseases such as tropical sprue—there is an increase in the transfer of albumin and other serum proteins from plasma to the intestine [118]. In these conditions, it has been estimated that as much as 25 percent of the average daily absolute degradation rate for albumin can be accounted for by loss in the stool [2].

In some instances, factors in addition to the mucosal disease play a role in altering albumin metabolism (see Table 13-3). In regional enteritis, involvement of lymphatics that results in obstruction may contribute to the protein loss [118]. In addition, the decreased availability of amino acids resulting from the malnutrition that may accompany chronic inflammatory diseases of the bowel or from the malabsorption that may be associated with mucosal diseases such as sprue [1] can affect the liver's synthesizing ability [1]. In one study of patients with tropical sprue and low serum albumin levels, the rate of albumin synthesis was found to be depressed in more than half of the patients [104].

Acute, transient, protein-losing gastroenteropathy lasting from a few weeks to a few months has been reported in a number of patients [118, 132, 133]. Most of these cases have been found in children in which the syndrome is usually associated with edema and hypoalbuminemia and generally follows episodes of gastroenteritis, acute upper respiratory infections, or allergic or infectious illnesses. Many of the patients have had a history of asthma, hay fever, or drug allergy, and peripheral eosinophilia is often present during the course of the illness.

Acute transient protein-losing gastroenteropathy is thought to be based on a hypersensitivity mechanism that results in a mucosal abnormality of the stomach. Roentgenographically, the rugal folds of the stomach may be very prominent. This latter feature, which is due to submucosal and mucosal edema [118], may lead to an erroneous diagnosis of hypertrophic gastritis (Menetrier's syndrome). The condition is self-limited.

INCREASED DEGRADATION OF ALBUMIN

As previously discussed, an increased level of albumin degradation is associated with several disease states that result in hypoalbuminemia. This is seen in diseases of such diverse causes as thyrotoxicosis, Cushing's syndrome, and protein-losing enteropathy (see Fig. 13-3). Even though it may contribute significantly to the overall problem, increased albumin degradation in these diseases plays only an ancillary role. There is a category of disorders in which an increased endogenous protein degradation rate exists as the primary mechanism that results not only in hypoalbuminemia but, in some instances, reduced levels of immunoglobulins as well.

Idiopathic edema. This is a disorder that usually affects women, and it is characterized by the occurrence of edema in the absence of liver or renal disease. The edema may vary in its severity, but it is generally present to some degree unless the patient is being treated with diuretic agents. In some patients, the edema may only appear while the patient is in the upright position. The cause of this state is unknown; however, a significantly reduced mean serum albumin concentration, mean plasma volume, and mean total circulating albumin level have been demonstrated in these patients. The total exchangeable albumin is also significantly reduced. Kinetic studies have indicated that an approximately 30 percent increase in the fractional degradation rate for albumin in these patients occurs in spite of the decreased albumin levels. The absolute degradation rate is only slightly reduced [90, 134] (see Fig. 13-3).

Familial idiopathic hypercatabolic hypoproteinemia. This condition has been described in patients having a significant reduction in the serum concentration of albumin and IgG. The levels of IgM are only slightly reduced, whereas those of IgA are normal or, in some instances, slightly elevated. The total albumin pool in these patients is less than 30 percent of normal with an IgG pool of less than 15 percent of normal. Synthesis rates for albumin are essentially normal, but the fractional degradation rate is considerably increased to more than twice the normal level.

In these patients, no loss of albumin or immunoglobulin can be detected, either renal or gastrointestinal. Other causes of a hypercatabolic state, such as thyrotoxicosis, are not present. The mechanisms by which this disease occurs are not known [135, 136].

Wiskott-Aldrich syndrome. The syndrome is characterized by thrombocytopenia, eczema, and recurrent infections with a variety of different types of organisms. The last feature appears to be due to an immunological deficiency affecting the afferent limb of the immune response [137]. The disease is inherited as a sex-linked recessive trait, and affected males seldom survive beyond ten years of age. Death usually results from infections or hemorrhagic complications.

Metabolic turnover studies in patients with the Wiskott-Aldrich syndrome have shown an increase in the fractional degradation rate for albumin to approximately twice normal. The fractional degradation rates for IgG, IgA, and IgM are significantly increased as well [135].

Investigations have shown a slight increase in the gastrointestinal loss of albumin but one that is not sufficient to account for the increased fractional degradation rate observed in the disease. No increase in the urinary loss of protein is seen, and no other cause for an increased catabolic state has been detected [135]. The exact mechanism for the increased degradation rate in this condition has yet to be defined.

References

1. Rothschild, M. A., Oratz, M., and Schreiber, S. S. Albumin synthesis. *N. Engl. J. Med.* 286:748, 816, 1972.
2. Rothschild, M. A., and Schreiber, S. S. Serum albumin. *Am. J. Dig. Dis.* 14:711, 1969.
3. Rothschild, M. A., Bauman, A., Yalow, R. S., and Berson, S. A. Tissue distribution of I-131 labeled human serum albumin following intravenous administration. *J. Clin. Invest.* 34:1354, 1955.
4. Reeve, E. V., and Chan, A. Y. Regulation of Interstitial Albumin. In M. A. Rothschild and T. Waldmann (Eds.), *Plasma Protein Metabolism.* New York: Academic, 1970. P. 89.

5. Yoffey, J. M., and Courtice, M. C. *Lymphatics, Lymph and the Lymphomyeloid Complex*. New York: Academic, 1970. P. 206.

6. Scatchard, G., Batchelder, A. C., and Brown, A. Osmotic pressure of plasma and of serum albumin. *J. Clin. Invest.* 23:458, 1944.

7. Ogston, A. G., and Phelps, C. F. The partition of solutes between buffer solutions and solutions containing hyaluronic acids. *Biochem. J.* 78:827, 1961.

8. Peters, T., Jr. Serum albumin. *Adv. Clin. Chem.* 13:37, 1970.

9. Bearn, A. G., and Cleve, H. Genetic Variation of Plasma Protein. In J. V. Stanbury, J. V. Wyngaarten, and D. S. Fredickson (Eds.), *The Metabolic Basis of Inherited Disease*. New York: McGraw-Hill, 1972. P. 1629.

10. Daughaday, W. H. Binding of corticosteroids by plasma protein. *J. Clin. Invest.* 37:519, 1958.

11. Putnam, F. W. Structure and Functions of the Plasma Proteins. In H. Neurath (Ed.), *The Proteins,* Vol. 3. New York: Academic, 1965. P. 153.

12. Moore, E. W. Ionized calcium in normal serum, ultrafiltrates and whole blood determined by ion-exchange electrodes. *J. Clin. Invest.* 49: 318, 1970.

13. Rothschild, M. A., Oratz, M., and Schreiber, S. S. Albumin Metabolism. In M. A. Rothschild and T. Waldmann (Eds.), *Plasma Protein Metabolism*. New York: Academic, 1970. P. 199.

14. Schultze, H. E., and Heremans, J. F. *Molecular Biology of Human Proteins,* Vol. 1. Amsterdam: Elsevier, 1966. P. 183.

15. Schultze, H. E., and Schwick, G. Quantitative immunologische Bestimmung von Plasmaproteinen. *Clin. Chim. Acta* 4:15, 1959.

16. Steinfield, J. Difference in daily albumin synthesis between normal men and women as measured with I[131] labeled albumin. *J. Lab. Clin. Med.* 55:904, 1960.

17. Störiko, K. Normal values for twenty-three different human plasma proteins determined by single radial immunodiffusion. *Blut* 16:200, 1968.

18. Keating, F. R., Jr., Jones, J. Z., Elveback, L. R., and Randall, R. V. The relation of age and sex to distribution of values in healthy adults of serum calcium, inorganic phosphorous, magnesium, alkaline phosphatase, total proteins, albumin and blood urea. *J. Lab. Clin. Med.* 73: 825, 1969.

19. Pollak, V. E., Mandema, E., Doig, A. B., Moore, M., and Karl, R. M. Observations on electrophoresis of serum proteins from healthy North American Caucasians and Negro subjects and from patients with systemic lupus erythematosus. *J. Lab. Clin. Med.* 58:353, 1961.

20. Rawnsley, H., Yonan, B. L., and Reinhold, J. G. Serum protein concentrations in the North American Negroid. *Science* 123:991, 1966.

21. Gordon, A. H., and Humphrey, J. H. Measurement of intracellular albumin in rat liver. *Biochem. J.* 78:551, 1961.

22. Beeken, W. L. In vitro metabolism of human serum albumin by subcellular fractions of hepatic tissue from man. *J. Lab. Clin. Med.* 65: 649, 1965.

23. Foster, J. F. Plasma Albumin. In F. W. Putnam (Ed.), *The Plasma Proteins,* Vol. 1. New York: Academic, 1960. P. 176.

24. Squire, P. G., Moser, P., and O'Konski, C. T. The hydrodynamic properties of bovine serum albumin monomer and dimer. *Biochemistry* 7:4261, 1968.

25. Hughes, W. L., Jr.   Interstitial Protein: The Proteins of Blood Plasma and Lymph. In H. Neurath and K. Bailey (Eds.), *The Proteins,* Vol. 2. New York: Academic, 1954. P. 663.
26. Hartley, R. W., Jr., Peterson, E. A., and Sober, H. A.   The relation of free sulfhydryl groups to chromatographic heterogeneity and polymerization of bovine plasma albumin. *Biochemistry* 1:60, 1962.
27. Hoch, H., and Morris, C. J. O. R.   Heterogeneity of human serum albumin. *Nature* 156:234, 1945.
28. Rejnek, J., Bedarik, T., and Koci, J.   Microheterogeneity of albumin. *Clin. Chim. Acta* 8:116, 1963.
29. Saifer, A., Robin, M., and Ventrice, M.   Starch gel electrophoresis of "purified" albumins. *Arch. Biochem. Biophys.* 92:409, 1961.
30. Scheurlen, P. G.   Über Serumeiweiss Veränderungen beim Diabetes Mellitus. *Klin. Wochenschr.* 33:198, 1955.
31. Wuhrmann, F.   Albumindoppelzacken als vererbbare Bluteiweissanomalie. *Schweiz. Med. Wochenschr.* 89:150, 1959.
32. Weitkamp, L. R., Salzano, F. M., Neel, J. V., Porta, F., Geerdink, R. A., and Tarnoky, A. L.   Human serum albumin: Twenty-three genetic variants and their population distribution. *Ann. Hum. Genet.* 36:381, 1973.
33. Kaarsalo, E., Melartin, L., and Blumberg, B. S.   Autosomal linkage between the albumin and Gc loci in humans. *Science* 158:123, 1967.
34. Blumberg, B. S., Martin, J. R., and Melartin, L.   Alloalbuminemia. Albumin Naskapi in Indians of the Ungava. *J.A.M.A.* 203:180, 1968.
35. Schultze, H. E., and Heremans, J. F.   *Physiology and Pathology of Plasma Proteins,* Vol. 2. Amsterdam: Elsevier, 1970. P. 321.
36. Warner, J. R., and Soeiro, R.   The involvement of RNA in protein synthesis. *N. Engl. J. Med.* 276:563, 675, 1967.
37. Hicks, S. J., Drysdale, J. W., and Munro, H. N.   Preferential synthesis of ferritin and albumin by different populations of liver polysomes. *Science* 164:584, 1969.
38. Redman, C. M.   Biosynthesis of serum proteins and ferritin by free and attached ribosomes of rat liver. *J. Biol. Chem.* 244:4308, 1969.
39. Glaumann, H., and Ericsson, J. L. E.   Evidence for the participation of the Golgi apparatus in the intracellular transport of nascent albumin in the liver cell. *J. Cell Biol.* 47:555, 1970.
40. Smallwood, R. A., Jones, E. A., Craigie, A., Raia, S., and Rosenoer, V. M.   The delivery of newly synthesized albumin and fibrinogen to the plasma in dogs. *Clin. Sci.* 35:35, 1968.
41. Woolley, G., and Courtice, F. C.   The origin of albumin in hepatic lymph. *Aust. J. Exp. Biol. Med. Sci.* 40:121, 1962.
42. Berson, S. A., and Yalow, R. S.   Distribution and metabolism of I[131] labeled proteins in man. *Fed. Proc.* 16(2)[Suppl.]:13, 1957.
43. Schreiber, S. S., Bauman, A., Yalow, R. S., and Berson, S. A.   Blood volume alterations in congestive heart failure. *J. Clin. Invest.* 33:578, 1954.
44. Zimmon, D. S., Oratz, M., Kessler, R., Schreiber, S. S., and Rothschild, M. A.   Albumin to ascites: Demonstration of a direct pathway bypassing the systemic circulation. *J. Clin. Invest.* 48:2074, 1969.
45. Takeda, Y., and Reeve, E. B.   Studies of the metabolism and distribution of albumin with autologous I[131] albumin in healthy men. *J. Lab. Clin. Med.* 61:183, 1963.
46. Tavill, A. S., Craigie, A., and Rosenoer, W. M.   The measurement of the synthetic rate of albumin in man. *Clin. Sci.* 34:1, 1968.

47. Hoffenberg, R., Black, E., and Brock, J. F. Albumin and gamma-globulin tracer studies in protein depletion states. *J. Clin. Invest.* 45: 143, 1966.

48. James, W. P., and Hay, A. M. Albumin metabolism: Effect of the nutritional state and the dietary protein intake. *J. Clin. Invest.* 47:1958, 1968.

49. Cohen, S., and Hansen, J. D. Metabolism of albumin and γ-globulin in kwashiorkor. *Clin. Sci.* 23:351, 1962.

50. Peters, T., Jr., and Peters, J. C. The biosynthesis of rat serum albumin. VI. Intracellular transport of albumin and rates of liver protein synthesis in vivo under various physiological conditions. *J. Biol. Chem.* 247:3858, 1972.

51. Rothschild, M. A., Oratz, M., Mongelli, J., and Schreiber, S. S. Amino acid regulation of albumin synthesis. *J. Nutr.* 98:395, 1969.

52. Munro, H. N. Factors in Regulation of Liver Protein Synthesis. In M. A. Rothschild and T. Waldmann (Eds.), *Plasma Protein Metabolism.* New York: Academic, 1970. P. 157.

53. Geffay, H., and Donnelly, J. S. The metabolism of serum proteins. II. The effect of dietary protein on the turnover of rat serum proteins. *J. Biol. Chem.* 231:111, 1958.

54. Bjørneboe, M., and Schwartz, M. Investigations concerning the changes in serum proteins during immunization; the case of hypoalbuminemia with high gamma globulin values. *J. Exp. Med.* 110:259, 1959.

55. Oratz, M. Oncotic Pressure and Albumin Synthesis. In M. A. Rothschild and T. Waldmann (Eds.), *Plasma Protein Metabolism.* New York: Academic, 1970. P. 233.

56. Rothschild, M. A., Oratz, M., Mongelli, J., and Schreiber, S. S. Albumin metabolism in rabbits during gamma globulin infusions. *J. Lab. Clin. Med.* 66:733, 1965.

57. Rothschild, M. A., Oratz, M., Mongelli, J., and Schreiber, S. S. Effect of albumin concentration on albumin synthesis in the perfused liver. *Am. J. Physiol.* 216:1127, 1969.

58. Rothschild, M. A., Oratz, M., Wimer, A., and Schreiber, S. S. Studies on albumin synthesis. The effects of dextran and cortisone on albumin metabolism in rabbits studied with I[131] albumin. *J. Clin. Invest.* 40:545, 1961.

59. Rothschild, M. A., Oratz, M., Evans, C., and Schreiber, S. S. Role of hepatic interstitial albumin in regulating albumin synthesis. *Am. J. Physiol.* 210:57, 1966.

60. Anderson, S. V., and Rossing, N. Metabolism of albumin and gamma-G-globulin during plasmapheresis. *Scand. J. Clin. Lab. Invest.* 30:183, 1967.

61. Hasch, E., Jarnum, S., and Tygstrup, N. Albumin synthesis rate as a measure of liver function in patients with cirrhosis. *Acta Med. Scand.* 182:83, 1967.

62. Rothschild, M. A., Oratz, M., Zimmon, D., Schreiber, S. S., Weiner, I., and Van Caneghem, A. Albumin synthesis in cirrhotic subjects with ascites studied with carbonate-14C. *J. Clin. Invest.* 48:344, 1969.

63. Dykes, P. W. The rates of distribution and catabolism of albumin in normal subjects and in patients with cirrhosis of the liver. *Clin. Sci.* 34: 161, 1968.

64. Kaitz, A. L. Albumin metabolism in nephrotic adults. *J. Lab. Clin. Med.* 53:186, 1969.

65. Garren, L. D., Richardson, A. P., Jr., and Crocco, R. M. Studies on

the role of ribosomes in the regulation of protein synthesis in hypophysectomized and thyroidectomized rats. *J. Biol. Chem.* 242:650, 1967.

66. Lewallan, C. G., Rall, J. E., and Berman, M.   Studies of iodo-albumin metabolism. II. The effects of thyroid hormone. *J. Clin. Invest.* 38:88, 1959.

67. Rothschild, M. A., Bauman, A., Yalow, R. S., and Berson, S. A.   The effect of large doses of desiccated thyroid on the distribution and metabolism of albumin I^{131} in euthyroid subjects. *J. Clin. Invest.* 32:422, 1957.

68. Bauman, A., Rothschild, M. A., Yalow, R. S., and Berson, S. A.   Distribution and metabolism of I^{131} labeled human serum albumin in congestive heart failure with and without proteinuria. *J. Clin. Invest.* 34:1359, 1955.

69. Takeda, Y.   Hormonal effects on metabolism and distribution of plasma albumin in the dog. *Am. J. Physiol.* 206:1229, 1964.

70. Sterling, K.   The effect of Cushing's syndrome upon serum albumin metabolism. *J. Clin. Invest.* 39:1900, 1960.

71. Cox, R. F., and Mathias, A. P.   Cytoplasmic effects of cortisol in liver. *Biochem. J.* 115:777, 1969.

72. Enwonwu, C. O., and Munro, H. N.   Changes in liver polyribosome patterns following administration of hydrocortisone and actinomycin D. *Biochim. Biophys. Acta* 238:264, 1971.

73. Rothschild, M. A., Oratz, M., Zimmon, G., Schreiber, S. S., and Weiner, I.   Normal albumin production in cirrhotic patients with ascites studied with 14C carbonate. *Strahlentherapie [Sonderb.]* 67:316, 1968.

74. Rubin, E., and Liber, C. S.   Alcohol-induced hepatic injury in non-alcoholic volunteers. *N. Engl. J. Med.* 278:869, 1968.

75. Rothschild, M. A., Oratz, M., Mongelli, J., and Schreiber, S. S.   Alcohol-induced depression of albumin synthesis: Reversal by trytophan. *J. Clin. Invest.* 50:1812, 1971.

76. Smuckler, E. A.   Studies on carbon tetrachloride intoxication. IV. Effects of carbon tetrachloride on liver slices and isolated organelles in vitro. *Lab. Invest.* 15:157, 1966.

77. John, D. W., and Miller, L. L.   Effect of whole body x-irradiation of rats on net synthesis of albumin, fibrinogen, alpha-1-acid glycoprotein, and alpha-2-globulin (acute phase globulin) by the isolated, perfused rat liver. *J. Biol. Chem.* 243:268, 1968.

78. Judah, J. D., and Nicholls, M. R.   Role of liver-cell potassium ions in secretion of serum albumin and lipoproteins. *Biochem. J.* 116:663, 1970.

79. Korner, A.   Regulation of the rate of synthesis of messenger ribonucleic acid by growth hormone. *Biochem. J.* 92:449, 1964.

80. Levin, L., and Leathem, J. H.   Relation of pituitary, thyroid and adrenal glands to maintenance of normal serum albumin and globulin levels. *Am. J. Physiol.* 136:306, 1942.

81. Curtain, C. C., Gajdusek, D. C., Kidson, C., Gorman, J., Champness, L., and Rodrique, R.   A study of the serum proteins of peoples of Papua and New Guinea. *Am. J. Trop. Med. Hyg.* 14:678, 1965.

82. Stransky, E., Dauis-Lawas, D. F., and Vicente, C.   On gamma-globulin levels in tropics. *J. Trop. Med. Hyg.* 54:182, 1951.

83. Schnakenberg, D. D., Krabitt, L. F., and Weiser, P. C.   The anorexic

effect of high altitude on weight gain, nitrogen retention and body composition of rats. *J. Nutr.* 101:787, 1971.

84. Fischer, C. L., Gill, C., Daniels, J. C., Cobb, E. K., Berry, C. A., and Ritzmann, S. E.   Effects of the space flight environment on man's immune system: I. Serum proteins and immunoglobulins. *Aerosp. Med.* 43:856, 1972.

85. Asen, P., Bottiger, L. E., Engstedt, L., Liljedahl, S. O., Zetterstrom, B., and Birke, G.   Studies on trauma. I. Intravascular aggregation of erythrocytes and changes in serum proteins and protein-bound carbohydrates. *Acta Chir. Scand.* 130:399, 1965.

86. Davies, J. W., Ricketts, C. R., and Bull, J. P.   Studies of plasma protein metabolism. I. Albumin in burned and injured patients. *Clin. Sci.* 23:511, 1962.

87. Malt, R. A., Wang, C. A., Yamazaki, Z., and Miyakuni, T.   Stimulation of albumin synthesis by hemorrhage. *Surgery* 66:65, 1969.

88. Neuhaus, O. W., Balegno, H. F., and Chandler, A. M.   Induction of plasma protein synthesis in response to trauma. *Am. J. Physiol.* 211:151, 1966.

89. Ragnotti, G., Cajone, F., and Bernelli-Zazzera, A.   Structural and functional changes in polysomes from ischemic livers. *Exp. Mol. Pathol.* 13:295, 1970.

90. Gill, J. R., Jr., Waldmann, T. A., and Bartter, F. C.   Idiopathic edema. I. The occurrence of hypoalbuminemia and abnormal albumin metabolism in women with unexplained edema. *Am. J. Med.* 52:444, 1972.

91. Rothschild, M. A., Oratz, M., Evans, C., and Schreiber, S. S.   Alterations in albumin metabolism after serum and albumin infusions. *J. Clin. Invest.* 43:1874, 1964.

92. Jensen, H., Rossing, N., Anderson, S. B., and Jarnum, S.   Albumin metabolism in the nephrotic syndrome in adults. *Clin. Sci.* 33:445, 1967.

93. Waterlow, J. C.   Observations on the mechanisms of adaptation to low protein intakes. *Lancet* 2:1091, 1968.

94. Radovich, J., Szentivanyi, A., and Talmage, D. W.   The lack of selective reincorporation into tissue protein of the amino acids derived from the catabolism of serum protein. *J. Gen. Physiol.* 47:297, 1963.

95. Kerr, R. M., DuBois, J. J., and Holt, P. R.   Use of I-125- and 51-Cr-labeled albumin for the measurement of gastrointestinal and total albumin catabolism. *J. Clin. Invest.* 46:2064, 1967.

96. Waldmann, T. A., Wochner, R. D., and Strober, W.   The role of the gastrointestinal tract in plasma protein metabolism. *Am. J. Med.* 46:275, 1969.

97. Gitlin, D., Janeway, C. A., and Farr, L. E.   Studies on the metabolism of plasma proteins in the nephrotic syndrome. Albumin, γ-globulin and iron binding globulin. *J. Clin. Invest.* 34:44, 1956.

98. Quincke, E., and Maurer, W.   Zur Frage nach den Ort des Serum-Eiweiss-Abbaues im Organismus. *Biochem. Z.* 329:392, 1967.

99. Wedeen, R. P., Goldstein, M., and Levit, M. F.   Mechanisms of edema and the use of diuretics. *Pediatr. Clin. North Am.* 18:561, 1971.

100. Klahr, S., and Slatopolsky, E.   Renal regulation of sodium excretion. *Arch. Intern. Med.* 131:780, 1973.

101. Baldus, W. P., Summerskill, W. J. J., Hunt, J. C., and Maher, F. T.   Renal circulation in cirrhosis: Observations based on catheterization of the renal vein. *J. Clin. Invest.* 43:1090, 1964.

102. Gordon, R. S., Jr., Barder, F. Z., and Waldmann, T. Idiopathic hypo-albuminemias. Clinical Staff Conference at the National Institutes of Health. *Ann. Intern. Med.* 51:553, 1959.
103. Fish, J. C., Remmers, A. R., Jr., Lindley, J. C., and Sarles, H. E. Albumin kinetics and nutritional rehabilitation in the home dialysis patient. *N. Engl. J. Med.* 287:478, 1972.
104. Jeejeebhoy, K. N., Samuel, A. M., Singh, B., Nadkarni, G. D., Desai, H. G., Borkar, A. V., and Mani, L. S. Metabolism of albumin and fibrinogen in patients with tropical sprue. *Gastroenterology* 56:252, 1969.
105. McFarlane, A. S. Measurement of synthesis rates of liver-produced plasma proteins. *Biochem. J.* 89:377, 1963.
106. Boyd, A. *A Textbook of Pathology.* Philadelphia: Lea & Febiger, 1970. P. 439.
107. Petermann, M. L. Alterations in Plasma Protein Patterns in Disease. In F. Putnam (Ed.), *The Plasma Proteins,* Vol. 2. New York: Academic, 1960. P. 309.
108. Bennhold, H., and Kallee, E. Comparative studies on the half-life of I¹³¹-labeled albumins and non-radioactive serum albumin in a case of analbuminemia. *J. Clin. Invest.* 38:863, 1959.
109. Waldmann, T. A., Gordon, R. S., Jr., and Rosse, W. Studies on the metabolism of the serum proteins and lipids in a patient with analbuminemia. *Am. J. Med.* 37:960, 1964.
110. Montgomery, D. A., Neill, D. W., and Dowdle, E. G. Idiopathic hypoalbuminemia. *Clin. Sci.* 22:141, 1962.
111. Beathard, G. A. Proteinuria and the nephrotic syndrome. *Tex. Med.* 69:51, 1973.
112. Pollak, V. E. Proteinuria. I. Mechanisms. *Hosp. Practice* 6:49, 1971.
113. Yssing, M., Jensen, H., and Jarnum, S. Albumin metabolism and gastrointestinal protein loss in children with nephrotic syndrome. *Acta Paediatr. Scand.* 58:109, 1969.
114. Marsh, J. B., and Drabkin, D. L. Metabolic channeling in experimental nephrosis. IV. Net synthesis of plasma albumin by liver slices from normal and nephrotic rats. *J. Biol. Chem.* 230:1073, 1958.
115. Birke, G. Regulation of Protein Metabolism in Burns. In M. A. Rothschild and T. A. Waldmann (Eds.), *Plasma Protein Metabolism.* New York: Academic, 1970. P. 415.
116. Hanback, L. D., and Rittenbury, M. S. Response of the reticuloendothelial system to thermal injury. *Surg. Forum* 16:47, 1965.
117. Ritzmann, S. E., Cobb, E. K., Mattingly, D., McClung, C., Goldman, A. S., Larson, D. L., and Daniels, J. C. Serum Protein Profiles in Burned Children. In P. Matter, T. L. Barclay, and Z. Konickova (Eds.), *Research in Burns, Transactions of the International Congress on Research in Burns.* Bern: Huber, 1970. P. 502.
118. Waldmann, T. A. Protein-losing enteropathy. *Gastroenterology* 50:422, 1966.
119. Petersen, V. P., and Hastrup, J. Protein-losing enteropathy in constrictive pericarditis. *Acta Med. Scand.* 173:401, 1963.
120. Petersen, V. P., and Ottosen, P. Albumin turnover and thoracic duct lymph in constrictive pericarditis. *Acta Med. Scand.* 176:334, 1964.
121. Waldmann, T. A., Steinfeld, J. L., Dutcher, T. F., Davidson, J. D., and Gordon, R. S., Jr. The role of the gastrointestinal system in "idiopathic hypoproteinemia." *Gastroenterology* 41:197, 1961.

122. Bookstein, J. J., French, A. B., and Pollard, H. M. Protein-losing gastroenterology: Concepts derived from lymphangiograph. *Am. J. Dig. Dis.* 10:573, 1965.

123. McGuigan, J. E., Purkenson, M. L., Trudeau, W. L., and Peterson, M. L. Studies of the immunologic defects associated with intestinal lymphangiectasia. *Ann. Intern. Med.* 68:398, 1968.

124. Pomerantz, M., and Waldmann, T. A. Systemic lymphatic abnormalities associated with gastrointestinal protein loss secondary to intestinal lymphangiectasia. *Gastroenterology* 45:703, 1963.

125. Gill, W. M., Jr., and Alfidi, R. J. Roentgenographic manifestations of lymphangiectasia. Report of a case. *Am. J. Roentgenol. Radium Ther. Nucl. Med.* 109:185, 1970.

126. Jeffries, G. H., Chapman, A., and Sleisenger, M. H. Low-fat diet in intestinal lymphangiectasia: Its effect on albumin metabolism. *N. Engl. J. Med.* 270:761, 1964.

127. Strober, W., Wochner, R. D., Carbone, P. P., and Waldmann, T. A. Intestinal lymphangiectasia: A protein-losing enteropathy with hypogammaglobulinemia, lymphocytopenia and impaired homograft rejection. *J. Clin. Invest.* 46:1643, 1967.

128. Griffen, W. O., Jr., Belin, R. P., Furman, R. W., Leiber, A., Schaeffer, J. W., and Dubilier, L. C. Colonic lymphangiectasia: Report of two cases. *Dis. Colon Rectum* 15:49, 1972.

129. Ivey, K., DenBeste, L., Kent, T. H., and Clifton, J. A. Lymphangiectasia of the colon with protein loss and malabsorption. *Gastroenterology* 47:709, 1969.

130. Schaefer, J. W., Griffen, W. O., Jr., and Dubilier, L. C. Colonic lymphangiectasia associated with a potassium depletion syndrome. *Gastroenterology* 55:515, 1968.

131. Butz, W. C. Giant hypertrophic gastritis. A report of fourteen cases. *Gastroenterology* 39:183, 1960.

132. Jones, E. A., Young, W. B., Morson, B. C., and Dawson, A. M. A study of six patients with hypertrophy of the gastric mucosa with particular reference to albumin metabolism. *Gut* 13:270, 1972.

133. Mahmoud, J., and McKechnie, J. Acute transient protein-losing gastroenteropathy in an adult. *Am. J. Gastroenterol.* 57:416, 1972.

134. Gill, J. R., Jr., Cox, J., Delea, C. S., and Bartter, F. S. Idiopathic edema. II. Pathogenesis of edema in patients with hypoalbuminemia. *Am. J. Med.* 52:452, 1972.

135. Strober, W., Blaese, R. M., and Waldmann, T. A. Abnormalities of Immunoglobulin Metabolism. In M. A. Rothschild and T. A. Waldmann (Eds.), *Plasma Protein Metabolism.* New York: Academic, 1970. P. 287.

136. Waldmann, T. A., Miller, E. J., and Terry, W. D. Hypercatabolism of IgG and albumin: A new familial disorder. *Clin. Res.* 16:45, 1968.

137. Cooper, M. D., Chase, H. P., Lowman, J. T., Krivit, W., and Good, R. A. Wiskott-Aldrich syndrome. *Am. J. Med.* 44:499, 1968.

Carrier Protein Abnormalities

14

Jerry C. Daniels

The maintenance of metabolic stability within the human body requires a rather complex series of transportation systems that interconnect different body compartments at all levels of biological organization. At the gross level, intertwining channels carry various biological fluids; at the cellular level, microtubular networks and transmembrane shuttle systems are evident; and, at the molecular level, there exist both molecular vehicles for various substances and specialized "electron transport" pathways.

The serum is a particularly important channel for the incessant transport and interchange of many metabolic entities. A number of proteins have been identified within normal human serum which function, either solely or partially, to carry specific substances from one body site to another within the intravascular compartment. Additionally, circulating albumin carries many substances "piggyback" in a rather nonspecific fashion, with its molecular passengers constantly boarding and unboarding as this protein travels the circulatory route (see Chap. 13).

The term *carrier protein* has been applied to those proteins whose primary function includes the specific attachment of a single molecular species and the delivery of that substance to an area of metabolic disposition. Such proteins have also been called *transport proteins, shuttle proteins,* and *conveyor proteins.* Many of these carrier proteins may perform concomitant functions, such as displaying acute-phase response to various stimuli (see Chap. 18). In certain clinical disorders, changes in carrier protein functions or concentrations may be important by consequence of alterations in the availability of passenger substances.

The carrier proteins to be considered are ceruloplasmin (copper carrier), haptoglobin (hemoglobin carrier), hemopexin (heme carrier), transferrin (iron carrier), and several less-understood proteins such as prealbumin (minor thyroxin carrier), thyroxin-binding globulin (major thyroxin carrier), transcobalamins (vitamin B_{12} carriers), transcortin (cortisol carrier), and albumin as a nonspecific shuttle mechanism (see Appendix). Undoubtedly, numerous other carrier proteins remain to be elucidated. Figure 14-1 illustrates the electrophoretic migration of carrier

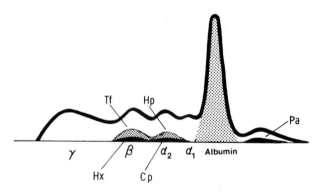

Figure 14-1
Electrophoretic
distribution of
major carrier pro-
teins and their
relative concen-
trations (for de-
tails, see text).

proteins in the α_2- and β-globulin fractions, where most carrier proteins are found with the exception of the rapidly migrating prealbumin (*Pa*) and the albumin fractions. Carrier protein ceruloplasmin (*Cp*) binds copper (*Cu*) for utilization in cellular enzyme systems; Figure 14-2 schematizes this physiological role of ceruloplasmin. Haptoglobin (*Hp*) carries free hemoglobin (Hb) to the reticuloendothelial system (RES) for degradation and iron rescue. When hemoglobin breakdown releases iron-containing heme moieties, these are taken up by circulating hemopexin (*Hx*). Free iron (Fe) is shuttled principally to the bone marrow for use in erythropoiesis by transferrin (*Tf*). Table 14-1 summarizes some of the properties of the carrier proteins.

Ceruloplasmin

PHYSIOLOGICAL ASPECTS
Ceruloplasmin is an α_2-globulin of 150,000 molecular weight, which is capable of reversibly binding eight atoms of copper to each molecule [1, 2] (see Fig. 14-2). This protein appears blue-green in the oxidized state, carries at least 95 percent of all copper in the body following gastrointestinal (GI) absorption of the metal, and exchanges bound copper with the surrounding medium for ultimate cellular incorporation into cytochrome oxidase (the terminal enzyme in the sequence of cellular oxygen consumption for energy production [3]) and possibly other copper-containing enzyme systems (e.g., tyrosinase, lysylamine oxidase, monoamine oxidase, ascorbic acid oxidase, and superoxide dismutase [4, 5]). Ceruloplasmin has recently been shown to possess histaminase activity [6], although the physiological significance of this finding is unclear.

PATHOPHYSIOLOGICAL ASPECTS

DECREASED SERUM CONCENTRATIONS
Acquired disorders. Since ceruloplasmin is produced in the liver, it is not surprising that decreased serum levels of this protein may occur in

Figure 14-2
Physiological role of ceruloplasmin
(for details, see text).

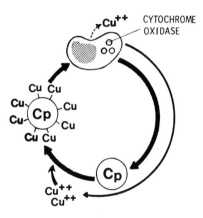

Ingestion

severe liver disease. The most extensive demonstration of such decreased levels has been in cases of primary biliary cirrhosis and primary biliary atresia [7]. Some feedback regulation of ceruloplasmin production in response to copper absorption must exist, since decreased ceruloplasmin levels have been documented in absorptive disorders where GI uptake of copper is impaired, notably in tropical and nontropical sprue and in scleroderma of the small bowel [3]. In these instances, the underlying clinical disorders account for the patient's symptoms, and the depressed ceruloplasmin level represents merely an associated laboratory finding rather than a primary pathophysiological mechanism.

Table 14-1.   Properties of Carrier Proteins

Protein	Binding Substance	Electro-phoretic Mobility	Molec-ular Weight	Normal Serum Concentration (mg/100 ml)
Ceruloplasmin	Copper	α_2	150,000	10–40
Haptoglobin	Hemoglobin	α_2	100,000	50–220
Hemopexin	Heme	β	70,000	70–130
Transferrin	Iron	β	80,000	200–400
Albumin	Ions, drugs, etc.	Albumin	69,000	3200–5000
Prealbumin	Thyroxine (260 μg/100 ml)	Prealbumin	61,000	10–40
Thyroxin-binding globulin	Thyroxine (21 μg/100 ml)	α_2	40,000	< 1
Transcortin	Cortisol (30 μg/100 ml)	α_1	–	~ 7
Cyanocobala-min I	Vitamin B_{12}	α_1	121,000	–
Cyanocobala-min II	Vitamin B_{12}	β	37,000	–

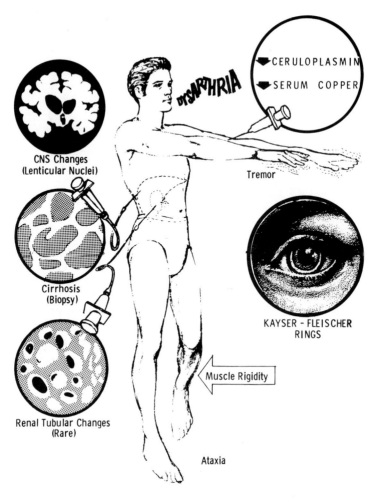

Figure 14-3
Clinical features of Wilson's disease (see Case Report 1).

Congenital disorders. An autosomal genetic defect of ceruloplasmin production exists in the form of Wilson's disease, which also is known as *hepatolenticular degeneration* [8]. The clinical features of this disease (Fig. 14-3), which may become manifest between ages 6 and 50 years but most commonly appear between late childhood and early adult life, are a result of the fact that copper in the free form exhibits considerable toxicity for certain tissues when it accumulates to excess levels, whereas ceruloplasmin-copper complexes are nontoxic.

Copper accumulation, with consequent tissue damage and malfunction, is common in the liver, brain, and cornea but rare in the kidney.

These accumulations are a direct result of the lack of the copper-carrier protein ceruloplasmin. In the liver, a 100-fold excess of copper is not unusual in patients with this disease. The result can appear either as hepatic parenchymal disease, often appearing as cirrhosis or masquerading as "chronic active hepatitis" [9], or as the complications of portal hypertension associated with postnecrotic cirrhosis (e.g., esophageal varices or hypersplenism). Copper levels in the brain may be 10 to 30 times normal. Copper tends to accumulate most often in the lenticular nuclei, and their degeneration leads to symptoms similar to those of parkinsonism or bizarre choreoathetoid movements. It may also be found in the cerebrum, cerebellum, thalamus, brain stem, and spinal cord, thus accounting for a wide variety of neurological symptoms ranging from psychoneurotic behavior to seizure disorders. Copper deposition in the cornea results in a golden-brown pigmentation encircling the cornea just within the corneoscleral junction, which must be confirmed by slit-lamp examination. This finding, which is virtually pathognomonic for Wilson's disease, is termed the *Kayser-Fleischer ring,* and it disappears with adequate treatment of the disease. Remarkably, there is a total lack of visual symptoms in patients exhibiting this sign. Renal involvement, primarily proximal tubular damage, is minor in Wilson's disease but may occasionally give rise to significant symptoms (including proteinuria and aminoaciduria). Hemolytic anemia has also been reported in Wilson's disease [10, 11] and may represent a direct toxic effect of copper on erythrocytes [12]. More subtle findings include an azure hue to the nailbeds and, infrequently, bone lesions. Figure 14-3 illustrates some of the clinical features of Wilson's disease. A typical case report is as follows:

Case Report 1
A 27-year-old man ceased employment because of a 2-year history of progressive tremor, ataxia, rigidity of skeletal muscles, incoordination, and dysarthria. Upon presentation for medical evaluation, the patient was found to be slightly cachectic. Peculiar greenish-brown rings of pigmentation were localized bilaterally at the periphery of the cornea that were best visualized by slit-lamp examination (i.e., Kayser-Fleischer rings). The liver edge was palpable about 2 cm below the right costal margin and was firm and not tender. Percutaneous liver biopsy revealed cirrhosis. Serum protein electrophoresis revealed polyclonal gammopathy. Radial immunodiffusion (RID) studies disclosed a severely diminished ceruloplasmin level (less than 1 mg per 100 ml), which correlated with a decreased total serum copper level. The patient responded satisfactorily to treatment with penicillamine (a chelating, copper-removing agent).
Final Diagnosis: Hepatolenticular degeneration (Wilson's disease).

The diagnosis of Wilson's disease rests on five cardinal points: first, the unequivocal demonstration of Kayser-Fleischer rings; second, the presence of less than 10 mg per 100 ml of serum ceruloplasmin as demonstrated by RID in patients with compatible clinical symptoms; third, if liver biopsy is possible in the face of clotting abnormalities, the demonstration of copper content in excess of 250 mg per gram of dry liver;

fourth, and less reliable, the urinary excretion of more than 100 μg per 100 ml copper in 24 hours; and fifth, and seldom used, a significant diminution of the incorporation of radioactive copper into ceruloplasmin. The most useful and practical of these approaches are the documentation of Kayser-Fleischer rings, which are found in about 70 percent of patients, and the deficiency of ceruloplasmin as demonstrated by RID, which is found in 95 percent of patients. It should be remembered, however, that an acute-phase increase in a deficient ceruloplasmin level, such as may occur with hepatitis or associated inflammatory complications, may transiently result in low normal ceruloplasmin levels, so that in some cases, serial determination of this protein may be necessary. It follows that although a low or absent serum ceruloplasmin may be diagnostic evidence of Wilson's disease, a ceruloplasmin concentration in the normal range does not necessarily rule out the presence of this disease [3, 8], particularly in its early stages [13].

Recent evidence for the existence of an abnormal storage protein (copperthionein) with a greatly increased affinity for copper in the liver of some patients with Wilson's disease [14] is of interest in view of an earlier suggestion [15] that such an abnormality would explain many of the defects of copper homeostasis in this disorder. Further studies are necessary before such a "magnet effect" can be considered as the genetic basis of Wilson's disease.

Treatment of Wilson's disease is directed toward the removal of excess copper from tissue depots. This may be accomplished quite satisfactorily by the administration of 1 to 2 gm daily of D-penicillamine, which provides urinary excretion of complexed copper and is usually associated with significant improvements of symptoms (Fig. 14-4). Concomitant pyridoxine administration (50 mg daily) will prevent the optic neuritis of vitamin deficiency that may accompany prolonged administration of this drug. After penicillamine administration, copper is removed rapidly from the kidneys, more slowly from the liver, and slowest from the central nervous system throughout a typical 12- to 14-month course of therapy [16]. Some cases have been treated continuously for up to 9 to 13 years, with complete clinical remission [17]. The toxicity of D-penicillamine, which is manifested primarily by nephrotoxicity, skin rash, and bone marrow suppression, may prohibit its use in a few patients. Use of the cupriuria produced by D-penicillamine as diagnostic evidence of Wilson's disease [9] is not advisable in the face of the recent evidence of the nonspecificity of this parameter [13].

Secondary drugs include the use of the chelating agent BAL (British antilewisite) in a dosage of 2.5 mg per kilogram twice daily in 5-day courses separated by 2-day intervals (GI toxicity may occur with this drug) in conjunction with potassium sulfide, 40 mg prior to meals. The latter drug prevents copper absorption and promotes fecal copper excretion. An oral chelating agent, carbacrylamine resin, has recently been reported to be effective in combination with a low copper diet [18]. Ethylenediaminetetraacetate (EDTA), another chelating agent, is curiously less reliable for copper removal than the other agents, but it may be

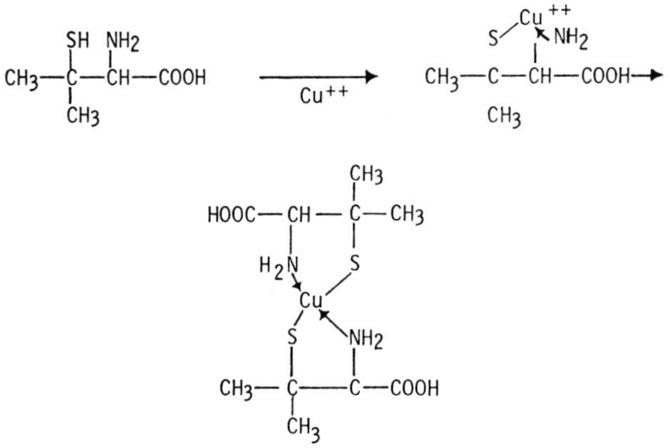

Figure 14-4
Mode of copper chelation by D-penicillamine.

used. Surgery for the CNS manifestations or portal hypertension of Wilson's disease has no place in the therapy of this disorder, and it may exacerbate the condition. Attempts at substitution therapy of ceruloplasmin are limited because of the expense and restricted supply of this substance [19].

Normal adult serum levels. Normal adult serum levels of ceruloplasmin are 10 to 40 mg per 100 ml, which are attained 3 to 6 months after birth following neonatal levels of 7 to 15 mg per 100 ml [20]. Ceruloplasmin is most conveniently assayed by RID, but it may be quantitated indirectly by its oxidative effect on a defined substrate or by chemical measurements of serum copper levels [21].

INCREASED SERUM CONCENTRATIONS
Ceruloplasmin levels may be elevated by a greatly increased plasma concentration of estrogen, as may occur in hepatitis, or by any of the numerous inflammatory stimuli that can elicit the "acute-phase" behavior of this protein (see Chap. 18).

Haptoglobin

PHYSIOLOGICAL ASPECTS
Haptoglobin is a system of closely related allotypic α_2-globulins with a mean molecular weight of about 100,000 that binds hemoglobin released into the circulation by intravascular hemolysis, such as that which occurs physiologically with erythrocyte senescence [1, 22]. Teleologically, such a "salvage" mechanism for retaining released hemoglobin ultimately serves as an "iron trap," which allows reutilization of iron in the synthesis of new hemoglobin for erythrocyte production. Iron represents a relatively precious commodity within the body economy, so that several backup systems exist for its conservation; haptoglobin, however,

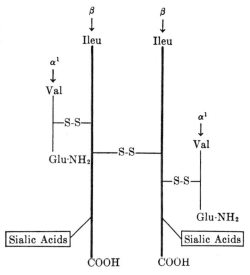

Figure 14-5
Proposed structure of Hp-1-1.
(Reproduced by permission.
From Shim, B. S., and Bearn,
A. G. *J. Exp. Med.* 120:
625, 1964.)

represents the first line of preservation. The large size of the hemoglobin-haptoglobin complex precludes renal loss of the hemoglobin. Free hemoglobin (Hb) combines with haptoglobin (Hp) to form stable hemoglobin-haptoglobin complexes (Hb-Hp), which are cleared from the circulation within minutes by the reticuloendothelial system (liver, bone marrow, and spleen). In the reticuloendothelial system (RES), further hemoglobin degradation occurs, and ultimate bone marrow erythropoiesis reutilizes the iron, eventually resulting in reticulocyte release. The proposed structure of Hp 1-1 (see discussion of phenotypes below) is depicted in Figure 14-5. It appears that the tetrameric α_2,β_2-hemoglobin molecule is split into the dimeric α,β form, which then complexes to the haptoglobin. The nature of the forces binding α,β-Hb to haptoglobin is unknown [23]. It is known that in a molar ratio of Hp to Hb of one, a tetramer of Hb (α_2,β_2, with a molecular weight of 64,500) is bound to one mole of Hp 1-1 (molecular weight 85,000). In a molar ratio of Hp to Hb greater than one, another complex is present in addition to the first one; it is formed by one dimer of Hb (α,β) and one mole of Hp 1-1 [24, 25]. By virtue of the rapid RES clearance mechanism, the amount of detectable Hb-Hp complexes at any given time is low (about 0.3 mg per 100 ml). Significant and rapid changes in serum haptoglobin concentrations obviously reflect rates of intravascular hemolysis. A postulated additional role for haptoglobin is that of an antiprotease [26] (see Chap. 15).

Starch-gel electrophoresis can separate haptoglobin into three phenotypes, which are designated Hp 1-1, Hp 2-2, and Hp 2-1, as expressions of two autosomal genes [33]. These phenotypes appear to arise by complex, and yet poorly understood, polymerization of basic subunits [1, 27]. They differ in molecular weight (Hp 1-1 is 80,000, Hp 2-1 is 120,000, and Hp 2-2 is 160,000) expressed as mean values for the vari-

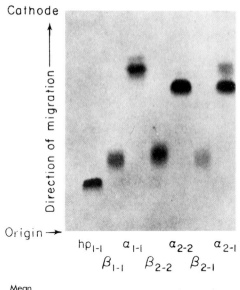

Figure 14-6
Electrophoretic separation patterns of the three haptoglobin phenotypes ($\beta_{1\text{-}1}$, $\beta_{2\text{-}2}$, $\beta_{2\text{-}1}$) and their molecular weights. (Modified from Gordon, S., Cleve, H., and Bearn, A. G. *Proc. Soc. Exp. Biol. Med.* 127:52, 1968.)

Cathode

Direction of migration

Origin →

$hp_{1\text{-}1}$ $\alpha_{1\text{-}1}$ $\alpha_{2\text{-}2}$ $\alpha_{2\text{-}1}$
$\beta_{1\text{-}1}$ $\beta_{2\text{-}2}$ $\beta_{2\text{-}1}$

Mean
Molecular Weights: (80,000)   (160,000)   (120,000)

ous polymers [1]. The haptoglobin molecule is comprised of α and β polypeptide chains. The physicochemical and immunological differences among these phenotypes appear to reside on the α chains of the haptoglobin molecule, while the β chains of all types appear identical [23]. Figure 14-6 shows the starch-gel electrophoretic separation patterns of the commonly encountered haptoglobin phenotypes.

Certain racial differences exist in the distribution of these phenotypes (Fig. 14-7). The frequency of Hp 1-1 in relation to the other haptoglobin phenotypes is highest among Africans, South and Central Americans, and the natives of several Pacific islands. It is lowest among Asians, especially East Indians, and among Europeans it has an intermediate frequency. The frequency of Hp 2-2 is highest among Asiatics and Europeans. Hp 2-1 occurs in approximately 10 percent of black Americans, but rarely in nonblacks [28]. Genetic polymorphism of haptoglobin types has been encountered in every population studied. Hp 2-2 occurs with an overall frequency which exceeds that of either Hp 1-1 or 2-1, and thus appears to be the genetically favored form. The advantage of this distribution is obscure, since no detectable difference in hemoglobin binding occurs among haptoglobin types. Since Hp 2-2 is considered to have developed from Hp 1-1, selection pressures leading to this event must have occurred very early in man's evolution [23]. The absence of detectable circulating haptoglobin has been defined as the Hp 0-0 state.

Attempts to relate haptoglobin phenotypes to disease processes have been numerous [23], but only the relations of Hp 1-1 to juvenile rheumatoid arthritis [29] and to leukemia [30] appear well founded at present. Further studies in this area may well clarify other associations.

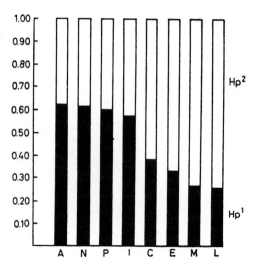

Figure 14-7
The frequencies of Hp alleles in the main human racial groups. *N:* Negroids, *A:* Australian aborigines, *L:* Lapps, *M:* Mongoloids, *C:* Caucasoids, *I:* Indians, *E:* Eskimos, *P:* Polynesians. (Reproduced by permission. From Walter, H., and Steegmuller, H. *Hum. Hered.* 19:209 [Basel: Karger, 1969].)

PATHOPHYSIOLOGICAL ASPECTS

DECREASED SERUM CONCENTRATIONS

Acquired disorders. Any disorder that is associated with significant intravascular hemolysis may result in diminished serum haptoglobin levels because of the accelerated removal of hemoglobin-haptoglobin complexes from the circulation without increased haptoglobin synthesis. Haptoglobin consumption effectively distinguishes intravascular hemolysis from extravascular hemolysis, as shown in Figure 14-8. Common acquired disorders include the autoimmune hemolytic anemias, whether idiopathic or associated with the broad spectrum of collagen-vascular disorders and other immunological derangements; the drug-induced hemolytic anemias (e.g., methyldopa); the macroangiopathic (i.e., large-vessel) hemolytic anemias, such as those that occur by the mechanical traumatization of erythrocytes by implanted prosthetic heart valves or vigorous prolonged blunt trauma to the extremities (e.g., swimming, karate exercises, or marching); the microangiopathic (i.e., small-vessel) hemolytic anemias, such as those that occur in disseminated intravascular coagulation; and such conditions as malarial infestation and paroxysmal nocturnal hemoglobinuria. Figure 14-9 summarizes common conditions in which intravascular fragmentation of erythrocytes leads to intravascular hemolysis with associated haptoglobin consumption; Figure 14-10 illustrates one means by which disseminated intravascular coagulation may lead to erythrocyte damage with hemolysis.

The clinical features of these disorders are quite variable, but the final common pathway of intravascular hemolysis may be accompanied by signs and symptoms of anemia, mild to moderate jaundice due to the accumulation of unconjugated bilirubin, and a brisk reticulocytosis. An illustrative case follows (see Fig. 14-11).

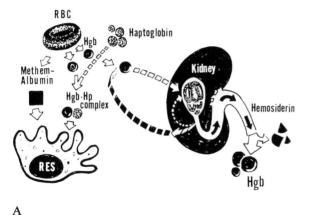

RBC

Haptoglobin

Hgb

Methem-
Albumin

Hgb·Hp
complex

Kidney

Hemosiderin

RES

Hgb

A

RBC

BILIRUBIN

Urobilinogen

REABSORBED

RES

Liver

G.I.

Fecal   Urine
UROBILINOGEN

B

Figure 14-8
A. Intravascular hemolysis. Erythrocyte in the process of hemolysis liberates free Hb and methemalbumin. The Hb is bound to the available circulating Hp to form firm Hb-Hp complexes. These are transported to the RES (e.g., liver), where they are phagocytosed and the iron is recycled in the process of erythropoiesis. If free Hb exceeds the available Hp, the Hb is then excreted into the urine. In this process, hemosiderin may be formed and excreted. *B.* Extravascular hemolysis without haptoglobin consumption. In contrast to intravascular hemolysis, extravascular hemolysis follows the usual pathways of red blood cell degradation and the formation of bilirubin and derivatives, which are excreted into the feces and urine.

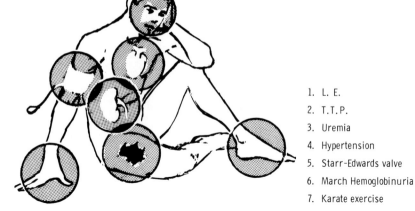

1. L. E.
2. T.T.P.
3. Uremia
4. Hypertension
5. Starr-Edwards valve
6. March Hemoglobinuria
7. Karate exercise

Figure 14-9
Conditions associated with intravascular hemolysis. *L.E.:* Lupus erythematosus. *T.T.P.:* thrombotic thrombocytopenic purpura.

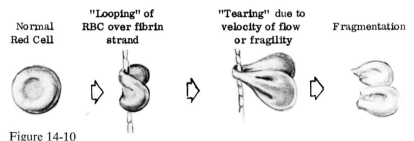

Normal Red Cell	"Looping" of RBC over fibrin strand	"Tearing" due to velocity of flow or fragility	Fragmentation

Figure 14-10
Mechanism of red blood cell fragmentation in disseminated intravascular coagulation (Modified from Bull, B. D., Rudenberg, M. L., Dacie, J. V., and Brain, M. C. *Br. J. Haematol.* 14:643, 1968.)

Case Report 2
A 21-year-old college student presented at the dispensary with a 2-month history of progressive fatigue, exertional dyspnea, fever, nausea, and severe weight loss. Physical examination revealed diffuse cervical lymphadenopathy, mild jaundice, hepatosplenomegaly, and a small pleural effusion on the left. The patient was hospitalized at the University Medical Center. Serum bilirubin was 6.5 mg per 100 ml, with 1.0 mg per 100 ml direct-reacting fraction. A blood count revealed 11,000 leukocytes per cubic millimeter with 60 percent lymphocytes and a normochromic normocytic anemia (hemoglobulin was 5.8 mg per 100 ml). Reticulocytes were 8.3 percent, and bone marrow aspiration revealed a reactive process with numerous erythrocytic precursors.

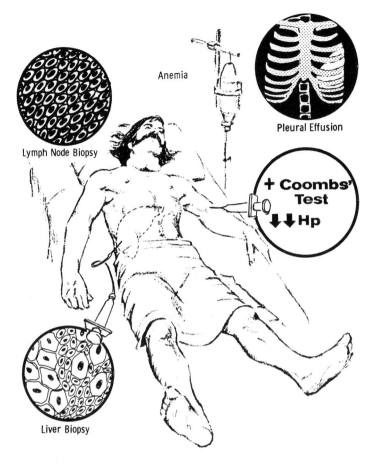

Anemia

Lymph Node Biopsy

Pleural Effusion

+ Coombs' Test
↓↓ Hp

Liver Biopsy

Figure 14-11
Clinical features of intravascular hemolytic state (see Case Report 2).

A direct Coombs' test was strongly positive. Serum haptoglobulin was 12 mg per 100 ml (normal is 50 to 220 mg per 100 ml). A lymph-node biopsy examination revealed the lymphocyte depletion-type of Hodgkin's disease. Results of a liver biopsy examination were positive, resulting in a IV-B staging. Despite chemotherapy, the patient underwent rapid deterioration and died of *Pseudomonas* pneumonia with sepsis on the 45th hospital day.

Final Diagnosis: Hodgkin's disease with intravascular autoimmune hemolysis.

The diagnosis of intravascular hemolysis—once the hemolytic state has been defined by reticulocytosis and, occasionally, by adjunctive measures (e.g., urinary hemosiderin, red-cell survival studies, or fecal urobilinogen)—as opposed to extravascular hemolysis, rests primarily on the demonstration of a decrease or absence of serum haptoglobin as measured by RID or electroimmunodiffusion (EID).

Treatment must be directed toward the underlying disorder (e.g., by drug therapy of autoimmune disease states, the removal of hemolytically active drugs, the cessation of mechanical trauma, or anticoagulation of disseminated intravascular coagulation), while supporting the patient by transfusion with packed red blood cells as warranted by hemoglobin levels.

Hepatic disorders have also been associated with acquired hypohaptoglobinemia [31].

Congenital disorders. A number of congenital defects that influence erythrocyte membrane stability may result under appropriate circumstances in significant intravascular hemolysis, with the removal of hemoglobin-haptoglobin complexes from the circulation by mechanisms identical to those in acquired disorders and the consequent depletion of serum haptoglobin. These include sickle-cell disease and other hemoglobinopathies, glucose-6-phosphate dehydrogenase deficiency, hereditary spherocytosis, thalassemia, and related disorders. Further, a congenital absence of haptoglobin (anhaptoglobinemia, which is actually a misnomer, since such cases most often represent a severe hypohaptoglobinemia) has been encountered in rare instances [32]. Figure 14-12 represents the family tree for propositus "L. B.," who was found to be in excellent health but with a virtually undetectable haptoglobin level (less than 1 mg per 100 ml). The possibility that the iron-salvage function of haptoglobin had been assumed by hemopexin has been considered, but L. B.'s hemopexin level was 75 mg per 100 ml (normal is 70 to 130 mg per 100 ml). A second case of anhaptoglobinemia in our files is that of N. C., whose haptoglobin was 3 mg per 100 ml with a hemopexin level that was diminished to 44 mg per 100 ml.

INCREASED SERUM CONCENTRATIONS

Haptoglobin may behave as an acute-phase reactant to a number of stimuli (see Chap. 18), showing a moderate to considerable rise in serum concentration in the presence of infection, neoplasia, trauma, and other inflammatory conditions characterized by tissue injury and repair. The possibility that haptoglobin may oppose, as a protective mechanism, the proteolytic activity of cathepsin-B [26] may be related to such increases (see Chap. 15). Hyperhaptoglobinemia is due to an enhanced hepatic synthesis of haptoglobin, which is induced by unknown factors that possibly include uncharacterized humoral influences, while the degradation rate of the protein remains unchanged [33]. It must, therefore, be kept in mind that the coexistence of inflammation and hemolysis may be associated with decreased, normal, or increased haptoglobin levels at the time of examination.

An example of the behavior of haptoglobin levels in the face of acute trauma is provided in Figure 14-13A, which shows the time-course profile of haptoglobin in 57 children sustaining acute thermal burn injury. The shaded zone represents the range of control levels determined in 141 burned children returning for reconstructive surgery at about 40 months postburn. Haptoglobin levels were significantly elevated as early as day

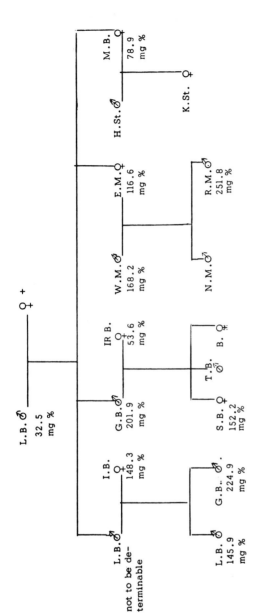

Figure 14-12
Family tree of propositus with anhaptoglobinemia, showing Hp concentrations of the different family members. (Reproduced by permission of Bonacker, L. H., Behring Diagnostics, Inc., Somerville, N.J.)

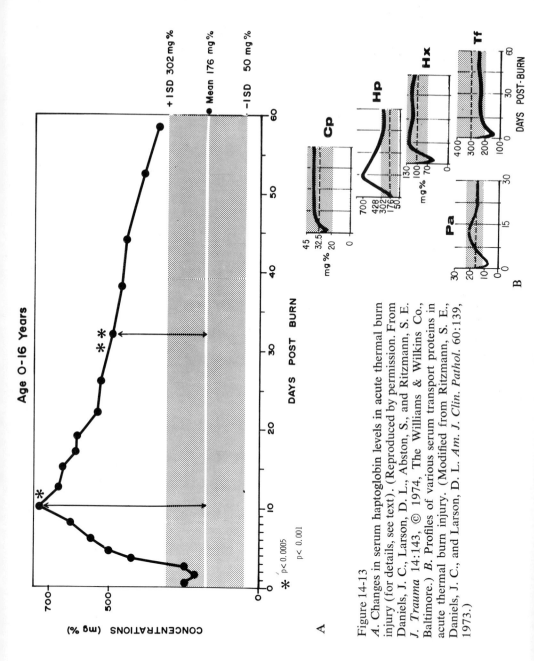

Figure 14-13

A. Changes in serum haptoglobin levels in acute thermal burn injury (for details, see text). (Reproduced by permission. From Daniels, J. C., Larson, D. L., Abston, S., and Ritzmann, S. E. *J. Trauma* 14:143, © 1974, The Williams & Wilkins Co., Baltimore.) *B*. Profiles of various serum transport proteins in acute thermal burn injury. (Modified from Ritzmann, S. E., Daniels, J. C., and Larson, D. L. *Am. J. Clin. Pathol.* 60:139, 1973.)

5 to 6, with a peak on day 12 at 701 mg per 100 ml ($p < .0005$). This elevation is greater than four standard deviations above the mean control level of 175 mg per 100 ml. Levels of this protein decreased slowly thereafter, but remained significantly elevated throughout the observation period, with a probability value of less than .001 as compared with the control mean shortly after one month postburn. Although an acute-phase reactant property of haptoglobin is the most likely explanation for this pattern, an alternative explanation may be offered. The hemoglobin liberated from the intravascular hemolysis that is associated with acute thermal burn injury should be readily cleared from the circulation as Hb-Hp complexes by the reticuloendothelial system. A blockade of the RES must be considered to be a logical result of overloading by tissue debris consequent to thermal trauma. Such a blockade could lead to decreased removal rates of Hb-Hp complexes from the circulation, thus accounting for the observed results [34].

TECHNIQUES OF QUANTITATION
Available haptoglobin can be quantitated by RID, within the normal levels of 50 to 220 mg per 100 ml, or by other techniques such as EID or colorimetry [35, 36]. However, the technical considerations of measuring the concentration of this protein by means of RID (see Chap. 4, pp. 61–68) must take into account the different haptoglobin types, since the molecular variations among the genetic types will affect diffusion rates. The values obtained for haptoglobin concentration by RID, with reference to standard human serum, must be multiplied by 0.6 for Hp 1-1, by 1.3 for Hp 2-1, and by 1.5 for Hp 2-2.

Hemopexin

PHYSIOLOGICAL ASPECTS
Hemopexin is a β-globulin with a molecular weight of 70,000 that specifically binds the iron-containing core of the hemoglobin molecule known as heme [1, 37]. When hemoglobin degradation occurs, dissociation into four heme subunits per molecule results. The iron within these heme shells then converts to the trivalent form from the bivalent state. In this oxidized form, the heme is bound by hemopexin and delivered to the hepatocytes of the liver, where the enzyme, heme oxygenase, initiates conversion of the heme to bilirubin. Thus, hemoglobin degradation, particularly that which occurs intravascularly, is normally accompanied by consumption of circulating hemopexin. A lesser amount of oxidized heme is bound by albumin, but this is eventually transferred to hemopexin for delivery to the liver [37].

PATHOPHYSIOLOGICAL ASPECTS

DECREASED SERUM LEVELS
Acquired disorders. In general, the same types of hemolytic disorders that result in haptoglobin utilization will affect hemopexin levels in

the same direction. The hemoglobin-haptoglobin complex will disintegrate into free haptoglobin and four heme moieties within richly vascular reticuloendothelial tissues [38]. To a lesser extent, such hemoglobin degradation occurs intravascularly with any degree of hemolysis; the iron-containing heme will be complexed with circulating hemopexin for delivery to the liver. Mild degrees of intravascular hemolysis, which are insufficient to exhaust the haptoglobin pool completely, may produce detectable changes in hemopexin. More importantly, depletion of the entire circulating haptoglobin pool by moderate intravascular hemolysis removes that index of hemolytic rate, and the "second line of defense" (i.e., hemopexin levels) becomes mandatory for quantitation of the erythrocyte destruction [37]. Thus, in those instances of brisk intravascular hemolysis, particularly in an acute episode in which haptoglobin removal is complete in the face of massive hemoglobin liberation, the excess of uncomplexed hemoglobin will undergo intravascular degradation to heme moieties, which will be complexed primarily to hemopexin and temporarily, and to a much lesser extent, to albumin. The albumin will later transfer its heme passengers to the higher affinity–specific carrier protein hemopexin as the latter becomes available after delivery of its initial heme saturation. The result is a significant and often prolonged decrease in circulating hemopexin. For these reasons, hemopexin levels are considered more sensitive and reliable in the quantitation of intravascular hemolysis than are those of haptoglobin. Hemopexin levels have found particular application as a monitor for the hemolytic component of prosthetic heart-valve replacement in cardiovascular surgery [39], where the hemolysis may be sufficient to render serum haptoglobin persistently undetectable [40]. Another recent application is the intrauterine detection of Rh disease by the measurement of hemopexin levels in amniotic fluid [41].

Low hemopexin levels may be associated with pathological conditions other than hemolytic disease. In certain renal diseases, nonspecific urinary excretion of low molecular weight proteins may lead to the loss of hemopexin. Similarly, loss of hemopexin due to the reduced synthesis by a failing liver may occur.

A case of the usefulness of hemopexin levels in intravascular hemolysis follows (Fig. 14-14).

Case Report 3

A 56-year-old executive presented with a 6-month history of chest pain and syncopal episodes. Physical examination revealed atherosclerotic changes by fundoscopy and early peripheral vascular disease. A loud systolic murmur was audible in the aortic area of the precordium, radiating to the neck. Cardiac catheterization confirmed a severe aortic stenosis. Accordingly, a Starr-Edwards ball-valve prosthesis, with a silicon rubber ball and bare metal cage, was inserted in place of the diseased valve. Postoperatively, the patient did well until about one year later, when he was hospitalized with exertional dyspnea, weakness, easy fatigability, and an obvious pallor. His prosthetic valve appeared to be functioning adequately. Hemoglobin was 8.0 gm per 100 ml, and the peripheral blood smear revealed anisocytosis, poikilocytosis,

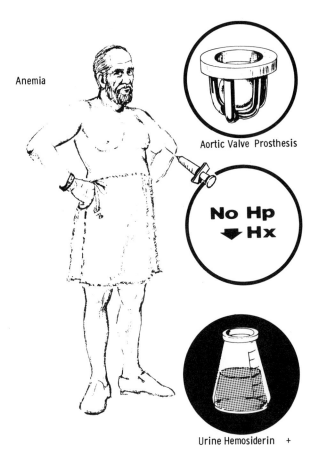

Anemia

Aortic Valve Prosthesis

No Hp
Hx

Urine Hemosiderin +

Figure 14-14
Application of hemopexin measurement to intravascular hemolysis (see Case Report 3).

and many schistocytes. The reticulocyte count was 11 percent. Serum hapto-globin levels were undetectable, and hemopexin levels were 40 mg per 100 ml. Based on these findings, a newer type of valve prosthesis, with a stellite ball and cloth-covered cage, was inserted in place of the original prosthesis. The patient has continued to do well, with no symptoms and with hemoglobin levels of about 12 gm per 100 ml. The same cardiovascular surgery team fol-lows its valve-replacement patients serially with a number of hematological parameters; it uniformly considers detectable haptoglobin levels to reflect an insignificant degree of intravascular hemolysis to warrant prosthesis replace-ment. Serum hemopexin levels are used to judge the severity of hemolysis and the necessity for revision in patients without serum haptoglobin.

Final Diagnosis: Hemolytic disease secondary to aortic valvular prosthesis.

Congenital disorders. The same congenital predispositions to hemo-lytic disease as discussed for haptoglobin apply to hemopexin. Again, hemopexin is a more sensitive and reliable indicator of active hemolysis, primarily because of total haptoglobin depletion [42].

INCREASED SERUM LEVELS

Increased hemopexin levels have been described in a wide variety of diseases, including multiple myeloma, Hodgkin's disease, acute myelocytic leukemia, diabetes mellitus, and various septic states [37, 43]. Extensive studies, which have attempted to ascertain whether such rises are of the acute-phase variety in response to the common denominator of tissue necrosis and inflammation, have revealed that such elevations are consistently modest and seldom more than twice normal. Serial sampling revealed no relation to severity or duration of inflammation, while known acute-phase proteins, including haptoglobin and lipoproteins (see Chap. 18), were significantly elevated in a correlated manner in the same patients [43]. Thus, the stability of homeostatic mechanisms that regulate hemopexin concentrations permits the use of serum levels of this protein to assess the severity of hemolysis in conditions concomitantly associated with acute-phase responses.

TECHNIQUES OF QUANTITATION

RID and EID are the most convenient methods for quantitating hemopexin, though other techniques are available [37]. Normal adult serum hemopexin levels as determined by RID are 70 to 130 mg per 100 ml.

Transferrin

PHYSIOLOGICAL ASPECTS

Transferrin is a β-globulin with 80,000 molecular weight that specifically binds two atoms of free (i.e., non-heme) iron to each molecule and subserves the transport of this metabolic commodity [1, 44]. Transferrin appears to be produced not only in the liver, but also in reticuloendothelial [45–47] and certain endocrine [48, 49] tissues. Free iron transport is required from its sites of generation by hemoglobin degradation (principally in the liver but to a lesser extent in the spleen) to the erythrocyte production sites within the bone marrow, as well as from the absorptive GI epithelial cells to sites of utilization in the bone marrow [50]. It is also transported in minute amounts to the liver and other tissues for incorporation into iron-containing enzyme systems (e.g., cytochromes). Physiological elevations of transferrin are seen during the second and third trimesters of pregnancy [51] and may be comparably induced by oral contraceptive agents [52].

PATHOPHYSIOLOGICAL ASPECTS

DECREASED SERUM LEVELS

Acquired disorders. A decrease in the circulating levels of transferrin is a rather nonspecific finding. Any acquired liver disease, especially portal cirrhosis and hemochromatosis, may result in diminished production of transferrin. Similarly, the "anemia of chronic disease" (sideropenia with reticuloendothelial siderosis), a veritable catch-all designation for a hypochromic microcytic anemia associated with chronic illness, may usually be differentiated from iron deficiency anemia by virtue of a decreased or normal serum transferrin level in the face of low serum iron levels. Special stains of bone marrow aspirates for iron are required to make this distinction definitively, however. Hypotransferrinemia is encountered in chronic infections [53], neoplasia, renal and hepatic diseases, and other categories of chronic debilitating illnesses, as well as by virtue of excessive loss in nephrosis. Figure 14-13B compares the serum profiles of various transport proteins following acute thermal burn injury; transferrin can be seen to be sharply depressed soon after the injury and remains at low normal values for up to 60 days [34].

The clinical importance of differentiating anemias that are characterized by low or normal serum transferrin from true iron deficiency anemia is that the former conditions will not respond to exogenous iron replacement. In such cases, iron therapy is not only futile, but it may result, over long periods of time, in iatrogenic hemochromatosis and is therefore contraindicated.

Congenital disorders. Congenital liver disease may result in hypotransferrinemia, and congenital atransferrinemia has occasionally been encountered. Heilmeyer [54] has reported the case of a 7-year-old girl with congenital atransferrinemia. She suffered from iron deficiency anemia in the face of excessive iron absorption due to the absence of plasma iron-binding activity. Features of hemosiderosis, including iron-laden macrophages and large depots of unutilized iron in the bone marrow, were present.

INCREASED SERUM LEVELS

Increased levels of transferrin, in contrast to the nonspecific decrease in chronic disease, reflect the body's attempt to enhance its iron stores by issuing abundant amounts of iron-carrying protein, which serves to amplify iron absorption from the GI tract. Thus, hypertransferrinemia has become almost synonymous with iron deficiency anemia. The underlying causes of iron deficiency anemia are numerous, but in the adult, they are more likely to be related to increased loss of iron stores (i.e., chronic hemorrhage) than to decreased iron ingestion. Defects of iron absorption may also occur (e.g., sprue).

Clinical manifestations of iron deficiency anemia are manifold, but they chiefly include pallor of the skin and mucosal surfaces, muscular weakness, easy fatigability, lack of ability to concentrate, restlessness, drowsiness, headaches, increased cold sensitivity, tinnitus, glossitis, and menstrual disturbances. Profound anemia may be associated with angina pectoris and electrocardiographic changes of coronary insufficiency. Splenomegaly may be encountered in some chronic states. A typical case of iron deficiency anemia follows, which is illustrated in Figure 14-15.

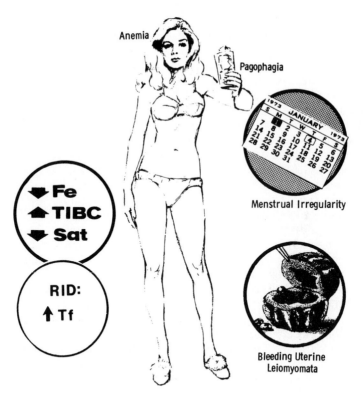

Figure 14-15
Clinical features of iron deficiency anemia (see Case Report 4).

Case Report 4

A 25-year-old laboratory technician complained of progressive fatigue and exertional dyspnea over a 6-month period. Additionally, she had recently noticed an increasing craving for ice cubes (pagophagia) [55]. Her menstrual history revealed slightly irregular menses with an increased flow over the previous 8 months. On physical examination, her nail beds and mucous membranes were pale. On pelvic examination she was found to have a large suprapubic mass, which was thought to be the uterus enlarged to nearly 12 cm in length. Laboratory studies revealed a leukocyte count of 3800 per cubic millimeter with an essentially normal differential, a hemoglobin of 9.6 gm per 100 ml, a hematocrit of 32 percent, and MCV of 65 cubic microns, an MCH of 20 pg per red cell, and an MCHC of 30 percent. Red cell morphology showed anisocytosis, poikilocytosis, and polychromatophilia. Serum iron was 66 μg per 100 ml, total iron-binding capacity (TIBC) was 437 mg per 100 ml, and iron saturation was 15 percent. A pregnancy test was negative. An upper GI roentgenographic series and an intravenous pyelogram were normal. She was referred to a surgeon, and exploratory laparotomy revealed a large leiomyoma of the uterus. On cut section, the tumor showed several areas of necrosis and hemorrhage. A myomectomy was performed, and postoperatively she was administered ferrous sulfate. Six weeks later, the patient's

Figure 14-16
Relationship between transferrin and plasma iron in health and disease expressed as percent of iron saturation of transferrin. Percent of transferrin bound with iron is shown in the dark areas.

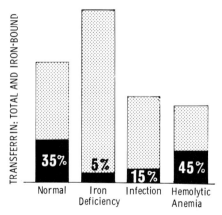

hemoglobin, hematocrit, and iron studies were normal, and she was without complaints.

Final Diagnosis: Iron deficiency anemia secondary to chronic blood loss.

Treatment of iron deficiency is most satisfactory with the oral administration of 300 mg of ferrous sulfate (or equivalent iron salts) three times daily. Treatment effectiveness may be gauged by appropriate reticulocytosis, and the duration of treatment should extend several months beyond the restoration of normal serum hemoglobin in order to replenish iron stores.

TECHNIQUES OF QUANTITATION

The serum transferrin concentration is most conveniently measured directly by RID or EID. Normal serum transferrin levels as measured by RID are 200 to 400 mg per 100 ml. The transferrin concentration reflects the so-called total iron-binding capacity (TIBC) that is utilized by hematologists as an index of iron metabolism and erythropoiesis (Fig. 14-16). Such techniques indirectly estimate the transferrin concentration by determining the ability of a given serum to combine with iron, as evidenced by colorimetric changes [56]. The results, then, represent the micrograms per 100 ml of iron that could be accommodated by the serum under test, as compared with the actual milligrams per 100 ml of transferrin as measured directly by RID.

The determination of increased serum transferrin concentrations is of paramount importance in identifying iron deficiency anemia, particularly in separating it from the previously mentioned iron-refractory anemias. Whether direct determination of transferrin by RID, EID, or indirect colorimetric assay by TIBC is used is without difference. With the increase in transferrin concentration (TIBC) in association with low serum iron, the percentage saturation of transferrin with iron falls to levels of 15 percent or less when iron deficiency is present, in contrast with normal (35 percent) states and other conditions (see Fig. 14-16). In general, the lower the serum iron levels, the higher the iron-binding capacity, and vice versa.

Table 14-2. Common Disorders and Drugs Influencing Thyroid-Binding Capacity of TBPA and TBG Proteins

Protein	Increase in Binding Capacity	Decrease in Binding Capacity
TBPA	Acromegaly Massive steroids Androgen treatment (slight effect)	Thyrotoxicosis Cirrhosis Severe illness or trauma Surgery Parturition Salicylates (massive doses[a])

TBG	Hypothyroidism
	Pregnancy
	Estrogen therapy
	Oral contraceptives
	Genetic and idiopathic
	  cirrhosis
	Acute intermittent
	  porphyuria
	Perphenazine therapy
	  (prolonged)
		Androgens and anabolic
		  steroids
		Acromegaly
		Nephrotic syndromes
		Marked hypoproteinemia
		Genetic and idiopathic
		  cirrhosis
		Uncompensated acidosis
		Dilantin[a]
		Prednisone therapy

[a] These agents affect capacity by displacing thyroxine from the protein, whereas the others result in actual changes in TBPA and TBG levels.

Abnormalities of Other Carrier Proteins

PREALBUMIN
Several minor serum components migrate electrophoretically ahead of the albumin fraction and constitute the prealbumin fraction [1]. One protein from this conglomerate is known to transport about one-third of the active thyroid hormone, thyroxin, in the serum and has accordingly been referred to as *thyroxin-binding prealbumin* (TBPA). The avidity of TBPA for thyroxin is estimated to be 260 μg per 100 ml serum, which is greater than that of thyroxin-binding globulin. Prealbumin may be readily quantitated by RID. Normal ranges are 10 to 40 mg per 100 ml by RID or EID. Table 14-2 enumerates disorders and other factors affecting the thyroxin-binding capacity of TBPA.

THYROXIN-BINDING GLOBULIN
The remaining two-thirds of the thyroid gland's thyroxin production is transported in the serum by an α_2-globulin, *thyroxin-binding globulin* (TBG) [1]. This protein is estimated to bind thyroxin at about 21 μg per 100 ml serum, which is with less avidity than TBPA. The measurement of the serum concentration of this protein is presently achieved by means other than immunodiffusion. The binding affinity of this protein for thyroxin is influenced by such factors as plasma estrogen levels, which appear to be as important as mere concentration of TBG in determining

the ratio of bound to unbound thyroxin in the serum. The minute amounts of unbound thyroxin represent the biologically active form of this potent hormone, which acts to regulate the general tempo of cellular function throughout the body. Defective TBG binding has been associated with a few cases of bisalbuminemia [57]. Table 14-2 indicates some of the more prominent factors influencing the thyroid-binding capacity of TBG.

TRANSCOBALAMINS

Vitamin B_{12} may be bound to a variety of serum proteins, but recent studies have supported specific carrier functions for only two: *transcobalamin I,* an α_1-globulin of molecular weight 121,000 [58, 59], appears to be the minor carrier and is inefficient in moving the vitamin into cells. *Transcobalamin II,* a β-globulin of molecular weight 35,000 to 38,000 [58, 59], is the major carrier [60]. A third B_{12}-binding protein has been postulated [61]. Transcobalamin II enters the blood after oral administration of vitamin B_{12}, binds the vitamin at the ileum, and rapidly moves from the plasma to tissues. A case of congenital absence of transcobalamin II has been described, which was manifested neonatally as fulminant megaloblastic anemia [62]. Transcobalamin I has been shown to increase in both chronic myeloproliferative states and leukemoid reactions. Transcobalamin II appears to decrease in myeloproliferative disorders, but not in leukemoid reactions, and may therefore offer diagnostic specificity. No direct measurement of these carrier proteins is currently available, but radioactive vitamin B_{12} isotope techniques have been developed for indirect estimation [63].

TRANSCORTIN

A specific cortisol-binding protein, termed *transcortin,* has been characterized as an α_1-globulin that is normally present in the serum at a level of about 7 mg per 100 ml. Its affinity for cortisol appears to be temperature dependent. Measurement is classically performed by column chromatography [1]. No specific pathogenic role has been identified for this carrier protein as yet.

ALBUMIN

Albumin molecules in the serum are laden at various times with a number of drugs, hormones, metallic ions, and other substances, many by a rather nonspecific attraction, in lieu of specific receptor mechanisms. Clinically important is the binding of various drugs (e.g., digoxin, diphenylhydantoin, and barbiturates), which is individualized for each drug. About 50 percent of the calcium in serum is bound to albumin. The hypocalcemia of hypoalbuminemia may result in the clinical symptoms of tetany (e.g., carpopedal spasm, positive Chvostek's sign, generalized seizures, and cardiac arrhythmias), particularly with serum albumin levels below 1.5 gm per 100 ml. The calcium binding of albumin is pH dependent, and only the unbound ionized calcium fraction is biologically active (see Chap. 13).

References

1. Schultze, H. E., and Heremans, J. F. *Molecular Biology of Human Proteins*, Vol. 1. Amsterdam: Elsevier, 1966.
2. Kasper, C. B., and Deutsch, J. F. Physicochemical studies of human ceruloplasmin. *J. Biol. Chem.* 238:2325, 1963.
3. Sternlieb, I., and Scheinberg, I. H. Ceruloplasmin in health and disease. *Ann. N.Y. Acad. Sci.* 94:71, 1961.
4. Evans, G. W. Copper homeostasis in the mammalian system. *Physiol. Rev.* 53:535, 1973.
5. Evans, G. W. Function and nomenclature for two mammalian copper proteins. *Nutr. Rev.* 29:195, 1971.
6. Hampton, J. K., Rider, L. J., Goka, T. J., and Preslock, J. P. The histaminase activity of ceruloplasmin. *Proc. Soc. Exp. Biol. Med.* 141:974, 1972.
7. Smallwood, R. A., Williams, H. A., and Rosenoer, V. M. Liver-copper levels in liver disease: Studies using neutron activation analysis. *Lancet* 2:1310, 1968.
8. Scheinberg, I. H., and Sternlieb, I. Wilson's disease. *Annu. Rev. Med.* 16:119, 1965.
9. Sternlieb, I., and Scheinberg, I. H. Chronic hepatitis as a first manifestation of Wilson's disease. *Ann. Intern. Med.* 76:59, 1972.
10. Cartwright, G. E., Hodges, R. E., Gubler, C. J., et al. Studies on copper metabolism. XIII. Hepatolenticular degeneration. *J. Clin. Invest.* 33: 1487, 1954.
11. McIntyre, N., Clink, H. M., Levi, A. J., et al. Hemolytic anemia in Wilson's disease. *N. Engl. J. Med.* 276:439, 1967.
12. Deiss, A., Lee, G. R., and Cartwright, G. E. Hemolytic anemia in Wilson's disease. *Ann. Intern. Med.* 73:413, 1970.
13. Lynch, R. E., Lee, G. R., and Cartwright, G. E. Penicillamine-induced cupriuria in normal subjects and in patients with acute liver disease. *Proc. Soc. Exp. Biol. Med.* 142:128, 1973.
14. Evans, G. W., Dubois, R. S., and Hambridge, K. M. Wilson's disease: Identification of an abnormal copper-binding protein. *Science* 181:1175, 1973.
15. Uzmaw, L. L., Iber, F. L., Chalmers, T. C., and Knowlton, M. The mechanism of copper deposition in the liver in hepatolenticular degeneration (Wilson's disease). *Am. J. Med. Sci.* 231:511, 1956.
16. Leu, M. L., Strickland, G., and Yeh, S. J. Tissue copper, zinc and manganese levels in Wilson's disease: Studies with the use of neutron activation analysis. *J. Lab. Clin. Med.* 77:438, 1971.
17. Deiss, A., Lynch, R. E., Lee, G. R., and Cartwright, G. E. Long-term therapy of Wilson's disease. *Ann. Intern. Med.* 75:57, 1971.
18. Strickland, G. T., Blackwell, R. O., and Watten, R. H. Metabolic studies in Wilson's disease. Evaluation of efficacy of chelation therapy in respect to copper balance. *Am. J. Med.* 51:31, 1971.
19. Bickel, H., Schultze, H. E., Grüter, W., and Göllner, I. Versuche zur Coeruloplasminsubstitution bei der hepatocerebralen Degeneration (Wilsonsche Krankheit). *Klin. Wochenschr.* 34:961, 1956.
20. Gitlin, D., and Biasuca, A. Development of γG, γA, γM, $\beta_1 C/\beta_1 A$, C_1-esterase inhibitor, ceruloplasmin, transferrin, hemopexin, haptoglobin, fibrinogen, plasminogen, α_1-antitrypsin, orosomucoid, β-lipoprotein, α_2-macroglobulin, and prealbumin in the human conceptus. *J. Clin. Invest.* 48:1433, 1969.

21. Beale, R. N., and Croft, D. The microdetermination of biological copper with oxalyldihydrazide. *J. Clin. Pathol.* 17:260, 1964.

22. Nyman, M. Serum haptoglobin. *Scand. J. Clin. Lab. Invest.* 11:39, 1959.

23. Sutton, E. The Haptoglobins. In A. G. Steinberg and A. G. Bearn (Eds.), *Progress in Medical Genetics,* Vol. 7. New York: Grune & Stratton, 1970. Pp. 163–216.

24. Waks, M., Alfsen, A., Schwaiger, S., and Mayer, A. Structural studies of haptoglobins. III. Interactions with hemoglobin. *Arch. Biochem. Biophys.* 132:268, 1969.

25. Lavialle, F., Rogard, M., and Alfsen, A. A Microcalorimetric Study of Haptoglobin-Hemoglobin Interaction. In H. Peeters (Ed.), *Proteins and Related Subjects. Protides of Biological Fluids,* Vol. 20. Amsterdam: Elsevier, 1972. Pp. 499–503.

26. Snellman, O., and Sylvén, B. Haptoglobin activity as a natural inhibitor of cathepsin-B activity. *Nature* 216:1033, 1967.

27. Smithies, A. Disulfide-bond cleavage and formation in proteins. *Science* 150:1595, 1965.

28. Giblett, E. R. The Haptoglobin System. In K. G. Jensen and S. A. Killman (Eds.), *Series Haematologica,* Vol. 1. Baltimore: Williams & Wilkins, 1968. Pp. 3–20.

29. Howard, A., and Ansell, B. B. Vertical starch-gel electrophoresis in some rheumatic diseases. *Ann. Rheum. Dis.* 23:232, 1964.

30. Wendt, G. G., Krüger, J., and Kindermann, I. Serumgruppen und Krankheit. *Humangenetik* 6:281, 1968.

31. Nandi, M., Lewis, G. P., Hershel, J., Slone, D., Shapiro, S., and Siskind, V. Evaluations of haptoglobin phenotype 0-0 in cirrhotic and non-cirrhotic hospital patients. *J. Clin. Pathol.* 23:695, 1970.

32. Bonacker, L. Congenital anhaptoglobinemia. Unpublished data, 1973.

33. Fink, D. J., Petz, L. D., and Black, M. B. Serum haptoglobin. *J.A.M.A.* 199:615, 1967.

34. Daniels, J. C., Cobb, E. K., Jones, J., Larson, D. L., Abston, S., and Ritzmann, S. E. Serum protein profiles in thermal burns. I. Serum electrophoretic patterns, immunoglobulins, and transport proteins. *J. Trauma* 14:137, 1974.

35. Owen, J. A., Better, F. C., and Hoban, J. A simple method for the determination of serum haptoglobin. *J. Clin. Pathol.* 13:163, 1960.

36. Veneziale, C. M., and McGuckin, W. F. A modified Owen method for the quantitative analysis of serum haptoglobin: The time method. *Mayo Clin. Proc.* 40:751, 1965.

37. Müller-Eberhard, U. Hemopexin. *N. Engl. J. Med.* 283:1090, 1970.

38. Müller-Eberhard, U., Bosman, C., and Liem, H. Tissue localization of the heme-hemopexin complex in the rabbit and the rat as studied by light microscopy with the use of radioisotopes. *J. Lab. Clin. Med.* 76:426, 1970.

39. Rubinsen, R. M., Morrow, A. G., and Gebel, P. Mechanical destruction of erythrocytes by incompetent aortic valvular prosthesis; clinical hemodynamic and hematologic findings. *Am. Heart J.* 71:179, 1966.

40. Eyster, M. E., Edgington, T. S., Liem, H., and Müller-Eberhard, U. Plasma hemopexin levels following aortic valve replacement: A valuable screening test for assessing the severity of cardiac hemolysis. *J. Lab. Clin. Med.* 80:112, 1972.

41. Müller-Eberhard, U., and Bashore, R. Assessment of Rh disease by

ratios of bilirubin to albumin and hemopexin to albumin in amniotic fluid. *N. Engl. J. Med.* 282:1163, 1970.

42. Müller-Eberhard, U., Javid, J., Liem, H., Hanstein, A., and Hanna, M. Plasma concentrations of hemopexin, haptoglobin and heme in patients with various hemolytic diseases. *Blood* 32:811, 1968.

43. Kushner, I., Edgington, T. S., Trimble, C., Liem, H. H., and Müller-Eberhard, U. Plasma hemopexin homeostasis during the acute phase response. *J. Lab. Clin. Med.* 80:18, 1972.

44. Bowman, B. H. Serum transferrin. In K. G. Jensen and S. A. Killman (Eds.), *Series Haematologica,* Vol. 1. Baltimore: Williams & Wilkins, 1968. Pp. 97–110.

45. Haurani, F. I., Meyer, A., and O'Brien, R. Production of transferrin by the macrophage. *J. Reticuloendothel. Soc.* 14:309, 1973.

46. Thorbecke, G. J., Hochwald, G. M., van Furth, R., Müller-Eberhard, H. J., and Jacobson, E. F. Problems in Determining the Sites of Synthesis of Complement Components. In G. E. W. Wolstenholme and J. Knight (Eds.), *Ciba Foundation Symposium: Complement.* Boston: Little, Brown, 1965. P. 99.

47. Stecher, V. J., and Thorbecke, G. J. Sites of synthesis of serum proteins. I. Serum proteins produced by macrophages in vitro. *J. Immunol.* 99:643, 1967.

48. Thorbecke, G. J., Liem, H. H., Knight, S., Cox, K., and Müller-Eberhard, U. Sites of formation of the serum proteins transferrin and hemopexin. *J. Clin. Invest.* 52:725, 1973.

49. Hochwald, G. M., Jacobson, E. B., and Thorbecke, G. J. C^{14}-amino acid incorporation into transferrin and B_{2A}-globulin by ectodermal glands in vitro. *Fed. Proc.* 23:557, 1964.

50. Levine, P. H., Levine, A. J., and Weintraub, L. R. The role of transferrin in control of iron absorption: studies on a cellular level. *J. Lab. Clin. Med.* 80:333, 1972.

51. Malkasian, G. D., Tauxe, W. N., and Hagedorn, A. B. Total iron-binding capacity in pregnancy. *J. Nucl. Med.* 5:243, 1964.

52. Jacobi, J. M., Powell, L. W., and Gaffney, T. J. Immunochemical quantitation of human transferrin in pregnancy and during the administration of oral contraceptives. *Br. J. Haematol.* 17:503, 1969.

53. Jarnum, S., and Lassen, N. A. Albumin and transferrin metabolism in infections and toxic diseases. *Scand. J. Clin. Lab. Invest.* 13:357, 1961.

54. Heilmeyer, L. Die Atransferrinämien. *Acta Haematol.* 36:40, 1966.

55. Coltman, C. A., Jr. Pagophagia and iron lack. *J.A.M.A.* 207:513, 1969.

56. Mandel, E. E. Serum iron and iron-binding capacity in clinical diagnosis. *Clin. Chem.* 5:1, 1959.

57. Sarcione, E. J., and Aungst, C. W. Bisalbuminemia associated with thyroxin-binding defect. *Clin. Chim. Acta* 7:297, 1962.

58. Hom, B., Olesen, H., and Louis, P. Fractionation of vitamin B_{12} binders in human serum. *J. Lab. Clin. Med.* 68:958, 1966.

59. Hom, B., and Olesen, H. Molecular weights of vitamin B_{12} binding proteins in human serum determined by Sephadex G-200 gel filtration. *Scand. J. Clin. Lab. Invest.* 19:269, 1967.

60. Rappazzo, M. E., and Hall, C. A. Transport function of transcobalamin II. *J. Clin. Immunol.* 51:1915, 1972.

61. Carmel, R., and Herbert, V. Vitamin B_{12}-binding of leukocytes as a

possible major source of the third vitamin B_{12}-binding protein of serum. *Blood* 40:542, 1972.

62. Hakami, N., Neiman, P. E., Canellors, G. P., and Lazerson, J. Neonatal megaloblastic anemia due to inherited transcobalamin II deficiency in two siblings. *N. Engl. J. Med.* 285:1163, 1971.
63. Hall, C. A. Vitamin B_{12}-binding proteins of man. *Ann. Intern. Med.* 75:297, 1971.

Abnormalities of Protease Inhibitors

15

Jerry C. Daniels

Life at the cellular level is regulated and perpetuated by a myriad of metabolic pathways that are intricately controlled by enzymes. One class of enzymes subserves the destruction of protein molecules of either endogenous or exogenous origin. Such enzymes, termed *proteases* (or proteinases), are ubiquitous, being both intracellular (within lysosomes) and extracellular (e.g., in pancreatic and salivary secretions). The proteolytic activity of these enzymes lacks the ability to distinguish isologous from homologous proteins, and it may be involved in such processes as autolysis, aging, and "innocent-bystander" injury to autologous tissue during protective immunological events. Proteases are particularly abundant in a mobile form by virtue of their lysosomal content in neutrophils. Lysosomal proteases in phagocytic cells are involved in the digestion of protein material engulfed by such cells.

These proteolytic activities are, in at least some instances, controlled by inhibitor molecules that antagonize or neutralize proteolysis. Such antagonism may involve specific receptor sites on the inhibitor molecule that combine directly with the enzyme; in some cases, however, the mechanism of antagonism is unknown. At times, a single inhibitor is capable of affecting, to different degrees, the activities of several types of proteases, which are often unrelated in function. These inhibitor molecules, termed *protease inhibitors* (antiproteases), are those proteins that combine with proteases, often forming strong reversible complexes to inhibit the activities of the proteolytic enzymes. Protease inhibitors may be assumed to regulate many of the processes of cellular metabolism by their engagement or disengagement of enzyme function. A protease-like activity may be required for malignant expression, and protection against carcinogenesis has been attributed to some protease inhibitors [1, 2].

The inhibitors to be discussed include α_1-antitrypsin, α_1-antichymotrypsin, inter-α-trypsin inhibitor, α_2-macroglobulin, and C1s inhibitor (see Appendix). These proteins migrate in the α_1-globulin or α_2-globulin regions on electrophoresis (Fig. 15-1). Some of the properties of protease inhibitors are summarized in Table 15-1.

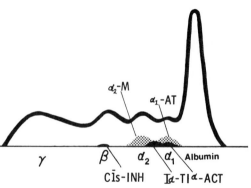

Figure 15-1
Electrophoretic distribution of protease inhibitors α_2-macroglobulin (α_2-M), α_1-antitrypsin (α_1-AT), α_1-antichymotrypsin (α_1-ACT), inter-α-trypsin inhibitor (I-α-TI), and C1s inhibitor ($C\bar{1}s$-INH), and their relative concentrations.

α_1-Antitrypsin

PHYSIOLOGICAL ASPECTS

Alpha-1-antitrypsin is an α_1-globulin of molecular weight 54,000 that is normally present in the serum at a concentration of 200 to 400 mg per 100 ml [3, 4] (see Table 15-1). This protein accounts for approximately 90 percent of the α_1-globulin fraction on serum protein electrophoresis. It inhibits the proteolytic activities of trypsin, chymotrypsin, plasmin, thrombin, collagenase, elastase, and pancreatic kallikrein; there is uncertainty as to its effect on plasma kallikrein [4]. The normal half-life of α_1-antitrypsin appears to be 5 to 6 days [5]. If normal human pancreas tissue is homogenized, two major enzymes may be isolated: trypsin (molecular weight 22,900) and chymotrypsin (molecular weight 27,000). Trypsin is inhibited strongly by α_1-antitrypsin and, to a lesser extent, by other protease inhibitors. It is also slowly inactivated at acid or alkaline pH ranges in the absence of inhibitors, but calcium ions will stabilize its activity. Trypsin acts to break the polypeptide chains of proteins by a very specific mechanism: it breaks the chain only at the carboxyl side of peptide bonds containing lysine or arginine in which the ϵ-amino or guanidino grouping is free. In concert with other proteolytic enzymes, trypsin converts dietary proteins in the gastrointestinal (GI) tract into amino acids, which are absorbed chiefly in the small intestine. Trypsin is also included among the proteolytic enzymes within lysosomes, particularly those of leukocytes. Thus, its liberation in association with cell death or inflammation poses a threat to the normal protein architecture of the body. It is in a protective capacity against such autodigestion that the inhibitory properties of α_1-antitrypsin are assumed to play a physiological role. It has been directly demonstrated that leukocytic proteases from purulent sputum are capable of digesting human lung tissue and that these enzymatic activities are strongly inhibited by the α_1-antitrypsin of normal serum [6]. Pregnancy and the use of oral contraceptives normally elevate serum α_1-antitrypsin levels [7].

The principal genetic allele for the phenotypic expression of α_1-antitrypsin has been termed the *Pi allele,* for "protease inhibitor" [8]. Vari-

Table 15-1. Properties of Protease Inhibitors

Protein	Inhibitory Target(s)	Electro-phoretic Mobility	Molec-ular Weight	Normal Serum Concentration (mg/100 ml)
α_1-Antitrypsin	Trypsin Chymotrypsin Plasmin Thrombin Collagenase Elastase Pancreatic kallikrein	α_1-Globulin	54,000	200–400
α_1-Antichymo-trypsin	Chymotrypsin	α_1-Globulin	69,000	40–60
Inter-α-trypsin inhibitor	Trypsin Chymotrypsin (weak)	α_1-, α_2-Globulin	160,000	~50
α_2-Macro-globulin	Trypsin Chymotrypsin Plasma kallikrein Thrombin Elastase	α_2-Globulin	820,000	200–350
C1s inhibitor	C1s	α_2-Globulin	104,000	20–30

ous alleles have been subgrouped on the basis of their differing electro-phoretic rates on starch-gel electrophoresis [9]; they are termed, in order of decreasing migration rates, Pi^F, Pi^I, Pi^M, Pi^S, Pi^V, Pi^X, and Pi^Z. The slowest moving electrophoretic variant, Pi^Z, has been associated with the most severe deficiency state. Thus, the phenotype ZZ represents the ho-mozygous state in which α_1-antitrypsin levels are lowest (10 to 15 per-cent), and phenotype MM is the most prevalent form. Thus, on a prac-tical clinical level, it becomes highly desirable (although technically arduous) to Pi type the α_1-antitrypsin as well as to quantitate its pres-ence. This may be accomplished by starch-gel electrophoresis followed by antigen-antibody crossed agarose electrophoresis, and the clinical significance of this approach has recently been reviewed [10, 11].

PATHOPHYSIOLOGICAL ASPECTS

DECREASED SERUM LEVELS
The decreased serum level of α_1-antitrypsin is the most commonly en-countered form of protease inhibitor abnormality. For all intents and purposes, the decreased state is always congenital. Since α_1-antitrypsin constitutes approximately 90 percent of the α_1-globulin fraction on se-rum electrophoresis, the conspicuous absence of this fraction led Laurell

Figure 15-2
Trimodal distribution of α_1-antitrypsin concentration in serum.

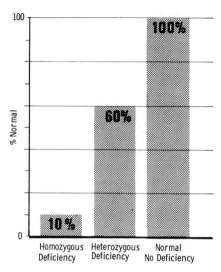

and Eriksson [12] to describe an α_1-antitrypsin deficiency in 5 of 1500 sera from hospitalized patients over a six-month survey. Trace or absent α_1-antitrypsin was demonstrated conclusively in each case by testing with specific anti-α_1-antitrypsin antisera to confirm those cases suspected from an electrophoretic determination. Additionally, 3 of the 5 patients with this deficiency had severe pulmonary disease. In examining relatives of α_1-antitrypsin-deficient patients, a trimodal distribution in α_1-antitrypsin levels was demonstrated [13]: normal, intermediate (60 percent of normal level), and low (10 percent of normal level). These distributions are graphically presented in Figure 15-2. This finding provided evidence for an autosomal recessive genetic inheritance of α_1-antitrypsin deficiency in homozygotes (low group) and in heterozygotes (intermediate group). Extensive studies, which incorporated the measurement of the trypsin inhibitory capacity (TIC), have confirmed and refined this congenital basis for α_1-antitrypsin distribution among the general population [14–17]. The frequency of this disorder among the general population is about 1 in 20 persons in the heterozygous form, and about 1 in 2000 in the homozygous form [18, 19]. This frequency is comparable to that of cystic fibrosis, which is considered to be one of the most prevalent congenital metabolic disorders.

The clinical consequences of homozygous α_1-antitrypsin deficiency [20–23] include most prominently a severe degenerative, emphysematous type of chronic obstructive pulmonary disease, which is marked by an early age of onset (20 to 30 years). It affects a disproportionate number of females and is invariably more pronounced in the lower lobes rather than throughout the lungs. Possible explanations for this predilection for the basal segments of the lungs [24] have been related to perfusion factors, such as decreased perfusion and ventilation of the lung bases of persons affected with α_1-antitrypsin deficiency, and an increased concentration of macrophages, with their proteolytic enzymes, in the bases of the lungs [25]. Environmental lung irritants appear to interact with this congenital susceptibility to aggravate the severity of the disease process [26, 27]. Whether heterozygotes are more susceptible to inhaled pollutants remains controversial [28], but it appears likely that they are [28a]. If so, they tend to develop the disorder at a later age than the homozygotes. It has been postulated that the pulmonary disease results from the autodigestion of lung tissue by the unopposed proteolytic activity of proteases that are released from leukocytes summoned by inflammatory stimuli [18, 19]. The question of whether trypsin, elastase, or other enzymes are the principal culprits provides considerable discussion [8, 29, 30]. The end result, in any case, is crippling respiratory insufficiency at a relatively early age. Some 30 percent of persons with α_1-antitrypsin deficiency also appear to suffer from peptic ulcer disease [28a], which again is possibly consequent to autoproteolysis due to the lack of an enzyme "brake."

A further, recently described, clinical feature of α_1-antitrypsin deficiency is a predisposition to hepatic cirrhosis in homozygous α_1-antitrypsin-deficient children [31]. Further studies of this relatively rare condition have shown the actual accumulation of α_1-antitrypsin in liver parenchyma in the face of severely deficient serum levels. More detailed investigations, which employed electron microscopy, have suggested that α_1-antitrypsin is synthesized normally within the hepatocytes, but that an undefined block to the release of this protease is present which results in engorgement of the hepatic parenchyma by α_1-antitrypsin [32, 33]. Most recently, cirrhosis accompanied by fluorescent-staining α_1-antitrypsin accumulation in the liver has been reported in one adult patient with homozygous α_1-antitrypsin deficiency [34] and in one adult with the heterozygous deficiency [35]. Clearly, this association may prove to be of far-reaching clinical significance. A typical case presentation of α_1-antitrypsin deficiency, depicted in Figure 15-3, follows:

Case Report 1
A 28-year-old man was referred to the clinic with a 7-year history of progressive, severe exertional dyspnea and cyanotic episodes. The patient lived in a rural community and denied having a smoking habit. He had a younger brother with a similar history of respiratory compromise. On physical examination, the patient was found to have an increased anteroposterior diameter of the chest with hypertrophy of the sternocleidomastoid musculature. Auscultation of the lungs revealed diffuse bilateral inspiratory and expiratory wheezes with scattered coarse rhonchi. The nailbeds were cyanotic and digital clubbing was present to a moderate degree. The chest roentgenogram revealed low, flat diaphragms, an elongated, thin cardiac silhouette, and hyperlucent lung fields. Radioisotope lung scans showed diffuse loss of parenchyma and vasculature predominantly in the lower lobes. The electrocardiogram revealed a right axis deviation. Blood gases indicated an elevated pCO_2 with a diminished pO_2. The blood pH was mildly acidic. Pulmonary function studies were compatible with the diagnosis of chronic obstructive pulmonary disease. Serum protein electrophoresis revealed a decreased α_1-globulin fraction and

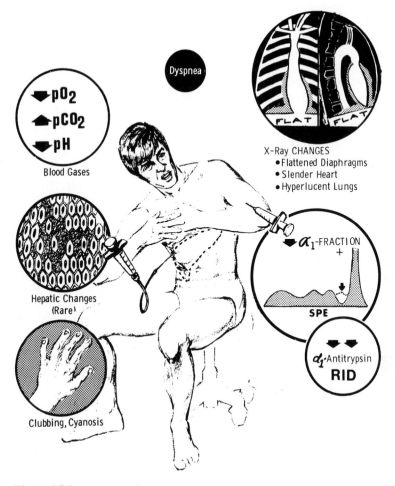

Figure 15-3
Clinical features of α_1-antitrypsin deficiency (see Case Report 1).

an almost absent level of α_1-antitrypsin. The patient was advised to avoid pulmonary irritants and was treated supportively with breathing exercises, intermittent positive-pressure breathing, and bronchodilators.

Final diagnosis: α_1-Antitrypsin deficiency with juvenile emphysema, homozygous variety.

At present, the only useful management of α_1-antitrypsin deficiency consists of the elimination of pulmonary irritants from the environment of the α_1-antitrypsin-deficient individuals, especially the homozygotes. Thus, the detection and characterization of α_1-antitrypsin deficiency among large populations is quite justified [8, 36, 37]. Susceptible individuals should be advised against smoking, exposure to air pollution, and inhalation therapy with proteolytic enzymes.

As with any of the biologically active proteins, particularly the protease inhibitors, measurement may be made of either the biological activity (i.e., functional activity) or the physical presence (i.e., concentration) of the protein in question. The detection of biological activity is made by measuring the trypsin-inhibiting capacity (TIC) or total antitryptic activity (TAT) as determined by the spectrophotometric analysis of trypsin-mediated colorimetric substrate reactions [14–17, 38].

Radial immunodiffusion (RID) and electroimmunodiffusion (EID) [39, 40] have been adeptly applied to the immunochemical measurement of the concentration of α_1-antitrypsin in serum and other biological fluids. The normal range found by RID is 200 to 400 mg per 100 ml. Talamo and associates [10, 41] have recently commented on the inadequacy of only immunochemical determinations in the clinical prognosis of deficiency states, since the genetic phenotype is of paramount importance. These investigators have developed phenotyping techniques for clinical application.

Initial screening of large populations may be accomplished by inspection of the α_1-globulin fraction on serum protein electrophoresis in apparently healthy persons, with mandatory confirmation by specific RID or EID tests for α_1-antitrypsin levels. However, it must be remembered that α_1-antitrypsin may behave as an acute-phase reactant in a variety of conditions, leading to a spuriously "normal" level at the time of sampling. This is a common reason for not diagnosing underlying α_1-antitrypsin deficiency in emphysematous patients when they are initially admitted to patient-care institutions, inasmuch as they are likely to harbor acute infections as the precipitating event for admission.

INCREASED SERUM LEVELS

Serum levels of α_1-antitrypsin may become nonspecifically increased during numerous disorders, particularly those involving inflammation or tissue breakdown [42]. Teleologically, this is logical since, with increased inflammation, there are large amounts of proteolytic enzymes being in need of neutralization in order to preserve the anatomical and functional integrity of the affected areas [43]. Such increases may mask true α_1-antitrypsin deficiency if the sampling is performed at the time of acute illness (see Chap. 18).

Figure 15-4 illustrates the acute-phase pattern of α_1-antitrypsin levels, which accompanied a similar pattern of haptoglobin levels, in an Apollo astronaut [44].

Case Report 2

A 36-year-old astronaut for the National Aeronautics and Space Administration Apollo program served as the lunar module pilot for launch program 13. This individual sustained fever, chills, dysuria, urinary frequency, pyuria, and lower back pain while in flight. On return, prompt medical attention revealed too-many-to-count white blood cells per high-powered field on microscopic examination of the urinary sediment. Urine culture and sensitivities

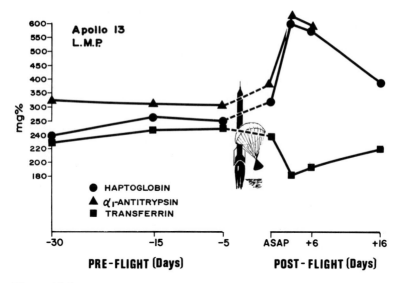

Figure 15-4
Acute-phase response of α_1-antitrypsin and haptoglobin in an Apollo lunar module pilot. The same stimuli failed to affect the serum concentrations of transferrin (see Case Report 2). (Reproduced by permission. From Fischer, C. L., et al. *Aerosp. Med.* 43:1122, 1972.)

revealed *Pseudomonas* species, which were also cultured from the blood. He responded uneventfully to appropriate antibiotic therapy.

Final diagnosis: Acute pyelonephritis (*Pseudomonas*) with septicemia.

α_1-Antichymotrypsin

PHYSIOLOGICAL ASPECTS

Alpha-1-antichymotrypsin is an α_1-globulin of molecular weight 69,000 that is normally present in the serum at levels of 40 to 60 mg per 100 ml (see Table 15-1). Its protease inhibitory capacity is highly specific for chymotrypsin alone [3, 4]. Chymotrypsin is a pancreatic enzyme that is involved in protein digestion in concert with trypsin and other proteolytic enzymes. It acts by specific cleavage of peptide bonds at the carboxyl side of tyrosine or phenylalanine. The enzyme is also found intracellularly in lysosomal packets, particularly in leukocytes. It is strongly inhibited by α_1-antichymotrypsin, which presumably provides a protective influence against the autodigestion of normal structural proteins.

PHYSIOLOGICAL ASPECTS

Disorders resulting from alterations in circulating antichymotrypsin levels may be only a subject of speculation, inasmuch as extensive human surveys have not yet been performed. Preliminary data suggest that α_1-antichymotrypsin may behave as an early acute-phase reactant [45]. The behavior of serum α_1-antichymotrypsin levels has been studied in

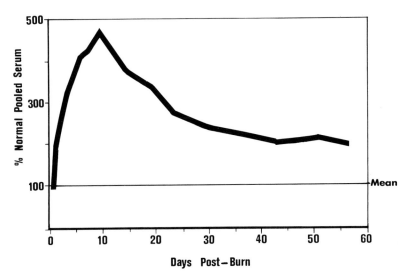

Figure 15-5
Profile of α_1-antichymotrypsin levels measured serially in children (ages 0–16) with acute thermal burn, as compared with normal levels. (Reproduced by permission. From Daniels, J. C., Larson, D. L., Abston, S., and Ritzmann, S. E. *J. Trauma* 14:153, © 1974, The Williams & Wilkins Co., Baltimore.)

162 children who sustained acute thermal burn injury. As shown in Figure 15-5, α_1-antichymotrypsin increased to a maximum (480 percent of normal) by day 10 after the injury and remained elevated throughout the observation period. It possibly functions as a protective mechanism that attempts to retard tissue necrosis by neutralizing destructive enzymes [46]. Excessive chymotrypsin activity could have GI consequences as a result of the pancreatic elaboration of this enzyme, as well as unpredictable diffuse effects due to its lysosomal concentrations.

This great initial increase of α_1-antichymotrypsin in burn injury is similar to that of haptoglobin in these same patients (see Chap. 14). It can only be speculated whether such increases are of a specific or nonspecific nature. The pattern follows that of an acute-phase response (see Chap. 18), but it could also represent an attempted neutralization of the increased proteolytic enzymes liberated in such patients. It is of interest that the peak α_1-antichymotrypsin levels are encountered simultaneously with the peak elevation in lysozyme, as a marker for the lysosomal enzyme package [47]. Specific antagonism (to cathepsins or plasmin, for example) may be involved, or other unknown mechanisms may be operative. A combination of factors is most likely the cause of this particular protein pattern.

TECHNIQUES OF MEASUREMENT
Functional measurements of α_1-antichymotrypsin are based on enzymatic methods [48, 49] and are similar to those used for determining the biological activity of α_1-antitrypsin.

For the immunochemical determination of α_1-antichymotrypsin concentrations, RID and EID provide rapid, sensitive, and reliable quantitative measurement.

Inter-α-trypsin Inhibitor

PHYSIOLOGICAL ASPECTS

Inter-α-trypsin inhibitor is an α-globulin of molecular weight 160,000 that migrates electrophoretically between the α_1- and α_2-globulin fractions (see Fig. 15-1). Its normal serum levels are about 50 mg per 100 ml (see Table 15-1). Inter-α-trypsin inhibitor primarily inhibits trypsin; it exhibits weak inhibition of chymotrypsin [3, 4]. It has the interesting characteristic of dissociating into a smaller molecular weight inter-α-trypsin inhibitor and an inhibitor polypeptide [3]. As with α_1-antitrypsin, the trypsin inhibitory properties of this protein may be protective against harmful proteolysis.

PATHOPHYSIOLOGICAL ASPECTS

Little information is available concerning specific abnormalities of the inter-α-trypsin inhibitor [50]. Serial measurements in 162 acutely burned children (Fig. 15-6) showed an early decline to a nadir (40 percent of normal) three days after the injury, with return to low normal ranges by the eighth day [46]. It is possible that the absence or diminution of inter-α-trypsin inhibitor could have clinical consequences due to a reduction in tryptic inhibitory activity throughout the body. This problem is yet to be studied.

TECHNIQUES OF MEASUREMENT

Functional measurements of inter-α-trypsin inhibitor are based upon the traditional enzymatic reactions providing for the quantitation of trypsin, thereby allowing indirect estimation of antitryptic activity. However, antitryptic activity is shared by a number of protease inhibitors, and the specific antitryptic contribution of this protein is difficult to establish in whole serum.

On the other hand, immunochemical quantitation by RID or EID is both rapid and specific.

α_2-Macroglobulin

PHYSIOLOGICAL ASPECTS

Alpha-2-macroglobulin is an α_2-globulin of molecular weight 820,000 that is present in normal serum at levels of 200 to 350 mg per 100 ml as measured by RID (see Table 15-1). It possesses inhibitory activity against trypsin, chymotrypsin, plasma kallikrein (but not pancreatic kallikrein), thrombin, and elastase [3, 4]. It is the most nonspecific of the protease inhibitors. Because of its multispecific activity, this protein is a key factor in the complex interrelationship between the coagulation,

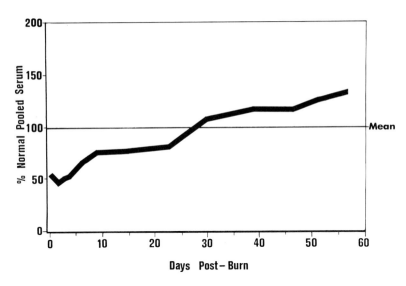

Figure 15-6
Serial measurements of inter-α-trypsin inhibitor in children (ages 0–16) with acute thermal burn, as compared with normal levels. (Reproduced by permission. From Daniels, J. C., Larson, D. L., Abston, S., and Ritzmann, S. E. *J. Trauma* 14:153, © 1974, The Williams & Wilkins Co., Baltimore.)

fibrinolytic, and kallikrein enzyme systems [51–53]. It is interesting that the linkage of small molecules, such as trypsin and chymotrypsin, to the 40-fold larger α_2-macroglobulin molecule appears to result in conformational changes, demonstrable by electron microscopy, which present to the reticuloendothelial system and are cleared as foreign bodies from the circulation [45]. In addition to its major protease-inhibitor functions, α_2-macroglobulin acts as a transport protein for certain hormones and contributes minimally to intravascular oncotic pressures. Pregnancy and estrogens are potent stimuli to elevations of circulating α_2-macroglobulin [54, 55].

PATHOPHYSIOLOGICAL ASPECTS

DECREASED SERUM LEVELS
Decreased serum levels of α_2-macroglobulin have been reported in several conditions, the pathophysiological significance of which remains unknown. Plasma levels of α_2-macroglobulin in rheumatoid arthritis have been shown to be low, in contrast to associated elevations of acute-phase reactants such as haptoglobin and C-reactive protein [56]. Preeclamptic females without proteinuria have decreased α_2-macroglobulin levels, which are possibly related to the proposed diminution of estrogen synthesis in this syndrome [57]; as noted earlier, estrogen is a known stimulant of α_2-macroglobulin levels. A nonspecific decrease in α_2-macroglobulin may occur in conditions of rapid synthesis of abnormal proteins

(e.g., multiple myeloma), presumably by usurpation of metabolic capacities vital to α_2-macroglobulin synthesis.

INCREASED SERUM LEVELS

Since estrogen is known to stimulate an increase in α_2-macroglobulin levels, it is not surprising that pregnancy leads to such increases, particularly during the third trimester [54, 55]. In contrast to the decreased α_2-macroglobulin levels in preeclampsia that is unaccompanied by proteinuria [57], the same condition in association with proteinuria results in elevated α_2-macroglobulin levels [58].

The most striking elevations of α_2-macroglobulin occur in the nephrotic syndrome [56, 58–60] (see Fig. 13-7 and Case Report 1, Chap. 13). The precise reason for this increase is not known, but it may be speculated that α_2-macroglobulin is increased in the neutralization of proteolytic enzymes in such patients. Lysosomal enzymes are known to be increased in renal failure patients. As shown in Figure 15-7, the increased lysozyme (muramidase) of chronic uremic patients falls with renal allotransplantation; this elevation appears to be a function of uremia [61]. Other mechanisms that possibly contribute to elevated α_2-macroglobulin include selective retention based on size-specific molecular sieving by "leaking" nephrotic glomerular basement membranes, enhanced hepatic synthesis to replace oncotic pressure losses associated with heavy proteinuria [58], and nonspecific acute-phase responses (see Chap. 18). Most likely, hyperalpha-2-macroglobulinemia in nephrosis is a multifactorial event [60]. Figure 15-8 compares the serum protein electrophoretic, ultracentrifugal, and RID characteristics of this increase.

Certain chronic liver diseases lead to α_2-macroglobulin elevations for obscure reasons, perhaps in part as a compensatory response to the hypoalbuminemia usually accompanying such disorders [56]. Elevations of α_2-macroglobulins have been reported in ataxia-telangiectasia [62] and diabetes mellitus [63]. Elevation in diabetes mellitus is of particular significance, since the binding of insulin has been proposed as a possible function of α_2-macroglobulin.

It is obvious from a number of studies [42, 56] that α_2-macroglobulin does not behave as an acute-phase reactant (see Chap. 18), but rather exhibits moderate to striking elevations in a defined number of conditions. Figure 15-4 illustrates this point in an Apollo lunar module pilot, who exhibited sharp increases in serum concentrations of haptoglobin and α_1-antitrypsin while α_2-macroglobulin remained within the normal range [44]. This dissociation of acute-phase reactants from α_2-macroglobulin is also seen in acute thermal burn injury (see Fig. 14-13B).

TECHNIQUES OF MEASUREMENT
Functional measurements of α_2-macroglobulin are based on the multifold protease inhibitory capabilities of this protein; most often its antitryptic function is employed [43]. Recently, it has been possible to separate α_2-macroglobulin into five components by means of polyacryl-

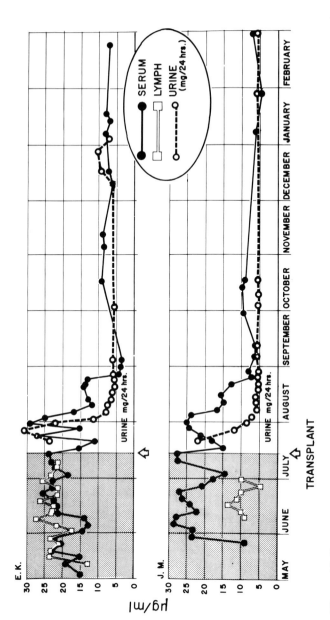

Figure 15-7
Lysozymal increase in two cases of renal failure, and the effect of allotransplantation. (Reproduced by permission. From Daniels, J. C., et al. *Tex. Rep. Biol. Med.* 30:9, 1972.)

Figure 15-8
Hyperalpha-2-macroglobulinemia in nephrosis—laboratory correlates. *SPE:* serum protein electrophoresis *UC:* ultracentrifugation; *RID:* radial immunodiffusion.

SPE:

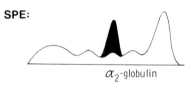

α_2-globulin

UC:

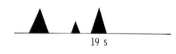

19 s

RID:

α_2M = 800 mg %

amide-gel electrophoresis, with differing enzyme-binding properties being found in each fraction [64].

Immunochemical quantitation of α_2-macroglobulin concentration is readily achieved by RID (the normal range is 200 to 350 mg per 100 ml) or EID, using specific antisera. RID is the most commonly employed mode of measurement for α_2-macroglobulin.

C1s Inhibitor

PHYSIOLOGICAL ASPECTS
C1s inhibitor is an α_2-globulin of molecular weight 104,000, and it is found in normal serum at levels of 20 to 30 mg per 100 ml (see Table 15-1). It is also known as *C1-esterase inhibitor, inhibitor of the activated first component of complement,* and *anti-C1s;* it has acquired the recognized abbreviation $C\bar{I}INH$. It specifically inhibits C1s, the activated form of the first component of the complement system, and thereby interrupts the cascade of complement interactions at a vulnerable point (see Chap. 16). The inhibitor also exhibits a negative influence on the proteolytic enzymes, plasmin and plasma kallikrein [3, 4]. Weak antitrypsin and antichymotrypsin activities have also been demonstrated. The primary function of C1s inhibitor, however, is to act as a regulatory "brake" on the complement activation process.

PATHOPHYSIOLOGICAL ASPECTS

CONGENITALLY DECREASED SERUM LEVELS
The rare congenital absence of the protease inhibitor of the first complement component (C1s) appears only in the heterozygous form, the homozygous state presumably being incompatible with life. Affected individuals display the syndrome of hereditary angioedema (angioneurotic edema, HANE), which is inherited as an autosomal dominant trait and

is directly associated with the absence of C1s inhibitor activity [65–68]. This disorder is marked by transitory, localized, painless swelling of the face, hands, feet, and genitals, or by more severe visceral edema of the GI tract resulting in nausea and emesis. Increased vascular permeability is seen in affected areas. Laryngeal edema is a frequent cause of death (in about 25 percent), which often culminates numerous recurrent attacks. Diagnosis is based on the clinical presentation, notably swelling in the absence of inflammatory characteristics, and the demonstration of decreased or absent inhibitor of C1s (C$\bar{1}$INH). Treatment with epinephrine and large doses of antihistamines is usually ineffective, and corticosteroid administration is indicated in all except the milder attacks (see Chap. 16). It is presently controversial whether the administration of fresh plasma restores the absent activity; recently, ε-aminocaproic acid administration has been reported to be a beneficial form of treatment. This has led to preliminary studies of other antifibrinolytic agents, such as tranexamic acid, as possibly beneficial therapeutic agents in this disorder [69]. A representative case, illustrated in Figure 15-9, follows:

Case Report 3
A 28-year-old housewife of Mediterranean descent noted a sudden onset of severe periorbital edema and swelling of the right hand, accompanied by wheezing and evidence of bronchial constriction, nausea, vomiting, and colicky abdominal pain. She had experienced annoying minor attacks of recurrent, transient, circumscribed subepithelial edema of the loose tissues for most of her life, which was accompanied by a faint serpiginous, maculopapular rash over the affected areas. Two siblings had died in early childhood of obscure precipitous respiratory distress syndromes. The patient sought medical attention for the symptoms described above. The edematous areas were nonpitting and nonpruritic. A special assay for the inhibitor of the first component of complement (C1-esterase inhibitor) by a consulting allergist revealed the absence of this inhibitor in the patient's serum. During the course of her evaluation, the patient developed severe laryngeal edema that was unresponsive to epinephrine and corticosteriods. Despite tracheostomy, the patient progressed to complete respiratory obstruction and sustained cardiopulmonary arrest; resuscitation was unsuccessful. Autopsy findings included severe submucosal edema of the larynx, diffuse edema and hemorrhage of the lung, and edema of the lamina propria of the jejunum. Leakage from postcapillary venules was pronounced in the electron microscopic examination of a section of edematous skin.
Final Diagnosis: Hereditary angioedema, with fatal laryngeal edema.

ACQUIRED DECREASED SERUM LEVELS
A secondary decrease in C$\bar{1}$INH has been reported recently in two patients with lymphosarcoma and circulating 7S IgM, both of whom exhibited unusual serum complement profiles. One had symptoms that were indistinguishable from hereditary angioedema [70].

TECHNIQUES OF MEASUREMENT
Measurement of the biological activity of C1s inhibitor is obtained by (1) the measurement of individual complement factors to demonstrate

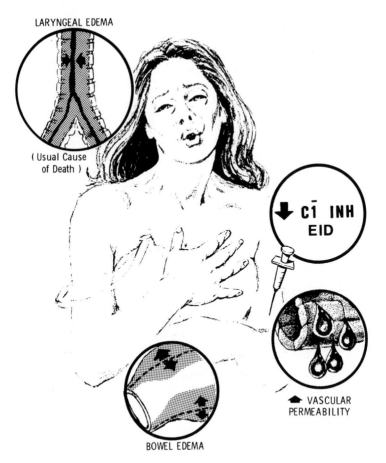

LARYNGEAL EDEMA

(Usual Cause
of Death)

C1̄ INH
EID

VASCULAR
PERMEABILITY

BOWEL EDEMA

Figure 15-9
Clinical features of hereditary angioedema (see Case Report 3).

the C1̄INH effect [66, 67], (2) specific antigen-antibody precipitin reactions on Ouchterlony plates between purified C1s and C1s-inhibitor-
containing plasma (see Chap. 4), or (3) the ultracentrifugation analysis
of material in serum that precipitates with isolated C1q [71, 72] (see
Chap. 16).

Quantitation of the physical presence of C1s inhibitor may be roughly
estimated by the size of the precipitin arc on immunoelectrophoresis
using antisera specific to C1̄INH. This semiquantitative approach allows only the gross determination of normal, increased, or decreased
categories. A technique for the hemolytic titration of C1̄INH has been
described [73].

References

1. Troll, W., Klassen, A., and Jancroft, A. Tumorigenesis in mouse skin: Inhibition by synthetic inhibitors of proteases. *Science* 169:1211, 1970.
2. Schnebli, H. P., and Burger, M. M. Selective inhibition of growth of transformed cells by protease inhibitors. *Proc. Natl. Acad. Sci. U.S.A.* 69:3825, 1972.
3. Schultze, H. E., and Heremans, J. F. *Molecular Biology of Human Proteins,* Vol. 1. Amsterdam: Elsevier, 1966.
4. Heimburger, N. Introductory Remarks: Proteinase Inhibition in Human Serum: Identification, Concentration, Chemical Properties, Enzymatic Specificity. In C. Mittman (Ed.), *Pulmonary Emphysema and Proteolysis.* New York: Academic, 1972. Pp. 307–310.
5. Makino, S., and Reed, C. E. Distribution and elimination of exogenous alpha$_1$-antitrypsin. *J. Lab. Clin. Med.* 75:742, 1970.
6. Leiberman, J., and Gawad, M. Inhibitors and activators of leukocytic proteases in purulent sputum. Digestion of human lung and inhibition by alpha$_1$-antitrypsin. *J. Lab. Clin. Med.* 77:713, 1971.
7. Lieberman, J., Mittman, C., and Kent, J. R. Screening for heterozygous α_1-antitrypsin deficiency. III. A provocative test with diethylstilbestrol and effect of oral contraceptives. *J.A.M.A.* 217:1198, 1971.
8. Fagerhol, M. K., and Laurell, C. B. The Pi System—Inherited Variants of Serum α_1-Antitrypsin. In A. G. Steinberg and A. G. Bearn (Eds.), *Progress in Medical Genetics,* Vol. 3. New York: Grune & Stratton, 1970. Pp. 96–111.
9. Fagerhol, M. K. The Pi system. Genetic variants of serum α_1-antitrypsin. *Semin. Hematol.* 1:153, 1968.
10. Talamo, R. C., Langley, C. E., Levine, B. W., and Kazemi, H. Genetic vs. quantitative analysis of serum alpha$_1$-antitrypsin. *N. Engl. J. Med.* 287:1067, 1972.
11. Lieberman, J., Gaidulis, M. S., Garoutte, B., and Mittman, C. Identification and characteristics of the common alpha$_1$-antitrypsin phenotypes. *Chest* 62:557, 1972.
12. Laurell, C. B., and Eriksson, S. The electrophoretic alpha$_1$-globulin pattern of serum in alpha$_1$-antitrypsin deficiency in patients with pulmonary emphysema. *Scand. J. Clin. Lab. Invest.* 15:132, 1963.
13. Eriksson, S. Studies in alpha$_1$-antitrypsin deficiency. *Acta Med. Scand.* 177[Suppl. 432]:1, 1965.
14. Hunter, C. C., Pierce, J. A., and LaBorde, J. B. α_1-Antitrypsin deficiency: A family study. *J.A.M.A.* 205:23, 1968.
15. Talamo, R. C., Allen, J. D., Kahan, M. G., and Austen, K. F. Hereditary α_1-antitrypsin deficiency. *N. Engl. J. Med.* 278:345, 1968.
16. Tarkoff, M. P., Kueppers, F., and Miller, W. F. Pulmonary emphysema and alpha$_1$-antitrypsin deficiency. *Am. J. Med.* 45:220, 1968.
17. Townley, R. G., Ryming, F., Lynch, H., and Brody, A. W. Obstructive lung disease in hereditary α_1-antitrypsin deficiency. *J.A.M.A.* 214:325, 1970.
18. Sharp, H. L. Alpha-1-antitrypsin deficiency. *Hosp. Practice,* May 1971. Pp. 83–96.
19. Guenter, C. A., Welch, M. H., and Hammersten, J. F. Alpha$_1$-antitrypsin deficiency and pulmonary emphysema. *Annu. Rev. Med.* 22:283, 1971.
20. Guenter, C. A., Welch, M. H., Russell, T. R., Hyde, R. M., and Ham-

mersten, J. F. The pattern of lung disease associated with alpha$_1$-antitrypsin deficiency. *Arch. Intern. Med.* 122:254, 1968.

21. Stein, P. D., Leu, J. D., Welch, M. H., and Guenter, C. A. Pathophysiology of the pulmonary circulation in emphysema associated with alpha$_1$-antitrypsin disease. *Circulation* 43:227, 1971.

22. Stevens, P. M., Hnilica, V. S., Johnson, P. C., and Bell, R. L. Pathophysiology of hereditary emphysema. *Ann. Intern. Med.* 74:672, 1971.

23. Meiers, H. G., Beisenherz, D., Bruster, H., Strassburger, D., and Gruel, H. α_1-Antitrypsin deficiency and emphysema. *Dtsch. Med. Wochenschr.* 93:1633, 1968.

24. Levine, B. W., Talamo, R. C., Shannon, D. C., and Kazemi, H. Alteration in distribution of pulmonary blood flow: An early manifestation of alpha$_1$-antitrypsin deficiency. *Ann. Intern. Med.* 73:397, 1970.

25. Eriksson, S., and Berven, H. Lung Function in Homozygous Alpha$_1$-Antitrypsin Deficiency: Studies in Patients with Severe Disease. In C. Mittman (Ed.), *Pulmonary Emphysema and Proteolysis.* New York: Academic, 1972. Pp. 7–23.

26. Resnick, H., Lapp, N. L., and Morgan, W. K. C. Serum trypsin inhibitor concentrations in coal miners with respiratory symptoms. *J.A.M.A.* 215:1101, 1971.

27. Hutchinson, D. C. S., Cook, P. J. L., Barter, C. E., Harris, H., and Hugh-Jones, P. Pulmonary emphysema and α_1-antitrypsin deficiency. *Br. Med. J.* 1:689, 1971.

28. Welch, M. H., Reinecke, M. E., Hammersten, J. F., and Guenter, C. A. Antitrypsin deficiency in pulmonary disease: The significance of intermediate levels. *Ann. Intern. Med.* 71:533, 1969.

28a. Lieberman, J. Heterozygous and homozygous alpha$_1$-antitrypsin deficiency in patients with pulmonary emphysema. *N. Engl. J. Med.* 281:279, 1969.

29. Talamo, R. C., et al. Symptomatic pulmonary emphysema in childhood, associated with hereditary alpha$_1$-antitrypsin and elastase inhibitor deficiency. *J. Pediatr.* 79:20, 1971.

30. Lieberman, J., and Kaneshiro, W. Inhibition of leukocytic elastase from purulent sputum by alpha$_1$-antitrypsin. *J. Lab. Clin. Med.* 80:88, 1972.

31. Sharp, H. L., Bridges, R. A., Krivit, W., and Freier, E. F. Cirrhosis associated with alpha$_1$-antitrypsin deficiency: A previously unrecognized inherited disorder. *J. Lab. Clin. Med.* 73:934, 1969.

32. Gordon, H. W., Dixon, J., Rogers, J. C., Mittman, C., and Lieberman, J. Alpha$_1$-antitrypsin (α_1AT) accumulation in livers of emphysematous patients with α_1AT deficiency. *Hum. Pathol.* 3:361, 1972.

33. Lieberman, J., Mittman, C., and Gordon, H. W. Alpha$_1$-antitrypsin in the livers of patients with emphysema. *Science* 175:63, 1972.

34. Cohen, K. L., Rubin, P. E., Echevarria, R. A., Sharp, H. L., and Teague, P. O. Alpha$_1$-antitrypsin deficiency, emphysema and cirrhosis in an adult. *Ann. Intern. Med.* 78:227, 1973.

35. Compara, J. L., Craig, J. R., Peters, R. L., and Reynolds, T. B. Cirrhosis associated with partial deficiency of alpha$_1$-antitrypsin in an adult. *Ann. Intern. Med.* 78:233, 1973.

36. Lieberman, J., Mittman, C., and Schneider, A. S. Screening for homozygous and heterozygous α_1-antitrypsin deficiency. Protein electrophoresis on cellulose acetate membranes. *J.A.M.A.* 210:2055, 1969.

37. Lieberman, J., and Mittman, C. Screening for heterozygous alpha$_1$-

antitrypsin deficiency. II. Effect of other serum protein abnormalities. *Ann. Intern. Med.* 73:9, 1970.

38. Erlanger, B. F., Kokowsky, N., and Cohen, W. The preparation and properties of two new chromagenic substrates of trypsin. *Arch. Biochem. Biophys.* 95:271, 1961.

39. Lopez, M., Tsu, T., and Hyslop, N. E., Jr. Studies of electroimmuno-diffusion: Immunochemical quantitation of proteins in dilute solutions. *Immunochemistry* 6:513, 1969.

40. Hyslop, N. E., Jr., Langley, C. E., Levine, B. W., and Talamo, R. C. Study of Methods of Measurement of the Alpha$_1$-Antitrypsin in Human Biological Fluids: Electroimmunodiffusion and Total Antitrypsin Activity. In C. Mittman (Ed.), *Pulmonary Emphysema and Proteolysis.* New York: Academic, 1972. Pp. 167–172.

41. Talamo, R. C., Langley, C. E., and Hyslop, N. E., Jr. A Comparison of Functional and Immunochemical Measurement of Serum Alpha$_1$-Antitrypsin. In C. Mittman (Ed.), *Pulmonary Emphysema and Proteolysis.* New York: Academic, 1972. Pp. 167–172.

42. Miesch, F., Bieth, J., and Metais, P. The α_1-antitrypsin and α_2-macroglobulin content and the protease-inhibiting capacity of normal and pathological sera. *Clin. Chim. Acta* 31:231, 1971.

43. Laurell, C. B. Comparison of Alpha$_1$-Antitrypsin and Alpha$_2$-Macroglobulin. In C. Mittman (Ed.), *Pulmonary Emphysema and Proteolysis.* New York: Academic, 1972. Pp. 349–354.

44. Fischer, C. L., Gill, C., Daniels, J. C., Cobb, E. K., Berry, C. A., and Ritzmann, S. E. Effects of the space flight environment on man's immune system. I. Serum proteins and immunoglobulins. *Aerosp. Med.* 43: 856, 1972.

45. Laurell, C. B. Variations of the Alpha$_1$-Antitrypsin Level of Plasma. In C. Mittman (Ed.), *Pulmonary Emphysema and Proteolysis.* New York: Academic, 1972. Pp. 161–166.

46. Daniels, J. C., Larson, D. L., Abston, S., and Ritzmann, S. E. Serum protein profiles in thermal burns. II. Protease inhibitors, complement factors, and C-reactive protein. *J. Trauma* 14:153,1974.

47. Daniels, J. C., Fukushima, M., Larson, D. L., and Ritzmann, S. E. Studies on muramidase (lysozyme). I. Serum and urine muramidase activity in burned children. *Tex. Rep. Biol. Med.* 29:13, 1971.

48. Rhodes, N. B., Bennett, N., and Feeney, R. E. The trypsin and chymotrypsin inhibitors from avian egg whites. *J. Biol. Chem.* 235:1686, 1960.

49. Elmore, D. T., and Smith, J. J. A new method for determining the absolute molarity of solutions of trypsin and chymotrypsin by using *p*-nitrophenyl N^2-acetyl-N^1-benzylcarbazate. *Biochem. J.* 107:103, 1968.

50. Heide, K., Heimburger, N., and Haupt, H. An inter-alpha trypsin inhibitor of human serum. *Clin. Chim. Acta* 11:82, 1965.

51. Harpel, P. C. Human plasma alpha$_2$-macroglobulin: An inhibitor of plasma kallikrein. *J. Exp. Med.* 132:329, 1970.

52. Harpel, P. C. Separation of plasma thromboplastin antecedent from kallikrein by the plasma α_2-macroglobulin, kallikrein inhibitor. *J. Clin. Invest.* 50:2084, 1971.

53. Szczeklik, A. Generation of the proteolytic activity bound with α_2-macroglobulin during plasma clotting. *Clin. Chim. Acta* 27:339, 1970.

54. Ganrot, P. O., and Bjerre, B. α_1-Antitrypsin and α_2-macroglobulin concentration in serum during pregnancy. *Acta Obstet. Gynecol. Scand.* 46: 126, 1967.

55. Horne, C. H. W., Mallinson, A. C., Ferguson, J., and Goudie, R. B. Effects of oestrogen and progestogen on serum levels of α_2-macroglobulin transferrin, albumin and IgG. *J. Clin. Pathol.* 24:464, 1971.

56. Housley, J. Alpha$_2$-macroglobulin levels in disease in man. *J. Clin. Pathol.* 21:27, 1968.

57. Horne, C. H. W., Howie, P. W., and Goudie, R. B. Serum alpha$_2$-macroglobulin, transferrin, albumin and IgG levels in preeclampsia. *J. Clin. Pathol.* 23:514, 1970.

58. Horne, C. H. W., Briggs, J. D., Howie, P. W., and Kennedy, A. C. Serum α_2-macroglobulins in renal disease and preeclampsia. *J. Clin. Pathol.* 25:590, 1972.

59. Steinis, W. J., and Mehl, J. W. The elevation of alpha$_2$-macroglobulin and trypsin-binding activity in nephrosis. *J. Lab. Clin. Med.* 67:559, 1966.

60. Kunkel, H. G. Macroglobulins and High Molecular Weight Antibodies. In F. W. Putnam (Ed.), *The Plasma Proteins,* Vol. 1. New York: Academic, 1960. Pp. 279–307.

61. Daniels, J. C., Fukushima, M., Fish, J. C., Tyson, K. R. T., Lindley, J. D., Remmers, A. R., Jr., Sarles, H. E., and Ritzmann, S. E. Studies on muramidase (lysozyme): II. Serum and urine muramidase patterns in chronic uremia, chronic hemodialysis, and renal allotransplantation. *Tex. Rep. Biol. Med.* 30:19, 1972.

62. James, K., Johnson, G., and Fudenberg, H. H. The quantitative estimation of α_2-macroglobulin in normal, pathological, and cord sera. *Clin. Chim. Acta* 14:207, 1966.

63. Müller, H., Kleine, N., Kaufmann, W., and Kluthe, R. α_2-Macroglobulinemia metabolism in diabetes mellitus. *Klin. Med. Wochenschr.* 48:1276, 1970.

64. Saunders, R., Dyce, B. J., Vannier, W. E., and Haverback, B. J. The separation of alpha-2-macroglobulin into five components with differing electrophoretic and enzyme-binding properties. *J. Clin. Invest.* 50:2376, 1971.

65. Donaldson, V. H., and Evans, R. R. A biochemical abnormality in hereditary angioneurotic edema: Absence of serum inhibitor of C'1-esterase. *Am. J. Med.* 35:37, 1963.

66. Donaldson, V. H., and Rosen, F. S. Action of complement in hereditary angioneurotic edema: The role of C'1-esterase. *J. Clin. Invest.* 43:2204, 1964.

67. Laurell, A. B., Lindegran, J., Malmos, I., and Martensson, H. Enzymatic and immunochemical estimation of C1 esterase inhibitor in sera from patients with hereditary angioneurotic edema. *Scand. J. Clin. Lab. Invest.* 24:221, 1969.

68. Rosen, F. S., Alper, C. A., Pensky, J., Klamperer, M. R., and Donaldson, V. H. Genetically determined heterogeneity of the C1 esterase inhibitor in patients with hereditary angioneurotic edema. *J. Clin. Invest.* 50:2143, 1971.

69. Blohmé, G. Treatment of hereditary angioneurotic oedema with tranexamic acid: A random double blind cross-over study. *Acta Med. Scand.* 192:293, 1972.

70. Caldwell, J. R., Ruddy, S., Schur, P. H., and Austen, K. F. Acquired C1 inhibitor deficiency in lymphosarcoma. *Clin. Immunol. Immunopathol.* 1:39, 1972.

71. Agnello, V., Winchester, R. J., and Kunkel, H. G. Precipitin reactions

of the C1q component of complement with aggregated γ-globulin and immune complexes in gel diffusion. *Immunology* 19:909, 1970.

72. Hannestad, K.   Presence of aggregated γG-globulin in certain rheumatoid synovial effusions. *Clin. Exp. Immunol.* 2:511, 1967.

73. Gigli, I., Ruddy, S., and Austen, K. F.   The stoichiometric measurement of the serum inhibitor of the first component of complement by the inhibition of immune hemolysis. *J. Immunol.* 100:1154, 1968.

Abnormalities of the Complement System **16**

Ernest S. Tucker, III, and Robert M. Nakamura

Multicomponent Nature of the Complement System

The importance of the complement system in the pathogenesis of human disease has been clearly defined by the work of many investigators during the past decade. Most notably, the complement system has been shown to be an important mediator in the pathogenesis of immunological tissue injury. The association of complement with immune phenomena has been observed since the turn of the century, but its role in immune disease remained obscure. During this time, the predominant focus was on its role in immune hemolysis. It was largely looked upon as a laboratory curiosity that provided a sensitive means for detecting antibody to a variety of antigens. It was not until the late 1950s and the 1960s that improved methods of biochemical purification allowed the isolation of the components of the complement system and a thorough study of their sequential interactions [1, 2].

Through the isolation and purification of individual components (see Appendix), it has been possible to reconstruct the entire sequence and to carry out physicochemical studies of the components and their modes of interaction. It is now recognized that a total of at least eleven individual proteins constitute the complement system [3] (Table 16-1). Each of these proteins is known to exist in human serum and the serum of other vertebrates in a precursor or inactive form. The components become activated in a sequential fashion following events that trigger the initial reaction. It has been shown that the immune reaction between antigen and certain types of antibody provides the necessary trigger mechanism for initial activation [4]. This activation by immune reactants has been demonstrated both in vivo and in vitro.

Following the initial activation, the subsequent reactions proceed in a cascade fashion with the production of molecules that possess significant biological activity [5] (Fig. 16-1). These activities will be discussed in more detail later, but it should be mentioned here that they range from

Table 16-1. Characteristics of Human Complement Components

Component[a]	Synonym	Electrophoretic Mobility	Cleavage Fragments	Molecular Weight (daltons)	Sedimentation Coefficient	Synthetic Inhibitors	Serum Concentrations ($\mu g/ml$)
C1q	⎫	γ_2	—	4×10^5	11.1	EDTA	170–200
C1r	C1	β	—	1.68×10^5	7.0	Organic phosphates (DFP)	60–80
C1s	⎭ C1 Esterase	α_2	—	7.9×10^4	4.0	Amino acid esters	30–60
C2	⎫	β_2	C2a, C2b C2 kinin	1.17×10^5	5.5	p-Chloromercuri-benzoate	20–40
C4	⎭ C3 Convertase β-1E-globulin	β_1	C4a, C4b	2.4×10^5	10.0	EDTA Hydrazine	170–200 390–470
C3	β-1C-globulin	β_1	C3a, C3b, C3c (β1A) C3d (α2D)	1.85×10^5 1.85×10^5	9.5	Aromatic amino acid esters Salicylaldoxime Phlorizin Hydrazine	800–1500
C5	⎫ β-1F-globulin	β_1	C5a, C5b	1.25×10^5	8.7	Glutamyltyrosine	60–90
C6	Trimolecular	β_2			5.6		40–80
C7	⎭ complex	β_2			6.7		40–80
C8		γ_1	—	1.5×10^5	8	—	1–10
C9		α_2	—	7.9×10^4	4.5	—	1–10

[a] The nomenclature of complement components in this chapter follows the protocol proposed by a committee on nomenclature of the World Health Organization in 1968. Each component is designated by the capital letter C, followed by the appropriate Arabic numeral, i.e., C1, C2, C3, and so on. C1 provides a slight exception. It consists of three proteins, designated as C1q, C1r, and C1s, which together form the trimolecular complex of C1. An activated component is denoted by a superscript bar above the symbol, thus C1 is activated C1. Cleavage products of the components are designated by a lower case letter following the component symbol; thus, C3 may give rise to fragments C3a, C3b, C3c, and C3d. Note that the prime mark (C′) is no longer used to denote complement. Reproduced by permission. From Committee report. *Bull. W.H.O.* 39:935, 1968.

neutralization of viruses to chemotaxis and the phagocytosis of particles by leukocytes. In addition to the active molecules, various inhibitors have been found in the serum of vertebrates [6]. These selectively suppress certain biological activities exerted by the active components. Indeed, it appears that in some instances there may be more than one inhibitor for each active component. The presence of such inhibitors provides a natural means of homeostatic regulation of the complement system. Only a few of these inhibitors have been isolated and defined as to their physicochemical characteristics and modes of action [7].

Considerable work remains before all of the steps in activation and suppression of the complement system are understood. The modes of activation of complement appear increasingly complicated as research in this area proceeds. In the past few years, it has become clear that two major pathways for the activation of the complement system exist [8, 9]. Before the discovery of the so-called alternate or bypass activation route, it was thought that the fixation of complement as the result of an immune reaction along a cell surface was the primary and singular mode of activating the complement sequence. It is now well recognized that activation of the terminal components can occur consequent to events in the fluid phase of the serum [8–10]. In the following discussion, the classic pathway of complement activation will be designated the *intrinsic pathway* and the alternate or bypass mechanism (now known to be composed of components of the properdin system) as the *extrinsic pathway*.

This chapter will discuss the variety of biological activities associated with activation of complement, the role of complement in immunological tissue injury, the effect on the host of inherited deficiencies of complement components, and abnormalities of complement associated with certain diseases.

THE INTRINSIC (CLASSIC) PATHWAY AND ITS MODE OF ACTIVATION

The manner in which complement components were first shown to be activated involved the use of an in vitro system that employed red blood cells coated with antibody [11]. The usual system employed is sheep red blood cells coated with rabbit antibody to the cells. These reactants provide both the immune phenomena and the surface of a cell membrane, which are necessary for the activation. The first component of complement is initially activated as a result of the binding of the molecule C1q to the antibody on the cell surface. It has been determined that this antibody must be either of the IgG or IgM class [12]. Other classes of antibody, including IgA, IgD, and IgE, do not fix complement by way of the intrinsic pathway [13]. The binding of C1q appears to result in the activation of the molecule by distortion (allosteric effect), so that certain chemical groupings located in the Fc portion of the antibody molecule are exposed [14]. This activation of C1q prepares a site for the activation of another component, C1r. This molecule then becomes bound to the C1q molecule, and a third site is thus prepared, where binding of another component, C1s, takes place in the presence of calcium. The bind-

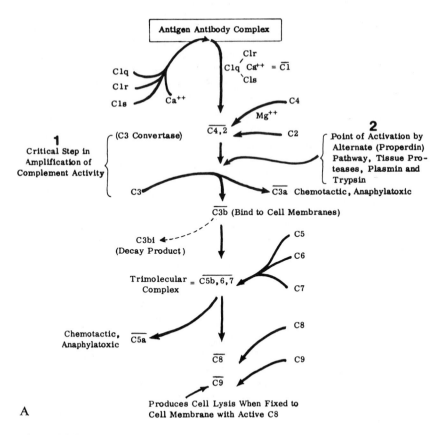

A

Figure 16-1

A. Classic, or intrinsic, pathway of complement activation initiated by immune reactants. (*1*) Note that cleavage of many C3 molecules by very little C3 convertase (C4,2) produces considerable amplification of complement activity. (*2*) The alternate (properdin) pathway; tissue proteases, trypsin, and plasmin produce activation of the complement system through C3 cleavage that is identical to that of C3 convertase.

B. Steps in immune hemolysis depicting the sequential activation of all of the serum complement components.

C. Extrinsic, or alternate (properdin), pathway of complement activation. (*1*) Note that the activation of C3PAse by C3 appears to be modulated by activated properdin (*2*). The cleavage of C3 also has an autocatalytic effect through the positive feedback of C3b on the activation of C3 proactivator convertase.

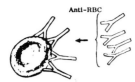

1 Sensitization of RBC by antibody (IgG or IgM)

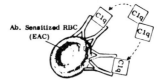

2. Initiation of complement activation by fixation of C1q to Fc portion of bound antibody.

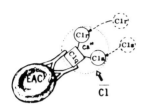

3. Subsequent formation of the active $\overline{C1}$ trimolecular complex (C1q, r, s) stabilized by Ca^{++} ligand.

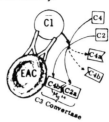

4. Activation of C4 and C2 to form the enzyme complex ($\overline{C4b}$, 2a) called C3 Convertase.

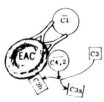

5. C3 Convertase cleaves serum C3 to C3b fragment that binds to the cell membrane and a small fragment (C3a) that does not.

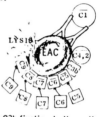

6. Following C3b fixation to the cell membrane, all of the terminal components are activated, thus producing hemolysis by the membrane lytic action of C9.

B

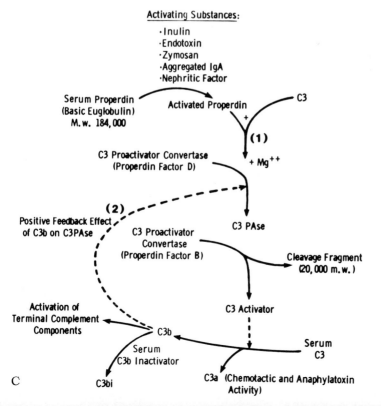

Activating Substances:
- Inulin
- Endotoxin
- Zymosan
- Aggregated IgA
- Nephritic Factor

Serum Properdin (Basic Euglobulin) M.w. 184,000 → Activated Properdin ← C3

(1) + Mg^{++}

C3 Proactivator Convertase (Properdin Factor D)

C3 PAse

(2)

Positive Feedback Effect of C3b on C3PAse

C3 Proactivator Convertase (Properdin Factor B) → Cleavage Fragment (20,000 m.w.)

C3 Activator

Activation of Terminal Complement Components ← C3b ← Serum C3

Serum C3b Inactivator

C3bi

C3a (Chemotactic and Anaphylatoxin Activity)

C

ing of this third component, C1s, results in a trimolecular complex bound by the calcium ion [15]. With activation, C1s exhibits esterase activity for its substrates, which are the precursors of both C2 and C4 in serum [16]. This activated trimolecular complex of C1qrs has been referred to as C1 esterase, although the actual esterolytic or proteolytic site is found in the C1s subunit [17]. The entirety of this trimolecular complex may be transferred from one binding site to another, and it may detach into the fluid phase [18].

Once there has been activation of C1, the subsequent steps in the sequence occur. The next reaction to follow is a cleavage of C4 by C$\bar{1}$, which releases a small peptide fragment, designated C4a, and a much larger residual fragment, C4b, which attaches to cell membrane receptors or transiently to the antibody C$\bar{1}$ complex on the cell surface [19]. However, most of the C4b remains in the fluid phase and may rapidly decay, thus becoming unable to bind to the cell membrane. Following cleavage of C4, there occurs cleavage of C2 in the serum so that two components, C2a and the smaller C2b, are produced [20]. In the presence of magnesium ion, the C2a combines with a C4b that has previously attached to the cell membrane [21]. This combination of C4b and C2a in their active state, held together by magnesium, results in an active proteolytic enzyme complex that is called *C3 convertase* [21]. The C2b fragment that is produced is relatively inert, and, along with a decay fragment of C2a, it becomes lost to the fluid phase of serum, unbound to the cell surface. The enzymatically active complex of C3 convertase has a relatively short in vitro half-life of between 12 and 15 minutes at 37°C [22]. Presumably, this short half-life also occurs in vivo. The C3 convertase that is fixed to the cell surface cleaves C3 from the serum into two fragments known as C3a and C3b [23]. The C3a fragment is of low molecular weight (7000 MW) and exhibits biological activities that have been characterized as anaphylatoxic (release of histamine from mast cells) and chemotactic (attraction of neutrophils and other polymorphonuclear leukocytes to a focus of activation) [24]. The C3b portion becomes attached to the cell membrane and also diffuses into the fluid phase of serum [25]. An inactivator that is present in plasma cleaves this fragment and renders it inactive [26]. Once there has been cleavage of C3 with the presence of C3b on the cell surface, subsequent activation of components C5, C6, and C7 occurs, which in turn leads to their attachment to the cell surface [25]. In the activation of C5, there is cleavage of the parent molecule into two fragments, one of which is designated C5a. The C5a fragment also demonstrates anaphylatoxic and chemotactic activity similar to the C3a fragment [27]. The trimolecular complex formed by C5, C6, and C7 may diffuse from the cell surface into the fluid phase and exhibit chemotactic activity for polymorphonuclear leukocytes [28].

The attachment of C8 to the cell membrane occurs following the fixation of C5, C6, and C7, and immediately a limited lytic reaction begins [29]. Shortly, with the binding of C9 to the cell surface there is increased erythrocyte damage, with acceleration of cell lysis [29]. The lysis appears to result from rupture of the plasma membrane, which is apparently due to a lytic effect on the phospholipid complex of the membrane [29, 30].

The complexity of the activation by the intrinsic, or classic, pathway is demonstrated by the diagram in Figure 16-1B.

THE EXTRINSIC (ALTERNATE) PATHWAY AND ITS MODE OF ACTIVATION

The concept of an alternate pathway of complement activation (Fig. 16-1C) developed from experiments that were undertaken to clarify the basis for spontaneous hemolysis in guinea pigs in the presence of certain activating factors [31]. One group of investigators has demonstrated a nonclassic mode of complement activation in humans in the disease known as *paroxysmal nocturnal hemoglobinuria* (PNH) [8, 32]. In other instances, investigators were intrigued by the hemolysis that resulted when guinea pig cells were exposed to substances such as zymosan (from yeast cell walls) and gram-negative bacteria [33]. The work has proceeded so that it is now clear that many of the activators of the terminal components of the complement system in the fluid phase are identical with components of the serum properdin system [34].

The initial triggering of the alternate system seems to occur as the result of activation by molecules such as agar, zymosan, inulin, bacterial polysaccharide, and aggregated immunoglobulins, notably IgA [35]. These substances seem to activate a molecule, which is possibly properdin itself, and, in turn, there then occurs activation of a precursor enzyme that is known as *C3 activator convertase* [35]. This convertase then produces an active enzyme, called *C3 activator,* which will cleave C3, producing the fragments C3a and C3b. These fragments are identical to those produced by C3 convertase cleavage in the classic system [35], and they also exhibit similar biological activity. The C3b fragment may attach to cell membranes and provide for the subsequent activation of the terminal complement components C5, C6, C7, C8, and C9, thus leading to cell lysis as in the classic system. It has also been noted that C3b produces a positive feedback effect by potentiating the activation of the C3 activator and thereby producing more cleavage products of C3 [36]. The limiting factor of this reaction appears to be a C3b inactivator (which was previously mentioned) that causes inactivation of C3b [26]. Without the inactivator, hypercatabolism of C3 occurs, which causes significant depletion of this important component [37].

The three parts of Figure 16-1 illustrate the composite interrelations of the properdin and classic systems of complement activation. Indeed, these diagrams, although they are complex, show the details of the major interrelations of these two systems. They are only a part of the numerous biochemical mediator systems that exist in the plasma of man and animals.

Biological Activities Associated with Activation of the Complement System

Research is revealing multiple biological activities associated with the complement system. Currently, there are a number of activities that have been shown to be associated with various complement components

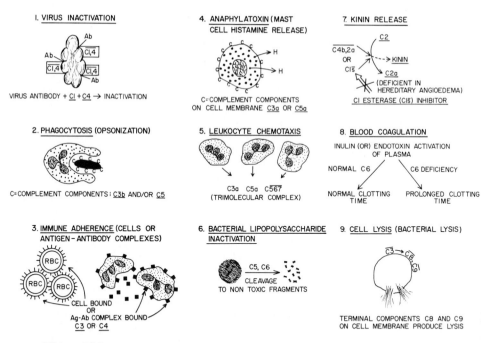

Figure 16-2
Biological activities of complement components.

in the activated state. These are shown in Figure 16-2. Generally, it can be seen that the biological effects are divided into those on cells and those affecting chemical systems in the plasma or animal tissues.

EFFECTS OF COMPLEMENT COMPONENTS ON CELLS

The majority of the direct effects of the activated components of complement are those on cell membranes. Chemical attraction for cells (chemotaxis) is exhibited by at least three components. The trimolecular complex of C$\overline{567}$ and the fragments C3a and C5a all exhibit potent chemotactic effects [24, 27, 28]. These are most pronounced for polymorphonuclear leukocytes, especially neutrophils. This activity appears to be due to the activation of esterases in the membranes of the cells undergoing the attraction [38]. The migration takes place against a concentration gradient to the focus where the active components are produced.

The well-known phenomenon of cell lysis is produced by activation of the terminal components, C8 and C9 [29, 30]. Lysis may involve not only red blood cells but also other cell types in the blood, cells of fixed tissues, and bacterial cells [39]. Bacterial lysis is a mechanism whereby the host defense is enhanced against infectious agents. On the other hand, lysis may cause widespread intravascular hemolysis in instances of hemolytic anemia of the newborn due to antibodies against the Rh antigens [40].

Phagocytosis is exhibited by many leukocytes of the peripheral blood, especially the polymorphonuclear leukocytes and the monocyte-macrophage group. These cells depend upon C5 or C3b for the facilitation of phagocytosis (which is also referred to as *opsonization*) [41, 42]. This facilitation by complement is demonstrated when microparticles of latex or bacteria are coated with C5 or C3b, and the amount of phagocytosis is determined. In such experiments where C5 or C3b is absent or depleted, there is no enchancement of phagocytosis. The enhancement mechanism appears to involve the binding of C5 or C3b to the particle surface, which then interacts with a complement receptor site on the phagocyte membrane, thereby promoting specific interaction between the particle and the phagocytic cell [41, 42]. This appears to enhance phagocytosis of the particle. The biochemistry and cellular physiology involved in this reaction remain to be clarified.

The production of anaphylatoxin is another effect of complement on cells. The fragments C3a and C5a both promote histamine release from mast cells (an event that has been referred to as *anaphylatoxic*) [24, 27]. C3a and C5a appear to behave similarly to other factors that are known to cause histamine release from basophils and mast cells. A two-step reaction, one step of which is calcium dependent, has been observed with each fragment. It is notable, however, that there is no cross reaction between C3a and C5a in producing this effect. This reaction was called *anaphylatoxic* because it was initially believed to be important in anaphylaxis. It has now been shown, however, that the contribution to anaphylaxis is not major, especially when it is compared to the atopic or reaginic mechanism, which appears considerably more important in clinical anaphylaxis [43].

A phenomenon that has been described as *immune adherence* is another effect of complement on cells [44]. The mechanisms of this reaction are similar to those in phagocytosis. The fixation of certain complement components (C3 or C4) to cell surfaces, either as the result of immune activation or consequent to activation by the extrinsic pathway, results in the preparation of a reactive site that can then react with receptors on the surface of other cells to produce an adherence between two or more cells [44, 45]. Formation of rosettes and cell clumps will occur due to this phenomenon.

EFFECTS OF COMPLEMENT COMPONENTS ON BIOCHEMICAL REACTIONS

Perhaps the most striking biochemical reaction that depends on complement is release of a permeability factor due to the action of C$\overline{1}$ on its natural substrate, C2. In this reaction, a polypeptide fragment is cleaved, and this fragment exhibits permeability activity along with other effects that identify it as a type of kinin [46]. It is not, however, identical with bradykinin, although it is similar in its pharmacological properties. Production of this kinin is suppressed by a natural inhibitor in plasma known as *Cl-esterase inhibitor* (C$\bar{1}$INH). There is a rare disease in humans known as *hereditary angioneurotic edema* in which there is deficiency of this serum inhibitor [47] (see Chap. 15). This deficiency appears to explain why episodes of tissue edema recur in these individuals. Often the site of the edematous reaction is in the respiratory tract, and if it involves the larynx, it can be a threat to life because of the potential airway obstruction. This disease will be discussed in more detail later.

The role of complement in virus neutralization can be demonstrated in vitro [48], and there are strong indications that it may be important in virus infections in vivo. The mechanism of inactivation is known to involve the first four complement components. It is thought that this inactivation occurs because of an effect on the surface protein-coating of the viral particles. It appears to be mostly dependent on C1 and C4, but the exact mechanism of inactivation is unclear [48]. C3 has also been considered important, since the ability of serum to neutralize virus can be destroyed by depleting C3 through prior cleavage of C3 with cobra venom factor.

The importance of certain complement components in blood coagulation has recently been investigated. It has been well established in a C6-deficient strain of rabbits that C6 is important in blood coagulation [49]. This effect was shown by demonstrating a difference in the inulin clotting time in C6-deficient rabbits compared to normal ones. Inulin was used as the activator of the clotting system, and in those animals who were C6 deficient, there was a significantly prolonged clotting time. In contrast, clotting times utilizing activators such as kaolin, glass, or diatomaceous earth showed no difference between the C6-deficient and the normal rabbits [49]. These data have not only shown a dependence on C6 in blood coagulation, but they have also shown a different pathway of coagulation that is complement dependent and distinct from the classic, intrinsic system of blood coagulation.

The ability of certain complement components to detoxify bacterial lipopolysaccharides has been reported. C5 appears to be of major importance in the cleavage, although C6 also appears to be involved. The role of C6 has been indicated by the effect of endotoxin on C6-deficient rabbits, who do not survive following injection of this material [50]. This ability to inactivate lipopolysaccharides may be of survival value for man and animals, since the adverse effects of endotoxin resulting from infections with gram-negative organisms are known to be life-threatening.

Role of the Complement System in Immunological Tissue Injury

With the foregoing description of the varied biological effects of the complement system, one can surmise that it is also important in the pathogenesis of immunological disease. Such significance can be demonstrated experimentally and by a comparative study in animals and man.

There are three major types of disease where complement bears a relationship to the development of tissue injury. These are immune hemolytic anemia, immune vasculitis, and different forms of immunological glomerulonephritis.

HEMOLYTIC ANEMIA

The pathogenesis of immune hemolytic anemia parallels the in vitro phenomenon of immune lysis of red blood cells [51]. A common type of immune hemolytic anemia in man is hemolytic disease in the newborn due to fetal-maternal blood incompatibility [40]. The most common antigens involved are those of the Rh system and the ABO system. The basis for the development of an immune reaction is the existence of fetal antigens on the red blood cells that provokes an antibody response in the mother (Fig. 16-3). A prior episode of sensitization during a previous pregnancy is an important factor in the subsequent development of high titers of antibody against the Rh and ABO antigens. The stimuli for increased antibody production are placental microhemorrhages, which allow mixing of the fetal and maternal blood. Once exposure has occurred, an increased antibody response on reexposure may be sufficient to cause severe hemolytic anemia in the newborn. Because the second response is of the anamnestic type, the antibody produced is of the IgG class and of a molecular size that will cross the placenta and enter the fetal circulation. Once the antibody enters the fetal circulation, it reacts with the antigens of the red blood cell membrane, and complement fixation ensues with lysis of the cells. Because of the hemolysis, the infant becomes severely anemic and accumulates bilirubin from the red blood cell breakdown, which can cause damage of the central nervous system. The blood of infants with hemolytic anemia characteristically exhibits a positive direct, and often a positive indirect, Coombs' antiglobulin reaction. This occurs with antiglobulin reagents that react primarily with immunoglobulins, as well as with complement components on the cell surface. Indeed, the presence of a positive Coombs' test in the presence of a rising serum bilirubin should lead one to suspect this as a possible diagnosis.

In other situations, the development of hemolytic anemia is less clearly defined. Often, the anemia may be related to drug therapy, where the drug functions as a hapten and becomes attached to the red blood cell surface [51]. The drug may provoke an antibody response in the host, thus causing production of complement-fixing antibodies that react with the drug [51, 52]. In other situations, the cause may be more obscure. Hemolytic anemia may be encountered as a result of immune-complex formation in the circulation, which produces activated complement components that become attached to the red blood cells and produce hemolysis. This has been referred to as an "innocent-bystander" type of reaction [53].

VASCULITIS

The contribution of complement to the development of immune vasculitis has been well studied in experimental animals [54]. Observations on the pathogenesis of vasculitis in humans appear to correlate well with the

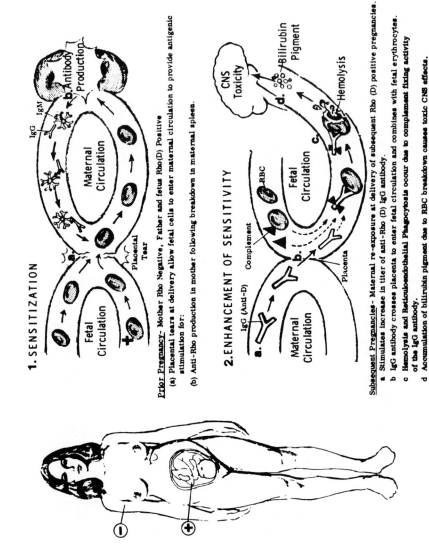

1. SENSITIZATION

IgG   IgM

b. Antibody Production

Maternal Circulation

Fetal Circulation

Placental Tear

Prior Pregnancy - Mother Rho Negative, Father and fetus Rho(D) Positive

(a) Placental tears at delivery allow fetal cells to enter maternal circulation to provide antigenic stimulation for:

(b) Anti-Rho production in mother following breakdown in maternal spleen.

2. ENHANCEMENT OF SENSITIVITY

CNS Toxicity

d. Bilirubin Pigment

c. Hemolysis

RBC

Fetal Circulation

Complement

IgG (Anti-D)

b.

a.

Maternal Circulation

Placenta

Subsequent Pregnancies - Maternal re-exposure at delivery of subsequent Rho (D) positive pregnancies.

a Stimulates increase in titer of anti-Rho (D) IgG antibody.

b IgG antibody crosses placenta to enter fetal circulation and combines with fetal erythrocytes.

c Hemolysis and Reticuloendothelial Phagocytosis occur due to complement fixing activity of the IgG antibody.

d Accumulation of bilirubin pigment due to RBC breakdown causes toxic CNS effects.

○ (I)

● (+)

Figure 16-3
Pathogenesis of Rho(D) hemolytic disease of the newborn.

data derived from experimental studies [55, 56]. The initial event in the development of vasculitis appears to be a localization of immune reactants within or surrounding the walls of the blood vessels. This localization can be produced in an animal that has been actively or passively sensitized to various antigens.

The prototype of this form of injury is exemplified in the Arthus reaction (see Chap. 17). In the Arthus reaction, the sensitized animal is injected with antigen into the subcutaneous tissue. On diffusion of the antigen from the injection site, it encounters antibody within the vessel wall as it contacts the blood plasma [57]. At optimal concentrations of antigen and antibody, a precipitate forms, and complement fixation occurs. As a consequence of complement fixation, chemotactic factors are produced and cause a heavy influx of leukocytes [58] into the blood vessel wall to the site of the antigen-antibody precipitate. On arrival, these leukocytes (mostly neutrophils) release their granules containing a variety of hydrolytic enzymes. These enzymes cause considerable destruction of the tissue. Histologically, the lesion exhibits extensive necrosis of the vessel wall and surrounding tissue.

Disseminated vasculitis can be induced experimentally following induction of circulating immune-complex formations [59]. This may be achieved by the injection of antigens into the circulating blood, which stimulate a significant antibody response. Approximately four to seven days following injection, the antibody appears in the circulation, and, when it combines with circulating antigen, immune complexes form. Usually, the antibody is of the IgM class and exhibits considerable complement-fixing activity. These circulating complexes are of varied molecular size. Some of the complexes may be much heavier than 23S, whereas others may be only slightly more than 7S in terms of their sedimentation coefficients. It has been found that a certain size of complex is optimal for localization of the complexes within the intima of blood vessels beneath the endothelium [60]. This critical size is in the range of 16S to 19S. Other factors are important in the localization of these complexes, such as those that affect the permeability of the endothelium [61, 62], e.g., histamine. The local increase of blood pressure on the endothelial surface also accounts for localization of complexes. Because of the permeability effects, more deposition occurs at points of bifurcation and at points of constriction, where the pressures are the greatest [62]. Once localization of the complex has occurred, it appears to be stationary and provides a focus for the chemotactic attraction of polymorphonuclear leukocytes. Leukocytes enter the vessel wall and release their hydrolytic enzymes, causing tissue destruction. When there has been widespread deposition of such complexes in many blood vessels throughout the body, there is also an accompanying widespread vasculitis. When such deposits localize within the glomerular tuft, this leads to one of the forms of acute glomerulonephritis [63].

GLOMERULONEPHRITIS

The majority of forms of glomerulonephritis appear to be complement dependent [64]. As mentioned in the preceding section, the localization of immune complexes that are capable of fixing complement may occur within the glomerular tuft along the basement membrane and cause one form of acute glomerulonephritis. The ensuing tissue destruction is produced by neutrophils emigrating to the glomerular basement and releasing their destructive enzymes [63]. In another form of glomerulonephritis, the event of neutrophil emigration with release of hydrolases is the same, but the initiating reaction is different (Fig. 16-4). In this type, the antigen is an intrinsic part of the tissue of the glomerular tuft (basement membrane), and the antibody reacts wherever the appropriate tissue is encountered [65]. These sites are usually along the basement membrane in the glomerulus, where complement fixation occurs and provides the focus for neutrophil chemotaxis and glomerular destruction.

In humans, both forms of glomerulonephritis have been recognized [66]. The acute nephritis that accompanies lupus erythematosus appears to result from the deposition of immune complexes formed by antinuclear antibody with DNA or DNA-nucleoprotein antigens. Such complexes have been shown to be potent in their ability to fix complement [67]. In other instances where an immune reaction with the basement membrane is the initiating factor, the resulting glomerulonephritis [68] due to anti-basement membrane antibody resembles that exhibited in the human disease known as *Goodpasture's syndrome*. Recently, there have been case reports of individuals with anti-basement membrane nephritis following exposure to hydrocarbon solvents [69].

There are many cases of glomerulonephritis that exhibit the presence of a granular deposition of γ-globulin and complement along the glomerular basement membrane. These findings suggest immune-complex deposition as a causative factor. Such granular deposit patterns outnumber those of the smooth linear deposition that is characteristic of anti-basement membrane glomerulonephritis. Forms of glomerulonephritis have recently been described in which the deposition of immunoglobulin is not a conspicuous feature, but the presence of complement, especially C3, and the deposition of properdin factors are notable [70]. Some of these cases have been referred to as *hypocomplementemic nephritis,* because of the significant lowering of complement activity in the blood of patients with this form of acute glomerulonephritis. In these cases, activity of the extrinsic system (alternate pathway) of complement activation has been found to be increased, and it is apparently important in the pathogenesis of this form of nephritis [70]. The factor (or factors) stimulating the activation of the alternate system have not yet been identified.

OTHER DISEASES

There has been considerable experimental work to establish a role of complement in the pathogenesis of acute arthritis and an attempt to relate complement activation to the morbidity of arthritis in humans. It has been possible to induce acute monoarticular arthritis experimentally by the direct injection of antigen into joint spaces [71], but acute arthritis as a feature of disseminated immune-complex disease appears to occur infrequently. The participation of complement in human arthritis remains

1. Mediated by Anti-Basement Membrane Antibody

a. Antibody combines with glomerular basement membrane antigen producing a uniform distribution along the glomerular loops. Immunofluorescence with anti-IgG exhibits a regular linear pattern outlining the capillary loops.

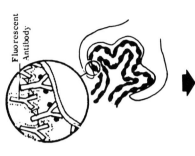

b. Subsequent fixation of complement by the immune reactants on the glomerular membrane produces a finely granular pattern on immunofluorescence with antisera to complement (C3)

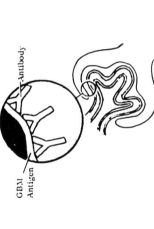

2. Mediated by Immune Complex Deposition

Immune complexes containing antigen, antibody and complement become deposited along the glomerular basement membrane producing an irregular (so called "lumpy-bumpy") pattern on immunofluorescence with antisera to immunoglobulins or complement components.

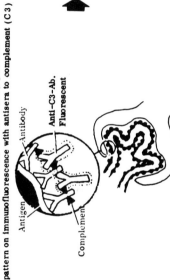

Due to complement activation both types exhibit neutrophilic infiltrates and variable patterns of glomerular destruction and repair associated with proteinuria.

Figure 16-4
Comparison of two types of immunological glomerulonephritis (for details, see text).

an open question, although the finding of cleavage products of complement components in the joint fluid of arthritic joints points to the likelihood of some role of complement [72].

Not all reactions that activate complement components are due to triggering by immune reactions. It has been shown that the release of proteases from damaged tissues and the activation of the fibrinolytic system are sufficient to produce active proteolytic enzymes that can cleave complement components to produce the biologically active fragments, which have been discussed [73]. In this regard, it appears that complement may have a ubiquitous role in the inflammatory process due to a variety of nonimmune mechanisms. It is thus important to keep in mind the possible overlap and confusion of assigning complement a definite role in the pathogenesis of disease unless it can be clearly shown that the activation of the complement system is a necessary prerequisite to tissue injury. Otherwise, complement activation may only be a secondary consequence of tissue damage due to other causes.

Inherited Deficiencies of Complement Components and Inhibitors

The previous discussions emphasize the role of complement in the development of tissue injury. In addition to its destructive potential, complement serves an important role in host defense, especially in the inactivation and the destruction of invasive microorganisms. This important role is clearly demonstrated in cases of hereditary deficiencies of certain critical complement components.

Recently, a case was reported that exemplifies the protective functions of complement [74]. The patient had severe, recurrent infections. In studies of the complement system, a significant decrease of the third component (C3) was found, and most of this was in the form of inactive C3b. When the catabolism of C3 was studied by injection of radiolabeled C3, it was found to be rapidly converted to the inactive C3b fragment. In addition, this patient's serum was shown to lack the ability to produce chemotactic factors. It did not enhance phagocytosis nor did it give rise to bacteriolysis when compared to the plasma of normal individuals. In addition, it was also found that this patient's serum was deficient in properdin factor B, or C3 activator, which has been discussed previously. It appears that this case represents an unusual instance where there is intense in vivo activity of the C3b inactivator [74].

Other types of complement deficiency have emphasized the importance of the complement system in host defense. A defect in the fifth component of complement (C5) has been identified in a family [75]. The initial discovery was prompted by examination of a young infant in the family who had recurrent infections with gram-negative organisms but who improved substantially after receiving transfusions of plasma. A deficiency of C2 [76] and deficiency of C1r [77] have been described, but neither of the patients in these instances exhibited a clinical problem of recurrent infection, although these patients appeared to have a significantly increased incidence of autoimmune hypersensitivity disease. Some observers have speculated that deficiencies of the early reacting components interfere with the ability of the host to neutralize viruses, and this would consequently allow for growth with dissemination of virus, accounting for the apparent hypersensitivity diseases noted in these patients. The properties of complement components that are important in the in vitro inactivation of viruses have been discussed.

Other abnormalities of the complement system have been described that are indirectly related to the impairment of host defense. In immune-deficiency syndromes, such as the classic form of sex-linked recessive agammaglobulinemia, the levels of C1q are often substantially below normal [78]. In these disorders, the assessment of the importance of C1q is limited by the associated immunological deficiency.

Electrophoretic variants of both C4 and C3 have received attention, but their significance remains unclear [79].

As mentioned previously, paroxsymal nocturnal hemoglobinuria (PNH) is associated with an abnormality of the complement system [8, 32]. On laboratory testing, the individuals who manifest this disease show an increased fragility of red blood cells with a tendency to spontaneous lysis. The defect appears to be due to the activation of the extrinsic (or bypass) system of complement activation with subsequent attachment of the terminal complement components, causing red blood cell lysis.

Deficiency of the inhibitor of C1 esterase is another disorder of the complement system which is inherited and which produces a functional problem [47]. This disease was mentioned briefly in an earlier section of this chapter. Because of the lack of this inhibitor, the affected individual will exhibit episodes of angioedema that may be life-threatening if it occurs in the larynx and trachea. This disease is inherited as an autosomal dominant form. The heterozygote appears to have a substantial decrease in the level of C1-esterase inhibitor (C1INH). Utilization of C4 and C2 as natural substrates of C1 esterase causes the levels of these complement components to be severely reduced during acute attacks. The trigger mechanisms of the reaction are unknown, but they seem to be based on the activation of C1 esterase by either a proteolytic enzyme or an allosteric mechanism. The mediator of the edematous reaction is shown in Figure 16-2, and is a polypeptide that exhibits the activity of a kinin. It has been shown to be different from bradykinin [80].

The occurrence of chemotactic inhibitors has been described. The presence of a chemotactic inhibitor has been reported in a number of patients with alcoholic cirrhosis [81], and a young child who manifested frequent skin and respiratory infections was found to have a serum inhibitor of chemotactic activity [82]. Other deficiencies of chemotaxis have been described in relation to some of the abnormalities of the complement system already mentioned, especially those involving C3. These, however, have not been due to an inhibitor, but rather to depletion or the lack of a component [74, 78].

Complement Levels in Disease

Methods are now available for the determination of complement components and complement activity on a routine basis in the clinical laboratory. Because of this, there is increasing information in the medical literature relating the levels of various components of complement and the total hemolytic activity of complement to various diseases. Much of the interest in complement has centered on diseases that are presumed to have an immunological basis. These include the so-called collagen diseases, rheumatoid arthritis, acute and chronic glomerulonephritis, and certain infectious diseases. The information relating to serum complement levels in disease often appears conflicting [83]. In clinical reports of the same or similar diseases, complement levels may be reported as decreased, normal, or increased; they often do not show a uniform change paralleling the disease process. Much of this variation occurs because of the time of sampling during the activity of the disease process. During periods when the disease process is active and complement activation is presumably at a maximum, the levels of complement components would be expected to be at a low level, in contrast to quiescent periods when normal levels might be encountered or during a recovery phase when there might be an increase in a particular component [84] (Fig. 16-5). Because of this time-course variation, there also appears to be confusion as to the merit of complement determinations in the clinical evaluation of various diseases. However, if one is sufficiently aware of this limitation and takes into account the time-course variation, complement levels can be useful in monitoring the activity of particular diseases, especially those due to immune reactions [85].

In the earlier discussion in this chapter on activation of the complement system, it is apparent that the activities of both the intrinsic and extrinsic pathways of complement activation may be monitored by the selective determination of individual components [86]. The activity of the intrinsic pathway can be determined by measuring the levels of C3 and C4. Activation of the complement system by this pathway would result in the lowering of the levels of these components. The activity of the extrinsic pathway, on the other hand, can be monitored by determining the levels of C3 and the C3 proactivator, since, with activity in the extrinsic pathway, the levels of these two factors will decrease substantially. There are currently available methods and materials for determining the levels of each of these factors by means of the radial immunodiffusion technique of Mancini (see Chap. 4). In those situations where tissue biopsy material may be available, an assessment of complement fixation by means of the fluorescent antibody technique can be carried out on frozen sections of the biopsied tissue [87]. Studies of this type would add confirmatory data to the determination of serum levels of the components.

It should always be remembered that a decrease in complement activity or a decrease in individual components does not necessarily imply the existence of an immunological disease or disorder. It is well recognized that the proteolytic enzymes that are released from various tissues as a

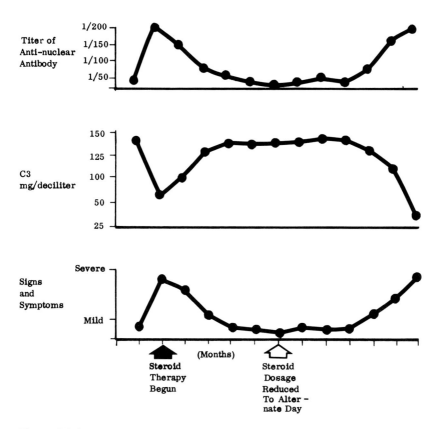

Figure 16-5
Time-course variation in serum complement (C3) levels in a case of dissemi-nated lupus erythematosus during recurrent exacerbations and remissions.

result of nonimmune injury, such as ischemia with coagulation necrosis or toxic necrosis, will produce cleavage of complement components simi-lar to that which is produced by the immune activation of the comple-ment sequence [73]. As the result of this nonimmune cleavage, the levels of hemolytic activity of complement and those of individual components may decrease. In this regard, it is important, if possible, to differentiate the onset of decreased complement levels in relation to the progress of disease. If the decrease follows tissue destruction due to trauma, isch-emia, or toxins, it is probable that the decrease is related to the release of tissue proteases. In contrast, low complement levels preceding the on-set of tissue damage point more directly to an immunological cause. Such decreases, however, may develop as a consequence of the activation of either the intrinsic (immunological) or extrinsic (nonimmunological) complement pathway. In those infectious diseases where complement levels are decreased, the explanation could be related to the release of tissue proteases as a result of damage by toxins from the organisms or by

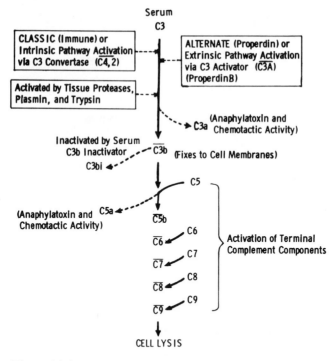

Serum
C3

CLASSIC (Immune) or
Intrinsic Pathway Activation
via C3 Convertase (C4,2)

ALTERNATE (Properdin) or
Extrinsic Pathway Activation
via C3 Activator (C̄3A)
(ProperdinB)

Activated by Tissue Proteases,
Plasmin, and Trypsin

→ C3a (Anaphylatoxin and Chemotactic Activity)

Inactivated by Serum
C3b Inactivator
C3bi ◄

C3b (Fixes to Cell Membranes)

C5

(Anaphylatoxin and   C5a
Chemotactic Activity)

C̄5b

C̄6 ◄ C6
C̄7 ◄ C7   } Activation of Terminal
C̄8 ◄ C8   Complement Components
C̄9 ◄ C9

CELL LYSIS

Figure 16-6
Biological activities associated with various modes of activation of the complement system through C3 cleavage by immune activation of the intrinsic pathway or through nonimmune pathways of the activated properdin system
(extrinsic pathway) or by proteolytic enzymes released in traumatic or inflammatory tissue injury.

complement fixation as a result of an immune response to the infectious
organism itself. In a severe infection, it is not always possible to differentiate between these two possibilities for an explanation of decrease in
complement activity. Figure 16-6 illustrates the various activity modes.

In the following pages of this chapter, the general aspects of complement activity in relation to certain diseases will be covered briefly.

ARTHRITIS
Reports in the literature are varied regarding the complement levels in
rheumatoid arthritis. Generally, it appears that complement levels are
normal or possibly elevated, with the exception of some rheumatoid-
factor positive patients who show low levels of total hemolytic complement [88]. The low complement levels appear to be associated with
severe, active disease, and they often indicate the development of vasculitis as a complication. During active disease, a decrease in complement
components in the synovial fluid has been reported. The presence of

cleavage products of complement components has been identified in synovial fluid, indicating complement depletion in relation to the inflammatory synovitis [72].

HEMOLYTIC ANEMIAS
Hemolytic anemias due to immune reactions are usually associated with evidence of the binding of complement components to the red blood cells [40, 51]. The presence of antibody and complement on the surface of the red blood cells gives a positive direct Coombs' reaction. The complement components are most abundant on the red blood cell surface when the antibody is of the IgM class. In contrast, in those hemolytic anemias that involve antibody of the IgG type, only small amounts of complement components are usually identified on the red blood cell [51]. Most characteristically, the hemolytic anemia associated with cold agglutinins are due to antibody of the IgM type [51].

RHEUMATIC FEVER
During episodes of activity in rheumatic fever, both hemolysis and the levels of individual complement components tend to be reduced. Presumably, the reduction is related to inflammation in the tissues and does not seem to bear a primary pathogenic relationship to the disease process [89]. By means of fluorescent antibody analysis, complement components have been identified in lesions of fibrinoid necrosis in rheumatic fever, but not in the giant cell reactions known as Aschoff's bodies.

INFECTIOUS DISEASE
Complement activity and the levels of various components may vary widely in infectious diseases. Decreased levels are frequently noted in bacterial endocarditis where there are complications of glomerulonephritis [90], in bacteremia [91], and in acute viral hepatitis [92].

HYPERSENSITIVITY AND AUTOIMMUNE DISEASE
In diseases such as lupus erythematosus [93], scleroderma [94], serum sickness [95], and acute vasculitis [96], the complement levels are reported as ranging from low to normal and, in rare instances, as increased. The decreased levels appear to be correlated with the active phases of the diseases. In lupus erythematosus with active nephritis, low levels of C3, low levels of other components, and a decrease in total hemolytic activity have been reported [93]. Presumably, the mechanism that accounts for the decrease is the fixation of complement by immune complexes of nuclear factors and antinuclear antibody. Determinations of C4 and IgG levels in cerebrospinal fluid (CSF) have been reported to be of value in differentiating active CNS involvement in lupus erythematosus from the encephalopathy due to steroid therapy. The specificity of low C4 and IgG in the CSF, however, has not yet been confirmed [67, 98]. In serum sickness, a similar mechanism seems to be operative [95].

The basis for decreased levels in other hypersensitivity diseases is less clear. Possibly the decreases are related to the inflammatory tissue destruction, but the possibility that the decrease in complement level has a pathogenic relationship cannot be dismissed. There have been studies that suggest a role of complement in the development of these hypersensitivity diseases, but the evidence is indirect and is mainly related to decreased serum complement levels and the evidence of complement deposition in the tissue lesions as found by fluorescent antibody techniques.

In addition to low levels of complement components, a decrease in the levels of components of the alternate or extrinsic pathway has also been reported in certain hypersensitivity diseases such as lupus erythematosus [93].

GLOMERULONEPHRITIS

The study of complement levels in glomerulonephritis has resulted in numerous clinical reports and studies attributing significance to their findings. In general, acute glomerulonephritis and the active phases of chronic glomerulonephritis are associated with low serum complement levels and, in some instances, with low levels of components of the extrinsic pathway [86]. In addition, renal biopsy material that has been studied by the fluorescent antibody technique has demonstrated the deposition of complement components and components of the properdin system in the glomeruli in glomerulonephritis [86].

The serum levels may return to normal after the acute phase subsides, but in some cases of chronic glomerulonephritis, a persistent decrease in levels of C3 has been noted. In fact, one form of chronic glomerulonephritis (hypocomplementemic nephritis) is persistently associated with low levels of C3 [70]. In this disease, normal levels of early reacting components are encountered in conjunction with decreased C3, and later reacting components; an associated decrease in properdin activity is also present and further decreases the level of C3 activator. The renal biopsy material in these cases has failed to demonstrate deposition of immunoglobulins, but it has demonstrated deposition of C3 and properdin factor B. A so-called nephritic factor has been identified in the serum of patients with this disease. This nephritic factor appears to be important in the activation of the alternate pathway and is presumably responsible for the decreased levels of the terminal complement components. In glomerulonephritis associated with lupus erythematosus (see Case Report and Fig. 16-7), there are decreases in the levels of both early and late complement components as well as a decrease in the levels of properdin factor B [93]. Renal biopsy specimens provide evidence of the deposition of properdin and complement in the glomeruli. These findings indicate that both the intrinsic and extrinsic pathways are important in this disease. It is of interest to note that the morphological form of lupus glomerulonephritis varies from membranous to diffuse proliferation and that it does not correlate with the pattern of deposition of immune reactants, complement components, or properdin factors.

In other reports, the serum of patients with membranoproliferative glomerulonephritis or acute poststreptococcal glomerulonephritis has ex-

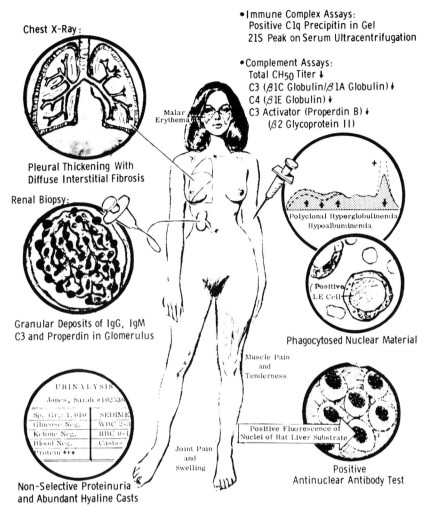

Chest X-Ray:

Malar Erythema

•Immune Complex Assays:
Positive C1q Precipitin in Gel
21S Peak on Serum Ultracentrifugation

•Complement Assays:
Total CH$_{50}$ Titer ↓
C3 (β1C Globulin/β1A Globulin) ↓
C4 (β1E Globulin) ↓
C3 Activator (Properdin B) ↓
(β2 Glycoprotein II)

Pleural Thickening With
Diffuse Interstitial Fibrosis

Polyclonal Hyperglobulinemia
Hypoalbuminemia

Renal Biopsy:

Positive
LE Cell

Granular Deposits of IgG, IgM
C3 and Properdin in Glomerulus

Phagocytosed Nuclear Material

Muscle Pain
and
Tenderness

URINALYSIS

Jones, Sarah #102530

Sp. Gr.: 1.010	SEDIME
Glucose Neg.	WBC 2-3
Ketone Neg.	RBC 0-1
Blood Neg.	Casts-
Protein +++	

Positive Fluorescence of
Nuclei of Rat Liver Substrate

Joint Pain
and
Swelling

Non-Selective Proteinuria
and Abundant Hyaline Casts

Positive
Antinuclear Antibody Test

Figure 16-7
Clinical manifestations and diagnostic findings in a case of lupus erythematosus with emphasis on the decreased levels of complement components (see Case Report, p. 288).

hibited normal levels of the early reacting complement components with decreases in the late reacting components and properdin factors [97]. On biopsy, depositions of properdin and C3 were identified in the glomeruli, but immunoglobulins and early reacting complement components were not found. These findings suggest that some mechanism other than the immunological activation of complement is active in the pathogenesis of these types of glomerulonephritis.

SYSTEMIC LUPUS ERYTHEMATOSUS

Case Report

A 34-year-old female who was seen for complaints of dull, aching pains in the muscles of the arms and legs (Fig. 16-7). A few months previously, she had had brief episodes of pain and swelling in the joints of the left hand, which subsided within a few days. Approximately one year previously, she had had an erythematous rash across the nose and in the malar regions.

The muscle pains developed insidiously with episodes of cramps, which later became persistent dull aches that were especially notable in the upper arms and in the thighs. On a few occasions, the patient had diffuse chest pain when taking a deep breath.

On physical examination, there was discoloration of the skin over the bridge of the nose and malar eminences in a "butterfly" distribution. On chest examination, faint breathing sounds and a decreased resonance on percussion were noted. The spleen was moderately enlarged to approximately 2 cm below the left costal margin. There was tenderness on palpation of the muscles in each arm and the thighs. Laboratory studies revealed a mild anemia and leukopenia with a total white blood cell count of 3200 per cubic millimeter with a normal differential. A mild thrombocytopenia of 120,000 platelets per cubic millimeter was found. On urinalysis, there was a 3+ reaction for protein, and on microscopic examination, the presence of hyaline casts was noted. Serum electrophoresis exhibited a pattern of polyclonal hyperglobulinemia. A lupus erythematosus (LE) cell preparation revealed numerous LE cells. A fluorescent antibody test on the patient's serum was positive in a serum dilution greater than 1:60. The staining pattern of the antinuclear reaction was described as homogeneous. Because of indications of renal disease, a renal biopsy was carried out, and fluorescent antibody studies revealed a granular deposition of immunoglobulins, complement, and components of the properdin system along the glomerular basement membrane in addition to morphological changes of acute membranoproliferative glomerulonephritis. A chest roentgenogram showed focal areas of pleural thickening and a fine diffuse interstitial fibrosis in both lungs.

Serum complement determinations revealed a substantial decrease in levels of the individual complement components C4 and C3 as well as a substantial decrease in the serum level of properdin factor B (C3 activator). Determination of the total hemolytic complement also exhibited a significant reduction in activity. The serum C3 levels on two occasions were reported at 20 and 33 mg per 100 ml (normal is 93 to 182 mg per 100 ml). C4 values were reported in the range of 250 μg per milliliter on two occasions (normal is 208 to 636 μg per milliliter). Levels of properdin factor B were in the range of 55 μg per milliliter (normal is 255 μg per milliliter [mean]).

Total hemolytic activity measured by the CH_{50} technique revealed results of 12 and 18 units per milliliter on two occasions (normal is 32 to 44 units per milliliter).

The diagnosis of disseminated lupus erythematosus was made, and therapy with high doses of steroid (60 mg prednisone) was begun, resulting in remission of the muscle pain, disappearance of the proteinuria, return of serum complement values to the normal range, and disappearance of the antinuclear antibody after one week of therapy.

Final Diagnosis: Disseminated lupus erythematosus (in remission following steroid therapy).

Conclusion

This chapter has focused on the complement system in relation to its roles as a protective system and as a potentially destructive system. These contrasting roles present the complement system as a two-edged sword that can counteract those factors which threaten the host, but, at the same time, can be subverted to a direct attack on the tissues of the host. In a way, this situation suggests an ethical analogy: that which works best for good also holds the most potential for evil.

References

1. Müller-Eberhard, H. J.   Complement. *Annu. Rev. Biochem.* 38:389, 1969.
2. Müller-Eberhard, H. J.   Chemistry and reaction mechanisms of the complement system. *Adv. Immunol.* 8:1, 1968.
3. Broom, D. H., Schultz, D. R., an Zarco, R. M.   The separation of nine components and two inactivators of components of complement in human serum. *Immunochemistry* 7:43, 1970.
4. Ishizaka, T., Tada, T., and Ishizaka, K.   Fixation of C'1 and C'1a by rabbit gamma G and gamma M. Antibodies with particulate and soluble antigen. *J. Immunol.* 100:1145, 1968.
5. Ward, P. A.   Biological activities of the complement system. *Ann. Allergy* 30:307, 1972.
6. Ruddy, S., and Austen, K. F.   Natural Control Mechanisms of the Complement System. In D. G. Ingram (Ed.), *Biological Activities of Complement*. Basel: Karger, 1972.
7. Tamura, N., and Nelson, R. A.   Three naturally occurring inhibitors of components of complement in guinea pig and rabbit serum. *J. Immunol.* 99:582, 1967.
8. Götze, O., and Müller-Eberhard, H. J.   Paroxysmal nocturnal hemoglobinuria: Hemolysis initiated by the C3 activator system. *N. Engl. J. Med.* 286:180, 1972.
9. Gewürz, H.   Alternate Pathways to Activation of the Complement System. In D. G. Ingram (Ed.), *Biological Activities of Complement*. Basel: Karger, 1972.
10. Gewürz, H., Shin, H. S., and Mergenhagen, S. E.   Interactions of the complement system with endotoxic lipopolysaccharide: Consumption of each of the six terminal complement components. *J. Exp. Med.* 128:1049, 1968.
11. Bordet, J.   Sur l'agglutination et la dissolution des globules rouges par le sérum d'animaux injectés de sang defibriné. *Ann. Inst. Pasteur* (Paris) 12:688, 1898.

12. Müller-Eberhard, H. J., and Calcott, M. A. Interaction between C'1q and gamma G globulin. *Immunochemistry* 3:500, 1966.
13. Isliker, H., Jocot-Guillarmod, H., Waldesduomalow, H. L., Fellenberg, N., Von, R., and Cerottini, J. C. Complement Fixation by Different IgG Preparations and Fragments. In P. A. Meischer and T. Grabar (Eds.), *Mechanisms of Inflammation Induced by Immune Injury. Sixth International Symposium, Immunopathology.* Basel: Schwabe, 1967.
14. Gigli, I., Kaplan, A. C., and Austen, K. F. Modulation of function of the activated first component of complement by a fragment derived from serum. *J. Exp. Med.* 134:1466, 1971.
15. Lepow, I. H., Nass, G. S., Todd, E. W., Pensky, J., and Hinz, C. F., Jr. Chromatographic resolution of the first component of human complement into three activities. *J. Exp. Med.* 117:983, 1963.
16. Gigli, I., and Austen, K. F. Fluid phase destruction of C2hu and C1hu. II. Unmasking by C4hu of C1hu specificity for C2hu. *J. Exp. Med.* 130:833, 1969.
17. Haines, A. L., and Lepow, L. H. Studies on human C'1 esterase. I. Purification and enzymatic properties. *J. Immunol.* 92:456, 1964.
18. Borsos, T., and Rapp, H. J. Hemolysin titration based on fixation of the activated first component of complement. Evidence that one molecule of hemolysin suffices to sensitize an erythrocyte. *J. Immunol.* 95:559, 1965.
19. Müller-Eberhard, H. J., and Lepow, I. H. C'1 esterase effect on activities and physico-chemical properties of the fourth component of complement. *J. Exp. Med.* 121:819, 1965.
20. Polley, M. J., and Müller-Eberhard, H. J. The second component of human complement: Its isolation fragmentation by C'1 esterase and incorporation into C'3 convertase. *J. Exp. Med.* 128:533, 1968.
21. Müller-Eberhard, H. J., Polley, M. J., and Calcott, M. A. Formation and functional significance of a molecular complex derived from the second and the fourth component of human complement. *J. Exp. Med.* 125:359, 1967.
22. Polley, M. J., and Müller-Eberhard, H. J. Enhancement of the hemolytic activity of the second component of human complement by oxidation. *J. Exp. Med.* 126:1013, 1967.
23. Müller-Eberhard, H. J., Dalmasso, A. P., and Calcott, M. A. The reaction mechanism of beta 1C-globulin (C'3) in immune hemolysis. *J. Exp. Med.* 123:33, 1966.
24. Dias Da Silva, W., Eisele, J. W., and Lepow, I. H. Complement as mediator of inflammation. III. Purification of the activity with anaphylatoxin properties generated by interaction of the first four components of the complement and its identification as a cleavage product of C'3. *J. Exp. Med.* 126:1027, 1967.
25. Cooper, N. R., and Becker, E. L. Complement associated peptidase activity of guinea pig serum. *J. Immunol.* 98:119, 1967.
26. Lachmann, P. J., and Müller-Eberhard, H. J. The demonstration in human serum of conglutinogen-activating factor and its effect on the third component of complement. *J. Immunol.* 100:691, 1968.
27. Cochrane, C. G., and Müller-Eberhard, H. J. The derivation of two distinct anaphylatoxin activities from the third and fifth components of human complement. *J. Exp. Med.* 127:371, 1968.
28. Ward, P. A., Cochrane, C. G., and Müller-Eberhard, H. J. Further studies on the chemotactic factor of complement and its formation in vivo. *Immunology* 11:141, 1966.

29. Manni, J. A., and Müller-Eberhard, H. J. The eighth component of human complement (C8): Isolation, characterization and hemolytic efficiency. *J. Exp. Med.* 130:1145, 1969.
30. Kolb, W. P., Haxby, J. A., Arroyave, C. M., and Müller-Eberhard, H. J. Molecular analysis of the membrane attack mechanism of complement. *J. Exp. Med.* 135:549, 1972.
31. Ballow, M., and Cochrane, C. G. Two anticomplementary factors in cobra venom: Hemolysis of guinea pig erythrocytes by one of them. *J. Immunol.* 103:944, 1969.
32. Götze, O., and Müller-Eberhard, H. J. Lysis of erythrocytes by complement in the absence of antibody. *J. Exp. Med.* 132:898, 1970.
33. Gewürz, H. Alternate Pathways to Activation of the Complement System. In D. G. Ingram (Ed.), *Biological Activities of Complement*. Basel: Karger, 1972.
34. Goodkofsky, I., and Lepow, I. H. Functional relationship of factor B in the properdin system to C3 proactivator of human serum. *J. Immunol.* 107:1200, 1971.
35. Götze, O., and Müller-Eberhard, H. J. The C3 activator system: An alternate pathway of complement activation. *J. Exp. Med.* 134:90, 1971.
36. Müller-Eberhard, H. J., and Götze, O. C3 proactivator convertase and its mode of action. *J. Exp. Med.* 135:1003, 1972.
37. Abramson, N., Alper, C. A., and Lachmann, P. J. Deficiency of C3 inactivator in man. *J. Immunol.* 107:19, 1971.
38. Becker, E. L. The relationship of the chemotactic behavior of the complement derived factors, C3A, C5A, and C567 and a bacterial chemotactic factor to their ability to activate the proesterase I of rabbit polymorphonuclear leukocytes. *J. Exp. Med.* 135:376, 1972.
39. Davis, S. D., Iannetta, A., and Wedgwood, R. J. Bactericidal Reactions of Serum. In D. G. Ingram (Ed.), *Biological Activities of Complement*. Basel: Karger, 1972.
40. Weiner, W. Hemolytic Disease of the Newborn and Other Conditions following Iso-Immunization. In B. G. H. Gell and R. R. A. Coombs (Eds.), *Clinical Aspects of Immunology* (2nd ed.). Philadelphia: Davis, 1968.
41. Miller, M. E. Demonstration of a major role in the fifth component of complement (C5) in the enhancement of phagocytosis. *Fed. Proc.* 29:433(abst.), 1970.
42. Gigli, I., and Nelson, R. A. Complement dependent immune phagocytosis. I. Requirements for C'1, C'4, C'2, C'3. *Exp. Cell Res.* 51:45, 1968.
43. Giertz, H. Pharmacology of Anaphylatoxin. In H. Z. Movat (Ed.), *Cellular and Humoral Mechanism in Anaphylaxis and Allergy*. Basel: Karger, 1969.
44. Nelson, D. S. Immune adherence. *Adv. Immunol.* 3:131, 1963.
45. Henson, P. M. Complement-Dependent Adherence to Cells of Antigen and Antibody, Mechanisms and Consequences. In D. G. Ingram (Ed.), *Biological Activities of Complement*. Basel: Karger, 1972.
46. Lepow, I. H. Permeability-Producing Peptide By-Product of the Interaction of the First, Fourth and Second Components of Complement. In K. F. Austen and E. L. Becker (Eds.), *Biochemistry of the Acute Allergic Reactions*. Oxford: Blackwell, 1971.
47. Donaldson, V. H., and Evans, R. R. A biochemical abnormality in hereditary angioneurotic edema: Absence of serum inhibitor of C'1 esterase. *Am. J. Med.* 35:37, 1963.

48. Notkins, A. L. Infectious virus-antibody complexes: Interaction with anti-immunoglobulins, complement and rheumatoid factor. *J. Exp. Med.* 134:415, 1971.
49. Zimmerman, T. S., and Arroyave, C. M. Participation of Complement in Initiation of Blood Coagulation and in the Normal Coagulation Process. In K. F. Austen and E. L. Becker (Eds.), *Biochemistry of the Acute Allergic Reactions.* Oxford: Blackwell, 1971.
50. Johnson, K. J., Ward, P. A., Osborn, M. J., and Arroyave, C. M. C5 as an inactivator of bacterial endotoxin. *Fed. Proc.* 31:736(abst.), 1972.
51. Levine, B. B., and Redmond, A. P. Immunochemical mechanisms of penicillin-induced Coombs' positivity and hemolytic anemia in man. *Int. Arch. Allergy Appl. Immunol.* 31:594, 1967.
52. Petz, L. D., and Fudenberg, H. H. Coombs-positive hemolytic anemia caused by penicillin administration. *N. Engl. J. Med.* 274:171, 1966.
53. Yachnin, S. Further studies on the hemolysis of human red cells by late acting complement components. *Immunochemistry* 3:505, 1965.
54. Cochrane, C. G. Immunologic Factors in Peripheral Vascular Disease. In J. L. Orbison (Ed.), *The Peripheral Blood Vessels.* International Academy of Pathology, IV. Baltimore: Williams & Wilkins, 1963.
55. Schroeter, A. L., Copeman, P. W. M., Jordan, R. E., Sams, W. M., Jr., and Winkelmann, R. K. Immunofluorescence of cutaneous vasculitis. *J. Clin. Invest.* 48:75A, 1969.
56. Gocke, D. J., Hsu, K., Morgan, C., Bombardieri, S., Lockshin, M., and Christian, C. L. Vasculitis in association with Australia antigen. *J. Exp. Med.* 134[Suppl.]:330, 1971.
57. Cochrane, C. G. Mediators of the Arthus and Related Reactions. In P. Kallos and B. H. Waksmann (Eds.), *Progress in Allergy,* Vol. 2. Basel: Karger, 1967.
58. Cochrane, C. G., Weigle, W. O., and Dixon, F. J. The role of polymorphonuclear leukocytes in the initiation and cessation of the Arthus vasculitis. *J. Exp. Med.* 100:481, 1959.
59. Dixon, F. J., Vazquez, J. J., Weigle, W. O., and Cochrane, C. G. Pathogenesis of serum sickness. *Arch. Pathol.* 65:18, 1958.
60. Cochrane, C. G., and Hawkins, D. Studies on circulating immune complexes. III. Factors governing the ability of circulating complexes to localize in blood vessels. *J. Exp. Med.* 127:137, 1968.
61. Henson, P. N., and Cochrane, C. G. Immunological induction of increased vascular permeability. I. A rabbit passive cutaneous anaphylactic reaction requiring complement, platelets and neutrophils. *J. Exp. Med.* 129:153, 1969.
62. Kniker, W. T., and Cochrane, C. G. The localization of circulating immune complexes in experimental serum sickness. The role of vasoactive amines and hydrodynamic forces. *J. Exp. Med.* 127:119, 1968.
63. Cochrane, C. G., and Dixon, F. J. Cell and Tissue Damage through Antigen-Antibody Complexes. In P. A. Miescher and H. J. Müller-Eberhard (Eds.), *Textbook of Immunopathology,* Vol. 1. New York: Grune & Stratton, 1969.
64. Unanue, E., and Dixon, F. J. Experimental glomerulonephritis, IV. Participation of complement in nephrotoxic nephritis. *J. Exp. Med.* 119:964, 1964.
65. Hawkins, D., and Cochrane, C. G. Glomerular basement membrane damage in immunological glomerulonephritis. *Immunology* 14:665, 1968.

66. Lewis, E. J., and Couser, W. G.   The immunologic basis of human renal disease. *Pediatr. Clin. North Am.* 18:467, 1971.
67. Petz, L. D., Sharp, G. C., Cooper, N. R., and Irvin, W. S.   Serum and cerebral spinal fluid complement and serum autoantibodies in systemic lupus erythematosus. *Medicine* (Baltimore) 50:259, 1971.
68. Lerner, R. A., Glassock, R. J., and Dixon, F. J.   The role of antiglomerular basement membrane antibody in the pathogenesis of human glomerulonephritis. *J. Exp. Med.* 126:989, 1967.
69. Beirne, G. J., and Brenman, J. T.   Glomerulonephritis associated with exposure to hydrocarbons: Mediated by antibodies to glomerular basement membrane. *Arch. Environ. Health* 25:365, 1972.
70. Vallota, E. H., Forristal, J., Davis, N. C., and West, C. D.   The C3 nephritic factor and membranoproliferative nephritis: Correlation of serum levels of the nephritic factor with C3 levels, with therapy and with progression of the disease. *J. Pediatr.* 80:947, 1972.
71. De Shazo, C. D., Henson, P. M., and Cochrane, C. G.   Acute immunologic arthritis in rabbits. *J. Clin. Invest.* 51:50, 1972.
72. Zvaifler, N. J.   Breakdown products of C'3 in human synovial fluids. *J. Clin. Invest.* 48:1532, 1969.
73. Ward, P. A.   Complement-Derived Chemotactic Factors and their Interactions with Neutrophilic Granulocytes. In D. G. Ingram (Ed.), *Biological Activities of Complement.* Basel: Karger, 1972.
74. Rosen, F. S., and Alper, C. A.   An enzyme in the alternate pathway to C3 activation (the properdin system) and its inhibition by a protein in normal serum. *J. Clin. Invest.* 51:80A, 1972.
75. Miller, M. E., and Nilsson, U. R.   A familial deficiency of the phagocytosis-enhancing activity of serum related to a dysfunction of the fifth component of complement (C5). *N. Engl. J. Med.* 282:354, 1970.
76. Agnello, V., de Bracco, M. M. E., and Kunkel, H. G.   Hereditary C2 deficiency with some manifestations of systemic lupus erythematosus. *J. Immunol.* 108:837, 1972.
77. Day, N. K., Geiger, H., and Stroud, R.   C1r deficiency: An inborn error associated with cutaneous and renal disease. *J. Clin. Invest.* 51:1102, 1972.
78. Köhler, P. F., and Müller-Eberhard, H. J.   Complement-immunoglobulin relations: Deficiency of C'1q associated with impaired immunoglobulin G synthesis. *Science* 163:474, 1969.
79. Alper, C. A., and Rosen, F. S.   Genetic Considerations. In D. G. Ingram (Ed.), *Biological Activities of Complement.* Basel: Karger, 1972.
80. Lepow, I. H.   Permeability-Producing Peptide By-Products of the Interaction of the First, Fourth and Second Components of Complement. In K. F. Austen and E. L. Becker (Eds.), *Biochemistry of the Acute Allergic Reactions.* Oxford: Blackwell, 1971.
81. DeNeo, A. N., and Andersen, B. R.   Defective chemotaxis associated with a serum inhibitor in cirrhotic patients. *N. Engl. J. Med.* 286:735, 1972.
82. Ward, P. A., and Schlegel, R. J.   Impaired leucotactic responsiveness in a child with recurrent infections. *Lancet* 2:344, 1969.
83. Townes, A. S.   Complement levels in disease. *Johns Hopkins Med. J.* 120:337, 1967.
84. Kohler, P. F., and Ten Bensel, R.   Serial complement component alterations in acute glomerulonephritis and systemic lupus erythematosus. *Clin. Exp. Immunol.* 4:192, 1969.

85. Perrin, L. H., Lambert, P. H., Nydegger, U. E., and Miescher, P. A. Quantitation of C3PA (properdin factor B) and other complement components in diseases associated with a low C3 level. *Clin. Immunol. Immunopathol.* 2:16, 1973.

86. Huhnsucker, L. D., Ruddy, S., Carpenter, C. B., Schur, P. H., Merrill, J. P., Müller-Eberhard, H. J., and Austen, K. F. Metabolism of third complement component (C3) in nephritis: Involvement of the classic and alternate (properdin) pathways for complement activation. *N. Engl. J. Med.* 287:835, 1972.

87. Lachmann, P. J., Müller-Eberhard, H. J., and Kunkel, H. G. Localization of the in vivo bound complement in tissue sections. *J. Exp. Med.* 115:63, 1963.

88. Franco, A. E., and Schur, P. H. Hypocomplementemia in rheumatoid arthritis. *Arthritis Rheum.* 14:231, 1971.

89. Ward, P. A., and Hill, J. H. Role of Complement in the Generation of Leukotactic Mediators in Immunologic and Non-Specific Tissue Injuries. In B. K. Forscher and J. C. Houck (Eds.), *Immunopathology of Inflammation.* Amsterdam: Excerpta Medica, 1971.

90. Williams, R. C., Jr., and Kunkel, H. G. Rheumatoid factor complement and conglutinin aberrations in patients with subacute bacterial endocarditis. *J. Clin. Invest.* 41:666, 1962.

91. McCabe, W. R. Serum complement levels in bacteremia due to gram negative organisms. *N. Engl. J. Med.* 288:21, 1973.

92. Alpert, E., Isselbacher, K. J., and Schur, P. H. The pathogenesis of arthritis associated with viral hepatitis: Complement-component studies. *N. Engl. J. Med.* 285:185, 1971.

93. Rothfield, N., Ross, A., Minta, J. O., and Lepow, I. H. Glomerular and dermal deposition of properdin in systemic lupus erythematosus. *N. Engl. J. Med.* 287:681, 1972.

94. Schur, P. H., and Austen, K. F. Complement in human disease. *Annu. Rev. Med.* 19:124, 1968.

95. Koffler, D., Agnello, V., Thoburn, R., and Kunkel, H. G. Systemic lupus erythematosus: Prototype of immune complex nephritis in man. *J. Exp. Med.* 134:169, 1971.

96. Gocke, D. J., Shu, K., and Morgan, C. Association between polyarteritis and Australia antigen. *Lancet* 2:1149, 1970.

97. Westberg, N. G., Naff, D. B., and Boyer, J. T. Glomerular deposition of properdin in acute and chronic glomerulonephritis with hypocomplementemia. *J. Clin. Invest.* 50:642, 1971.

98. Levin, A. S., Fudenberg, H. H., Petz, L. D., and Sharp, G. C. IgG levels in cerebrospinal fluid of patients with central nervous system manifestations of systemic lupus erythematosus. *Clin. Immunol. Immunopathol.* 1:1, 1972.

Immune-Complex Diseases 17

Robert M. Nakamura and Ernest S. Tucker, III

Immune complexes are macromolecular complexes of varying sizes that consist of antigen and antibody molecules bound specifically together. The immune complexes may be insoluble or soluble, depending upon the ratio of antibody to antigen. Soluble complexes form in the presence of excess antigen, and insoluble precipitates may form in the equivalence zone of the antigen-antibody interaction.

Von Pirquet [1] in 1911 postulated the presence of foreign serum antigens and homologous antibodies in the circulation that form toxic compounds responsible for lesions in organs and tissues that do not have a specific immunological relationship to the injected antigen. Approximately half a century later, definite evidence was presented that antigen-antibody complexes unrelated to the specific tissue may mediate pathological mechanisms with injury [2–5]. Today, the role of antigen-antibody complexes in the pathogenesis of vasculitis and glomerulonephritis in human disease has been well established (Fig. 17-1). The glomerulonephritis associated with serum sickness, poststreptococcal infection, systemic lupus erythematosus, and certain infectious diseases is believed to be mediated by immune complexes [6–10]. Australia antigen-antibody complexes have been found to be localized in the vascular lesions of human cases of polyarteritis nodosa [11]. Also, immune complexes probably play a significant role in the pathogenesis of lesions in rheumatoid arthritis [12].

Cryoglobulins are serum proteins that are insoluble at 4°C and usually redissolve on heating to 37°C. These reversibly cold-precipitable globulins have been described in many clinical conditions, including lymphoproliferative disorders [13, 14], collagen diseases [14–16], and viral infections [14, 17]. Patients with cryoglobulinemia exhibit a wide variety of conditions, such as glomerulonephritis, vasculitis, and purpura, which suggests that many of these patients demonstrate an immune-complex type of autoimmune disorder.

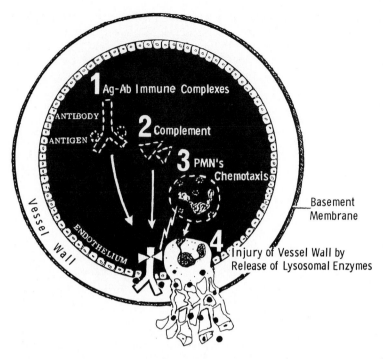

Lesion: Vasculitis–Glomerulonephritis

Figure 17-1
Immune complex injury.

Physiological Aspects of Immune Complexes

Immune complexes, especially those of smaller size, may persist in the circulation and equilibrate between the intravascular and extravascular fluid compartments, as do serum proteins [18]. The amount of protein in the extravascular fluid spaces after equilibration may be correlated exponentially with the effective hydrodynamic diffusion radius of the protein molecule or immune complex [18]. The larger complexes localize along the vascular and glomerular basement membranes. The localization of the complexes depends upon the size of the complexes as well as upon the presence of vascular permeability factors, such as vasoactive amines [2, 5, 19]. The following steps are involved in the deposition of immune complexes [5, 19]:

1. Immune complexes of varying size must be in the circulation.
2. In the presence of basophilic leukocytes with adherent IgE immunoglobulin antibody, the antigen reaction with cell-fixed IgE induces the release of a soluble intermediate, platelet agglutinating factor (PAF).
3. The PAF activates platelets to clump and release serotonin and vasoactive amines.

4. The amines cause an increased permeability of blood vessels, mainly in areas of platelet agglutination along the blood vessel wall.
5. With the increased permeability, immune complexes greater than 19S become lodged along the basement membrane. The fixation of complement with the release of chemotactic factors and the attraction of polymorphonuclear leukocytes may result in injury to the basement membrane.

The vascular injury results from complement activation with the release of proteolytic enzymes from lysosomes and from the membranes of polymorphonuclear leukocytes. The deposition of soluble immune complexes, as in serum sickness disease, may be inhibited with the use of antihistamines and serotonin antagonists [5, 20].

Very little is known about the relationship of immune complexes to the kinin-forming and intrinsic clotting systems in inflammatory injury [21]. The Hageman factor has been found to be involved in the pathway of activation of the clotting system and the kinin-forming system [22]. Extensive in vitro laboratory studies showed no evidence of interaction between the Hageman factor and immune complexes [21]. The immunoglobulins did not activate the Hageman factor; on the other hand, bacterial contaminants did activate the Hageman factor and initiated the intrinsic clotting system [21].

Pathophysiology of Immune Complexes and Cryoglobulins

The pathogenic role of antigen-antibody complexes in autoimmune disorders is unquestioned. Cryoglobulins are seen in a wide variety of conditions, such as glomerulonephritis, vasculitis, and purpura, which suggests that these proteins are involved in an immune-complex type of autoimmune disorder [14, 23–25]. Many autoantibodies have been found in the cryoprecipitates, and this supports the theory that cryoglobulins represent antibodies formed to specific antigen-antibody complexes that lead to new complexes with cryoprecipitable properties. The mixed cryoglobulins can fix complement and have been shown to possess biological properties similar to those of specific antigen-antibody complexes [5, 14, 23]. Significant evidence, which will be discussed later, has been obtained over the past few years to indicate that mixed cryoglobulins play an in vivo pathogenic role in lesions of glomerulonephritis [5, 14, 23] and vasculitis [14, 23].

INSOLUBLE IMMUNE COMPLEXES
Immune complexes may be insoluble or soluble, depending upon the ratio of antibody to antigen. An example of tissue injury resulting from insoluble immune complexes is the Arthus reaction [2–5, 26]. A local Arthus reaction with vasculitis is produced when antigen is injected into a previously sensitized host (Fig. 17-2). Insoluble immune complexes are formed that precipitate and localize along the vascular basement mem-

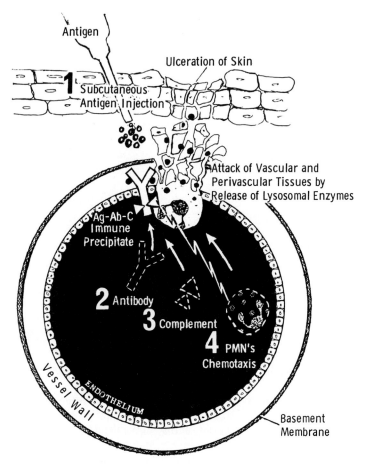

Figure 17-2
Arthus reaction. When horse γ-globulin antiserum to snake venom is given by local subcutaneous injection to a person for snake bite treatment, a local Arthus reaction may result if the patient is previously sensitized to horse γ-globulin. Circulating antibody to horse γ-globulin will form deposits of immune precipitates along the vascular walls of the skin and initiate a topical immune-complex reaction.

brane. The complexes fix complement, and chemotaxis of the polymorphonuclear leukocytes, phagocytosis of immune precipitates, destruction of lysosomes, release of proteolytic enzymes, and resultant tissue injury ensue. In the pathogenesis of the reaction, the fixation of complement with polymorphonuclear leukocyte infiltration is necessary for tissue injury.

SOLUBLE IMMUNE COMPLEXES
An example of soluble immune complexes is observed in serum sickness [2, 3, 27]. When a large amount of foreign serum protein is injected,

there is an initial induction period before the production of antibodies to the injected foreign protein occurs. The antibody that is produced combines with antigen in serum, and at first there is an extreme excess of antigen resulting in the formation of soluble antigen-antibody complexes. With the appearance of antigen-antibody complexes, there is a simultaneous lowering of serum complement and the appearance of inflammatory lesions in the kidneys, heart, arteries, and joints that are similar to the lesions found in acute glomerulonephritis, systemic lupus erythematosus, polyarteritis nodosa, and rheumatoid arthritis. Immunofluorescent studies have provided evidence for the deposition of circulating complexes, with the localization of IgG and C3 in the affected organs [2–5, 26, 28, 29].

In 1905, Von Pirquet and Schick first recognized that arthritis, glomerulonephritis, and vasculitis appeared 10 days to 2 weeks following passive immunization with horse antitetanus toxin [30]. The disease was the result of production of circulating antibody to the injected horse serum, and it represents the syndrome of serum sickness. Rich and Gregory [31] experimentally produced serum sickness in rabbits with large injections of bovine serum albumin (BSA). Dixon and others [2–4, 27] described the pathogenic events in experimental serum sickness in rabbits. By following the elimination of radiolabeled BSA, Dixon and co-workers [2, 27] observed that lesions of arthritis, glomerulonephritis, and vasculitis appeared at the time of immune elimination of the labeled antigen when soluble complexes in antigen excess were demonstrable in the serum (Fig. 17-3). The soluble antigen-antibody complexes may initiate tissue damage by reacting with various serum components. They can activate part of the C1q component of complement to an active esterase. In addition, they will cause the formation of fibrinolysin, anaphylatoxin, and active vasoactive peptides. At the cellular level, the following reactions may be seen [2–5]:

1. Degranulation of mast cells with liberation of various amines.
2. Attachment of complexes to leukocytes and platelets with agglutination.
3. Contraction of smooth muscle.
4. Increase of vascular permeability.
5. Endothelial proliferation.
6. Chemotactic attraction of mature granulocytes in the presence of complement.
7. Production of degenerative, hyaline changes in various tissues.

CRYOGLOBULINS AND THEIR RELATIONSHIP TO IMMUNE COMPLEXES

The cryoglobulins consist of complexes of immunoglobulins or single immunoglobulins that may have been altered by some unknown process. They are insoluble at 4°C, but they may aggregate at temperatures as high as 30°C [32, 33]. Such a temperature can be reached in peripheral capillaries [34]. Many of the cryoglobulins have the ability to fix com-

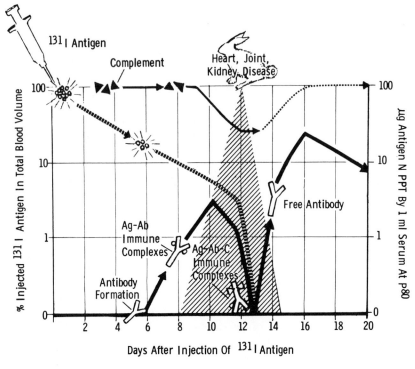

Figure 17-3
Immunological and morphological events transpiring after the injection of
131I-labeled bovine serum albumin into a rabbit in the dose of 250 mg/kg,
simultaneous with the appearance of detectable antigen-antibody complexes
in the circulation. (1) There is a decrease in serum complement levels. (2)
Lesions that represent the hallmark of immune-complex disease are seen:
(a) vasculitis in various zones including the heart, (b) glomerulonephritis,
and (c) serositis. (3) Free antibody appears in the circulation and the inflammatory lesions of serum sickness disappear rapidly after elimination of all
antigen-antibody complexes.

plement and initiate an inflammatory reaction similar to that of the classic antigen-antibody complexes, and thus they probably play a significant role in the pathogenesis of viral diseases and in the production of
the lesions of vasculitis and glomerulonephritis [14, 17, 23].

CLASSIFICATION OF CRYOGLOBULINS
The majority of the cryoglobulins are either intact monoclonal immunoglobulins or mixed cryoglobulins in which one component, usually IgM,
exhibits antibody activity to IgG [23]. There are other cryoproteins distinct from immunoglobulins such as cryofibrinogens. In this chapter, the
term *cryoglobulin* will be considered to be similar in meaning to the
more precise term *cryoimmunoglobulin*.

Table 17-1. Classification of Cryoglobulins (Cryoimmunoglobulins)

Type	Nature of Immunoglobulins[a]	Diseases[b]
Pure monoclonal cryoglobulin	IgG IgM IgA Bence Jones proteins	Myeloma Waldenström's macroglobulinemia Lymphoma Other malignancy Cold-agglutinin disease
Mixed monoclonal cryoglobulin (one component is a monoclonal immunoglobulin)	IgM and IgG IgA and IgG IgG and IgG	Primary or secondary Waldenström's macroglobulinemia Multiple myeloma Lymphoma
Polyclonal cryoglobulin (single or mixed cryoprecipitate)	One or more polyclonal immunoglobulins	Rheumatoid arthritis Systemic lupus erythematosus Bacterial or viral infections

[a] Any of the immunoglobulins may or may not have rheumatoid factor (RF) activity.
[b] In some cases, the cryoglobulin is not associated with a specific disease and is called *essential* or *idiopathic* cryoglobulin.

In the various studies reported, many of the cryoprecipitates contain proteins other than immunoglobulins. Some of the different combinations of immunoglobulin and serum proteins that have been noted [14, 23] are (1) IgG, IgM, and C3; (2) IgG, C3, and fibrinogen; (3) IgG, IgM, and α-macroglobulin; and (4) lipoprotein and immunoglobulins.

Three types of cryoglobulins or cryoimmunoglobulins can be described on the basis of immunoglobulin homogeneity according to Grey and Kohler [23] (Table 17-1). Each of the three categories listed below can be further subdivided on the basis of whether or not one of the immunoglobulins in the cryoprecipitate has anti-γ-globulin or rheumatoid factor activity.

Pure monoclonal cryoglobulin. Pure monoclonal cryoglobulin is found most frequently in patients with Waldenström's macroglobulinemia, lymphomas, and myelomas. The monoclonal immunoglobulin may be either IgG, IgM, IgA, or Bence Jones proteins. In certain cases, the monoclonal cryoglobulin is not associated with a specific disease and is called *essential* or *idiopathic*. Some of the patients considered to have essential or idiopathic pure cryoglobulinemia may later develop a malignant lymphoma. The monoclonal cryoglobulin may or may not possess anti-γ-globulin or rheumatoid factor activity.

Mixed monoclonal cryoglobulin. In mixed monoclonal cryoglobulin two or more immunoglobulins are found in the cryoprecipitate and one component is a monoclonal immunoglobulin. This complex may or may not demonstrate rheumatoid factor activity. Mixed cryoglobulins are seen in Waldenström's macroglobulinemia; in lymphomas, myelomas, and other tumors; and in collagen vascular diseases and certain viral infections [14, 23]. In such conditions, the patients demonstrate associated autoantibodies. The cryoglobulins may fix complement in vitro and in vivo [14, 23]. Besides precipitating in the cold in vitro, the cryoglobulin complexes may precipitate in vessels and kidney glomeruli in vivo and produce syndromes of purpura, arthritis, and glomerulonephritis [5, 14, 23, 25, 35–37].

Many of the mixed cryoglobulins have been studied and found to contain specific antigens, antibodies, and complement. Cryoglobulins are often associated with some unusual infections [14]. Wager et al. [17] have studied cryoglobulins in cases of cytomegalovirus infection and infectious mononucleosis and have detected the following antibodies in the cryoprecipitates: antiglobulin rheumatoid factor, antinuclear antibodies, heterophile antibody, and cold agglutinins.

Polyclonal cryoglobulins. In this category, one or more immunoglobulins may be seen in the cryoprecipitate that are polyclonal in nature. There are very few data on the polyclonal cryoglobulins, since they are usually seen in very low concentrations [23]. A mixed polyclonal cryoglobulin in the cryoprecipitate contains a polyclonal rheumatoid factor along with a polyclonal IgG. An example of polyclonal cryoglobulins is found in rheumatoid arthritis in which the rheumatoid factor observed is polyclonal in nature [38].

ROLE OF CRYOGLOBULINS IN GLOMERULONEPHRITIS
AND OTHER DISEASES

Cryoglobulins play a role in the pathogenesis of glomerulonephritis in a manner similar to that of immune complexes. The role of cryoglobulins in the pathogenesis of the nephritis of systemic lupus erythematosus (SLE) is discussed below. Cryoglobulins also play a role in the pathogenesis of joint lesions in rheumatoid arthritis, which is discussed further in the section on rheumatoid arthritis.

Cryoglobulins have been found in patients with poststreptococcal and nonpoststreptococcal glomerulonephritis [25, 37]. IgG, IgM, and C3 globulins were observed in the cryoprecipitates in several of the patients, and the proteins were observed to be localized in the glomerular basement membrane upon immunofluorescence studies. No evidence of streptococcal antigen was found in the cryoprecipitates, and attempts to localize the streptococcal antigen on the glomeruli of the patients were unsuccessful [25]. In one case of glomerulonephritis, fibrinogen was noted with immunoglobulin and complement in the cryoprecipitate [39].

Cryoglobulins associated with glomerulonephritis have been noted in cytomegalovirus infection [17] and infectious mononucleosis. Such cryoproteins have been demonstrated to possess biological properties similar to those of immune complexes [25]. The cryoprotein complex is able to fix complement components and to initiate the inflammatory reaction with basement membrane damage and possible deposition of fibrinogen products. The cryocomplexes may aggregate at temperatures as high as 30°C [32], and there is evidence that this temperature is regularly reached in the peripheral capillaries, which may cause vasculitis [34].

Immune-Complex Diseases

DIAGNOSIS OF IMMUNE-COMPLEX DISEASE AND CRYOGLOBULINEMIA

HISTORY AND PHYSICAL EXAMINATION

Immune complexes or cryoglobulins may be suspected to play a role in the pathogenesis of diseases that show the clinical signs and symptoms of (1) glomerulonephritis; (2) vasculitis with multisystem involvement; (3) synovitis with joint swelling and pain; (4) polyserositis with pleural effusion and pain; (5) purpura; (6) Raynaud's phenomenon; (7) anemia; (8) deficient exocrine function, e.g., Sjögren's syndrome; (9) lymphoproliferative disorders such as leukemia or lymphoma; (10) certain bacterial or viral diseases such as subacute bacterial endocarditis, infectious mononucleosis, cytomegalic inclusion disease, syphilis, and leprosy; (11) malignant tumors; and (12) cirrhosis.

FINDINGS ON COMMON LABORATORY TESTS

Proteinuria and hematuria found by urinalysis may indicate glomerulonephritis. The findings of a complete blood count may show evidence of hemolytic anemia, pancytopenia, lymphoproliferative disorder, or infectious mononucleosis. Protein electrophoresis may demonstrate abnormal globulins or the presence of monoclonal proteins.

SPECIFIC LABORATORY TESTS IN THE WORK-UP OF SUSPECTED IMMUNE COMPLEX DISEASES

The following tests are helpful in the evaluation of an immune-complex disorder (see also Chap. 9):

1. Serum protein analyses, including electrophoresis and immunoelectrophoresis [40–42].
2. Semiquantitative serum cryoglobulin determination and tests for the formation of cryoprecipitate at 4°C [32, 40].
3. Tests for immune complexes in the serum and joint fluid with the C1q component of complement [43, 44], monoclonal rheumatoid factor [38], or the platelet aggregation test [45, 46].
4. Biopsy of kidney, muscle, or synovium for routine histological, electron microscopic, and immunofluorescence studies.
5. Measurement of complement levels in the serum, joint fluid, or both [22, 47, 48].

RECOMMENDED LABORATORY TESTS IN CASES OF CRYOGLOBULINEMIA

If the serum tests are positive for cryoglobulins, further tests should be conducted to determine whether there is a monoclonal protein with rheumatoid factor activity. Further tests may include serum protein immuno-electrophoretic studies, the quantitation of immunoglobulins, the quantitation of cryoglobulins, and the analysis of serum for the presence of rheumatoid factor, antinuclear factor activity, cold agglutinin activity, and autoimmune antibody by Coombs' test.

CASE STUDY OF IMMUNE-COMPLEX DISEASE WITH
GLOMERULONEPHRITIS AND DISSEMINATED ARTERITIS

This case concerns a 23-year-old female who had been seen by her physician during the previous year because of intermittent joint pain and swelling. On her initial examination, the right elbow and wrist exhibited swelling and warmth, and pain occurred on movement. No other joints were involved at that time, but subsequently swelling and pain occurred in the left wrist and elbow as well as the right foot and the metacarpophalangeal and proximal interphalangeal joints of both hands. Initial laboratory studies revealed mild anemia, slight leukocytosis with increased lymphocytes, and a significantly elevated erythrocyte sedimentation rate (ESR). Latex tests for rheumatoid factor and C-reactive protein were positive in high titer. Cardiac enlargement was noted on a chest roentgenogram, and minimal changes were found on electrocardiography, which were nonspecific T wave changes and a prolonged PR interval. A lupus erythematosus (LE) cell preparation exhibited erythrophagocytosis, but no LE cells were found. The tentative diagnosis was acute rheumatic fever, and she was treated with salicylates and penicillin. Within the week following therapy, the pain and swelling in the joints subsided, but the ESR continued to be significantly elevated. Urinalysis during this period revealed no proteinuria.

Approximately three months after this initial episode, she returned to her physician on an emergency visit with fever, pain in her wrists and phalangeal joints, and a swollen right foot that was warm and painful. Axillary and inguinal lymphadenopathy were detected on physical examination. Laboratory studies revealed persistence of the anemia and lymphocytosis as well as the elevated erythrocyte sedimentation rate. Urinalysis at that time showed 3+ proteinuria, hyaline casts, and minimal microscopic hematuria. Tests of LE cell preparations were negative; however, fluorescent antinuclear antibody study exhibited a pattern of combined nucleolar and cytoplasmic staining on human renal substrate tissue that could be abolished by prior absorption with human γ-globulin.

Rheumatoid factor continued to be detected in high titer. At this time, she was hospitalized for further diagnostic studies and treatment. Biopsy of one of the enlarged axillary nodes, along with biopsy of skin and muscle, was performed. The node exhibited diffuse follicular hyperplasia of the cortical and medullary zones. In the skin biopsy, many of the small blood vessels exhibited necrotizing vasculitis with fibrinoid destruction of the vessel wall and a heavy infiltrate of neutrophils (Fig. 17-4). Immunofluorescence studies showed extensive deposits of γ-globulin and complement within the vascular walls. A percutaneous renal biopsy was performed, and the specimen exhibited the changes of membranous

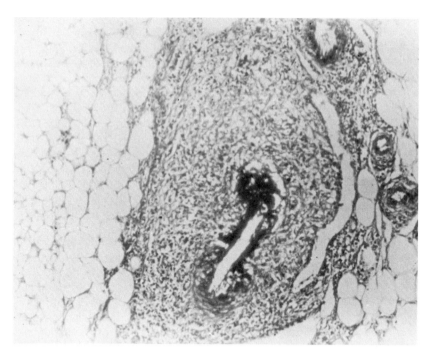

Figure 17-4
Necrotizing vascultis. Section of arterial vessel in subcutaneous tissue of skin shows fibrinoid necrosis of the vessel wall with heavy infiltrate of polymorphonuclear inflammatory cells. (H & E section, ×40.)

glomerulonephritis with focal fibrinoid necrosis. Immunofluorescence studies revealed the abundant deposition of γ-globulin and complement in a granular, so-called "lumpy-bumpy" pattern along the glomerular basement membrane. The electron microscopic examination showed the presence of granular deposits in the glomerular basement membrane and infiltration of neutrophils under the endothelium against the basement membrane. Studies of the serum complement activity by immunodiffusion and immunoelectrophoresis revealed a significant decrease in β-1C globulin (C-3) and evidence of the conversion of β-1C to β-1A globulin (C-3 breakdown product).

The diagnosis of immune-complex disease was made on the basis of the immunopathological studies. The patient was started on treatment with high initial doses of steroids (80 mg prednisone every other day) with subsequent tapering to a maintenance dosage (15 mg per day). The patient's complaints of joint pain, fever, and generalized aching abated temporarily on this therapeutic regimen. However, the proteinuria and elevation of the ESR persisted.

Seven months later, the patient was seen for complaints of chest pain, which was diagnosed as pleural in origin and associated with pleural effusion. The pleural fluid was removed by thoracentesis, which yielded normal cytological features and no growth on culture. Also noted at this time was a large, circumscribed area of necrosis and ulceration in the left lateral thigh that progressively enlarged to a diameter of 7 cm and became deeply eroded. Biopsy specimens of the margins of the lesion revealed necrotizing vasculitis.

During this hospitalization, she began to complain of more intense fatigue and shortness of breath. Edema developed in the face and hands along with hypoalbuminemia, hypercholesterolemia (370 mg per 100 ml), and persistent proteinuria. Progressive elevation of blood urea nitrogen was also noted. The shortness of breath became more severe with the onset of cough and sputum production. A *Pseudomonas* species was found on culture that was resistant to most antibiotics except gentamicin. She improved with gentamicin therapy; however, diminished pulmonary function persisted, and there was evidence of impaired diffusion capacity and hypoxemia.

A determination of homoreactant antibody (rheumatoid factor) revealed an extremely high titer of 1:20,480. On this basis, treatment with penicillamine (1.5 gm per day) was begun. Low-dose steroid therapy was also continued. After beginning this therapy, her joints have remained asymptomatic, and there has been no further cough or complaints of pleural pain. Healing of the large ulcer in the left thigh occurred gradually, and there has been remission of the edema of the hands and face. The proteinuria and hypoalbuminemia have continued.

SYSTEMIC LUPUS ERYTHEMATOSUS (SLE)–PRIMAL MODEL OF IMMUNE-COMPLEX DISEASE IN HUMANS

ROLE OF IMMUNE COMPLEXES IN THE PATHOGENESIS OF SLE

Great progress has been made in the understanding of the pathogenic events during the disease course of lupus erythematosus; however, as in many of the autoimmune diseases, the exact cause of the disorder is unknown [49]. SLE may be classified under the category of non-organ-specific autoimmune disease, along with rheumatoid arthritis and other collagen diseases. In the general theories of autoimmunity, lupus erythematosus (LE) may come under the category of abnormal immune mechanisms in which there is some disturbed tolerance or failure of self-recognition. There is production of antibodies to many cellular constituents and native DNA. Antibody production to specific native DNA has not been induced experimentally, although experimental animals such as mice [50] and dogs [51] have been shown to demonstrate a spontaneous lupus-like disease similar to the human disease. There is a wide spectrum of overlap between pure discoid and classic SLE, and a small percentage of discoid lupus patients may eventually develop SLE.

The clinical manifestations of SLE involve multiple organ systems. The disease may be diagnosed when multisystem involvement with glomerulonephritis is seen in the presence of LE-cell or antinuclear antibodies [52]. It has been shown that when a lupus erythematosus patient is exposed to excessive sunlight, there may be an exacerbation of symp-

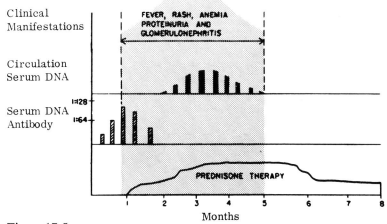

Figure 17-5
Correlation of circulating DNA antibody and free serum DNA with the clinical course in a case of systemic lupus erythematosus.

toms. The patient will develop fever, skin lesions, pleuritis, anemia, and antibodies to DNA. The alteration of nuclear DNA by ultraviolet light has been well documented recently [53–56]. Tan and co-workers [6] have demonstrated that during the exacerbation of a clinical case of lupus erythematosus, DNA appears in the circulation. DNA in serum was detected by the agar-gel double-diffusion technique. With the appearance of DNA in the serum, there is fever with proteinuria, and prednisone treatment results in a gradual disappearance of the free DNA or DNA-anti-DNA immune complexes (Fig. 17-5). Free serum DNA is only rarely seen in other disease conditions. In the pathogenesis of lupus erythematosus, it is felt that the antigen-antibody complexes of DNA and anti-DNA are the important toxic immune complexes that cause diffuse membranous and proliferative glomerulonephritis or focal glomerulonephritis (see Chap. 9).

The distribution of C3 and IgG in an irregular "lumpy-bumpy" pattern, as visualized by immunofluorescence, is in marked contrast to the linear type of fluorescent pattern that is seen in Goodpasture's syndrome, which shows basement membrane antibodies (Fig. 17-6). The evidence for the role of antigen-antibody complexes in the nephritis of SLE is as follows [57]:

1. The deposition of immunoglobulins and complement within the membrane of glomeruli is similar to the findings of serum sickness.
2. Antinuclear antibodies can be specifically eluted from glomeruli in greater concentrations than in serum.
3. Serum complement levels are depressed during periods of active nephritis.
4. DNA and other nuclear antigens have been demonstrated in the glomeruli by immunofluorescence.

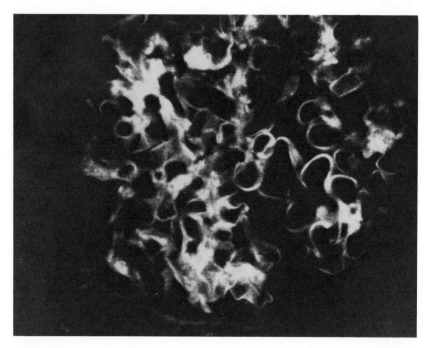

Figure 17-6
Kidney lesion of systemic lupus erythematosus. The section of glomerular lesion shows irregular deposits of IgG and C3 along the epithelial side of the basement membrane, which were revealed by fluorescent antibody studies. (×400.)

The cutaneous manifestations of SLE are varied. Fluorescence studies of the skin have demonstrated the fixation of immunoglobulins and complement along the basement membrane. Also, immune complexes of DNA in the upper part of the dermis have been observed. In addition, antibodies have been seen in the nuclei of squamous epithelial cells [58, 59].

Ultraviolet radiation has been shown to cause alteration of the DNA of human skin in vivo [54]. The in vivo changes were demonstrated by immunofluorescence, using antibodies specific for DNA that had been altered by exposure to ultraviolet light. Therefore, the skin of SLE patients may be a potential source of nuclear antigens that are released into the circulation during tissue damage. These antigens combine with circulating antinuclear antibodies to form immune complexes that are potentially harmful to other organs.

ROLE OF CRYOGLOBULINS IN SLE
In SLE, circulating cold-insoluble complexes were observed in a significant number of patients. The cryoglobulins in SLE may possess biological properties similar to those of immune complexes, and they were observed along with other circulating immune complexes in active cases of lupus nephritis [5, 7, 44] (Fig. 17-7).

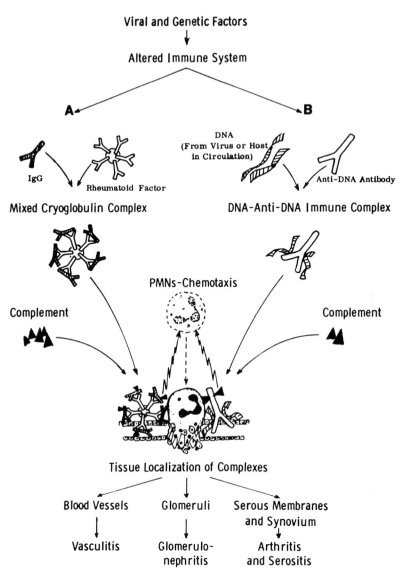

Viral and Genetic Factors

Altered Immune System

A **B**

DNA
(From Virus or Host
in Circulation)

IgG
Rheumatoid Factor
Anti-DNA Antibody

Mixed Cryoglobulin Complex   DNA-Anti-DNA Immune Complex

PMNs-Chemotaxis

Complement   Complement

Tissue Localization of Complexes

Blood Vessels   Glomeruli   Serous Membranes
and Synovium

Vasculitis   Glomerulo-   Arthritis
nephritis   and Serositis

Figure 17-7
Pathogenesis of systemic lupus erythematosus.

Stastny and Ziff [60] observed circulating cold-insoluble complexes of cryoglobulins in one-third of the cases of SLE observed. These complexes consisted mainly of IgG and the C1q component of complement, but significant amounts of DNA antibodies were not found. The presence of cryoglobulins is associated with a decrease of C3 in 90 percent of the cases, whereas in SLE without the pressence of cryoproteins, only 12 percent of the cases demonstrated a decrease in serum C3 concentration. The isolated cryoprotein that contained IgG and C1q produced a significant reduction in the in vitro hemolytic activity of human complement. Hanauer and Christian [16] first demonstrated that serum from SLE patients contains cryoprecipitates with C1q and rheumatoid factor.

Recent evidence has been obtained that a high molecular weight immune complex (greater than 19S) that is independent of the DNA-anti-DNA system may play a role in the nephritis process of SLE [43, 44]. In SLE patients, this system is mediated by the in vivo interaction of rheumatoid factor and the C1q component of complement with circulating complexes. Such patients demonstrate serum cryoglobulins [5, 7, 44]. These cryoglobulins can be classified as a polyclonal type, since the rheumatoid factor and other immunoglobulins are not homogeneous. Rheumatoid factor has been detected in the cryoprecipitates from patients with SLE, and, in addition, fluorescence localization studies with fluorescein-labeled aggregated γ-globulin demonstrated the presence of rheumatoid factor in the glomeruli of SLE patients [7]. Thus, cryoglobulin complexes containing rheumatoid factor may play a role in the pathogenesis of the renal injury in SLE.

In addition to large cryoglobulin complexes that can react with rheumatoid factor and C1q in SLE patients, Agnello et al. [44] have demonstrated low molecular weight (approximately 7S) C1q reactants in the sera of such patients. Both the large complexes and unidentified low molecular weight reactants are associated with the active state of the disease.

ROLE OF COMPLEMENT AND PROPERDIN IN SLE

Total serum complement levels are decreased in active cases of SLE, largely due to the action of immune complexes and cytotoxic antibodies. Properdin [61] is a distinct protein that is involved in the alternate pathway of complement activation that is not antibody mediated [22]. Properdin was demonstrated by indirect immunofluorescence in the kidneys of SLE patients [62]. One patient showed localization of properdin in both the kidney and skin [62]. The presence of properdin suggests that the alternate pathway of complement activation is involved in the pathogenesis of SLE [9, 62]. The low C3 levels observed in cases of SLE were found to be due largely to its decreased synthesis [63]. Perhaps cytotoxic antibodies may be partly responsible for the decreased synthesis of C3.

CELLULAR IMMUNITY AND LYMPHOCYTOTOXIC ANTIBODIES IN SLE

There have been conflicting reports as to the status of cellular sensitivity in SLE [64, 65]. One group of investigators observed that cellular immunity is depressed during the early stages prior to treatment [66]. A recent report indicates that in many cases of SLE patients, the cellular immunity mechanisms are not depressed as demonstrated by conventional skin-test antigens and in vitro lymphocyte transformation tests [64]. Delayed cellular sensitivity to nuclear antigens has been observed in certain cases of SLE [49]. SLE patients have a high incidence of lymphocytotoxic antibodies [67]. The presence of cytotoxic antibodies was definitely related to the presence of clinical symptoms and correlated inversely with the white blood count and serum C3 levels [68]. The action of lymphocytotoxic antibodies on cell membranes may lead to complement-mediated cell injury, which in turn results in the release of nuclear antigens and other intracellular antigens [68].

EVIDENCE FOR GENETIC AND OTHER CAUSATIVE FACTORS IN SLE

For a long time, many investigators have probed the genetic predisposition to SLE. Grumet and co-workers [69] have shown that patients with SLE have a high frequency of the human leukocyte antigens HL-A8 (33 percent) and W15 (40 percent) as compared to the control population frequencies of 11 and 10 percent, respectively. The association of histocompatibility-linked immune response genes (Ir genes) is similar to the association observed in mice [70].

More recently, in various kidney biopsy specimens from patients with SLE, virus-like bodies have been demonstrated [71–73]. These bodies are tubuloreticular structures, and at first they were believed to have a superficial resemblance to a myxovirus. In biopsy specimens from SLE cases, distinctive particles were also noted by electron microscopy [73]. These so-called virus-like structures have been demonstrated in the cytoplasm of endothelial cells in many cases of SLE. A thorough electron microscopic study incorporating blind controls demonstrated the virus-like tubuloreticular structures (TRS) in the buffy coat of lymphocytes of patients with SLE, discoid lupus erythematosus, and other connective tissue diseases [73]. The clinical evaluation of SLE patients demonstrated no significant differences between those with TRS-positive and those with TRS-negative lymphocytes. The possible etiological explanation of SLE may be compared to the explanation of autoimmunity and malignancy in the spontaneous disease of New Zealand mice (the counterpart of human lupus) [74]. The mouse disease probably results from a genetic defect in which there may be a lysogenic or defective virus that may initiate an immunological imbalance. The immunological imbalance is manifested by an abnormal antibody response, with the production of autoantibodies to nuclear antigens and resulting immune-complex disease, and a depression in cellular immunity, with impaired immune surveillance resulting in a malignancy [74].

SLE also occurs in dogs and, like its counterpart in man, it is a multisystem disease that usually affects young adult females [51]. The results of a genetic analysis of an established breeding colony were consistent with the concept that canine SLE can be explained by the vertical transmission of an infectious agent in genetically susceptible individuals [51]. The cause of SLE in humans, however, is still largely unknown. The role of viruses in the mediation of immunological mechanisms in genetically prone individuals still remains to be investigated.

LABORATORY TESTS FOR THE DIAGNOSIS OF SLE

SLE is a disease that involves multiple systems and is often accompanied by glomerulonephritis, although destructive arthritis is rare. The clinical findings, along with the presence of LE cells or antinuclear antibodies, help in reaching the diagnosis [52].

In a laboratory test for the diagnosis of SLE, one would prefer a very sensitive test that could detect the presence or absence of antinuclear antibodies in patients' sera and still have a low incidence of false-positive tests in an "apparently normal" population [75]. The absence of antinuclear antibodies for practical purposes would rule out the possibility of SLE if the patient had not been treated with corticosteroids or immunosuppressive drugs.

In the various collagen diseases, antibodies to many different nuclear antigens are seen. The significant nuclear antigens are:

1. native DNA or double-stranded DNA
2. denatured DNA or ultraviolet denatured DNA
3. nucleoprotein (DNA-histone)
4. saline-extractable antigens (one of the antigens has been identified as Sm antigen [carbohydrate-containing protein] [76]; also, ribonucleoproteins have been identified in this fraction [77, 78])
5. nucleolar (RNA) antigens (antibody to nucleolar RNA may be frequently seen in systemic scleroderma) [79]

The various diagnostic tests for antinuclear antibodies that are available in the clinical laboratory are:

1. LE cell test [80]
2. antiglobulin consumption test [81]
3. complement-fixation tests
4. precipitin tests [6]
5. agglutination tests [82–85]
6. radiolabeled DNA with antigen-binding capacity [86–88]
7. indirect immunofluorescence [89]
8. peroxidase enzyme-conjugated antibody technique [90, 91]

The *LE cell test* is quite insensitive and only positive in 50 to 80 percent of the cases [92–96]. The LE cell reaction occurs in three phases [92]: (1) There is a reaction of the LE cell humoral factor with extracted nuclear material. (2) The humoral factor has been identified as a 7S, complement-fixing antibody. After combining with extracted nuclei, there is a modification of the nuclear material, with the formation of hematoxylin bodies. (3) The last phase consists of phagocytosis of the hematoxylin body by living polymorphonuclear leukocytes.

In the performance of the LE cell test, there should be traumatization of the cellular material with extrusion of the nuclei. The nuclear material then reacts with the antibody, causing the formation of the hematoxylin body. Phagocytosis of the hematoxylin body by polymorphonuclear leukocytes occurs in the presence of complement. The LE cell shows a neutrophilic leukocyte that is distended with a homogeneous hematoxylin body in which the pattern of the nuclear membrane structure is absent [95, 96] (see Chap. 16).

The *"Tart" cell* was first described in a patient named Tart, and it is normally produced by the phagocytosis of a nucleus, usually by a monocyte [96]. The Tart cell may be seen in cases of drug sensitivity and antileukocyte antibodies.

In the presence of leukocytic antibodies (HLA) that react with the antigens along the nuclear membrane, the Tart cell may form [97]. In the Tart cell, the outline of the nuclear chromatin patterns is seen, and it is not homogeneous as in the true LE cell.

The *antiglobulin consumption test* [81] is a cumbersome test in which nuclear stroma is first reacted with the patient's serum. Antinuclear antibodies in the serum adhere to the nuclear stroma. After repeated washing, the antinuclear antibodies are eluted from the nuclear stroma and quantitated by inhibition of the Coombs' test.

The *complement-fixation test* is a sensitive test and is useful in that specific nuclear antigens may be utilized. However, these tests are unwieldy in the clinical laboratory, and the patients' sera often contain anticomplementary substances.

The *precipitin test* depends upon a secondary manifestation of the antigen-antibody reaction and is relatively insensitive. However, when large agar plates are used, DNA may be detected in the very low concentrations of 1 to 5 μg per milliliter [6]. DNA has been found in patients' sera just prior to the detection of DNA-anti-DNA antigen-antibody complexes in cases of SLE with exacerbation of the disease syndrome. Often, one can detect different antibodies to either native, single-stranded, or heat-denatured DNA.

Several different *agglutination tests* for the detection of antinuclear antibodies have been published, which include techniques based on the passive hemagglutination of DNA-coated red blood cells and the agglutination of coated latex particles or coated bentonite particles. A latex agglutination test for anti-DNA histone is available commercially*† and has been proved to be fairly specific in routine use, but it has the great disadvantage of poor sensitivity [82, 98]. A modified assay for antibodies against DNA that utilizes formalized and tanned red blood cells has been developed [84, 85]. The hemagglutination technique was found to be a useful method for detecting antibodies to photo-oxidized DNA, ultraviolet-irradiated DNA, and single-stranded DNA, as well as to native DNA. Positive hemagglutinating DNA antibodies have been demonstrated in patients who show no detectable precipitating antibodies by the agar-gel double-diffusion test. Sharp et al. [78, 99] have used the

* Hyland Division, Travenol Laboratories, Inc., P.O. Box 2214, Costa Mesa, Calif. 92626.
† Behring Diagnostics, Inc., Rt. 202-206 North, Somerville, N.J. 08876.

hemagglutination technique for the detection of antibodies to DNA and extractable nuclear antigens. The agglutination tests for the detection of DNA antibodies are of great value in definitive diagnosis and in following patients undergoing therapy.

The *radiolabeled DNA antigen-binding capacity* technique, in which DNA is labeled by incorporation with tritiated actinomycin D or tritiated dimethylsulfate, is the most sensitive test available today for the detection of free DNA or anti-DNA antibody [88]. If the serum contains any antibody to DNA, it will bind with the DNA. The DNA that is complexed with antibody is insoluble in 50 percent ammonium sulfate, while free DNA is found in the supernate. One can also demonstrate the presence of free DNA in the serum by this technique. The concentrations of DNA or DNA antibody may be determined by the ratio of binding to radiolabeled DNA in comparison with a standard curve.

The *indirect immunofluorescence test* is the most practical one in the clinical laboratory today [89]. Patient serum is reacted with a section of substrate that contains nuclei, and, after washing the section, it is reacted with fluoresceinated antihuman globulin. The existence of a wide variety of antibodies in SLE has been demonstrated by this technique. Evidence of a monoclonal type of antinuclear antibody has not been found [100]. Various IgM, IgA, and IgG antibodies have been noted in cases of SLE. IgG is almost always present in the presence of other classes of antibodies. The fluorescence test is very sensitive, and it can be developed to the point where a negative test may, for all practical purposes, rule out the diagnosis of SLE if the patient is not being treated with corticosteroids or immunosuppressive drugs. From the pattern of fluorescence and titer, one can obtain some idea as to the type of antinuclear antibody involved [101, 102]. When the serum is tested in various dilutions, the antibody with the strongest titer will show a characteristic fluorescent pattern. A *membranous ring or shaggy pattern* is seen with antibodies to coarse, insoluble DNA and deoxyribonucleoproteins. The rim pattern is often seen in cases with a high titer of antinuclear antibody. A *homogeneous pattern* is seen with antibodies to nucleoproteins and ribonucleoproteins. The *speckled pattern* is often seen with antibodies to saline-extractable antigens, which include soluble nucleoproteins, Sm antigen, and ribonucleoproteins. An extremely high-titer speckled pattern, sometimes greater than 1:256, may be seen in an SLE-related disorder, called the *mixed connective tissue syndrome,* which is characterized by a scleroderma-like syndrome and myositis with Raynaud's phenomenon [78]. This disease has a good prognosis and responds extremely well to corticosteroid therapy. A *nucleolar pattern* is seen with antibodies to nucleolar RNA; this antibody is most easily detected by the indirect immunofluorescent test [79].

There is much confusion concerning the results of indirect fluorescent nuclear antibody tests, since there are numerous substrates being utilized [103]. The common substrates used today are chicken erythrocytes [104], human leukocytes [105], human skin tissue [106] (hemorrhoidal tissue is often used), tissue culture cells and tumor cells [107], and rat or mouse kidney [101].

We have demonstrated with recent experiments that chicken nuclei are poor for demonstration of the speckled pattern that is caused by antibodies to saline-extractable antigen or soluble nucleoproteins [108]. This is understandable, since mammalian and nonmammalian proteins usually do not cross-react. Human leukocytes are readily available and very commonly used; however, interference by blood-group antibodies and anti-leukocyte antibodies occurs. With human leukocytes, the test is very sensitive and often results in false-positive reactions. Human tissue, such as skin, may suffer a disadvantage resulting from the presence of blood-group antibodies if tissue from other than type O patients is used. We prefer the use of rat or mouse kidney, in which there is no interference from blood-group antibodies. Sera are screened at 1:4 and 1:16 dilutions. The incidence of positive fluorescence at a 1:4 dilution is about 2 percent in an apparently normal population [109]. If the serum shows a positive result at the 1:16 titer, then it is further tested at 1:64 and 1:256 dilutions.

In the fluorescence test, one should be careful that the substrate is fixed in acetone, since failure to fix the substrate will result in the elution of some of the nuclear constituents. Nonfixation of the substrate may yield a negative fluorescence test even though there is a positive LE cell phenomenon. We have observed two cases that have been referred by other laboratories in which the initial findings were positive LE cell tests and negative indirect fluorescent antibody tests [108]. Both cases showed a positive speckled pattern with fixed rat kidney substrate. One case showed a decreased fluorescence titer with unfixed rat kidney, and the second case was negative when tested with chicken red blood cell nuclei.

A titer of 1:16 or greater in the antinuclear fluorescent antibody test is usually present before there is evidence of a positive LE cell test [110]. The various patterns of fluorescence are (1) homogeneous, (2) rim and fibrillar, (3) combined rim and homogeneous, (4) speckled, and (5) nucleolar [101]. In infectious mononucleosis, there is often a low titer and an irregular, shaggy type of pattern. The antinuclear antibodies are of the IgG and IgM class. They appear in the cryoprecipitates when sera are stored at 4°C, but they do not give rise to the LE cell phenomenon [111].

In collagen disease, the incidence of various antinuclear antibodies has been found in SLE to be 99 percent or greater; in Sjögren's syndrome, 68 percent; in scleroderma, 40 percent; and in adult rheumatoid arthritis, 22 percent [112]. The incidence of antinucleolar antibodies in systemic sclerosis is 54 percent; SLE, 26 percent; rheumatoid arthritis, 9 percent; and rheumatoid syndrome, 8.3 percent. In general, the higher the titer of antinuclear antibodies, the more likely is the diagnosis of SLE. The reciprocal titers in SLE are often high, usually being in the range of 164 to 256. In other diseases, such as rheumatoid arthritis, Addison's disease, and pernicious anemia, the reciprocal antibody titers are often 64 or less.

The *peroxidase enzyme-conjugated antibody technique* may be used to test for the presence of antinuclear antibody [90, 91]. Antibody to human IgG is conjugated to horseradish peroxidase and is used to demonstrate the adherence of antinuclear antibodies to substrate nuclei. Localization of the enzyme is shown by reactions with 3,3′-diaminobenzidine, which yields an insoluble main reaction product. Patterns of nuclear staining are observed with this technique, and these correlate with the patterns seen by the fluorescence method. Comparison of the titers of antinuclear antibody showed the peroxidase method to be as sensitive as the fluorescence technique. A conventional microscope may be used in the peroxidase enzyme method, and no special equipment is necessary.

TESTS FOR MONITORING THE THERAPY OF SLE

Tests for the definitive evaluation of SLE therapy may be different from those used for screening purposes. In the initial screening tests for diagnosis, one would prefer a very sensitive test for all types of antinuclear antibodies, such as the indirect fluorescence test for the peroxidase enzyme method.

The important pathogenic antibody is presumably the DNA antibody. When DNA is released from tissues into the circulation and combines with DNA antibody, immune complexes are formed and clinical symptoms develop [5–7]. Almost all cases of active SLE nephritis show antibodies to double-stranded DNA as well as antibody to denatured DNA [6]. Antibodies to DNA may be detected by agar-gel double-diffusion, hemagglutination, complement-fixation, or radiolabeled DNA antigen-binding capacity tests. When patients with SLE respond to treatment with prednisone, immunosuppressive agents, or both, the DNA antibody level will decrease and eventually disappear. Thus, the specific test for antibodies to native DNA is more useful for monitoring the clinical course of SLE. After treatment, antinuclear antibodies other than DNA antibody may still be present and detectable by the immunofluorescence test. Therefore, antinuclear antibody titers as determined by the indirect immunofluorescence test may not be as useful as specific tests for DNA antibody to monitor therapy. Recently, Sharp et al. [99] have reported that individuals with SLE and renal disease who will respond to treatment show antibodies to DNA that decline with treatment, and 86 percent of patients have antibodies to the extractable nuclear antigen, which is believed to be nuclear ribonucleoprotein. In cases of SLE with renal disease that fail to respond to therapy, antibodies to DNA are persistent, and the incidence of antibodies to extractable nuclear antigen is only 8 percent.

Other laboratory procedures that should be considered in the evaluation of SLE are tests for serum cryoglobulins, serum complement, or serum immune complexes by C1q precipitation, as well as immunofluorescence studies on kidney biopsy specimens to evaluate any existing glomerulonephritis.

CASE STUDY OF SLE

A 34-year-old white housewife complained of fever and weakness of several months' duration. Within the past two months, she had tired easily and developed swelling of the ankles with fever, chills, and malaise. Several days prior to admission, her fever rose to 103°F, with some response to aspirin, and she developed a vesicular erythematous facial rash.

On physical examination, the vesicular erythematous eruption was evident on the malar prominences, nose, and lips. The joints did not show any significant swelling. Her temperature was 102°F and her blood pressure was 98/60 mm Hg. Urinalysis showed a specific gravity of 1.016 with a 4+ albumin, and the sediment contained some granular and hyaline casts with a few red and white blood cells. The hemoglobin was 9.8 gm, and the white blood cell count was 4400 per cubic millimeter with 73 percent neutrophils, 20 percent lymphocytes, 4 percent band forms, 2 percent monocytes, and 1 percent atypical lymphocytes. The total serum protein was found to be 7 gm per 100 ml, and fractionation showed an albumin level of 4.2 gm per 100 ml and a globulin level of 2.8 gm per 100 ml. The total hemolytic serum complement activity was 54 percent of normal control. The alkaline phosphatase level was 4.5 Bodansky units per 100 ml, and the SGOT was 14 units. The latex test for rheumatoid factor was negative, as was the heterophil test. Tests for serum cryoglobulins were negative. The antistreptolysin titer was less than 100 Todd units. The roentgenograms of the chest and hand, as well as the electrocardiogram, showed no significant abnormality. Cultures of the throat were negative for beta-hemolytic streptococci.

The fluorescent antinuclear antibody test was positive, with a homogeneous pattern at a titer of 1:256. The indirect immunofluorescence test for antinuclear antibody was performed with use of acetone-fixed rat kidney substrates [101]. The LE cell test was positive. The patient was diagnosed as having systemic lupus erythematosus, and treatment with prednisone was begun. Subsequently, the fluorescent antinuclear antibody titer decreased to 1:16.

She was followed over a period of several months with the determinations of titers of antinuclear antibodies by the fluorescence method and DNA antibodies by a hemagglutination method [85] and a double-diffusion technique [6]. One year later, the fluorescent antinuclear antibody titer was 1:128, and antibodies to DNA were noted by the red blood cell hemagglutination method up to a titer of 1:16. During an exacerbation of the disease that was characterized by general skin rash, high fever, and increased proteinuria, DNA appeared in the serum with the disappearance of antibody.

A biopsy of the kidney was performed, and fluorescent antibody studies revealed glomerular fixation of IgG, IgM, and β_1C-globulin in an irregular "lumpy-bumpy" pattern. A diagnosis of lupus immune complex nephritis was made. The serum β_1C-complement level was decreased.

The diagnosis of SLE is based on the presence of multisystem involvement and the demonstration of LE cells or positive antinuclear antibodies, or both. Except after administration of corticosteroid or immunosuppressive therapy, the absence of antinuclear antibodies excludes the diagnosis of SLE. SLE is often accompanied by glomerulonephritis and nonerosive arthritis. The coexistence of rheumatoid arthritis with SLE, SLE with erosive arthritis, or rheumatoid arthritis with glomerulonephritis is extremely rare.

The levels or the presence of nuclear antigen-antinuclear antibody complexes in the circulation may be correlated with the complement level, since complement is decreased during the active phase of the disease. The important antigen-antibody complex appears to be DNA-anti-DNA, and the antibody levels to DNA, as determined by agar-gel diffusion or the hemagglutination test, are useful for following the clinical course and prognosis of the disease. In contrast, the indirect fluorescent antinuclear antibody test detects a wide variety of nuclear antigens and is a sensitive test for diagnosis, but it is not the ideal test for monitoring the course of the disease.

RHEUMATOID ARTHRITIS (RA)

PATHOGENESIS OF JOINT LESIONS IN RA

Polyarthritis with pannus formation and the destruction of the joint spaces is the hallmark of rheumatoid arthritis. Other features include diffuse vasculitis, but glomerulonephritis is usually absent in rheumatoid arthritis. Glomerulitis characteristically occurs in most immune-complex diseases. There is abundant evidence that γ-globulin complexes are involved in the immunopathological mechanisms associated with the synovial lesions of rheumatoid arthritis [12, 38, 113, 114]. Some of the findings follow [12, 38, 47, 48, 114]: (1) depression of complement in the synovial fluid, (2) high concentration of γ-globulin complexes, (3) deposition of immunoglobulin and complement in the synovium (as detected by immunofluorescence studies), (4) deposition of immunoglobulins and complement in leukocytes, and (5) synthesis of immunoglobulins in the synovium.

In addition, cryoprecipitable complexes with varying amounts of IgG, IgM, and DNA have been found in the joint fluid of patients who have detectable rheumatoid factor in their serum [114, 115]. The cryoproteins found in the joint were not seen in the companion serum samples [115] (Fig. 17-8).

ETIOLOGY AND ROLE OF RHEUMATOID FACTOR (RF)

The rheumatoid factor (RF) includes both 7S and 19S immunoglobulins with antibody specificity to certain determinants on the γ-globulin molecule. The determinants may be exposed by physical aggregation of γ-globulin or by immune complex formation. Thus, rheumatoid factor may be an antibody directed against a γ-globulin determinant which is ordinarily hidden in the intact molecule but which becomes exposed after an antigen-antibody reaction. RF is detected in the serum of 80 percent of patients with rheumatoid arthritis [12].

The exact mechanism of production of the RF factor in rheumatoid arthritis is unknown. The RF factor in rheumatoid arthritis is usually polyclonal in nature and may be produced as an antibody to an antigen-

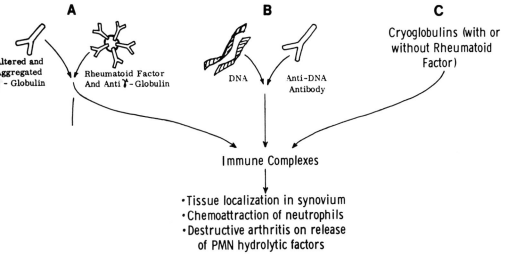

Figure 17-8
Various immune complexes in joint lesions of rheumatoid arthritis.

antibody complex. The γ-globulin is altered in the reaction with a specific antigen, such as a bacteria or virus, and may initiate production of RF. The presence of RF is found in a wide variety of diseases [116, 117]. RF may be produced by the host in an attempt to inactivate the so-called viral-antibody complex, with subsequent complement fixation. There is some evidence to support this possibility. Notkins and co-workers [118, 119] have reported some interesting experiments with viral antibody complexes and RF. They demonstrated that interaction of antiviral antibody with virus can still result in the formation of infectious viral-antibody complexes. Such complexes may be recovered from chronically infected animals. In vitro experiments have shown that RF itself failed to induce neutralization of *herpes simplex* viral-antibody complexes, but it increased the susceptibility of the complexes to neutralization by complement [119].

The RF factor is found in diseases other than rheumatoid arthritis, and, conversely, cases of rheumatoid arthritis may not demonstrate RF. The presence of high titers of RF, however, correlates with the more active, severe cases of rheumatoid arthritis [116]. In this disorder, RF will interact with antigen-antibody complexes as well as with aggregates of γ-globulin, and it has the capability to fix complement and initiate a destructive Arthus reaction type of inflammation in the joint space. The polymorphonuclear leukocytes that are attracted will release lysosomal enzymes, producing proteolytic destruction of tissues [120]. The complexes can, in turn, activate plasma kallikrein, lead to kinin formation, and initiate synovitis. The rheumatoid synovial fluid characteristically demonstrates low total hemolytic complement levels during the active stages of the disease [47, 48] (Fig. 17-9).

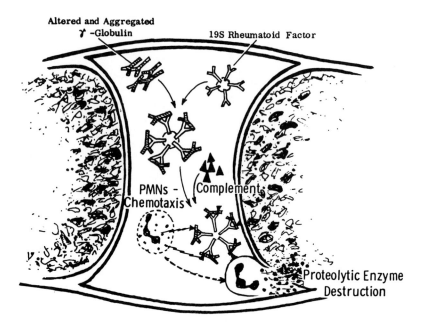

Figure 17-9
Role of rheumatoid factor in the pathogenesis of joint lesions in rheumatoid arthritis.

Currently, viruses are suspected in the causation of a wide variety of collagen vascular diseases. Viruses are known to induce the alteration of host tissue, with the formation of neoantigens. An immune reaction can occur against the altered host tissue, with formation of autoantibodies and immune complexes. The concept that rheumatoid arthritis is due to a virus has been investigated. So far in a study of 187 specimens from 142 subjects with rheumatoid arthritis by a variety of sensitive methods [121], there is no definite evidence of virus infection.

REACTIVITY OF γ-GLOBULIN COMPLEXES IN SERUM AND JOINT FLUID
Rheumatoid arthritis patients have γ-globulin complexes in both serum and joint fluid. The rheumatoid factor involved is usually polyclonal in nature and combines with γ-globulin to form immune complexes [38]. The complexes found in the serum and joint fluid differ in their immunochemical properties. The γ-globulin complexes from the joint fluid of patients react readily in vitro with C1q and polyclonal or monoclonal RF to form a precipitate [38, 43]. The joint fluid complexes are pathogenic and contribute to the inflammatory destruction of the joint space.

Winchester et al. [38] demonstrated that the γ-globulin complexes in the serum and joint fluid of patients with rheumatoid arthritis differed in their reactivity to C1q and monoclonal RF. Serum complexes from patients with rheumatoid arthritis consisted mainly of high molecular

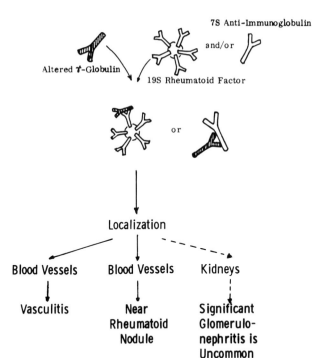

Figure 17-10
Serum immune complexes in rheumatoid arthritis.

weight but acid-dissociable 7S γ-globulin molecules. The exact nature of the complex is unknown, although 7S γ-globulin rheumatoid factors play a role in the formation of the complex. The serum complexes do not precipitate with C1q, but they demonstrate an in vitro precipitin reaction on gel diffusion with monoclonal RF. The serum complexes in rheumatoid arthritis are not associated with an in vivo depression of serum complement, and their different properties help explain the low incidence of glomerulonephritis in patients with this affliction (Fig. 17-10).

ROLE OF CRYOGLOBULINS IN RA
Cryoprecipitates have been observed in the synovial fluid of patients with rheumatoid arthritis [14, 23, 115]; however, such patients had no detectable cryoglobulin in their sera. In one study, the synovial fluid of all 21 patients with rheumatoid arthritis studied showed evidence of cryoprecipitates. Twelve of the 21 patients exhibited mixed polyclonal cryoglobulins with IgG-IgM and both κ and λ light chains. Ten of the 12 mixed synovial cryoprecipitates had antiglobulin RF activity. Three contained antinuclear antibody activity of the IgG class, and IgM antinuclear antibody was found in two. One patient with Reiter's syndrome had synovial cryoglobulin with the presence of denatured DNA and RF activity.

The most commonly employed tests in the clinical laboratory for the detection of RF are the human IgG-coated latex agglutination test and the sensitized sheep agglutination test.

Human IgG-coated latex agglutination test. This test was first described by Singer and Plotz [122]. It uses latex particles coated with human γ-globulin that are reacted against various dilutions of test serum. The latex test is most likely to react with an IgM rheumatoid factor [12, 123]. The greatest problem with this test is the lack of standardization of different latex tests for rheumatoid factors [123, 124]. A recent study has shown that the latex tests can be standardized with a reference standard [125].

In a quantitative study of the latex fixation test, Cats and Klein [124] noted that male and female patients fulfilling five or more of the American Rheumatoid Association Criteria [126] often had titers greater than 1:160.

Sensitized sheep cell agglutination test (Waaler-Rose). Sheep cells are coated with subagglutinating amounts of rabbit anti-sheep red cell antibody, and these provide the test reagent for rheumatoid factor [127, 128]. The test does not have the sensitivity of the latex test, but it is probably more specific for the detection of RF. A titer of greater than 1:16 is considered to be significant. Research reference standards are available for the sensitized sheep cell test [129].

The latex test and the sensitized sheep cell agglutination tests are, in general, more sensitive for the detection of 19S RF. When the above agglutination tests for RF are negative or positive, the rheumatoid arthritis patients are called *seronegative* or *seropositive*. Normal, healthy people may show evidence of RF by the agglutination test. They usually have low titers, and the frequency of positive reactions increases with age [130, 131]. In one study, the incidence of RF in elderly people correlated with a history of chronic infection, and it did not demonstrate a direct correlation with age or sex [131].

There are numerous other procedures available for the detection of rheumatoid factor. In general, the laboratory tests for RF are not of a diagnostic nature, but they are helpful in prognosis, since patients with active disease tend to have high levels of RF. In the early stages of rheumatoid arthritis, RF might not be seen in 15 to 25 percent of the cases [132]. Within the past few years, investigators have shown the presence of serum IgM, IgA, and IgG antiglobulins in RA by sensitive immunoadsorbent methods [133]. These various antiglobulins have been noted to correlate with disease activity. Thus, in a strict sense, the term *seronegative* does not mean a complete absence of existing antiglobulins.

There are several joint diseases in which RF is usually absent, and therefore the serum test for RF may be helpful in differential diagnosis. An absence of RF is usually found in osteoarthritis, ankylosing spondylitis, gout, rheumatic fever, suppurative arthritis, psoriatic arthritis, colitic arthritis, and Reiter's syndrome [116, 134].

The RF test is usually positive in a high percentage of cases of rheumatoid disease, adult rheumatoid arthritis, Sjögren's syndrome, systemic lupus erythematosus, scleroderma, juvenile rheumatoid arthritis, and Still's disease [116, 134].

RF can often be detected in the sera of patients with subacute bacterial endocarditis, tuberculosis, syphilis, infectious hepatitis, kala-azar, leprosy, sarcoidosis, and other conditions associated with hypergammaglobulinemia [116, 134].

References

1. Von Pirquet, C. E.   Allergy. *Arch. Intern. Med.* 7:259, 1911.
2. Dixon, F. J.   The role of antigen-antibody complexes in diseases. *Harvey Lect.* 58:21, 1963.
3. Weigle, W. O.   Fate and Biological Action of Antigen-Antibody Complexes. In W. H. Taliaferro and J. H. Humphrey (Eds.), *Advances In Immunology.* New York: Academic, 1961. P. 283.
4. Cochrane, C. G., and Dixon, F. J.   Cell and Tissue Damage Through Antigen-Antibody Complexes. In P. Miescher and H. J. Müller-Eberhard (Eds.), *Textbook of Immunopathology,* Vol. 1. New York: Grune & Stratton, 1969. P. 94.
5. Cochrane, C. G., and Koffler, D.   Immune Complex Disease in Experimental Animals and Man. In F. J. Dixon and H. G. Kunkel (Eds.), *Advances in Immunology,* Vol. 16. New York: Academic, 1973. P. 183.
6. Tan, E. M., Schur, P. H., Carr, R. I., and Kunkel, H. G.   Deoxyribonucleic acid (DNA) and antibodies to DNA in the serum of patients with systemic lupus erythematosus. *J. Clin. Invest.* 45:1732, 1966.
7. Koffler, D., Agnello, V., Thoburn, R., and Kunkel, H. G.   Systemic lupus erythematosus: Prototype of immune complex nephritis in man. *J. Exp. Med.* 134[Suppl.]:169, 1971.
8. Churg, J., and Grishman, E.   Ultrastructure of immune deposits in renal diseases. *Ann. Intern. Med.* 76:479, 1972.
9. Hunsicker, L. G., Ruddy, S., Carpenter, C. B., Schur, P. H., Merrill, J. P., Müller-Eberhard, H. J., and Austen, K. F.   Metabolism of third complement component (C3) in nephritis. *N. Engl. J. Med.* 287:835, 1972.
10. Roy, L. P., Fish, A. J., Michael, A. F., and Vernier, R. L.   Etiologic Agents of Immune Deposit Disease. In R. S. Schwartz (Ed.), *Progress in Clinical Immunology,* Vol. 1. New York: Grune & Stratton, 1972. P. 1.
11. Gocke, D. J., Hsu, K., Morgan, C., Bombardieri, S., Lockshin, M., and Christian, C. L.   Vasculitis in association with Australian antigen. *J. Exp. Med.* 134[Suppl.]:330, 1971.
12. Broder, I., Urowitz, M. B., and Gordon, D. A.   Appraisal of rheumatoid arthritis as an immune complex disease. *Med. Clin. North Am.* 56: 529, 1972.
13. Ritzmann, S. E., and Levin, W. C.   Cryopathies: a review. Classification, diagnostic and therapeutic considerations. *Arch. Intern. Med.* 107: 754, 1961.
14. Barnett, E. V., Bluestone, R., Cracchiola, A., Goldberg, L. S., Kantor, G. L., and McIntosh, R. M.   Cryoglobulinemia and disease. *Ann. Intern. Med.* 73:95, 1970.

15. Meltzer, M., and Franklin, E. C. Cryoglobulins, rheumatoid factor and connective tissue disorders. *Arthritis Rheum.* 10:489, 1967.
16. Hanauer, L. B., and Christian, C. L. Studies of cryoproteins in systemic lupus erythematosus. *J. Clin. Invest.* 46:400, 1967.
17. Wager, O., Rasanen, J. A., Hageman, A., and Klemola, A. Mixed cryoglobulinemia in infectious mononucleosis and cytomegalovirus mononucleosis. *Int. Arch. Allergy Appl. Immunol.* 34:345, 1968.
18. Nakamura, R. M., Spiegelberg, H. L., Lee, S., and Weigle, W. O. Relationship between molecular size and intra- and extravascular distribution of protein antigens. *J. Immunol.* 100:376, 1968.
19. Cochrane, C. G. Initiating Events in Immune Complex Injury. In B. Amos (Ed.), *Progress in Immunology, First International Congress of Immunology.* New York: Academic, 1971. P. 144.
20. Cochrane, C. G. Mechanisms involved in the deposition of immune complexes in tissues. *J. Exp. Med.* 134[Suppl.]:75, 1971.
21. Cochrane, C. G., Wuepper, K. D., Aiken, B. S., Revak, S. D., and Spiegelberg, H. L. The interaction of Hageman factor and immune complexes. *J. Clin. Invest.* 51:2736, 1972.
22. Ruddy, S., Gigli, I., and Austen, K. F. The complement system of man. *N. Engl. J. Med.* 287:489, 545, 591, 641, 1972.
23. Grey, H. M., and Kohler, P. F. Cryoimmunoglobulins. *Semin. Hematol.* 10:87, 1973.
24. Seligmann, M., and Bronet, J. C. Antibody activity of human myeloma globulins. *Semin. Hematol.* 10:163, 1973.
25. McIntosh, R. M., Kulvinskas, C., and Kaufman, D. B. Cryoglobulins. II. The biological and chemical properties of cryoproteins in acute poststreptococcal glomerulonephritis. *Int. Arch. Allergy. Appl. Immunol.* 41:700, 1971.
26. Cochrane, C. G. Mediators of the Arthus and related reactions. *Prog. Allergy* 11:1, 1967.
27. Dixon, F. J., Vazquez, J. J., Weigle, W. O., and Cochrane, C. G. The pathogenesis of serum sickness. *Arch. Pathol.* 65:18, 1958.
28. McCluskey, R. T. Evidence for immunologic mechanisms in several forms of human glomerular diseases. *Bull. N.Y. Acad. Med.* 46:769, 1970.
29. McCluskey, R. T. The value of immunofluorescence in the study of human renal disease. *J. Exp. Med.* 134[Suppl.]:242, 1971.
30. Von Pirquet, C. F., and Schick, B. *Serum Sickness.* B. Schick (Trans.). Baltimore: Williams & Wilkins, 1951.
31. Rich, A. R., and Gregory, J. E. The experimental demonstration that polyarteritis nodosa is a manifestation of hypersensitivity. *Bull. Johns Hopkins Hosp.* 72:63, 1943.
32. Peetoom, F., and Van Loghem-Langereis, E. IgM-IgG (β_2M-7s γ) cryoglobulinemia. An autoimmune phenomenon. *Vox Sang.* 10:281, 1965.
33. Ritzmann, S. E., Daniels, J. C., and Levin, W. C. Paralymphomatous Disease: The Syndrome of Macroglobulinemia. In *Leukemia and Lymphoma.* (A collection of papers presented at the 14th Clinical Conference on Cancer, 1969, at the University of Texas M. D. Anderson Hospital and Tumor Institute, Houston.) Chicago: Year Book, 1970. Pp. 169–221.
34. Swisher, S. S., and Vaughan, J. H. Acquired Hemolytic Diseases. In M. Samter (Ed.), *Immunological Diseases* (2nd ed.). Boston: Little, Brown, 1971.

35. Meltzer, M., Franklin, E. C., Elias, K., McCluskey, R. T., and Cooper, H. Cryoglobulinemia—a clinical and laboratory study. *Am. J. Med.* 40:837, 1969.

36. Whitsed, H. M., and Penny, R. IgA/IgG cryoglobulinemia with vasculitis. *Clin. Exp. Immunol.* 9:183, 1971.

37. McIntosh, R. M., Kaufman, D. B., and Kulinskas, C. Cryoglobulins. I. Studies on the nature, incidence and clinical significance of serum cryoproteins in glomerulonephritis. *J. Lab. Clin. Med.* 75:566, 1970.

38. Winchester, R. J., Kunkel, H. G., and Agnello, V. Occurrence of γ-globulin complexes in serum and joint fluid of rheumatoid arthritis patients: Use of monoclonal rheumatoid factors as reagents for their demonstration. *J. Exp. Med.* 134[Suppl.]:286, 1971.

39. McIntosh, R. M., and Grossman, B. IgG, β_1C, fibrinogen and cryoprotein in acute glomerulonephritis. *N. Engl. J. Med.* 285:1521, 1971.

40. Cawley, L. P. *Electrophoresis and Immunoelectrophoresis.* Boston: Little, Brown, 1969.

41. McKay, G. G. Practical Applications of Immunoelectrophoresis. In H. Dettelbach and S. E. Ritzmann, *Lab Synopsis,* Vol. 2 (2nd ed.). Somerville, N.J.: Behring Diagnostics, 1969. Pp. 1–8.

42. Ritzmann, S. E., Lawrence, M. C., and Daniels, J. C. Serum Protein Analysis—Immunoelectrophoresis. In J. B. Fuller (Ed.), *Selected Topics in Clinical Chemistry* (3rd ed.). Chicago: American Society of Clinical Pathologists' Commission on Continuing Education. 1972. P. 148.

43. Agnello, V., Winchester, R. J., and Kunkel, H. G. Precipitin reactions of the C1q component of complement with aggregated γ-globulin and immune complexes in gel diffusion. *Immunology* 19:909, 1970.

44. Agnello, V., Koffler, D., Eisenberg, J. W., Winchester, R. J., and Kunkel, H. G. C1q precipitins in the sera of patients with systemic lupus erythematosus and other hypocomplementemic states: Characterization of high and low molecular weight types. *J. Exp. Med.* 134[Suppl.]: 228, 1971.

45. Penttinen, K., Vaheri, A., and Myllylä, G. Detection and characterization of immune complexes by the platelet aggregation test. I. Complexes formed in vitro. *Clin. Exp. Immunol.* 8:389, 1971.

46. Myllylä, G., Vaheri, A., and Penttinen, K. Detection and characterization of immune complexes by the platelet aggregation test. II. Circulating Complexes. *Clin. Exp. Immunol.* 8:399, 1971.

47. Britton, M. C., and Schur, P. H. The complement system in rheumatoid synovitis. II. Intracytoplasmic inclusions of immunoglobulins and complement. *Arthritis Rheum.* 14:87, 1971.

48. Franco, A. E., and Schur, P. H. Hypocomplementemia in rheumatoid arthritis. *Arthritis Rheum.* 14:231, 1971.

49. Estes, D., and Christian, C. L. The natural history of systemic lupus erythematosus by prospective analysis. *Medicine* (Baltimore) 50:85, 1971.

50. Burnet, M. Implications for autoimmune disease in man. Studies on NZB mice and their hybrids. II. Renal and thymic disease. *R. Inst. Public Health Hyg. J.* 29:95, 1966.

51. Lewis, R. M., and Schwartz, R. S. Canine systemic lupus erythematosus. Genetic analysis of an established breeding colony. *J. Exp. Med.* 134:417, 1971.

52. Dubois, E. L. *Lupus Erythematosus.* New York: McGraw-Hill, 1966.

53. Tan, E. M. Antibodies to deoxyribonucleic acid irradiated with ultra-

violet light: Detection by precipitin and immunofluorescence. *Science* 161:1353, 1968.

54. Tan, E. M., and Stoughton, R. B. Ultraviolet light induced damage to desoxyribonucleic acid in human skin. *J. Invest. Dermatol.* 52:537, 1969.

55. Tan, E. M., Freeman, R. G., and Stoughton, R. B. Action spectrum of ultraviolet light induced damage to nuclear DNA in vivo. *J. Invest. Dermatol.* 55:439, 1970.

56. Freeman, R. G., Knox, J. M., and Owens, D. W. Cutaneous lesions of lupus erythematosus induced by monochromatic light. *Arch. Dermatol.* 99:677, 1969.

57. Barnett, E. V., Kantor, G., Bickel, Y. B., Forsen, R., and Gonick, H. C. Systemic lupus erythematosus. *Calif. Med.* 11:467, 1969.

58. Percy, J. S., and Smyth, C. J. The immunofluorescent skin test in systemic lupus erythematosus. *J.A.M.A.* 208:485, 1969.

59. Tan, E. M., and Kunkel, H. G. An immunofluorescent study of the skin lesions in systemic lupus erythematosus. *Arthritis Rheum.* 9:37, 1966.

60. Stastny, P., and Ziff, M. Cold-insoluble complexes and complement levels in systemic lupus erythematosus. *N. Engl. J. Med.* 280:1376, 1969.

61. Pensky, J., Hinz, C. F., Todd, E. W., Wedgwood, R. J., Boyer, J. T., and Lepow, I. H. Properties of highly purified human properdin. *J. Immunol.* 100:142, 1968.

62. Rothfield, N., Ross, H. A., Menta, J. O., and Lepow, I. H. Glomerular and dermal deposition of properdin in systemic lupus erythematosus. *N. Engl. J. Med.* 287:681, 1972.

63. Sliwinski, A. J., and Zvaifler, N. J. Decreased synthesis of the third component of complement (C3) in hypocomplementic systemic lupus erythematosus. *Clin. Exp. Immunol.* 11:21, 1972.

64. Goldman, J. A., Litwen, A., Adams, L. E., Krueger, R. C., and Hess, E. V. Cellular immunity to nuclear antigens in systemic lupus erythematosus. *J. Clin. Invest.* 51:2669, 1972.

65. Horwitz, D. A. Impaired delayed hypersensitivity in systemic lupus erythematosus. *Arthritis Rheum.* 15:353, 1972.

66. Bitter, T., Bitter, R., Silberschmidt, R., and Dubois, E. L. In vivo and in vitro study of cell mediated immunity (CMI) during the onset of systemic lupus erythematosus (SLE). *Arthritis Rheum.* 14:152 (abst.), 1971.

67. Terasaki, P. I., Mottironi, V. D., and Barnett, E. V. Cytotoxins in disease—autocytotoxins in lupus. *N. Engl. J. Med.* 283:724, 1970.

68. Butler, W. T., Sharp, J. T., Rossen, R. D., Lidsky, M. D., Mittal, K. K., and Gard, D. A. Relationship of the clinical course of systemic lupus erythematosus to the presence of circulating lymphocytoxic antibodies. *Arthritis Rheum.* 15:231, 1972.

69. Grumet, F. C., Coukell, A., Bodmer, J. E., Bodmer, W. F., and McDevitt, H. O. Histocompatibility (HL-A) antigens associated with systemic lupus erythematosus. *N. Engl. J. Med.* 285:193, 1971.

70. McDevitt, H. O., and Benacerraf, B. Genetic Control of Specific Immune responses. In F. J. Dixon, Jr., and H. G. Kunkel (Eds.), *Advances in Immunology,* Vol. 11. New York: Academic, 1969. P. 31.

71. Kavano, K., Miller, L., and Kimmelstill, P. Virus-like structures in lupus erythematosus. *N. Engl. J. Med.* 281:1228, 1969.

72. Grausz, H., Earley, L. E., Stephens, B. E., Stephen, B. G., Lee, J. C., and Hopper, J., Jr. Diagnostic import of virus-like particles in the glomerular endothelium of patients with systemic lupus erythematosus. *N. Engl. J. Med.* 283:506, 1970.

73. Andres, G. A., Spiele, H., and McClusky, R. T. Virus-like Structures in Systemic Lupus Erythematosus. In R. S. Schwartz (Ed.), *Progress in Clinical Immunology*, Vol. 1. New York: Grune & Stratton, 1972. P. 23.

74. Talal, M. Immunologic and viral factors in the pathogenesis of systemic lupus erythematosus. *Arthritis Rheum.* 13:887, 1970.

75. Nakamura, R. M., and Allen, H. J. Laboratory tests for the diagnosis of systemic lupus erythematosus and related disorders. *Cutis* 11:655, 1973.

76. Tan, E. M., and Kunkel, H. G. Characteristics of a soluble nuclear antigen precipitating with sera of patients with systemic lupus erythematosus. *J. Immunol.* 96:464, 1966.

77. Koffler, D., et al. Antibodies to polynucleotides in human sera: Antigenic specificity and relation to disease. *J. Exp. Med.* 134:294, 1971.

78. Sharp, G. C., Irvin, W. C., Tan, E. M., Gould, R. G., and Holman, H. R. Mixed connective tissue disease: An apparently distinct rheumatic disease syndrome associated with a specific antibody to an extractable nuclear antigen (ENA). *Am. J. Med.* 52:148, 1972.

79. Ritchie, R. F. Antinucleolar antibodies. *N. Engl. J. Med.* 282:1174, 1970.

80. Hargraves, M. M., Richmond, H., and Morton, R. Presentation of two bone marrow elements: the "Tart" cell and the "LE" cell. *Mayo Clin. Proc.* 23:25, 1948.

81. Miescher, P. Mise an evidence du facteur LE par la réaction de consommation d'anti-globuline. *Vox Sang.* 5:116, 1955.

82. Dubois, E. L., Drexler, E., and Arterberry, J. D. A latex nucleoprotein test for diagnosis of systemic lupus erythematosus: A comparative evaluation. *J.A.M.A.* 177:141, 1961.

83. Lawlis, J. F. Serological detection of desoxyribonucleic acid (DNA) adsorbed to formalized erythrocytes. *Proc. Soc. Exp. Biol. Med.* 98:300, 1958.

84. Koffler, D., Carr, R., Agnello, V., Thoburn, R., and Kunkel, H. G. Antibodies to polynucleotides in human sera: Antigenic specificity and relation to disease. *J. Exp. Med.* 134:294, 1971.

85. Inami, Y. H., Nakamura, R. M., and Tan, E. M. Microhemagglutination test for the simultaneous detection of antibodies to native and denatured DNA and for the determination of circulating serum DNA. *J. Immunol. Methods* 3:287, 1973.

86. Wold, R. T., Young, F. E., Tan, E. M., and Farr, R. S. Deoxyribonucleic acid antibody: A method to detect its primary interaction with deoxyribonucleic acid. *Science* 161:806, 1968.

87. Pincus, T., Schur, P., Rose, J. A., Decker, J. L., and Talal, N. Measurement of serum DNA-binding activity in systemic lupus erythematosus. *N. Engl. J. Med.* 281:701, 1969.

88. Carr, R. I., Koffler, D., Agnello, V., and Kunkel, H. G. Studies on DNA antibodies using DNA labeled with actinomycin-D (3H) or dimethyl (3H) sulfate. *Clin. Exp. Immunol.* 4:527, 1969.

89. Beck, J. S. Antinuclear antibodies: Methods of detection and significance. *Mayo. Clin. Proc.* 44:600, 1969.

90. Benson, M. D., and Cohen, A. S.   Antinuclear antibodies in systemic lupus erythematosus. *Ann. Intern. Med.* 73:943, 1970.
91. Dorling, J., Johnson, G. D., Webb, J. A., and Smith, M. E.   Use of peroxidase conjugated antiglobulin as an alternative to immunofluorescence for the detection of antinuclear factor in serum. *J. Clin. Pathol.* 24:501, 1971.
92. Beerman, H.   The L.E. cell and phenomenon in lupus erythematosus. *Am. J. Med. Sci.* 222:473, 1951.
93. Haserick, J. R.   Evaluation of three diagnostic procedures for systemic lupus erythematosus. *Ann. Intern. Med.* 44:497, 1956.
94. Hargraves, M. M.   The LE cell phenomenon. *Adv. Intern. Med.* 6:133, 1954.
95. Hargraves, M. M.   The discovery of the LE cell and its morphology. *Mayo Clin. Proc.* 44:579, 1969.
96. Hargraves, M. M., Richmond, H., and Morton, R.   Presentation of two bone marrow elements: The "Tart" cell and the LE cell. *Proc. Staff Mayo Clin.* 23:25, 1948.
97. Miale, J. B.   *Laboratory Medicine: Hematology* (4th ed.). St. Louis: Mosby, 1972. P. 919.
98. Dubois, E. L., and Strain, L.   SLE latex test kit. *J.A.M.A.* 14:205, 1974.
99. Sharp, G. C., Irvin, W. S., LaRoque, R. L., Velez, C., Daly, V., Kaiser, A. D., and Holman, H. R.   Association of autoantibodies to different nuclear antigens with clinical patterns of rheumatic disease and responsiveness to therapy. *J. Clin. Invest.* 50:350, 1971.
100. Barnett, E. V., Condemi, J. J., Leddy, J. P., and Vaughan, J. H.   Gamma 2, gamma 1A, and gamma 1M antinuclear factors in human sera. *J. Clin. Invest.* 43:1104, 1964.
101. Tan, E. M.   Relationship of nuclear staining patterns with precipitating antibodies in systemic lupus erythematosus. *J. Clin. Lab. Med.* 70: 800, 1967.
102. Tan, E. M., Northway, J. D., and Pinnas, J. L.   The clinical significance of antinuclear antibodies. *Postgrad. Med.* 54:143, 1974.
103. Hijmans, W., Schmit, H. R. E., Mandema, E., Niehuis, R. L. F., Feltkamp, T. E. W., Holborow, E. J., and Johnson, G. D.   Comparative study of the detection of antinuclear factors with the fluorescent antibody technique. *Ann. Rheum. Dis.* 23:73, 1964.
104. TenVeen, J. H., and Feltkamp, T. E. W.   Formalized chicken red cell nuclei as a simple antigen for standardized antinuclear factor determination. *Clin. Exp. Immunol.* 5:673, 1969.
105. Alexander, W. R. M., Bremner, J. M., and Duthie, J. J. R.   Incidence of the antinuclear factor in human sera. *Ann. Rheum. Dis.* 19:338, 1960.
106. Blundell, G. P.   Fluorescent Antibody Methods. In M. Stefanini (Ed.), *Progress in Clinical Pathology,* Vol. 3. New York: Grune & Stratton, 1970. P. 211.
107. Muna, N. M., Verner, J. L., and Hammond, D. F.   Fluorescent antibody technique as a routine procedure in the diagnosis of lupus erythematosus using stored tissue culture cells. *Am. J. Clin. Pathol.* 45:117, 1966.
108. Cleymaet, J. E., and Nakamura, R. M.   Indirect immunofluorescent antinuclear tests: Comparison of sensitivity and specificity of different substrates. *Am. J. Clin. Pathol.* 58:388, 1972.

109. Tan, E. M.   Personal communication, 1972.
110. Barnett, E. V.   Diagnostic aspects of lupus erythematosus cells and antinuclear factors in disease states. *Mayo Clin. Proc.* 44:645, 1969.
111. Kaplan, M. E.   Antinuclear antibodies in infectious mononucleosis. *Lancet* 1:561, 1966.
112. Beck, J. S.   Autoantibodies to cell nuclei. *Scott. Med. J.* 8:373, 1963.
113. Zvaifler, H. J.   Immunoreactants in rheumatoid synovial lesions. *J. Exp. Med.* 134[Suppl.]:276, 1971.
114. Zvaifler, H. J.   The Immunopathology of Joint Inflammation in Rheumatoid Arthritis. In F. J. Dixon and H. G. Kunkel (Eds.), *Advances in Immunology*, Vol. 16. New York: Academic, 1973. P. 256.
115. Marcus, R. L., and Townes, A. S.   The occurrence of cryoproteins in synovial fluid; the association of a complement-fixing activity in rheumatoid synovial fluid with the cold precipitable protein. *J. Clin. Invest.* 50:282, 1971.
116. Freyberg, R. H.   Differential diagnosis of arthritis. *Postgrad. Med.* 51:20, 1972.
117. Lawrence, J. S., Locke, G. B., and Ball, J.   Rheumatoid serum factor in population in the U. K.   I. Lung disease and rheumatoid serum factor. *Clin. Exp. Immunol.* 8:723, 1971.
118. Ashe, W. K., Daniels, C. A., Scott, G. S., and Notkins, A. L.   Interaction of rheumatoid factor with infectious herpes simplex virus-antibody complexes. *Science* 172:176, 1971.
119. Notkins, A. L.   Infectious virus-antibody complexes. *J. Exp. Med.* 134[Suppl.]:41, 1971.
120. Chayen, J., and Bitensky, L.   Lysosomal enzymes in inflammation. *Ann. Rheum. Dis.* 30:522, 1971.
121. Phillips, P. E.   Virologic studies in rheumatoid arthritis and other connective tissue diseases. *J. Exp. Med.* 134[Suppl.]:313, 1971.
122. Singer, J. M., and Plotz, C. M.   The latex fixation test. I. Application to the serologic diagnosis of rheumatoid arthritis. *Am. J. Med.* 21:888, 1956.
123. Waller, M.   Methods of measurement of rheumatoid factor. *Ann. N.Y. Acad. Sci.* 168:5, 1969.
124. Cats, A., and Klein, F.   Quantitative aspects of the latex fixation and Waaler-Rose test. *Ann. Rheum. Dis.* 29:663, 1970.
125. Jones, W. L., and Wiggins, G. L.   A study of rheumatoid arthritis latex kits. *Am. J. Clin. Pathol.* 60:703, 1973.
126. Ropes, M. W., Bennett, G. A., Cobb, S., Jacox, R. F., and Jessar, R. A.   Proposed diagnostic criteria for rheumatoid arthritis. *Bull. Rheum. Dis.* 9:175, 1958.
127. Rose, H. M., Ragan, C., Pearce, E., and Lipman, M. O.   Differential agglutination of normal and sensitized sheep erythrocytes by sera of patients with rheumatoid arthritis. *Proc. Soc. Exp. Biol. Med.* 68:1, 1948.
128. Waaler, E.   On the occurrence of a factor in human serum activating the specific agglutination of sheep blood corpuscles. *Acta Pathol. Microbiol. Scand.* 17:172, 1940.
129. Anderson, S. G., Bentzon, M. W., Houba, V., and Krage, B.   International reference preparation of rheumatoid arthritis serum. *Bull. W. H. O.* 42:311, 1970.
130. Dequeker, J., Van Noyen, R., and Vandipitte, J.   Age-related rheuma-

toid factors: Incidence and characteristics. *Ann. Rheum. Dis.* 28:431, 1969.

131. Hooper, B., Whittingham, S., Mathews, J. D., MacKay, I. R., and Curnow, D. H. Autoimmunity in a rural community. *Clin. Exp. Immunol.* 12:79, 1972.

132. Sharp, J. T., Calkins, E., Cohen, A. S., Schubart, A. F., and Calabro, J. J. Observations on the clinical, chemical and serological manifestations of rheumatoid arthritis based on the course of 154 cases. *Medicine* (Baltimore) 43:41, 1964.

133. Panush, R. S., Bianco, H. E., and Schur, P. H. Serum and synovial fluid IgG, IgA and IgM antiglobulins in rheumatoid arthritis. *Arthritis Rheum.* 14:737, 1971.

134. Hollingsworth, J. W. *Local and Systemic Complications of Rheumatoid Arthritis.* Philadelphia: Saunders, 1968.

Acute-Phase Proteins

18

Craig L. Fischer and Charles W. Gill

Although many more elaborate indicators of inflammatory disease have been described, the clinical findings of fever, leukocytosis, and an increased erythrocyte sedimentation rate (ESR) are the acute-phase phenomena most often relied upon to define the active state of inflammation. Fever has been almost synonymous with disease for centuries, whereas the laboratory-oriented measurements are of more recent origin. At present, the acute-phase proteins (acute-phase protein reactants) are being utilized to assess certain disease states.

The acute-phase proteins (see Appendix) constitute an electrophoretically heterogeneous group of glycoproteins that migrate between the albumin and γ-globulin fractions (Fig. 18-1). They are functionally diverse and consist of a protease inhibitor (α_1-antitrypsin), carrier proteins for hemoglobin (haptoglobin) and copper (ceruloplasmin), a protein that is essential in the clotting mechanism (fibrinogen), and proteins whose functions are less well defined, such as C-reactive protein and α_1-acid glycoprotein (Table 18-1). These acute-phase proteins are valuable in the detection, diagnosis, prognosis, and therapeutic monitoring of diseases involving tissue damage and inflammation. They offer a more specific approach to the assessment of certain disease processes than the acute-phase phenomena of fever and leukocytosis alone. When placed in perspective, a typical acute-phase reaction has a configuration as shown in Figure 18-2.

Fever

Fever is a common response to tissue injury and inflammation. It is now known that phagocytic cells, such as polymorphonuclear leukocytes and fixed tissue macrophages, have the ability to elaborate a substance called *endogenous pyrogen* (EP) [1]. This substance in turn is sensed by the anterior hypothalamus and a sequence of events is initiated that results in fever. Various stimuli can cause the phagocytes to elaborate EP, such as bacteria, endotoxins, antigen-antibody complexes, and tissue necrosis [1]. Febrile states may also exist that are unassociated with these usual stimuli (e.g., pheochromocytoma, hyperetiocholanolonism, thyroid storm, certain brain lesions, and heat stroke).

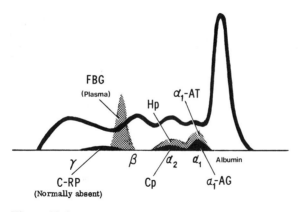

Figure 18-1
Electrophoretic distribution of the acute-phase proteins—α_1-acid glycoprotein, α_1-antitrypsin, ceruloplasmin, C-RP, and fibrinogen—and their relative contributions. α_1AG: α_1-acid glycoprotein; α_1AT: α_1-antitrypsin; Cp: ceruloplasmin; C-RP: C-reactive protein; FBG: fibrinogen.

Leukocytosis

Secondary leukocytosis, as indicated by a white blood cell count of more than 10,000 per cubic millimeter, is a common accompaniment of inflammation and, in the acute-phase process, is usually secondary to an absolute increase in neutrophilic granulocytes (see Fig. 18-2). The stimuli for leukocytosis are diverse and rather nonspecific. Strenuous exercise, toxicity, alterations in cardiac rhythm (paroxysmal tachycardia), pregnancy, localized inflammation, and acute bleeding are a few of the many clinical entities associated with leukocytosis. In overwhelming infection (e.g., septicemia) and certain specific infectious diseases (e.g., typhoid, paratyphoid, or viral diseases), leukopenia (a white blood cell count of less than 4000 per cubic millimeter) rather than leukocytosis is often found [2]. Patients with bone marrow depression and profound leukocytopenia are unable to exhibit a leukocytic response to infection, and therefore white blood cell counts are of little aid in monitoring these individuals. These factors combined tend to limit the usefulness of leukocytosis as an overall reliable indicator of disease processes involving tissue necrosis and inflammation.

Erythrocyte Sedimentation Rate (ESR)

ESR has been used clinically to assess the activity of some diseases that involve inflammation, tissue necrosis, or both. The sedimentation rate is directly related to red cell aggregates and the number of erythrocytes per aggregate [3]. Haptoglobin has an augmenting effect on the ESR (particularly the haptoglobin 2-2 species), as do IgG and ceruloplasmin [4]. However, the principal protein constituent that is responsible for an accelerated ESR is fibrinogen [5]. The interactions among ESR, fibrino-

Table 18-1. Characteristics of Acute-Phase Proteins

Protein	Molecular Weight	$S_{20,w}$	Electrophoretic Mobility	Peptide Content (%)	Carbohydrate Content (%)	Normal Median (mg/100 ml)	Serum Content Range[a] (mg/100 ml)	Biological Function
C-Reactive protein	135,000–140,000	7.5	α_1-Globulin	100	0	0.5	0	Opsonin; acute-phase reactant
α_1-Acid glycoprotein	44,100	3.1	α_1-Globulin	62	41.4	72	55–120	Inactivation of progesterone; acute-phase reactant
α_1-Antitrypsin	45,000	3.4	α_1-Globulin⁻	86	12.4	245	180–305	Protease inhibitor of trypsin and chymotrypsin; acute-phase reactant
Ceruloplasmin	160,000	7.1	α_2-Globulin	89	8.0	35	10–40	Copper-binding oxidase activity; acute-phase reactant
Haptoglobin 1-1 Haptoglobin 2-1 Haptoglobin 2-2	85,000	4.4 4.3–6.5 7.5	α_2-Globulin	81	19.3	160	85–213	Hemoglobin-binding peroxidase; acute-phase reactant
Fibrinogen	341,000	7.6	β_2-Globulin	97	2.5	300	200–450	Coagulable protein; acute-phase reactant

[a] $N = 274$; age range, 35–65 years.

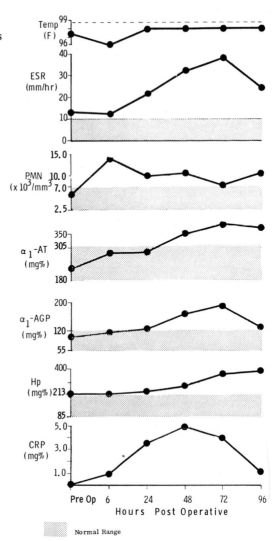

Figure 18-2
Acute-phase protein levels
in uncomplicated surgery.

gen, α-globulins, C-reactive protein, and the white blood cell count are seen in Table 18-2. From these simultaneously acquired data it can be concluded that a significant intercorrelation exists among the ESR, α-globulins (i.e., fractions containing ceruloplasmin and haptoglobin), and fibrinogen. The C-reactive protein, does not correlate significantly with any of these parameters, which suggests that C-reactive protein either responds to different stimuli or responds in a different time frame. Unfortunately, many other factors that are independent of inflammation affect the ESR. Macrocytosis, spherocytosis, hypercholesterolemia, cryo-globulinemia, polycythemia, anemia, and age are but a few of the com-plexing variables encountered when using ESR as a guide to the presence of active inflammation and tissue necrosis [5].

Table 18-2. Intercorrelation of Acute-Phase Phenomena[a]

	ESR	WBC	α-Proteins	C-RP	Fibrinogen
ESR	1.00	—	—	—	—
WBC	0.05	1.00	—	—	—
α-Proteins	0.58[b]	0.18	1.00	—	—
C-RP	0.34	0.17	0.41	1.00	—
Fibrinogen	0.73[b]	0.048	0.77[b]	0.00	1.00

[a] Linear regression analysis correlating ESR, WBC count, α-globulins, C-RP, and fibrinogen in 18 patients.
[b] Significant correlation. Positive correlation at the 0.5 level is denoted by a coefficient of correlation greater than 0.468.

Acute-Phase Proteins

α_1-ACID GLYCOPROTEIN

The biological properties of α_1-acid glycoprotein are little understood; however, this protein is associated with the inactivation of progesterone and it participates in the acute-phase protein response to inflammation. This protein is normally elevated in the last trimester of pregnancy [6]. It is suspected that α_1-acid glycoprotein is polymorphic in man [7], and it is probable that its sialic acid content varies in certain disease states [7]. Genetic studies are not yet complete; however, types 1, 2, and 3 have been described, based on the electrophoretic properties of α_1-acid glycoprotein at pH 4.8 [7, 8]. It is also probable that α_1-acid glycoprotein exhibits variant molecular forms depending on the body site where it is found [4]. α_1-acid glycoprotein is found in sputum samples in trace amounts; however, in alveolar carcinoma, it is reported to be present in relatively high amounts [4]. α_1-acid glycoprotein is known to be produced primarily by the liver, and it is always present at birth [16]. The plasma half-life has been determined to be 5.2 days with 11.5 to 14 percent of the body pool degraded per day [16]. As interesting and potentially informative as these facts are for the protein chemist and geneticist, one must not lose sight of the fact that α_1-acid glycoprotein, as measured immunologically [9], can serve as a responsive indicator of inflammation or tissue necrosis, or both.

α_1-ANTITRYPSIN

α_1-Antitrypsin is a protease inhibitor (see Chap. 15) that protects against autodigestion of body tissues by the enzymes trypsin and chymotrypsin [4]. This protease inhibitor plays a particularly important role in the protection of lung tissue against damage by endogenously released trypsin. The lung is the site of significant leukocyte degradation with the subsequent release of leukocyte-derived proteases, particularly trypsin. In the condition of congenital α_1-antitrypsin deficiency, lung damage by endogenously produced trypsin does occur and can result in juvenile emphysema. α_1-antitrypsin is known to be produced by the liver; however, other important sources, which have not yet been delineated, may also produce significant amounts of this protein [10, 4]. This protein is present in the serum of term babies and even premature infants [4].

CERULOPLASMIN

Ceruloplasmin is an α_2-globulin that has oxidase activity and is responsible for transporting copper (see Chap. 14). Although chromatographic and electrophoretic heterogeneity have been demonstrated [4], the natural lability of this protein has always cast some doubt on these findings [11]. Ceruloplasmin is found in small quantity in the 17-week-old fetus; it is easily demonstrated in the plasma of 24-week-old fetuses, and, at term, approximately one-third of the normal adult level is present [16]. The concentration of ceruloplasmin is significantly increased by estrogen and estrogen-containing medications [12]. Because of the number of women on oral contraceptives, pregnant women, and elderly patients on therapeutic regimens of estrogen, the diagnostic and prognostic usefulness of ceruloplasmin as an acute-phase protein is limited. It may still be of some service, however, if applied appropriately to male patients.

HAPTOGLOBIN

Haptoglobin is the hemoglobin-binding protein (see Chap. 14). When hemoglobin is released intravascularly from erythrocytes, it is bound by haptoglobin, forming haptoglobin-hemoglobin complexes. These complexes are then removed by the reticuloendothelial system, specifically by the Kupffer's cells of the liver [13], thereby effecting a conservation of the body's iron stores. Three genetically determined forms (sequential primary allomeres) of haptoglobin have been described [16]. These phenotypes have been designated 1-1, 1-2, and 2-2, with the allomere 1-1 the most common form. Functionally, the hemoglobin-binding properties vary among these phenotypes [14], and the commercial antibody reagents used in quantitative haptoglobin determinations have their greatest specificity for the 1-1 form. These facts suggest that both the hemoglobin-binding and immunological analytical methods could yield spurious values; however, this does not appear to be a practical problem in assessing haptoglobin in the acute-phase protein response. Haptoglobin is produced primarily in the liver, although some authors have suggested that the spleen and bone marrow also participate in its synthesis [4]. Haptoglobin is not detected in 14- to 23-week-old fetuses, and is found only in small amounts in 10 percent of babies at term [4]. The plasma half-life has been determined to be 3.5 to 4.0 days [4].

FIBRINOGEN

Fibrinogen is of primary importance as a clotting factor (Factor I), and, although it responds as an acute-phase protein, several points detract from its routine use in evaluating inflammatory disease states. Fibrinogen can only be evaluated in plasma samples, whereas the other acute-phase proteins can be assayed in both serum and plasma. Hemorrhage and certain coagulopathies (e.g., disseminated intravascular coagulopathy or consumptive coagulopathy) may also present confounding factors when using fibrinogen determinations in the evaluation of an acute-phase response. Because of the significance of fibrinogen in the ESR, any variable that affects fibrinogen can likewise impair the reliability of the ESR as a measurement of acute-phase phenomena.

C-REACTIVE PROTEIN (C-RP)
C-reactive protein holds a unique position among the acute-phase proteins. The usual methods employed for C-RP detection (e.g., latex agglutination and radial immunodiffusion) are insensitive to the amounts found in normal individuals. The C-polysaccharide of *Pneumococcus* was described first by Tillet and Francis in 1930 [15]. However, it was not until 1941, that MacLeod and Avery [16] noted that in certain patients with acute inflammation, a serum protein was found that reacted with this C-polysaccharide. This protein was termed *C-reactive protein,* and at first it was thought to be specific for patients with pneumococcal infections. This contention has subsequently been dispelled, and the relative nonspecificity of C-RP is now recognized. C-RP is known to exhibit microheterogeneity, and it therefore probably represents a family of closely related proteins [4]. In patients free of inflammation or tissue necrosis, C-RP is either absent from the serum or present in concentrations below 0.5 mg per 100 ml. Neonates born with inflammatory disease processes can show elevations in C-RP; however, maternal infections associated with elevated C-RP values will not be reflected in the sera of the newborn [4]. C-RP values in cerebrospinal fluid may be reflections of the serum levels at the time of sampling; therefore, serum values must be determined simultaneously with those in the CSF. Skin bullae often closely reflect the serum protein patterns, and it is therefore common to find C-RP in bullous fluid aspirated from patients with thermal burns, pemphigus vulgaris, and other bullous lesions [4].

Physiological and Pathophysiological Aspects

MECHANISMS OF THE ACUTE-PHASE RESPONSE
The mechanisms leading to an increase of acute-phase proteins have been the subject of considerable debate. The notion that these glycoproteins are released locally from affected tissues in the area adjacent to acute inflammation has been discussed [17]. More recently, by using isotope-labeling techniques and isolated perfused liver preparations, it has been demonstrated that the proteins are produced in the liver and released into the hepatic circulation [18]. These studies have also shown conclusively that the increase of acute-phase proteins is the result of an increased synthesis rate. Beyond the fact that the acute-phase proteins are produced in the liver and that their increased serum concentrations reflect increased synthesis, the exact details are little understood. Although the levels of these glycoproteins rise after tissue necrosis and inflammation, additional factors may modify their kinetics. Regulators

such as adrenal steroids [19, 20], as well as the possible role of inhibitors and hormones such as insulin, growth hormone, parathyroid extracts [21], and thyroid-stimulating hormone [22] must be considered.

Irrespective of the complexities involved in the modulation of individual acute-phase proteins, the inciting cause appears to be inflammation and tissue damage; however, the role of leukocytosis in the acute-phase protein response is controversial [23]. It is possible that inflammation is only a sequel or an additive factor to the acute-phase protein phenomenon. At the ultrastructural organelle and biochemical levels, the lysosomes and their enzymes appear to be instrumental in eliciting an acute-phase protein response. Recent data suggest that disruption of the cellular lysosomes is an early step in a series of events leading to the eventual stimulation of acute-phase protein synthesis [24]. Although incompletely investigated, a connection between prostaglandins (PGA_1) and acute-phase protein response warrants consideration, since injured tissue it known to release prostaglandins that are also leukotactic [25, 26]. Additionally, the possible effects of endotoxins must be considered, since endotoxin shock may be associated with an acute-phase protein response and increased amounts of PGA_1 [27].

In general, the response of the acute-phase proteins as a class remains obscure. It has been suggested that these proteins serve as inhibitors or neutralizing agents for lysosomal enzymes that are released during tissue necrosis and acute inflammation [24]. Such an action would provide a feedback mechanism relating lysosomal enzyme production and the ensuing acute-phase reactants in general body defense against cell injury. Recently, evidence has been presented that C-RP is an opsonin that can bind to certain bacteria in the presence of calcium ion, and thereby enhance the phagocytosis of several bacterial species [28].

TIME-COURSE PROFILES
The time-concentration profiles of the acute-phase response vary for the different proteins as seen in Figure 18-2 [29, 30]. In general, when tissue necrosis (with or without inflammation) has become established, the serum concentrations of C-RP and α_1-acid glycoprotein begin to increase rapidly within 6 to 8 hours and reach maximum levels between 48 and 72 hours. This is followed by increases in the concentration of haptoglobin, ceruloplasmin, and α_1-antitrypsin as early as 12 to 24 hours, with maximum levels usually occurring between 72 and 96 hours. It is this "time-phasing" that led to the designation of *acute-phase protein* response.

As long as active tissue destruction is present, C-RP and α_1-acid glycoprotein will remain elevated and in proportional concentration to the extent of tissue damage. C-RP levels closely parallel the clinical course, and therefore it is presumed that this protein has a relatively short biological half-life. This in turn suggests a large reserve capacity for synthesis of this protein. As the disease process resolves, the C-RP and α_1-acid glycoprotein levels decrease rapidly, whereas the haptoglobin, ceruloplasmin, and α_1-antitrypsin levels decrease at a slower rate.

The maximum amplitudes of the acute-phase protein response vary somewhat from patient to patient, but they usually will reach the maxima between 2 and 4 days after a definite inciting episode [31]. Prolonged elevation of acute-phase proteins is a clue that the tissue injury process is still active.

Clinical Implications and Diagnostic and Prognostic Aspects

PRINCIPLES OF CLINICAL APPLICATION
Several general principles relating to the specific uses of acute-phase proteins in clinical medicine must be considered:

1. Single or widely-spaced determinations of acute-phase proteins are of limited help. The presence or absence of an inflammatory process can be assessed by isolated measurements, but in dynamic clinical situations, serial determinations at appropriate times (i.e., acute-phase protein profiles; see Figure 18-2) can provide important diagnostic and prognostic information that would be unobtainable by single, random determinations.
2. It is important to quantitate precisely the acute-phase proteins, since small incremental changes can be of clinical significance. Frequently employed semiquantitative methods are inadequate for proper utilization of the informational content inherent in acute-phase protein profiles.
3. The significance of acute-phase proteins is best evaluated in terms of a group, e.g., α_1-acid glycoprotein, α_1-antitrypsin, haptoglobin, and C-RP.

DETERMINATION OF ACUTE-PHASE PROTEINS

IMMUNOLOGICAL TECHNIQUES
Immunological methods for the quantitation of proteins have allowed widespread investigation of acute-phase reactants in clinical medicine (see Chap. 4). With the advent of radial immunodiffusion (RID) and electroimmunodiffusion (EID), precise and accurate quantitation of acute-phase proteins has become possible. It is important to note that the EID method lends itself best to the quantitation of acute-phase protein phenomena, since the time interval between sample acquisition and reporting is considerably shorter than with RID (e.g., 30 minutes versus 6 to 24 hours) [9]. The rapidity of EID permits the physician to utilize the acute-phase phenomena for the solution of timely clinical problems within a time frame approaching that of the white blood cell and differential counts (see Table 18-1 for normal values).

OTHER ASSAYS
C-RP has, for many years, been detected by means of a latex agglutination test or a precipitation test. The latter test is time-consuming and only

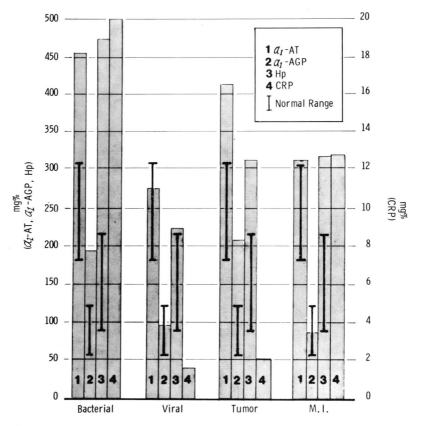

Figure 18-3
Acute-phase protein responses to four different categories of inflammation:
bacterial infection with inflammation, viral infection (exclusive of viral hepatitis), tumor with necrosis and inflammation (without bacterial infection),
and a sterile inflammatory process without tumor necrosis. *M.I.:* myocardial
infarction.

marginally quantitative, whereas the former test, although rapid, can
be capricious and is only semiquantitative at best.

INDICATIONS FOR ACUTE-PHASE PROTEIN PROFILES
Acute-phase protein evaluations can be utilized effectively to answer
several clinical questions: Is an active inflammatory process (or tissue
necrosis) ongoing? If inflammation is present, what is the trend? Although the acute-phase protein responses are nonspecific phenomena,
when used quantitatively they are relatively precise indicators of active
inflammation. As a group, they appear to show fewer spurious or unin-
terruptable vacillations than the often utilized indicators for inflammation, e.g., the ESR and white blood cell count (WBC). Patients with

Table 18-3. Analysis of Variance between Highest Mean Values of Acute-Phase Proteins in Three Types of Inflammation[a]

Protein	Bacterial (N = 20)	Viral (N = 20)	Tumor (N = 10)
α_1-Antitrypsin			
Bacterial	< .05	—	—
Viral	> .05[b]	< .05	—
Tumor	< .05	> .05[b]	> .05[b]
α-Acid Glycoprotein			
Bacterial	> .05[b]	—	—
Viral	< .05	> .05[b]	—
Tumor	> .05[b]	< .05	> .05[b]
Haptoglobin			
Bacterial	< .05	—	—
Viral	< .05	> .05[b]	—
Tumor	> .05[b]	> .05[b]	> .05[b]
C-RP			
Bacterial	< .05	—	—
Viral	< .05	< .05	—
Tumor	> .05[b]	> .05[b]	< .05

[a] Student T-test analysis of variance.
[b] Probability (P) value greater than .05 represents a significant difference.

profound neutropenia can be monitored with acute-phase protein assays even though the WBC count remains unresponsive. In situations involving septicemia, the WBC count may remain in the low range of normal, whereas the acute-phase proteins respond in a manner consistent with the seriousness of this disease process. Postsurgical patients (particularly those cases in which bacterial contamination is known to be a factor) can be effectively monitored by acute-phase protein assay for abscess formation or other septic complications. Indeed, these proteins may be more reliable indicators in these circumstances than the WBC count. Rheumatic processes can be followed with acute-phase protein determinations in lieu of the ESR, thereby obviating some of the complexing factors, unrelated to the inflammation, that influence the ESR.

SPECIFIC APPLICATIONS OF ACUTE-PHASE PROTEINS
It is possible to distinguish among major categories of inflammatory disease by utilizing selected acute-phase proteins as a panel (Fig. 18-3, Table 18-3). We have established a panel that includes C-RP, α_1-acid glycoprotein, α_1-antitrypsin, and haptoglobin, although other combinations of the acute-phase reactants may also yield discriminating values. In general, bacterial infections yield the highest levels of all four acute-phase reactants that we routinely study (see Case Report 1 and Fig. 18-4), whereas viral infections are most often characterized by relatively low levels of C-RP and α_1-acid glycoprotein with moderately elevated levels of α_1-antitrypsin and haptoglobin. Tumors that are associated with

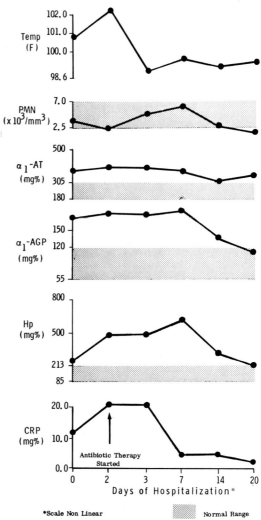

Figure 18-4
Acute-phase protein levels in bacterial infection (septicemia). (See Case Report 1.)

necrosis and inflammation often show a response pattern characterized by a low C-RP, disproportionately elevated α_1-acid glycoprotein [32] and moderately elevated α_1-antitrypsin and haptoglobin. Myocardial infarctions show a relatively high C-RP, low α_1-acid glycoprotein, and moderately elevated haptoglobin and α_1-antitrypsin levels. The statistical analysis supporting these statements is shown in Table 18-3. These patterns, although typical, are not diagnostic and must be interpreted with care and knowledge of the clinical circumstances (see Fig. 18-3). Certain disease entities, which are unrelated to inflammation or tissue necrosis, can alter the acute-phase protein pattern(s), as summarized in Table 18-4.

Table 18-4.   Sources of Error in Interpretation of Acute-Phase Proteins

Protein	Cause	Relative Error
C-RP	?	?
α_1-Acid glycoprotein	Pregnancy (3rd trimester)	Increased
α_1-Antitrypsin	Genetic	Decreased
Ceruloplasmin	Genetic (Wilson's disease)	Decreased
	Severe liver disease	Decreased
	Estrogen	Increased
	Birth control pills	Increased
	Pregnancy	Increased
Haptoglobin	Intravascular hemolysis	Decreased
	Severe liver disease	Decreased
Fibrinogen	Consumptive coagulopathies	Decreased
	Severe liver disease	Decreased

CASE REPORTS

BACTERIAL INFECTIONS
Certain patients with fever or those suspected of having an occult septicemia or other overwhelming infection may be afflicted with disease states in which the WBC count may be depressed and may therefore not reflect the underlying pathology. The use of acute-phase proteins in evaluating patients with leukopenia is exemplified in the following case study (see Fig. 18-4):

Case Report 1
A 64-year-old female was admitted to the Eisenhower Medical Center with a 3-day history of abdominal pain, stiffness of the neck, right facial tenderness, myalgia, nausea, and vomiting. On admission her temperature was 101°F (oral). A complete blood count revealed a WBC count of 4500 with 74 percent polymorphonuclear leukocytes, 5 percent band forms, 11 percent lymphocytes, and 10 percent monocytes. Blood cultures were taken upon admission, and by the second day of hospitalization *Staphylococcus aureus* (coagulase-positive) was identified in all blood cultures taken. Appropriate antibiotic therapy was instituted, and the patient improved dramatically over the next five days. By the 20th hospital day she had almost completely recovered and was discharged.

This case study demonstrates the potential vagary of WBC counts as opposed to the more consistent reflection of the underlying disease process that is provided by the acute-phase protein reactants.

The clinical course of patients with serious infections can be monitored by acute-phase protein profiles, and therapy can be effectively guided by their responses. This next case depicts a typical application of acute-phase proteins in such a setting (see Fig. 18-5):

Figure 18-5
Acute-phase protein levels in serious bacterial infection (see Case Report 2).

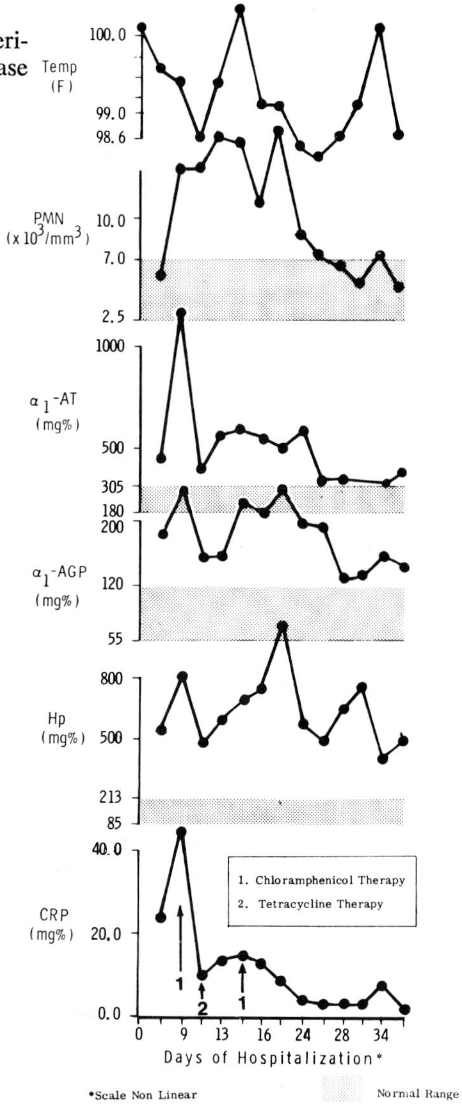

Case Report 2
A middle-aged female was admitted to the Eisenhower Medical Center with fever, generalized malaise, myalgia, and tachycardia. On the third day of hospitalization, she developed multiple joint effusions from which gram-negative, intracellular diplococci were found by gram stain. Immunofluorescence and standard culture procedures proved the organism was *Neisseria meningitidis*. Because of multiple drug allergies, chloramphenicol therapy was instituted on the third day of hospitalization with good response. On the tenth hospital day, she was placed on tetracycline therapy, but exacerbation of her fever and malaise occurred. Chloramphenicol therapy was reinstituted on the thirteenth hospital day, again with good effect. On the thirty-first day

of hospitalization, the patient developed an upper respiratory infection that abated without specific therapy. By the fortieth day of hospitalization, the patient had recovered and was discharged.

RESPONSE PATTERNS FOLLOWING SURGERY

The surveillance of postsurgical patients subsequent to procedures complicated by contamination (such as perforated diverticulum, infarcted bowel, or other surgical complications) is significantly enhanced by serial determinations of acute-phase proteins. These proteins as indicators are more sensitive and responsive than many clinical signs, and these indicators can be less confusing than the commonly employed WBC count. The acute-phase protein profile in Figure 18-6 shows a typical response to an uncomplicated herniorrhaphy in the great majority of surgical patients, the C-RP and α_1-acid glycoproteins should begin a downward trend around the third postsurgical day [33]. A definite increase in these parameters by the fourth or fifth postoperative day definitely suggests that a process involving significant tissue damage or inflammation has intervened, as illustrated by the following case reports.

Case Report 3

A 44-year-old female, who had a long history of ulcerative colitis and was on steroid therapy, experienced a sudden onset of cramping abdominal pain and distention (see Fig. 18-7). Her usually frequent stools ceased. After 36 hours her symptoms abated, only to return as a generalized abdominal pain with radiation to her right shoulder. A diagnosis of perforated viscus was made, and at surgery, a perforated gastric ulcer was found. The immediate postoperative course was uneventful; however, the C-RP failed to continue its trend toward normal by the ninth postoperative day. Upon reevaluation, it was determined that a subphrenic abscess existed. The abscess was drained on the thirteenth postoperative day, and a subsequent, uneventful recovery resulted, with C-RP returning to normal by the third day after the drainage procedure.

Case Report 4

A 16-year-old girl was admitted with a three-day history of migratory arthralgias and fever, which developed about two weeks after an untreated acute pharyngitis (see Fig. 18-8). On admission, the patient had an acute arthritis of the right knee and left ankle. Arthrocentesis produced sterile fluid with decreased levels of complement components C3 (β_1C/A-globulin) and C4 (β_1E-globulin). A systolic murmur of mitral regurgitation was present. A prolonged P-R interval was seen on the electrocardiogram (ECG). The antistreptolysin-O (ASO) titer was 666 Todd units, the ESR was 42 mm per hour (corrected), and the C-RP was 4+. The patient was begun on acetylsalicylic acid therapy, and subsequent salicylate levels revealed therapeutic serum concentrations. The joint symptoms resolved, the fever disappeared, the mitral murmur abated, and the ECG reverted to a normal pattern. The ASO titer was 333 Todd units and the ESR fell to 28 mm per hour; however, the C-RP persisted at 4+ reactivity. Two weeks later, the patient was still asymptomatic, the ASO titer was 166 Todd units, and the ESR was 18 mm per hour, but the CRP was still 4+. Radial immunodiffusion quantitation of C-RP showed this to correspond to 2 mg per 100 ml. Just prior to

Figure 18-6
Clinical values in acute-phase reaction following an uncomplicated herniorrhaphy.

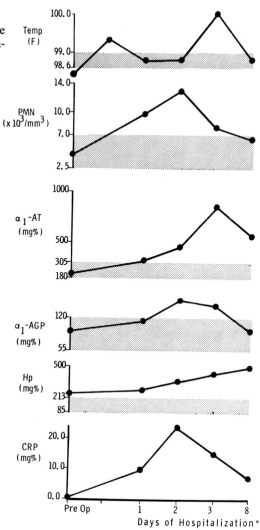

Figure 18-7
Acute-phase protein levels in surgical complication (infection). (See Case Report 3.)

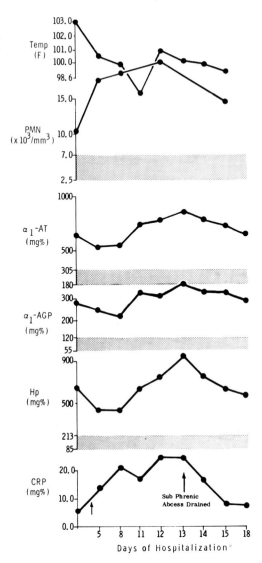

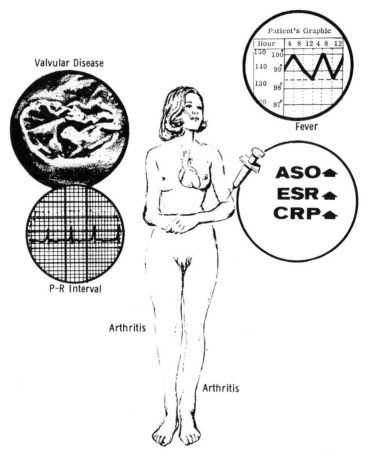

Figure 18-8
Clinical features of a patient with rheumatic fever (see Case Report 4).

a planned discharge from the hospital, acute arthritis and a carditis reappeared. More vigorous salicylate therapy to the upper limits of acceptable serum salicylate concentrations resulted eventually in complete disappearance of these symptoms. When the C-RP became nonreactive, the patient was discharged on salicylates and penicillin prophylaxis for subacute bacterial endocarditis. She has remained asymptomatic since then.

Summary

In this section on acute-phase proteins, an attempt has been made to highlight the few basic facts known about them and to emphasize their use in clinical medicine. Although the nonspecificity of their reaction is recognized, their usefulness in certain clinical situations should not be underestimated. The elevation of C-RP or characteristic changes in the other acute-phase reactants indicates tissue damage, inflammation, or both, with great reliability. If acute-phase protein evaluations are used sequentially, they can provide excellent means of assessing disease activity and of guiding therapy.

References

1. Atkins, E., and Bodel, P.   Fever. *N. Engl. J. Med.* 286:27, 1972.
2. Wintrobe, M. M.   The Leukocytes. In M. M. Wintrobe (Ed.), *Clinical Hematology* (6th ed.). Philadelphia: Lea & Febiger, 1967. P. 271.
3. Fagraeus, R.   The suspension-stability of the blood. *Acta Med. Scand.* 55:1, 1921.
4. Schultze, H. E., and Heremans, J. F.   *Molecular Biology of Human Proteins,* Vol. 1. Amsterdam: Elsevier, 1966. P. 149.
5. Diggs, L. W.   Blood Techniques. In S. F. Miller (Ed.), *Textbook of Clinical Pathology* (5th ed.). Baltimore: Williams & Wilkins, 1955. P. 69.
6. Shetlar, M. R., Bullock, J. A., Shetlar, C. L., and Payne, R. W.   Comparison of serum C-reactive protein, glycoprotein and seromucoid in cancer, arthritis, tuberculosis and pregnancy. *Proc. Soc. Exp. Biol. Med.* 88:107, 1955.
7. Schmid, K., Binnette, J. P., Tokita, K., Moroz, L., and Yoshizaki, H.   The polymorphic forms of alpha-1-acid glycoprotein of normal Caucasian individuals. *J. Clin. Invest.* 43:2347, 1964.
8. Tokita, K., and Schmid, K.   Variants of alpha-1-acid glycoprotein. *Nature* 200:266, 1963.
9. Gill, C. W., Fischer, C. L., and Holleman, C. L.   Rapid method for protein quantitation by electroimmunodiffusion. *J. Clin. Chem.* 17:501, 1971.
10. Asofsky, R., and Thorbecke, G.   Sites of formation of immune globulins and of a component of c_3. *J. Exp. Med.* 114:471, 1961.
11. Deutsch, H. F., and Fisher, G. B.   Studies of human ceruloplasmin fractions separated by chromatography on hydroxylapatite. *J. Biol. Chem.* 239:3325, 1964.
12. Sternlieb, I., and Scheinberg, I. H.   Ceruloplasmin in health and disease. *Ann. N.Y. Acad. Sci.* 94:71, 1951.
13. Peters, J. H., and Alper, C. A.   Haptoglobin cellular localization studies. *J. Clin. Invest.* 45:314, 1966.
14. Shim, B., and Beam, A.   Immunological and biochemical studies in serum haptoglobin. *J. Exp. Med.* 120:611, 1964.
15. Tillet, W. S., and Francis, R.   Serological reaction in pneumonia with a non-protein somatic fraction of pneumococcus. *J. Exp. Med.* 52:561, 1930.
16. MacLeod, C. M., and Avery, O. T.   The occurrence during acute infections of a protein not normally present in the blood. *J. Exp. Med.* 73:183, 1941.
17. Bole, G., and Leutz, J.   The participation of inflammatory connective tissue in synthesis of acute serum glycoproteins. *J. Lab. Clin. Med.* 70:880, 1967.
18. Hurlimann, J., Thorbecke, G., and Hochwald, G.   The liver as the site of C-reactive protein formation. *J. Exp. Med.* 123:365, 1966.
19. Weimer, H., and Coggshell, G.   Divergent responses of serum glyco-

protein fractions to tissue injury in adrenalectomized rats. *Con. Physical Pharma.* 45:767, 1967.

20. Heim, W. G., and Ellenson, S. R. Adrenal cortical control of the appearance of rat slow alpha-2-globulin. *Nature* 213:1260, 1967.

21. Shetlar, M., Howard, R., Joel, W., Cartwright, C., and Reifenstein, E. The effects of parathyroid hormone on serum glycoprotein and seromucoid levels on the kidney of the rat. *Endocrinology* 59:532, 1952.

22. Boas, N., and Ludwig, A. Endocrine regulation of serum hexosamine levels. *J. Clin. Endocrinol. Metab.* 12:965, 1952.

23. Darcy, D. A. Response of a serum glycoprotein to tissue injury and necrosis. *Br. J. Exp. Pathol.* 46:155, 1965.

24. Koj, A. Synthesis and turnover of acute phase reactants. *Ciba Found. Symp.*, 1970. Pp. 79–101.

25. Brocklehurst, W. E. Role of kinins and prostaglandins in inflammation. *Proc. R. Soc. Med.* 64:4, 1971.

26. Giroud, J. P., and Willoughby, D. A. The interrelations of complement and a prostaglandin-like substance in acute inflammation. *J. Pathol.* 181:241, 1970.

27. Kessler, E., Hughe, R., Bennett, E., and Nadela, S. Evidence for the presence of prostaglandin-like material in the plasma of dogs with endotoxin shock. *J. Lab. Clin. Med.* 81:85, 1973.

28. Kindmark, C. O. In vitro binding of human C-reactive protein by some pathogenic bacteria and zymosan. *Clin. Exp. Immunol.* 11:283, 1972.

29. Ritzmann, S. E., and Daniels, J. C. Serum Protein Analysis. In J. B. Fuller (Ed.), *ASCP Workshop Manual, Selected Topics in Clinical Chemistry* (3rd ed.). Chicago: American Society of Clinical Pathologists' Commission on Continuing Education, 1972. P. 175.

30. Werner, M. Serum protein changes during the acute phase reaction. *Clin. Chim. Acta* 25:299, 1969.

31. Werner, M., and Odenthal, D. Serum protein changes after gastrectomy as a model of acute phase reaction. *J. Lab. Clin. Med.* 70:302, 1967.

32. Cleve, H., and Strohmeyer, G. Quantitative Variationen von Serum Alpha-1-Glycoprotein, Gc und Alpha-2-Macroglobulin mit der Radialen Immunodiffusion. *Klin. Wochenschr.* 20:1051, 1967.

33. Crockson, R., Payne, C., Ratcliff, A., and Soothill, J. Time sequence of acute phase reactive proteins following surgical trauma. *Clin. Chim. Acta* 14:435, 1966.

Immunoglobulin Abnormalities   **19**

Stephan E. Ritzmann

Developmental Aspects of B- and T-Cell Systems of Immunity

Studies of the developmental aspects of immunity in animals and humans have provided some understanding of the mechanisms governing the immune systems. Much of this information provides the basis for the clinical approach to immunoglobulin abnormalities.

PHYLOGENY

Based on phylogenetic, ontogenetic, and experimental evidence, two related immune systems, or lymphoid divisions, have been recognized: the *thymus (T) system,* with the thymus as its cradle, and the *bursa or bone marrow (B) system,* which is primarily represented by the bursa of Fabricius in fowls or its equivalent in other species. Both the thymus and bursa are gut-associated organs (Fig. 19-1). The T-lymphocyte system is principally responsible for cellular immunity (e.g., delayed hypersensitivity and transplantation immunity). The B-lymphocyte system, with its plasma cells, chiefly provides humoral defense by means of immunoglobulins that function as antibodies.

Phylogenetically, the lymphoid system emerged approximately 450 to 500 million years ago in primitive fish (i.e., elasmobranchs, as exemplified by the guitarfish). The subsequent organization of the thymus gradually evolved to its final complexity in man (Fig. 19-2). The human lymphoid system has been divided into a central component (equivalent to the thymus and bursa) and a peripheral component (spleen and lymph nodes). The spleen first appeared as an organ in the elasmobranchs, but the lymph nodes first appeared in the amphibians. The human thymus, which is derived from the third and fourth pharyngeal pouches, may be considered the pacemaker of the T-lymphocyte system.

Approximately 400 million years ago in the evolutionary scheme, immunoglobulin precursors and the capacity for antibody response emerged in vertebrates, such as the cyclostomes (e.g., the hagfish and lamprey). These vertebrates produce a primordial immunoglobulin consisting of

Figure 19-1

Phylogenesis of the immune system. The primitive thymus of certain fish is organized and located near the gills. In addition to the thymus, the chicken has a bursa of Fabricius (*right arrow*). The rabbit has both a thymus and Peyer's patches (*right arrow*) as organized lymphoid tissue. (Modified from Good, R. A. *Hosp. Practice* 2:39, 1967.)

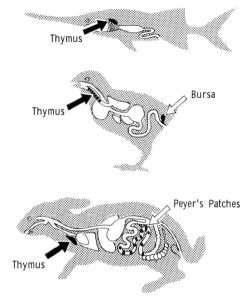

a tetrameric configuration of polypeptide chains with a molecular weight (MW) of approximately 70,000 and subunits linked by noncovalent bonds; however, these molecules are devoid of light chains [1]. The gradual phylogenetic evolution of immunoglobulins has led to their final molecular complexity and diversity in man. Immunoglobulins that are composed of heavy and light polypeptide chains are present in the ancient placoderms. The heavy polypeptide chains of these immunoglobulins resemble those of the mammalian μ chains, and the heavy and light chains are linked by disulfide bridges. The heavy and light chains contain regions of variable amino-acid sequence (V region; 10,000 MW) and constant amino-acid sequence (G region; 12,000 MW) that are similar to those of human immunoglobulins (see Fig. 19-13). The amino-acid sequences in the N-terminal portion of the light and heavy chains reveal homologies with the κ light chains in man. In general, the molecular form of the IgM class of immunoglobulin molecules has been, according to Good and Finstad [1], "remarkably constant through the eons of history."

A second immunoglobulin class emerges with the lungfishes. This class has heavy chains similar to those of the IgG molecules in reptiles and avian species (38,000 MW) but which are distinct from the amphibian and mammalian IgG (50,000 MW). The phylogenetic evolution of IgM involves polymerization, perhaps due to duplication of precursor genes, whereas the evolution of IgG may have resulted from variations of the number of C regions [1, 2].

The class specificity for the various heavy chains, which reside in the constant (i.e., C_H) regions, represents the evolutionary divergence of the immunoglobulin structure to provide functions auxiliary to the specific

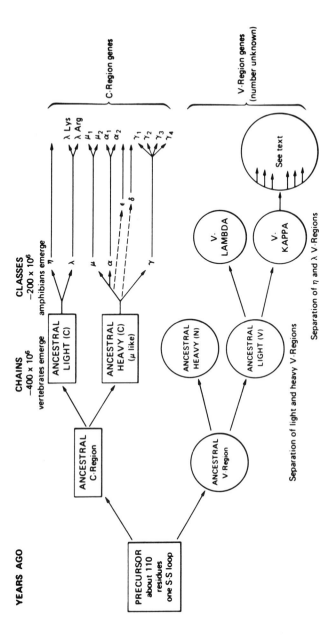

Figure 19-2

Possible scheme for the evolution of human immunoglobulins. The evolution of the ancestral V regions of λ and heavy chains is not shown, but it probably follows the general pattern of that of κ chains. (Reproduced by permission. From Fudenberg, H. H., Pink, J. R. L., Stites, D. P., and Wang, A. C. *Basic Immunogenetics*. New York: Oxford University Press, 1972.)

antigen-binding (e.g., complement fixation) that serves different effector functions [3, 4] (see Figs. 19-11 and 19-14). The final diversity of the immunoglobulins allows the expression of more than 100,000 different antibody specificities [5]; thus, the immunoglobulins provide antibody activity against an almost infinite number of antigens, including certain synthetic substances without natural counterparts.

Since all antibodies appear to differ from one another within their variable polypeptide regions as to their primary amino-acid sequence, the immunoglobulins present an extreme degree of heterogeneity that is unique among the serum proteins [6]. Among the mechanisms responsible for such diversity, two approaches have been primarily considered. The *instructive theory of antibody formation* postulates that antigens induce the synthesis of new and specific antibodies within the B cells. On the other hand, the *selection theory* [4] of antibody formation postulates the preexistence of cells with the potential of responding to any antigen and producing its corresponding antibody by clonal expansion. In this latter view, the role of the antigen is that of a selector of the appropriate antibody-producing cell clone, which causes it to divide and induce antibody synthesis. The site of the immunoglobulin molecule involved in antigen binding probably occupies not more than 1 percent of the total molecule; it is located near the amino terminal end of the variable region (see Fig. 19-13). It is not clear whether the required diversity of B-cell clones is present at the level of the germ cell, which contains a large number of genes coded for specific antibodies, or whether somatic mutation of a smaller number of such genes is instrumental.

There is controversy regarding the genetic control of immunoglobulin synthesis, but it appears likely that at least one gene exists for each class or subclass of heavy chains and one for each type of light chains. Thus, there are at least ten genes coding for heavy chains and three for light chains. The structure of variable regions could result from somatic mutations or other mechanisms to provide for the diversity of antibody functions [8]. The qualitative nature of the antibody response is genetically determined, but the quantitative aspects are also subject to environmental factors, such as the exposure to and the nature of the antigen. For instance, germ-free animals demonstrate hypogammaglobulinemia, but after exposure to the normal environment, normal immunoglobulin levels ensue.

ONTOGENY

The developmental factors of the lymphoid system in mammals, including man, are depicted in *Figure 19-3* [9]. In the embryo, hematopoietic and lymphoid stem cells originate in the blood islets of the area vasculosa in the yolk sac and, subsequently, in the fetal liver and bone marrow. Descendants of these lymphoid stem cells migrate through the thymus, where they undergo maturational changes by certain hormone-like factors. After such a change, these T-lymphoid cells are endowed with immunological competence. They emigrate to the peripheral lymphoid organs, including the lymph nodes and spleen, where they "homestead"

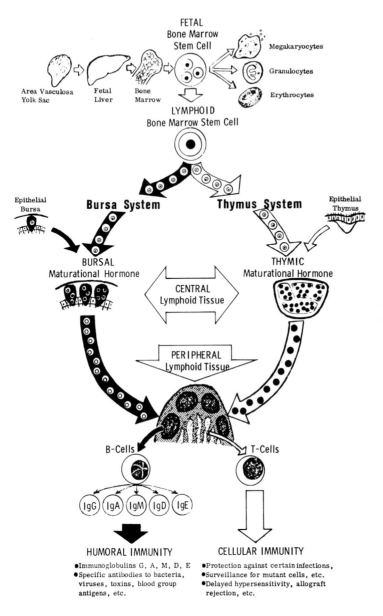

FETAL
Bone Marrow
Stem Cell

Megakaryocytes

Granulocytes

Erythrocytes

Area Vasculosa
Yolk Sac

Fetal
Liver

Bone
Marrow

LYMPHOID
Bone Marrow Stem Cell

Epithelial
Bursa

Bursa System

Thymus System

Epithelial
Thymus

BURSAL
Maturational Hormone

CENTRAL
Lymphoid Tissue

THYMIC
Maturational Hormone

PERIPHERAL
Lymphoid Tissue

B-Cells

T-Cells

(IgG) (IgA) (IgM) (IgD) (IgE)

HUMORAL IMMUNITY

●Immunoglobulins G, A, M, D, E
●Specific antibodies to bacteria,
viruses, toxins, blood group
antigens, etc.

CELLULAR IMMUNITY

●Protection against certain infections,
●Surveillance for mutant cells, etc.
●Delayed hypersensitivity, allograft
rejection, etc.

Figure 19-3
Simplified, schematic diagram of the ontogeny of the human immune systems
(for details, see text). (Modified from Good, R. A. *Hosp. Practice* 2:39,
1967. Reproduced with permission from Ritzmann, S. E., Sakai, H., and
Daniels, J. C. In G. J. Race (Ed.), *Laboratory Medicine*. New York: Harper
& Row, 1975.)

in specific regions, namely, the deep cortical or paracortical areas of the lymph nodes and the periarteriolar areas of the spleen. These areas are referred to as the *thymus-dependent* or *T areas*. T cells provide cellular immunity, which encompasses delayed skin hypersensitivity, protection against viral, fungal, and intracellular bacterial pathogens, immunological surveillance against oncogenesis, and transplantation immunity. The mobilizable fractions of the T-cell populations constitute the recirculating lymphoid cell pool, which are immunologically competent, but are unsensitized and virgin (T_2 cells). They are, however, capable of specific interactions with antigens, proliferative expansion, blastoid transformation, and subsequent participation in inflammation and lymphokine production. Such specifically sensitized lymphocytes become killer (T_3) cells, which lose their capacity for recirculation. Related cells transform into memory (T_4) cells, which allow a potentiated response to the reintroduction of the same antigen. Such a secondary immune response results in the rapid reversion of specific memory cells into killer cells [10] (Fig. 19-4).

Additional descendants of bone-marrow lymphoid stem cells migrate through the bursal regions in birds and the bursa-equivalent in man. The exact nature of the bursa-equivalent in humans remains in doubt, but the elusive equivalent system is probably the bone marrow itself [11]. Within this bursa-equivalent system, the B cells are modified, probably by the effects of maturational hormones, whereby they become immunologically competent. They subsequently emigrate to the lymphoid organs, where they are found preferentially in the germinal centers, far cortical areas, and the medullary cords of the lymph nodes, as well as the red pulp of the spleen. These are the *thymus-independent areas* (bursa or bone-marrow dependent) or, simply, *B areas*.

The B cells are responsible for humoral immunity, which is manifested by the production of the immunoglobulins IgG, IgA, IgM, IgD, and IgE by mature B cells (i.e., plasma cells). B cells with IgG, IgA, or IgM surface immunoglobulins and the potential for immunoglobulin production are found in the spleen and peripheral blood of 14½-week-old fetuses in relative numbers that are similar to those found in the blood of term infants, normal children, and adults [12]. The order of appearance of these cells is probably (1) IgM, (2) IgG, and (3) IgA [13]. Prebursal immunologically incompetent stem cells undergo modifications resulting in postbursal (B_1) cells. In the peripheral lymphoid organs, these cells are further differentiated and expanded into mature (B_2) cells. These postbursal B cells are predominantly found in the B areas of the peripheral lymphoid organs, the lamina propria of the gastrointestinal (GI) tract and secretory glands, the bone marrow, and the lymph and blood. Newer analytical techniques (e.g., immunofluorescence tests for detection of immunoglobulin surface markers [14–17] and rosette techniques [17, 18] have established that approximately 20 to 25 percent of peripheral blood lymphocytes are B cells. This ratio is significantly altered in several disease states (e.g., chronic lymphocytic leukemia) [17]. Mature B cells that are capable of producing and secret-

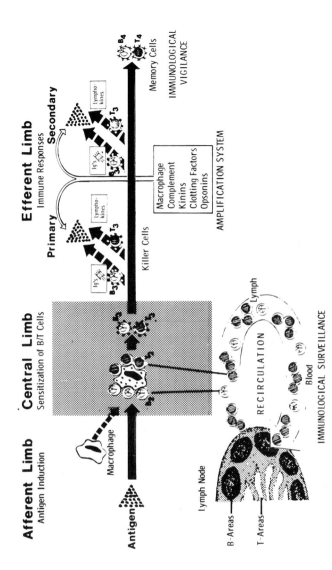

Figure 19-4

Immunodynamics. Simplified diagrammatic presentation of the various steps involved in the afferent, central, and efferent limbs of immunity (for explanation see p. 358). (Reproduced by permission. From Ritzmann, S. E., Sakai, H., and Daniels, J. C. In G. J. Race (Ed.), *Laboratory Medicine*. New York: Harper & Row, 1975.)

ing immunoglobulins may be termed *killer* (B₃) *cells;* these elaborate the specific antibodies that are depicted at the antigenic target. Memory (B₄) cells provide the anamnestic, secondary response to the same antigen (see Fig. 19-4).

By careful morphological analysis of the structure of lymph nodes and the spleen in humans and experimental animals, one can define the deficiency of lymphoid populations in terms of T-cell or B-cell depletion. Furthermore, many immunological diseases can be viewed in this context, i.e., either as B-cell, T-cell or combined B-T-cell abnormalities [19].

The recent trend toward the use of symbols such as T_{1-4} cells, B and A (accessory) cells, the objectification of the terminology, and the implied clarity of our concepts of immunology should not, however, conceal the considerable degree of conscious over-simplification in this approach [10]. *Figure 19-4* presents a simplified diagram of the various steps thought to be involved in the afferent, central, and efferent limbs of immunity. Lymphoid stem cells from the bone marrow give rise to the B- and T-cell systems. A prethymic, immunologically incompetent stem cell enters the thymus, where it undergoes proliferation that eventuates in a postthymic T_1 *cell.* Further proliferative expansion occurs under the humoral influence of the thymus. Once in the periphery, the T_1 cell populations are further differentiated and expanded into a second stage, i.e., T_2 *cells,* by a process that presumably also involves humoral influences of the thymus. The long-lived T_2 cells in man seem to have a life span exceeding five years. T_2 cells are found in the blood, lymph, and peripheral lymphoid organs (T areas). These immunologically competent (but yet unsensitized) virgin T_2 cells represent a rapidly mobilizable recirculating lymphoid cell pool capable of specific interactions with antigen, proliferative expansion, blastoid transformation, and subsequent participation in inflammation and lymphokine production. After the interaction of T_2 cells with specific antigens, specifically sensitized lymphocytes will result. Some of these become *killer cells,* i.e., T_3 *cells,* which lose their capacity for recirculation and become short-lived end-stage cells. The T_3 cells selectively traffic to the inflammatory sites, and they accumulate at the sites of the specific antigenic targets. Most sensitized lymphocytes, however, become or evoke *memory cells,* i.e., T_4 *cells,* allowing a potentiated response to the reintroduction of the same antigen. Such a secondary immune response results in the rapid reversion of specific T_4 memory cells into T_3 killer cells. T_4 cells are radioresistant and are found in the peripheral lymphoid organs. Similarly, prebursal, immunologically incompetent stem cells arise in the bursa equivalent in man (presumably the bone marrow), where they undergo proliferation resulting in postbursal B_1 *cells.* Further proliferative expansion occurs under the influence of the microenvironment and, presumably, humoral factors of the bursa equivalent. In the peripheral lymphoid organs, these are further differentiated and expanded into B_2 *cells.* These postbursal B_2 cells (i.e., plasma cell-like) are predominantly found in the B areas of the peripheral lymphoid organs, the lamina propria of the gastrointestinal tract and secretory glands, the bone marrow, and the peripheral blood and lymph. They are capable of producing immunoglobulins. In analogy to the T_3 and T_4 cells, these may be termed B_3 *killer* and B_4 *memory* cells. In contrast to the T_3 cells, however, the B_3 cells exert their killer effect indirectly by the production and release of specific antibodies.

The host's response to an antigen varies in type and intensity. It depends upon the host's immunological maturity and age, genetic make-up, and previous exposure to the antigen. The immune response is often a combined B-T-response that consists of an extremely complex chain of events. These can be classified as belonging to three functional stages: *the afferent limb of immunity* (i.e., antigen acceptance and processing), *the central limb of immunity* (i.e., antigen-sensitive lymphocytes become committed to participate in the responses against the specific antigen), and *the efferent limb of immunity* (i.e., the effector side of the immune response).

IMMUNODYNAMICS–PRIMARY AND SECONDARY ANTIBODY RESPONSES

The classic immunological reaction by B cells involves two major processes which differ qualitatively and quantitatively (Fig. 19-5). The *primary immune response* results from the first exposure to a foreign antigen. It requires a certain period of time to occur (i.e., a lag phase). The chief immunoglobulin produced by the primary immune response is IgM. The *secondary immune response* to an antigen, on the other hand, involves the reexposure of the same sensitized host that has previously undergone a primary immune response to the same foreign antigen. It is marked by a much more rapid production of larger quantities of specific antibodies. Prolonged exposure to antigens (e.g., chronic infections), however, often results in an overlapping of both the primary and secondary immune responses. The chief immunoglobulin class produced by the secondary immune response is IgG. This sequence of occurrence of first IgM and then IgG antibodies following antigenic stimulation reflects a recapitulation of the phylogenetic and ontogenetic order of the immunoglobulin synthesis in man of IgM to IgG to IgA [4, 20].

In *Figure 19-5,* the primary and secondary responses are contrasted. There are four phases of antibody response.

Primary Responses: (1) *Lag (latent or inductive) phase:* This occurs between contact of target cells with antigen and the beginning of antibody production, lasting a few days. RNA synthesis takes place and ribosomes accumulate in differentiating B cells. (2) *Log (production or synthetic) phase:* Following the induction period, there is a logarithmic increase in the amount of antibody in the serum for approximately 5 to 10 days until it reaches a peak. (3) *Plateau phase:* The log phase is followed by a transitory plateau phase of 1 to 3 days. (4) *Decline phase:* The final stage is a gradual decline of the antibody levels. The log phase is characterized by an excess of antibody synthesis over catabolism; the plateau phase, by equal rates of synthesis and catabolism; and the de-

PRIMARY ANTIBODY RESPONSE   SECONDARY ANTIBODY RESPONSE

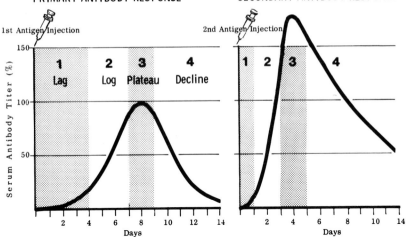

Figure 19-5
Primary and secondary serum antibody response following antigen injection
(for explanation see pp. 359–360).

cline phase, by an excess of catabolism over synthesis. The chief antibody produced during the primary immune response is of the IgM class.

Secondary Responses: A second administration of the same dose of
this antigen produces an accelerated and exaggerated antibody response.
The lag phase is shorter (hours), the log phase is steeper, and the peak
titer is higher than in the primary response. The principal antibody produced as a result of the secondary immune response is of the IgG class.

Tertiary responses usually do not differ significantly from secondary
responses.

An example of this shift in antibody classes is the antibody response
to Rh-positive fetal cells crossing into the Rh-negative maternal blood.
During the first Rh incompatible pregnancy (i.e., primary immunization), the maternal antibody response is reflected by the occurrence of
saline Rh antibodies of the IgM class. Subsequent incompatible pregnancies (i.e., secondary, tertiary, etc., immune responses) lead to the
production of IgG-class Rh antibodies, which (in contrast to the IgM
Rh antibodies) cross the placenta into the fetal circulation and cause
hemolysis and erythroblastosis fetalis (see Chap. 16).

SENESCENCE OF IMMUNITY
The lymphoid system undergoes immunological aging and involution.
This is reflected by morphological changes (e.g., thymic involution and
lymphocyte depletion in the peripheral lymphoid organs) as well as
functional changes (e.g., a decline of immunological vigor due to decreased antigenic responsiveness). An example of senescence of the
B-cell system is shown in Figure 19-6 [13, 21]. The biological effects of
the age-related decline in immunological functions are profound. Diseases

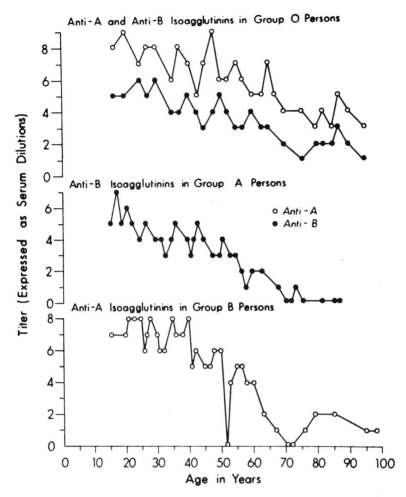

Figure 19-6
Relationship of anti-A and anti-B isoagglutinin titers to age. Decrements in anti-A and anti-B antibody titers are correlated with increasing age. (Reproduced by permission. From Somers, H., and Kuhns, W. J. *Proc. Soc. Exp. Biol. Med.* 141:1104, 1972.)

occurring with advanced age, disordered immune functions, and impaired immunosurveillance include autoimmunity, malignancies, amyloidosis, monoclonal gammopathies, and others.

Physiological Aspects of Immunoglobulins

Tiselius in 1937 separated serum proteins electrophoretically into albumin and α-, β-, and γ-globulins [22]. It was subsequently demonstrated that most proteins with antibody properties (i.e., the capacity to react specifically with some foreign substances or antigens) resided in the

Figure 19-7
Normally, light and heavy polypeptide chains are produced in a synchronous fashion (i.e., a light chain to heavy chain ratio of 1:1) on the ribosomes within the endoplasmic reticulum of the plasma cells (i.e., B-lymphocytes). Subsequently, these light and heavy chains are assembled into complete immunoglobulin molecules (e.g., IgG), which are then secreted. (Reproduced by permission. From Ritzmann, S. E., and Daniels, J. C. In G. J. Race (Ed.), *Tice's Practice of Medicine,* Vol. 2. New York: Harper & Row, 1974.)

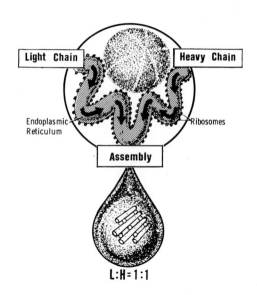

γ-globulin fraction. The term γ-*globulin* was initially equated with those proteins possessing antibody characteristics. The application of immunoelectrophoresis [23] resulted in the demonstration of the electrophoretic migration ranges of antibody proteins within the entire γ-, β-, and α_2-globulin ranges (see Fig. 1-13, Chap. 1). Consequently, the functional term *immunoglobulin* was suggested [24, 25] for those proteins possessing either antibody characteristics or the characteristic structure of antibodies. Normal human serum contains five classes of immunoglobulins: IgG, IgA, IgM, IgD, and IgE, each with different physical, chemical, and immunological properties [26, 27] (see Appendix).

CELLULAR SOURCES OF IMMUNOGLOBULINS
Although plasma cells were described by Ramon y Cajal [28] in 1894 and a correlation between plasmocytosis and myelomatosis was suggested by Wright [29] in 1900, these cells were first implicated in γ-globulin synthesis by Bing and Plum [30] in 1937 and Kolouch [31] in 1939. Direct evidence for the elaboration of γ-globulins by plasma cells was provided subsequently [32–34], and clinical correlations were established [35]. Many of the intracellular events associated with synthesis, transport, and secretion of immunoglobulins by plasma cells have been elucidated [36]. This relationship is depicted in Figure 19-7. The human bone marrow may be a major site for IgG synthesis [37].

IMMUNOGLOBULIN CLASSES IgG, IgA, IgM, IgD, AND IgE
Most immunoglobulins have been discovered in patients with immunoglobulin abnormalities. These "experiments of nature," as Good [1] has termed them, have led to the detection of IgM, a macroglobulin in the serum of patients with macroglobulinemia, which was previously termed

β_2M-, γ_1M-, and γM-*globulin,* among other designations. Waldenström [38] first detected it, and it was subsequently characterized by Burtin et al. [39]. IgA, which was previously termed β_1A-, γ_1A-, and γA-*globulin,* among other designations, was found by Heremans et al. in patients with IgA myeloma [25, 40]. IgD, formerly termed γD-globulin, was described by Rowe and Fahey [41, 42] in a patient with IgD myeloma. IgE, formerly termed γE-globulin, was reported by Ishizaka et al. [43, 44] in patients with allergic disorders and, subsequently, in a patient with IgE myeloma [45].

Likewise, subunits of immunoglobulins have been discovered in patients with immunoglobulin abnormalities. The Bence Jones proteins were discovered in the first patient reported with myeloma [46, 47]. The free heavy chains associated with γ-chain disease were reported by Franklin et al. [48] and Osserman and Takatsuki [49]. The α heavy-chain disease was reported by Seligmann et al. [50], and μ heavy-chain disease by Forte et al. [51]. Low molecular weight IgM was discovered by Solomon and Kunkel [52] in a patient with monoclonal gammopathy. Half molecules of IgG were found in a patient with plasmocytoma [53], and deleted heavy- and light-chain disease was first noted with malignant lymphoma [54]. Continued vigilance for immunoglobulin abnormalities will likely lead to the recognition of additional immunoglobulins or subunits and their associated disorders.

Based on the reactivity of these proteins with specific antisera as well as on other criteria, five classes of human immunoglobulins have been described. In normal serum, there are three quantitatively major immunoglobulins: immunoglobulin G, or IgG; immunoglobulin A, or IgA; and immunoglobulin M, or IgM; and two quantitatively minor immunoglobulins: immunoglobulin D, or IgD; and immunoglobulin E, or IgE. (According to a recent World Health Organization Report [27], the terms γG-globulin, γA-globulin, γM-globulin, γD-globulin, and γE-globulin should be discarded.) Together, the immunoglobulins constitute 20 to 25 percent of the total serum proteins. Some of the properties of these immunoglobulins are listed in Table 19-1. The various classes of normal immunoglobulins are characterized by a remarkable degree of heterogeneity with respect to structure (i.e., antigenic characteristics), function (i.e., antibody properties), and genetic characteristics (i.e., allotypes or heritable γ-globulin groups). Each immunoglobulin molecule consists of a multichain structure (Figs. 19-8 and 19-9).

The basic structure of the immunoglobulins consists of four polypeptide chains linked by hydrogen and disulfide bonds. Two of the chains, each with a molecular weight of 20,000 to 25,000, contain no carbohydrates and are termed *light chains* or *L chains.* They are linked to two carbohydrate-containing *heavy chains* or *H chains* with a molecular weight of 50,000 to 70,000 each. The normal IgG, IgD, and IgE molecules and the majority of serum IgA molecules consist of monomers. In contrast, the normal IgM molecule is a pentamer (19S; 900,000 MW) that is composed of five monomeric IgM moieties, $(\mu_2\kappa_2)_5$ and $(\mu_2\lambda_2)_5$, which are linked by interchain disulfide bridges. The star-like or spider-

Table 19-1. Characteristics of Human Immunoglobulins[a]

A. Structural and Physicochemical Properties

Immunoglobulin Classes and Subclasses	Polypeptide Chains — Heavy	Polypeptide Chains — Light	Immunoglobulin Types (κ)	Immunoglobulin Types (λ)	Light Chain Ratios (κ/λ)	Molecular Formulas	Association with — Secretory Piece	Association with — J Chain	Total Carbohydrate (% per weight)	Molecular Weight	Sedimentation Coefficients ($S_{20,w}$)	Electrophoretic Mobility (Relative)
1. IgG	γ	κ,λ	IgG	IgG		$\gamma_2\kappa_2$ & $\gamma_2\lambda_2$	−	−	~2.5	150,000	7	γ_2-α_2-globulin
A. IgG$_1$	γ_1	κ,λ	IgG$_1$	IgG$_1$	2.4	$(\gamma_1)_2\kappa_2$ & $(\gamma_1)\lambda_2$	−	−	~2.5	H chains 50,000		Slow
B. IgG$_2$	γ_2	κ,λ	IgG$_2$	IgG$_2$	1.1	$(\gamma_2)_2\kappa_2$ & $(\gamma_2)\lambda_2$	−	−	~2.5			Slow
C. IgG$_3$	γ_3	κ,λ	IgG$_3$	IgG$_3$	1.4	$(\gamma_3)_2\kappa_2$ & $(\gamma_3)\lambda_2$	−	−	~2.5	L chains 22,500		Slow
D. IgG$_4$	γ_4	κ,λ	IgG$_4$	IgG$_4$	8.0	$(\gamma_4)_2\kappa_2$ & $(\gamma_4)\lambda_2$	−	−	~2.5			Fast
2. Serum IgA	α	κ,λ	IgA	IgA		$\alpha_2\kappa_2$ & $\alpha_2\lambda_2$	−	+[b]	~7.5	160,000 (320,000)[b] (480,000)[b] (640,000)[b]	7 (9)[b] (11)[b] (13)[b]	γ_1-β_1-globulin
A. IgA$_1$	α_1	κ,λ	IgA$_1$	IgA$_1$	1.4	$(\alpha_1)_2\kappa_2$ & $(\alpha_1)_2\lambda_2$	−	−	~7.5	H chains 60,000		
B. IgA$_2$	α_2	κ,λ	IgA$_2$	IgA$_2$	1.6	$(\alpha_2)_2\kappa_2$ & $(\alpha_2)_2\lambda_2$	−	−	~7.5	L chains 22,500		
Secretory IgA	α	κ,λ	IgA-SP	IgA-SP		$(\alpha_2\kappa_2)_2$-SP & $(\alpha_2\lambda_2)_2$-SP	+	+	~12	390,000	11.4	
3. IgM	μ	κ,λ	IgM	IgM	3.2	$\mu_2\kappa_2$ & $\mu_2\lambda_2$	−	+	~12	900,000 H chains 70,000 L chains 22,500	19 (24)[b]	γ_1-β_1-globulin
4. IgD	δ	κ,λ	IgD	IgD	0.3	$\delta_2\kappa_2$ & $\delta_2\lambda_2$	−	−	~13	180,000	7	γ-β-globulin
5. IgE	ϵ	κ,λ	IgE	IgE		$\epsilon_2\kappa_2$ & $\epsilon_2\lambda_2$	−	−	~11	200,000	8	γ-β-globulin

B. Body Distribution, Concentrations, and Metabolic Properties

Immuno-Globulin Classes and Sub-Classes	Primary Body Distribution	Serum Concentrations (90th percentile ranges)		Rate of Synthesis (mg/kg/day)	Total Circulating Pool (mg/day)	Rate of Catabolism (%/day)	Fractional Catabolic Rate (% of vascular pool)	Half-Life in Serum (days)
		(mg/100 ml)	(IU/ml)					
1. IgG	45% Intravascular	800–1800 (average)	90–210	~30	500	3	6.7	23
A. IgG₁		~850	~100					23
B. IgG₂		~300	~35					23
C. IgG₃		~100	~12					8
D. IgG₄		<50	<6					23
2. Serum IgA	40–45% Intravascular	90–450 (average)	55–270	25	90	12	25	6
A. IgA₁		~300	~180					6
B. IgA₂		~40	~24					6 (?)
Secretory IgA A. IgA₁ B. IgA₂	Secretions of breast, salivary, respiratory, intestinal epithelium	Saliva: ~10 mg/100 ml Colostrum: ~450 mg/100 ml						
3. IgM	75% Intravascular	60–280	70–320	~6	35	14	18	5
4. IgD	75% Intravascular	0.3–40	2–280	0.4	1.1		37	2.8
5. IgE	50% Intravascular, present in mucinous exocrine secretions	10–1000 (ng/ml)	5–500	0.02	0.02		89	2.4

[a] Data from references [5, 26, 55, 60, 75, 85, 88, 90, 98].
[b] Polymer values.

Table 19-1 (*continued*)

C. Biological Properties

Immunoglobulin Classes and Sub-Classes	Complement Fixation	Agglutination Activity	In Vitro Opsonization	Passage Across Placenta	Arthus Reaction	Binding to Macrophages	Reaginic, Homocytotropic Activity[c]	Passive Cutaneous Anaphylaxis[d]	Allotypes H Chain	Allotypes L (κ) Chain
1. IgG	+	+	+	+	+	+	−	+	Gm 1–23	Inv 1–3
A. IgG$_1$	++			+		++	−	+	Gm	Inv
B. IgG$_2$	+			±		++	−	−	Gm	Inv
C. IgG$_3$	++			+		++	−	+	Gm	Inv
D. IgG$_4$	−[e]			+		±	−	+	Gm	Inv
2. Serum										
IgA	−	±	−	−	−		−	−	Am 1–2	Inv
A. IgA$_2$	−			−			−	−	Am 1	Inv
B. IgA$_2$	−			−			−	−	Am 2	Inv
Secretory IgA										
3. IgM	+++	+++	+++	−	+	−	−	−	−	Inv
4. IgD	−			−	−		−	−	−	Inv
5. IgE	−			−	−		+	−	−	Inv

[c] Binding to mast cells.

[d] Anaphylactic reaction with guinea-pig skin.

[e] IgG$_4$ can activate complement via alternate pathway.

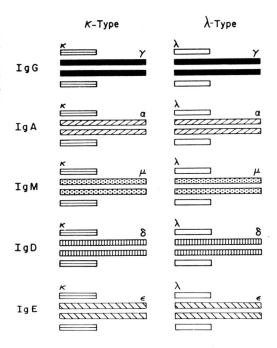

Figure 19-8
Basic structure of IgG, IgA, IgM (only monomeric moiety shown), IgD, and IgE. (Modified from Osserman, E. F., and Fahey, J. L. *Am. J. Med.* 44:256, 1968.)

like molecular configuration of such IgM molecules can be visualized by electronmicroscopy [56]. The H chains of a human IgG_1 myeloma protein have been found to be composed of 446 amino-acid residues, and the L chains of 214 amino-acid residues [57].

LIGHT (L) CHAINS
L chains are common to all immunoglobulins and are responsible for the common properties and the cross-reactivity between the various immunoglobulin classes. Two types of structurally and antigenically distinct light chains, designated *kappa* (κ) and *lambda* (λ), are recognized (see Fig. 19-8). The immunoglobulin "type" refers to the L chains, which determine whether an immunoglobulin is either κ-type or λ-type. (According to a World Health Organization recommendation [27], the terms *type K* and *type L* light chains should be replaced by κ- and λ-*types,* i.e., $IgG(\kappa)$, $IgA(\lambda)$, and so on.) Individual immunoglobulin molecules possess κ *or* λ light chains but not both, and normal human serum generally contains a mixture of about twice as many κ-type IgG molecules as λ-type molecules [7, 58].

Approximately half of the peptides of each L chain are individually specific (i.e., idiotypic), and the other half are type-specific (i.e., κ or λ chain type-specific) [59]. The first 107 amino-acid residues at the amino (NH_2) terminal end of the polypeptide chain constitute the variant region (V_L); the sequence of the V_L is unique for each protein. The remaining 107 amino-acid residues constitute the constant region (C_L) of the L chains. There are two different basic sequences of the constant

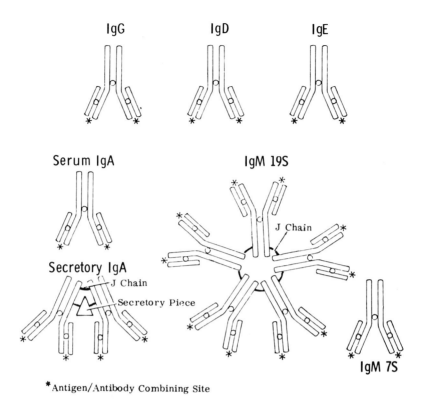

IgG   IgD   IgE

Serum IgA   IgM 19S

J Chain

Secretory IgA

J Chain

Secretory Piece

IgM 7S

*Antigen/Antibody Combining Site

Figure 19-9
Molecular configurations of IgG, IgD, IgE, serum and secretory IgA, and IgM.

regions of the L chains: C_κ is common to all κ light chains, and the distinct C_λ is common to all λ light chains (Fig. 19-10). Within the V_L regions, there are certain specific sequence similarities that allow the separation of subgroup designations [60, 61]. Presently, three subgroups of κ light chains ($V_{\kappa I}$, $V_{\kappa II}$, and $V_{\kappa III}$) and five subgroups of λ light chains ($V_{\lambda I}$, $V_{\lambda II}$, $V_{\lambda III}$, $V_{\lambda IV}$, and $V_{\lambda V}$) have been recognized [5, 60] (see Fig. 19-10).

Free L chains of both type κ and type λ (i.e., polyclonal L chains) appear in normal urine in trace amounts. L chains consist of an NH_2 terminal portion (V_L), which is variable in amino-acid sequence, and a carboxyl (COOH) terminal portion (C_L), which is essentially constant in sequence. The V portion is a determinant of antibody specificity. The heavy (H) chain is thought to be organized in a manner similar to the L chain, with analogous V_H and C_H portions (see Fig. 19-13).

HEAVY (H) CHAINS
The H chains are distinctive for each class of immunoglobulin. Differences between the various classes of H chains include their amino acid composition and sequence, molecular weight, carbohydrate contents,

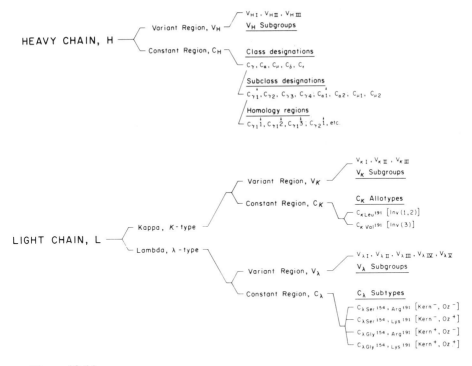

Figure 19-10
Terminology of the heavy and light chains of human immunoglobulins. (Reproduced by permission. From Solomon, A., and McLaughlin, C. L. *Semin. Hematol.* 10:3, 1973.)

electrophoretic mobility, and antigenic and allotypic specificity. This heterogeneity of structure is related to the diversity of antibody functions. H chains of IgG, IgA, IgM, IgD, and IgE are termed *gamma* (γ), *alpha* (α), *mu* (μ), *delta* (δ), and *epsilon* (ϵ) chains, respectively. At least four subclasses of IgG (IgG$_{1,2,3,4}$) have been identified (Fig. 19-11), and they differ in certain biological properties (see Table 19-1). Two subclasses of IgA (IgA$_1$ and IgA$_2$) and IgM (IgM$_1$ and IgM$_2$) have been described (see Fig. 19-11). Any one molecule of immunoglobulin consists of only one class or subclass of H chains in addition to one type of L chains. The immunoglobulin "class" (or "subclass") refers to the H chain, which determines whether an immunoglobulin is of the IgG (IgG$_1$, IgG$_2$, and so on) class, IgA (IgA$_1$ or IgA$_2$) class, or IgM (IgM$_1$ or IgM$_2$) class.

Data obtained from amino acid sequence analysis of γ [57] and μ heavy chains [62] demonstrate that the H chains also consist of variable (V_H) and constant (C_H) regions. The first 121 amino-acid residues constitute the V_H region, and the remaining 325 amino-acid residues, the C_H regions of the H chains. The C_H region can be subdivided into three equal homologous regions, termed $C_H{}^1$, $C_H{}^2$, and $C_H{}^3$. The C_H regions provide the molecular basis for the different characteristics of the

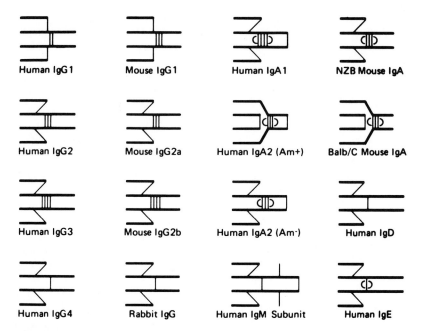

Figure 19-11
Distributions of interchain disulfide bridges (*thin lines*) joining light and heavy chains (*short* and *long thick lines*) in different immunoglobulin classes and subclasses. The positions of the bridges are taken by comparison with homologous sequences in human IgG$_1$ molecules. In some cases, it is not ruled out that the marked bridges are labile intrachain rather than interchain bridges.

The exact number of inter-heavy-chain disulfide bridges (*bracketed*) in IgA molecules is uncertain, as are the positions in the heavy chain of the bridges in mouse IgA and IgE. The bridge involved in covalent dimerization of IgA molecules has not been established. Am+ and Am− are allotypic forms of human IgA$_2$ molecules. (Reproduced by permission. From Fudenberg, H. H., Pink, J. R. L., Stites, D. P., and Wang, A. C. *Basic Immunogenetics.* New York: Oxford University Press, 1972.)

various immunoglobulin classes and subclasses. These constant regions are therefore termed Cγ, Cα, Cμ, Cδ, and Cϵ for the immunoglobulins IgG, IgA, IgM, IgD, and IgE, respectively. Further distinctions are Cγ_1, Cγ_2, Cγ_3, and Cγ_4 for the immunoglobulin subclasses IgG$_1$, IgG$_2$, IgG$_3$, and IgG$_4$, respectively, and Cα_1 and Cα_2 for the C$_H$ region of the IgA$_1$ and IgA$_2$ subclasses, respectively. Within the variable region of the H chain, there are three subgroups: V$_{HI}$, V$_{HII}$, and V$_{HIII}$ [5] (see Fig. 19-10).

IgG AND IgG SUBCLASSES
Four distinct subclasses of IgG [63], each of which is under separate genetic control, have been defined. They are designated *IgG$_1$, IgG$_2$, IgG$_3$,*

and *IgG₄* [64, 65]. Their approximate relative distribution among the IgG class is 70 to 75 percent, 10 to 20 percent, and 5 to 10 percent, and 3 to 5 percent, respectively. These proteins of the IgG subclasses possess characteristic bonds [5] (see Fig. 19-11 and Table 19-1). The various IgG subclasses are associated with distinctive genetic (Gm) factors [5, 60]. The physicochemical properties of IgG and its subclasses are summarized in Table 19-1.

SERUM IgA AND IgA SUBCLASSES
Most serum IgA molecules consist of one pair of identical κ or λ light chains and one pair of identical α heavy chains. Serum IgA has a molecular weight of approximately 170,000 daltons. A small portion (less than 10 percent) of serum IgA molecules exists in polymeric forms, which may be dimers (9S; 320,000 MW), trimers (11S; 480,000 MW), tetramers (13S; 640,000 MW), and probably also pentamers (15S; 820,000 MW). Serum IgA tends to form complexes with other proteins, especially with albumin [66]. Almost half of the total body pool of serum IgA is intravascular [30, 66–68]. The two IgA subclasses, IgA₁ and IgA₂, reveal significant structural differences and variations in the interchain disulfide bonds linking the H and L chains (see Fig. 19-11). The ratio of IgA₁ and IgA₂ molecules in normal serum is approximately 9 to 1.

SECRETORY IgA
In addition to serum IgA, secretory IgA also exists. Its synonyms are exocrine IgA [66] and external IgA [69]. It consists of two IgA molecules linked by a polypeptide chain, termed the *secretory* or *transport piece,* with 60,000 MW (see Fig. 19-9), as well as another polypeptide chain, the *joining (J) chain,* with 25,000 MW. The total molecular weight of the secretory IgA unit is 390,000 (11.8S) (see Table 19-1). Secretory IgA is formed in plasma cells, which are abundantly present in the lamina propria of the mucosa (400,000 per cubic millimeter) [66] (Fig. 19-12). These cells are present mainly in the mucous membranes of the respiratory and GI tracts. The secretory piece, which is produced by the epithelial cells, is joined to the IgA molecules during their transit through the epithelial layer; it may provide resistance of the IgA molecule to the action of proteolytic enzymes in the succus [66, 67] or it may provide an "anchoring" mechanism of IgA to the luminal surface of the epithelial cells to prevent its rapid washout [70]. The J piece is probably synthesized by plasma cells, and its biological function may be associated with the propensity of IgA molecules to form aggregates and polymers. Some of the IgA (without the secretory piece) that is produced by plasma cells in the lamina propria of the gut may reach the circulation [66] (see Fig. 19-12).

IgM
The serum IgM is a pentamer composed of five IgM monomers that are linked by disulfide bridges and J chains (see Fig. 19-9). The molecular

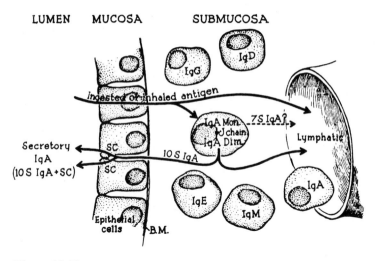

LUMEN   MUCOSA   SUBMUCOSA

Figure 19-12
Sites of synthesis and routes of transport of immunoglobulins from the submucosal areas of a secretory organ such as the gastrointestinal tract. It has
been shown that IgA is synthesized in the plasma cells and then moves in two
directions: one fraction goes into the general circulation via the lymphatics
as serum IgA and another fraction passes through the cells of the epithelial
lining, where the secretory piece is acquired. On leaving the epithelial cells
and entering the secretory tract, the protein is now secretory IgA. (From
Tomasi, T. B., Jr. *N. Engl. J. Med.* 287:500, 1972. Reprinted by permission
from the *New England Journal of Medicine.*)

weight of this spider-like structure is approximately 900,000 (19S). Two
subclasses of IgM, IgM_1 and IgM_2, have been demonstrated immunochemically [71]. The pentameric IgM molecule can be reduced and de-
polymerized by sulfhydryl or mercaptan reagents into subunits [72–74],
which are prevented from reaggregating by alkylation of the sulfhydryl
groups. The IgM antibody has ten potential combining sites, but ordinarily only five are expressed. The IgM molecule contains approximately
10 percent carbohydrates (hexose, fucose, hexosamine, and sialic acid),
which are associated with the Fc_μ fragment.

LOW MOLECULAR WEIGHT IgM
In addition to the high molecular weight 19S IgM, a low molecular
weight 7S IgM has been demonstrated in trace amounts in the serum
from healthy persons and, in higher concentrations, in that of patients
with a variety of disorders [60]. This naturally occurring 7S IgM is composed of two light chains and two μ heavy chains. The presence of 7S
IgM in human serum may be due to a deficiency of the synthesis of J
chains [60], which prevents the assembly of these monomeric IgM moieties into the complete pentameric 19S IgM molecule.

IgD

This immunoglobulin is composed of one pair of L chains (either κ or λ) and one pair of δ heavy chains. Its biological function remains elusive. The physicochemical properties of IgD are listed in Table 19-1.

IgE

This class of immunoglobulins [75, 76] was discovered in reagin-rich sera from atopic patients. The IgE molecule consists of one pair of L chains (either κ or λ) and one pair of ϵ heavy chains. The physicochemical properties of IgE are summarized in Table 19-1.

CLEAVAGE PRODUCTS OF IMMUNOGLOBULINS

Further insight into the structure of immunoglobulins was obtained by cleavage experiments with proteolytic enzymes, mercaptans, and other substances [45, 77, 78]. Papain hydrolyzes IgG molecules into three fragments, each with a molecular weight of approximately 50,000: the *Fc fragment* (crystallizable and complement-binding), and two *Fab fragments* (antigen-binding). Similar cleavage products are obtained from the other immunoglobulin classes.

Figure 19-13 summarizes the enzymatic cleavage properties of IgG. In solution, IgG maintains a T-shaped configuration (lower portion of central diagram), but it assumes a Y-shape on combination with antigen (upper portion of the central diagram). This movement occurs at the "hinge region" of the heavy chains. Light (L) chains (22,000 molecular weight) are of at least two types, κ and λ, represented by kappa and lambda polypeptide chains in higher vertebrates. Heavy (H) chains (55,000 molecular weight) of IgG are termed gamma (γ) chains. The L and H chains are bound by noncovalent bonds and one disulfide bond, whereas two to five inter-heavy-γ-chain disulfide bonds are present, varying with the IgG subclasses. Four subclasses of human γ chains are recognized (IgG_1, IgG_2, IgG_3, and IgG_4), and another subclass, IgG_5, has recently been proposed. The subclasses vary in peptide and amino acid composition as well as in biological properties. Both of the γ chains of an IgG molecule are of the same subclass. The variable (V) portion of the light (V_L) and heavy (V_H) chains is located on the amino terminal end of these chains and is responsible for specific interaction with antigen. The constant (C) portion of light (C_L) and heavy (C_H) chains constitutes the remainder of these polypeptides. The C_H consists of three homologous regions almost equal in length; they are designated C_H^1, C_H^2, and C_H^3. The hinge region is located between C_H^1 and C_H^2. They determine the polymorphism of these chains—that is, the light chain types and subtypes and the heavy chain subclasses—but they are constant within each type, subtype, or subclass and do not vary with antibody specificity, as does the variable portion. Inv (inhibitor V) and Gm (gamma) are heritable loci present on kappa C_L of all immunoglobulin classes and the gamma C_H of IgG, respectively. Each light chain possesses one Inv marker or "nonmarker" (the absence of a detectable marker), whereas each heavy chain has two allelic Gm markers or "non-

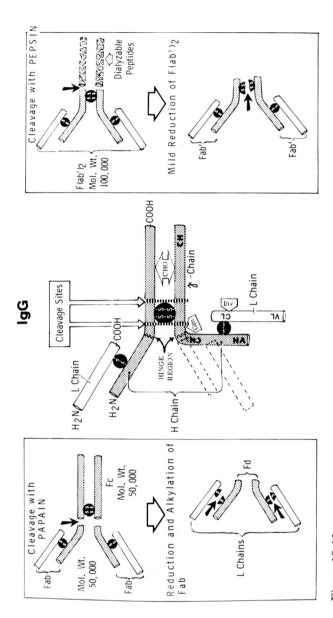

Figure 19-13

The IgG molecule and products of classic enzymatic cleavage (for explanation see pp. 374–375). (Modified from Wolf, R. E., and Deicher, H. *New Physician* 17:335, 1968.)

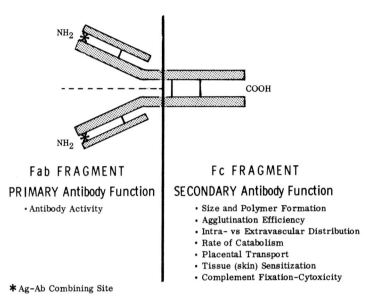

NH$_2$ ✱

COOH

NH$_2$ ✱

Fab FRAGMENT	Fc FRAGMENT
PRIMARY Antibody Function	SECONDARY Antibody Function
• Antibody Activity	• Size and Polymer Formation
	• Agglutination Efficiency
	• Intra- vs Extravascular Distribution
	• Rate of Catabolism
	• Placental Transport
	• Tissue (skin) Sensitization
	• Complement Fixation-Cytoxicity

✱ Ag–Ab Combining Site

Figure 19-14
Functional aspects of the IgG molecule. *: Ag-Ab combining site.

markers": one on the Fd fragment and one on the Fc portion. The Fc fragment, produced by papain cleavage of IgG (*left side*) consists of the carboxyl terminal halves of the two gamma heavy chains. It is crystallizable and is responsible for auxiliary biological properties of the molecule other than interaction with antigen, e.g., complement fixation, interaction with rheumatoid factors or receptors on cell membranes, placental transfer, catabolic properties, and passive cutaneous anaphylaxis. The Fc-like portion of IgG is split into small, dialyzable, inactive peptides during pepsin cleavage (*right side*). Each Fab fragment produced by papain cleavage is composed of one light chain and the amino terminal portion of one gamma heavy chain (Fd). It contains the antibody-active site of the IgG molecule. Fab may be split into component light chains and Fd fragments by reduction and alkylation. F(ab′)$_2$ is a 5S, bivalent antibody fragment produced by pepsin cleavage and is similar to two Fab fragments bound by a disulfide linkage. The Fab′ fragment is produced by the mild reduction of F(ab′)$_2$ and is similar to the Fab fragment. Cleavage sites are indicated by arrows in Figure 19-13.

The Fc fragment of IgG consists of the carboxyl terminal portion of the two γ heavy chains (including the constant homology regions C_H^2 and C_H^3) that are joined by a disulfide link, and it contains no L chains. It possesses no antibody activity, but it provides auxiliary functions and is responsible for placental transfer, skin binding, metabolic properties (e.g., biological survival), gut transfer, opsonization, anaphylaxis, the complement fixation of IgG, and other functions [79] (Fig. 19-14).

The Fab fragments (including the V_L and C_L regions) are composed of an L chain and the amino terminal portion of one H chain (i.e., the Fd fragment, including the V_H and C_H^1 regions) connected by disulfide bonds (see Fig. 19-13). They retain antibody activity. Reduction and alkylation of Fab fragments separate the L chains from the Fd fragments. Pepsin digestion of IgG yields 5S divalent antibody fragments with an approximate molecular weight of 100,000, which are referred to as $F(ab')_2$. These divalent fragments are capable of precipitating with antigens. Further reduction with mercaptans leads to the production of 3.5S univalent Fab' fragments with a molecular weight of 56,000. The full expression of antibody activity requires both the H and L chains; the almost unlimited diversity of antibodies resides in the V_L and V_H regions.

IMMUNOGLOBULIN ALLOTYPES

Two major groups or allotypes with distinctive genetic markers are known to contribute further to the heterogeneity of human immunoglobulins (see Figs. 19-10, 19-11, and 19-13). One group, the *Gm factor,* is associated with IgG and reflects the allelic genes that regulate the composition of the C region of the γ-polypeptide ($C\gamma$) chains. More than 25 different Gm factors (Gm 1, 2, 3, and so on) are known [5]. The IgG 1, 2, 3, and 4 subclasses possess distinctive genetic Gm factors [5]. These allotypic differences are the result of amino acid replacements that occur as genetic variants in the constant portion of the molecule of IgG subclasses (C_1, C_2, and so on).

The other major genetic marker, the *Inv factor* [5], is found only on the κ light chains of all immunoglobulin classes. Three different Inv factors (Inv 1, 2, and 3) are recognized. As with hemoglobins, the constituent polypeptide chain is considered to be under the control of a distinct structural gene. The Inv marker is expressed in the constant region of the residue at position 191 of the κ light chain. The Inv 1 and Inv 2 allotypes are associated with a leucyl residue at position 191, and Inv 3, with a valyl residue at this position in the C region (i.e., $C\kappa$ $Leuc^{181}$ and $C\kappa$ Val^{191}).

Another genetic factor, termed *Am2* [5], has been found in IgA_2 molecules; it is located on the C_α^2 chain. IgA_1 molecules are termed *Am2(−)* (see Figs. 19-10, 19-11, and 19-13). Comparable genetic markers on μ, δ, and ϵ heavy chains or on λ light chains have not been observed.

IMMUNOGLOBULIN CONCENTRATIONS

The levels of serum immunoglobulins are age-dependent, including both the intrauterine and extrauterine periods of life (Fig. 19-15; see also Figs. 4-5 to 4-7).

IgG

The fetal IgG is derived mostly from the maternal circulation by selective placental transfer mechanisms. During the first 20 weeks of gestation, IgG levels are approximately 10 percent of adult normal levels, and they remain low even in the presence of fetal infections such as rubella

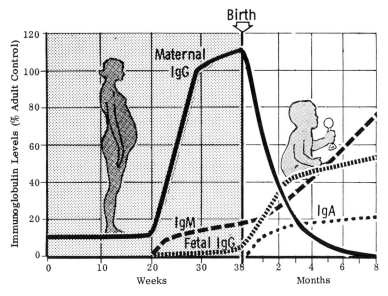

Figure 19-15
Intrauterine development of serum immunoglobulin levels. Data are expressed as the geometrical mean percent of adult control values. The line labeled *maternal IgG* signifies serum levels thought to be derived primarily from placental transfer, whereas other lines, including those referring to IgM and IgG, indicate serum levels believed to result from the fetus' or infant's own production. (Modified from Alford, C. A., Jr. *Pediatr. Clin. North Am.* 18:99, 1971.)

[80, 81] (see Fig. 19-15). Between the 22nd and 28th week of gestation, however, there is a sharp increase in the ability of the placenta to pass IgG from the maternal circulation. By the 26th or 27th week of gestation, the level of IgG in the fetus is usually the same as that in the mother. After delivery, maternal IgG, in both premature and mature infants, is catabolized in an approximate half-life of 30 days, and the maternal IgG disappears from the serum of the infant during the latter half of the first year. The fetal serum levels of the IgG subclasses are similar to those of the maternal levels, with the exception of lower fetal IgG$_2$ concentrations [82]. This supply of the mother's IgG antibody store provides the newborn with an efficient mode of "passive" immunization against a wide spectrum of infectious agents.

The level of serum IgG decreases rapidly after birth from the adult level in umbilical cord serum to a low level, at 3 to 4 months of age, of approximately 350 to 400 mg per 100 ml (40 to 45 international units [IU] per milliliter), which indicates that little synthesis occurs during this period. Thereafter, it gradually increases to 700 to 800 mg per 100 ml (80 to 90 IU per milliliter) by the end of the first year, and it attains an average adult level before 16 years of age (1250 mg per 100 ml or 145 IU per milliliter). The relative concentrations of the four subclasses, IgG$_1$, IgG$_2$, IgG$_3$, and IgG$_4$, in young male adults is 60.9, 29.6, 5.3, and 4.2 percent, respectively [83].

IgA

There is no placental transfer of maternal serum IgA. In about the second week of life, a low level of IgA can usually be detected. The breast-fed newborn is supplied with the maternal antibody store of secretory IgA contained in the colostrum, which is extraordinarily rich in secretory IgA. This transfer provides an effective "passive" immunization of the newborn against most GI infections.

The serum IgA level increases slowly during infancy and childhood. It reaches about 25 percent of the adult value at the end of the first year and 50 percent at age 3½ years. The average adult level is approached at age 16 years (210 mg per 100 ml or 125 IU per milliliter). The developmental profile of secretory IgA levels is not known.

IgM

Maternal IgM does not cross the placenta, and it cannot be detected in fetal serum before the 20th week of gestation. Average fetal serum levels between the 20th and 30th week of gestation are approximately 10 percent of normal adult serum concentrations in both premature and term infants. The IgM levels subsequently rise rapidly; the fetus and the newborn apparently can produce IgM earlier and at higher rates than IgG and IgA. Consequently, demonstration of increased IgM in cord sera is employed increasingly to indicate fetal antigenic stimulation, such as intrauterine infections. The normal distribution of cord blood IgM levels is shown in Figure 19-16. The IgM that is detectable in small quantities in umbilical cord serum is apparently produced by the fetus [84]. The serum level of IgM increases rapidly after birth and reaches an average adult level before IgG or IgA do; 50 percent of adult levels are present at 4 months of age, and adult levels (140 mg per 100 ml or 160 IU per milliliter) are obtained between 8 and 15 years of age.

IgD AND IgE

IgD and IgE are either absent or of low concentration in cord blood, but they also gradually reach adult serum levels by 2 to 5 years of age (an IgD level of 4 mg per 100 ml or 30 IU per milliliter). The newborn mean IgE level is approximately 1 percent of the adult normal mean concentration [85, 86]. The adult serum IgE levels (approximately 10 to 1000 ng per 100 ml or 5 to 500 IU per milliliter) are only about 1/40,000 of those of IgG.

BODY DISTRIBUTION OF IMMUNOGLOBULINS

IgG

At least half of the total body IgG resides in the interstitial fluids, and the remainder is found in the plasma [63]. The maternal IgG also traverses the placenta and results in comparable fetal IgG levels. There

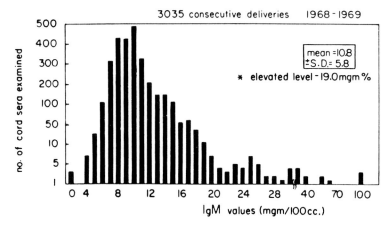

Figure 19-16
Distribution of IgM levels in 3035 specimens of cord sera collected over a one-year period. The geometrical mean level is approximately 11 mg per 100 ml. IgM was considered to be increased to more than 19.0 mg per 100 ml in 2 percent of the cases (69 cases). *: according to log normal probability chart. (Reproduced by permission. From Alford, C. A., Jr. *Pediatr. Clin. North Am.* 18:99, 1971.)

occurs some selection for the IgG subclasses, however, since concentrations of IgG$_1$, IgG$_3$, and IgG$_4$ subclasses are present in similar amounts in both the mothers and infants, but IgG$_2$ is considerably lower in the fetal than in the maternal circulation [82]. The transport of IgG across the placenta against a concentration gradient is a saturable process. A suggested mechanism for the transport of IgG across the placenta may be similar to that for the intestinal crossing of IgG in neonatal rats [87], which involves the initial attachment of an IgG molecule to IgG-Fc-specific membrane receptors on enterocytes, with subsequent invagination of the membrane to form pinocytic vesicles that migrate to the base of the cell and release the IgG into microvillous lacteals. Furthermore, such a mechanism may also be instrumental in the normal IgG catabolism that results in the characteristic concentration-catabolism relationship [87].

IgA
The body distribution of serum IgA is similar to that of IgG. Secretory IgA is the principal form of antibody secretions. It is the predominant immunoglobulin in human saliva, tears, colostrum, and nasal, tracheobronchial, and GI secretions, as well as in bile and secretions from the urinary passages [3, 66–68].

IgM
Approximately 75 to 80 percent of 19S IgM remains in the intravascular compartment [4].

IgD AND IgE
The body distribution of IgD is similar to that of IgM [5, 88], and the distribution of IgE, to that of IgA [76, 88].

SYNTHESIS AND CATABOLISM OF IMMUNOGLOBULINS
The serum and tissue concentrations of the immunoglobulins reflect a balance between the production rates and catabolic properties [87, 89] (see Table 19-1). Each of the immunoglobulin classes has a unique pathway of synthesis and rate of catabolism. Radiolabeling techniques have led to the clarification of most metabolic aspects of immunoglobulins.

A number of factors control immunoglobulin synthesis, including the age of the person, the functional state of the central and peripheral lymphoid organs, antigen stimulation, and antibody activity as a self-regulator. The administration of certain immunosuppressive drugs (e.g., corticosteroids and 6-mercaptopurine) results in decreased immunoglobulin levels. The catabolism of the immunoglobulins is determined by factors that affect all serum proteins as well as factors that affect only one or more immunoglobulin classes or subclasses. These distinctive properties are attributed to the different H chains, particularly to areas on the Fc fragments, and consequently they vary for the different immunoglobulin classes and subclasses. The metabolism of the Fc fragment is similar to that of the intact immunoglobulin, whereas that of the Fab fragment and free L chains is less than 1/50 of that of the Fc fragment [90]. Nonspecific factors affecting immunoglobulin catabolism are poorly understood. Hypermetabolism of immunoglobulins, which is associated with shortening of the IgG half-life and an increase in the fractional catabolic rate [88], is observed in patients with fever or during the administration of corticosteroids or thyroxin [87]. Thus, a general increase in the total body metabolic tempo, the final common pathway of these factors, is likely to be expressed in the immunoglobulins as in other body constituents.

IgG
In healthy adults, approximately 2 gm of IgG are synthesized and catabolized each day [91]. The rate of synthesis of IgG is approximately 30 mg per kilogram of body weight per day in the older child and adult. The synthesis rate of IgG is similar to that of IgA, but 5 times that of IgM, about 80 times that of IgD, and over 2000 times that of IgE [90]. The biological half-life of IgG is approximately 25 days, and the survival time seems to be inversely related to serum IgG levels. All four subclasses of IgG are subject to this concentration-catabolism effect [87] (see Figs. 19-17 and 19-18). Agammaglobulinemic patients or patients with IgA or IgM monoclonal gammopathies and decreased IgG levels show a prolonged half-life of IgG [92]. Conversely, the rate of catabolism of IgG in individuals with elevated IgG levels, due either to infections (polyclonal IgG increase) or to IgG myeloma (monoclonal IgG increase), is increased and this probably contributes to the low levels of normal,

Figure 19-17
Relationship between survival (T½) of IgG and the serum concentration obtained from turnover studies performed in patients with a wide range of IgG concentrations. The structural configurations of the γ-globulin molecules determining the effect of concentration on catabolism are restricted to the Fc fragment of the heavy chains. This concentration-catabolism relationship has clinical implications with regard to γ-globulin therapy. (Modified from Waldmann, T. A., Blaese, R. M., and Strober, W. In M. A. Rothschild and T. Waldmann (Eds.), *Plasma Protein Metabolism. Regulation of Synthesis, Distribution and Degradation.* New York: Academic, 1970.)

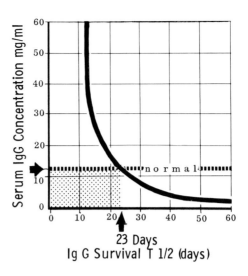

Ig G Survival T 1/2 (days)

residual IgG in these patients [91, 92]. The rates of catabolism of IgG_1, IgG_2, and IgG_4 myeloma proteins are similar to those of normal IgG, but IgG_3 myeloma proteins are catabolized more rapidly than the normal IgG [93]. It must be realized that the concentration of the different subclasses of IgG also affects the survival of the other subclasses. For instance, elevated IgG_1 concentrations result in a shortened survival of the IgG_2, IgG_3, and IgG_4 subclasses [88]. The mechanisms responsible for this IgG concentration-catabolism relationship are unknown, but they may be similar to those that govern the selective transport of IgG across the placenta, yolk sac, or intestinal epithelium; that is, there may be a saturable protective system that is specific for IgG [94].

SERUM IgA
The rate of synthesis of serum IgA in adults is approximately 8 to 10 mg per kilogram of body weight per day [95]. The half-life of serum IgA is between 6 and 8 days, and it appears to be independent of the serum concentrations of IgA. The precise metabolic properties of secretory IgA are unknown.

IgM
19S IgM remains predominantly within the intravascular compartment (approximately 75 to 88 percent) [96]. The average rate of synthesis of IgM in normal subjects is 6 to 7 mg per kilogram of body weight per day. The average biological half-life of IgM is approximately 5 days.

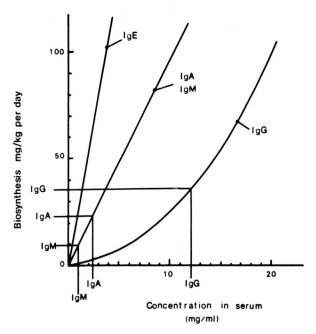

Figure 19-18
Relationship between the concentrations of IgE, IgA, IgM, and IgG in the serum and the rate of biosynthesis of these proteins. (Reproduced by permission. From Heremans, J. F., and Masson, P. L. *Clin. Chem.* 19:294, © 1973, *Clinical Chemistry.*)

There appears to be no relationship between the fractional catabolic rate and the serum levels.

IgD
The IgD is predominantly located within the vascular compartment (approximately 75 percent) [97]. The median synthetic rate is 0.4 mg per kilogram of body weight per day, and the median biological half-life is 2.8 days. The fractional catabolic rate of IgD appears to be inversely related to its serum concentration in that subjects with high serum IgD levels tend to have lower fractional catabolic rates than those with low serum levels. This concentration-catabolism relationship for IgD is the opposite of that for IgG.

IgE
The serum IgE concentration may not fully reflect the "effective" IgE levels in a given patient, since it is preferentially produced in regional areas, including the respiratory and gastrointestinal mucosa as well as in the regional lymph nodes [98]. Furthermore, it has an affinity for mast cells. Its catabolic rate is rapid, and its half-life is about 2.3 days.

In general, there are three different catabolic patterns that affect the various immunoglobulin classes. For instance, IgM and IgA have catabolic rates that are independent of their serum concentrations (see Fig. 19-18). IgD (like some other serum proteins, such as haptoglobin and transferrin) has an inverse relationship between the catabolic rate and the serum concentration; the catabolic rate of IgD tends to be low in relation to the high serum concentration of that protein. A third pattern of the concentration-catabolism relationship is observed with IgG (see Figs. 19-17 and 19-18). The catabolic rates of IgG vary in direct proportion to the serum concentrations of IgG. Thus, the catabolic rate of IgG is reduced (and survival is prolonged) in patients who have low serum γ-globulin concentrations secondary to decreased synthesis, and its half-life may be as long as 70 days. Conversely, with increasing serum IgG concentrations, the survival half-life time decreases from the normal 23 to 25 days progressively until a limit is approached of 10 to 11 days and a serum concentration of approximately 30 mg per milliliter [90].

BIOLOGICAL FUNCTIONS OF IMMUNOGLOBULINS

GENERAL ASPECTS

The various immunoglobulin classes possess numerous individual antibody functions, and each class exhibits variable specificities of antibodies. Carry-over terms for differing antibody expressions are still in use; these include *complete antibodies, saline antibodies, cold antibodies,* and so forth, which reflect the various facets of IgM reactivity. Such terms as *incomplete antibodies, warm antibodies, blocking antibodies,* and so forth reflect those of IgG. These various functional denominations are summarized in Table 19-2 for blood-group antibodies. IgM "complete" antibodies agglutinate certain red blood cells in saline suspension, but, in contrast, IgG "incomplete" antibodies do not directly agglutinate saline-suspended red blood cells. These IgG antibodies are not large enough to "bridge the gap" between the adjacent red blood cells, in contrast to the larger, complete IgM molecules (Fig. 19-19).

The red blood cells can be brought close enough together to allow IgG molecules to agglutinate them by altering the electrical forces that repel any two cells (the zeta potential). This can be done by adding bovine albumin or enzymes such as trypsin. Another way of detecting incomplete IgG antibodies is by means of the *antiglobulin (Coombs') test* (see Fig. 19-19). Blood-group antibodies, which are added to the red blood cells and combined with them without producing agglutination, are detected by subsequent washing of the mixture of coated red blood cells and serum to remove all serum proteins, followed by addition of a rabbit antiglobulin antiserum to human globulin. The last reagent reacts with the human globulin on the red blood cells and causes agglutination. The Coombs' test is a very important diagnostic test in clinical immunology. It is essential for the detection of numerous autoimmune antibodies (e.g., acquired autoimmune hemolytic anemias), isoimmune antibodies (e.g., erythroblastosis fetalis due to Rh antibodies in Rh-positive in-

Table 19-2. Blood-Group Antibodies

Functional Denomination	Definition	Immuno-globulin Class
Naturally occurring antibodies	Present without any known antigenic stimulants (e.g., anti-A, B, I, etc.).	IgM
Immune antibodies	Formed as a result of exposure to foreign antigens (e.g., transfusion, pregnancy).	IgG
Complete antibodies	Agglutinate saline-suspended red cells (e.g., anti-A, B, H, I, etc.).	IgM
Incomplete antibodies	Do not agglutinate saline-suspended red cells.	IgG
Cold antibodies	React maximally with red cells at 4°C.	IgM
Warm antibodies	React maximally with red cells at 37° C.	IgG
Blocking antibodies	Thought to block the reaction with red cells.	IgG
Saline antibodies	See *complete antibodies* above.	IgM
Coombs' antibodies	Agglutinate red cells in the presence of Coombs' serum; see *immune antibodies,* above.	IgG

fants), or drug-induced immune hemolytic disorders (e.g., by penicillin, quinine, α-methyldopa, or cephalothin).

SPECIFIC ANTIBODY FUNCTIONS

The various immunoglobulin classes subserve a wide variety of specific antibody functions.

IgG contains the majority of antibacterial, antiviral, and antitoxic antibodies. It comprises antinuclear antibodies, incomplete Rh antibodies, immune ABO blood-group antibodies, as well as antibodies to insulin, ragweed, and many others [66]. The IgG subclasses possess similar antibody functions, as well as several individual characteristics [99]. Notably, IgG_4 fails to fix complement, in contrast to the other IgG subclasses, but it activates complement via the alternate pathway. The IgG_2 subclass contains predominantly antidextran and antilevan antibody activity. IgG_3 proteins have a propensity to aggregate, and rheumatoid factors react poorly with this subclass.

Serum IgA also subserves numerous antibody functions, and it includes antitoxins as well as certain antiviral and antibacterial antibodies [66]. Secretory IgA provides a protective "antibody paint" [100] that coats mucous surfaces, thus providing a first line of regional defense [67]. The tendency of IgA to form complexes with other protein sub-

"Complete" antibodies

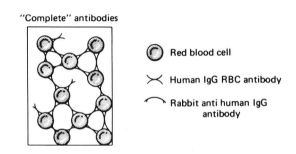

◉ Red blood cell

✕ Human IgG RBC antibody

⌒ Rabbit anti human IgG
      antibody

"Incomplete" antibodies

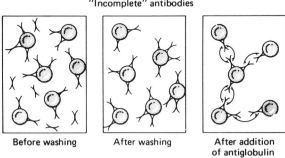

Before washing   After washing   After addition
                                           of antiglobulin

Figure 19-19

Detection of complete antibodies: No Coombs' test needed. *Detection of incomplete antibodies:* Coombs' test needed to "enlarge" the IgG anti-red cell antibody to "bridge the gap" between two adjacent cells, leading to agglutination. The so-called "non-γ" type of Coombs' test is based on the same principle, with the substitution of antibody to human complement components for the anti-human IgG antibody as the "bridging" antibody. This test may be positive in patients whose red cells carry such complement components as a reflection of immune sensitization.

Indirect Coombs' test: Detects incomplete antibodies in the serum. *Direct Coombs' test:* Detects incomplete antibodies on red cells. (Reproduced by permission. From Fudenberg, H. H., Pink, J. R. L., Stites, D. P., and Wang, A. C. *Basic Immunogenetics.* New York: Oxford University Press, 1972.)

stances may aid its protective functions. IgA antibodies do not fix complement; however, they may activate complement via the alternate pathway. IgA possesses numerous specific antibody functions [66], including isoagglutination, antibacterial activity, poliovirus neutralization, and other antiviral activities. Prior to their elucidation, secretory IgA antibodies were termed *mucoantibodies* and *coproantibodies*.

IgM contains most natural antibodies: the ABO blood-group isohemagglutinins, cold agglutinins (i.e., anti I or i antibodies), anti-IgG autoantibodies (i.e., rheumatoid factors), Wassermann antibodies, heterophil antibodies, saline Rh antibodies, and others [66]. IgM antibodies against gram-negative bacteria appear to be more effective than IgG antibodies.

Numerous specific antibodies are provided by all three major immunoglobulin classes, such as antibodies to insulin, *Brucella,* diphtheria, gram-negative bacteria, ragweed, antinuclear factors, incomplete Rh antibodies, isohemagglutinins, and others.

The antibody functions of IgD are unknown. They may carry certain autoimmune activity in selected patients (such as antinuclear, antithyroid activity [101]). Using immunofluorescence, they are frequently found as B-cell surface immunoglobulins, which perhaps suggests a recognition function for antigens [102, 103].

IgE possesses reaginic activity and carries Prausnitz-Küstner (PK) antibody activity. IgE antibodies are synonymous with allergic, homocytotropic, anaphylactic, reaginic, atopic, and skin-sensitizing antibodies. IgE is found to carry the reaginic activity to numerous antigens, such as ragweed, grass pollen, horse dandruff, egg white, house dust, and penicillin [75]. Additionally, it is related to antiparasitic immunity (see Chap. 6).

Pathophysiological Aspects of Immunoglobulins

IMMUNOGLOBULIN DEFICIENCIES

Immunoglobulin abnormalities can be classified according to their pathogenesis into immunoglobulin deficiencies, immunoglobulin overproduction (e.g., polyclonal and monoclonal gammopathies), and immunoglobulin interactions (e.g., immune complexes, hyperviscosity). Immunoglobulin interactions are discussed separately (see Chap. 17 and Chap. 20).

Immunoglobulin deficiency disorders may be due to (1) defective synthesis of all classes, several classes, or selective classes or subclasses of immunoglobulins, e.g., X-linked congenital agammaglobulinemia, selective IgA deficiency, IgG subclass deficiency (see Table 19-4 and Fig. 19-20); (2) pathological loss of immunoglobulins, e.g., nephrotic syndrome, protein-losing gastroenteropathies, thermal burns (see Table 19-5); (3) *increased degradation of immunoglobulins,* e.g., myotonia congenita (see Table 19-6); or (4) *hypocatabolism* [119] (see Table 19-6), leading to increased L-chain levels and other aberrations.

Overproduction states of immunoglobulins are ordinarily associated with increased levels of the immunoglobulin classes, especially IgG, IgA, and IgM in various relative concentrations. Polyclonal gammopathy is usually due to prolonged antigenic stimulation, e.g., chronic infections (see Table 19-7 and Figs. 19-24 and 19-25). It reflects a secondary, reversible plasmocytosis analogous to leukocytosis due to infections. *Monoclonal gammopathies* are characterized by the overproduction of one homogeneous immunoglobulin—i.e., M protein of one class, one subclass, one type, such as IgG_2 (κ)—by one clone of plasma cells which proliferates selectively within the wide spectrum of B-cell clones (Fig. 19-24). Often, there is an inverse relationship between the M-protein level and the concentration of the residual (normal, background) immunoglobulins (i.e.,

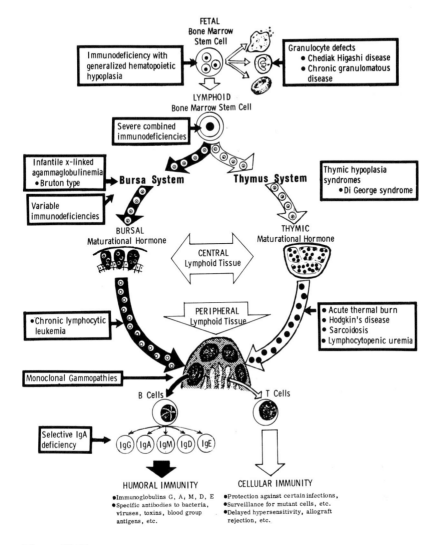

FETAL
Bone Marrow Stem Cell

Immunodeficiency with generalized hematopoietic hypoplasia

Granulocyte defects
- Chediak Higashi disease
- Chronic granulomatous disease

LYMPHOID
Bone Marrow Stem Cell

Severe combined immunodeficiencies

Infantile x-linked agammaglobulinemia
- Bruton type

Bursa System

Thymus System

Thymic hypoplasia syndromes
- Di George syndrome

Variable immunodeficiencies

BURSAL
Maturational Hormone

THYMIC
Maturational Hormone

CENTRAL
Lymphoid Tissue

PERIPHERAL
Lymphoid Tissue

- Chronic lymphocytic leukemia

- Acute thermal burn
- Hodgkin's disease
- Sarcoidosis
- Lymphocytopenic uremia

Monoclonal Gammopathies

B Cells

T Cells

Selective IgA deficiency

IgG IgA IgM IgD IgE

HUMORAL IMMUNITY
- Immunoglobulins G, A, M, D, E
- Specific antibodies to bacteria, viruses, toxins, blood group antigens, etc.

CELLULAR IMMUNITY
- Protection against certain infections,
- Surveillance for mutant cells, etc.
- Delayed hypersensitivity, allograft rejection, etc.

Figure 19-20
Immunological blocks associated with various hereditary and acquired immunodeficiency disorders based upon the ontogenetic dichotomy into B and T systems. A spectrum of primary and secondary immunodeficiency disorders can be correlated with aberrations at various levels of immunological developmental stages. Most of these disorders may be viewed as being characterized by certain complete or partial "immunological blocks" within this framework. Some of the suggested sites of immunological blocks are depicted. These include chronic lymphocytic leukemia (which may be viewed as a nonsecretory, monoclonal proliferative B-cell disorder), monoclonal gammopathies (i.e., secretory, proliferative B-cell diseases), and impaired synthesis of B cells, such as infantile X-linked agammaglobulinemia and variable immunodeficiencies associated with a decrease of most immunoglobulin classes, as well as those associated with selective decreases of immunoglobulin classes (e.g., selective IgA deficiency).

the higher the M-protein level, the lower the residual immunoglobulin concentrations), thus presenting a combination of overproduction and deficiency states.

DIAGNOSTIC APPROACHES TO IMMUNOGLOBULIN DISORDERS

Inasmuch as most immunoglobulin aberrations reflect B-cell disorders, various aspects of the B-cell system require analysis in such patients, often in conjunction with an examination of the T-cell system. These tests, which are modified from Good et al. [19], are summarized in Table 19-3.

HISTORY OF INFECTIONS [19, 104]

Significant degrees of B-cell deficiencies are often associated with increased susceptibility to infections with high-grade, extracellular, encapsulated pyogenic pathogens, including pneumococci, streptococci, *Hemophilus influenzae,* meningococci, and *Pseudomonas aeruginosa.* Other infecting organisms pose either less of a problem (e.g., staphylococci, other enterobacteria, some fungi, and certain viruses) or no problem (e.g., certain viruses, fungi, and other bacterial pathogens). In contrast, patients with isolated T-cell deficiency (e.g., DiGeorge's syndrome or Hodgkin's disease) (Fig. 19-20) are most susceptible to infections with fungi (especially cryptococci), certain viruses (e.g., herpes and vaccinia), mycobacteria, atypical acid-fast organisms, some of the so-called lower-grade pathogens, and intracellular bacterial pathogens (e.g., *Listeria*). Patients with combined B-T-cell deficiencies (e.g., Swiss-type agammaglobulinemia) are most susceptible to infections that begin early in life, such as those due to fungi, *Pneumocystis carinii,* viruses, atypical acid-fast bacteria, and low-grade or high-grade encapsulated bacteria. The clinical course of B-T-cell deficiency is inexorably progressive, leading to early death.

SERUM PROTEIN ELECTROPHORESIS

The finding of a decreased γ-globulin fraction usually indicates the presence of hypo- or even agammaglobulinemia brought about by a severe reduction of IgG. (IgG accounts for approximately 90 percent of the γ-globulin fraction on serum protein electrophoresis.) Deficiencies of the other immunoglobulin classes are not reflected by serum protein electrophoresis (see Chap. 2).

QUANTITATION OF THE IMMUNOGLOBULINS

IgG, IgA, IgM, and IgD can be readily quantitated by radial immunodiffusion (RID) or electroimmunodiffusion (EID) (see Chap. 4). IgE can be quantitated by RID or radioimmunoassay (RIA) (see chap. 6). Salivary secretory IgA can be semiquantitatively determined by Ouchterlony double-diffusion tests or immunoelectrophoresis (IEP) (see Chap. 5). In any patient, the mechanism leading to hypogammaglobulinemia must be considered, and the increased loss or accelerated degradation of immunoglobulins must be specifically ruled out.

Table 19-3.   Diagnostic Approach to B- and T-Cell System Disorders

I. *B-Cell Deficiencies*
   A. *Clinical information:* History of infections and specific identification of bacteria causing frequent pneumonia, sepsis, conjunctivitis, and meningitis
   B. *In vitro assays*
      1. Serum protein electrophoresis for evidence of hypogammaglobulinemia
      2. Quantitation of IgG, IgA, and IgM. In selected cases, additional assays may be needed for:
         a. IgD and IgE
         b. Secretory IgA
         c. IgG subclasses
         d. Fractional catabolic rates and/or synthetic rates for individual immunoglobulins
         e. Quantitation of blood B cells (immunofluorescence, B rosettes, etc.)
      3. Quantitation of antibody concentrations to antigens widely distributed in nature, e.g., isohemagglutinins, ASO, Schick test, antiviral antibodies, etc.
   C. *In vivo procedures*
      1. Quantitation of antibody response to killed polio virus vaccines, diphtheria or tetanus toxoids, and polysaccharide antigens from pneumococcal, meningococcal, and hemophilic microorganisms
      2. Lymph node biopsy and evaluation of histological state of B areas, especially after antigenic stimulation

II. *T-Cell Deficiencies*
   A. *Clinical information:* History of infections and specific identification of fungi, viruses, and facultative intracellular bacterial pathogens
   B. *In vitro assays*
      1. Blood lymphocyte counts for evidence of quantitative T-cell deficiency (i.e., lymphocytopenia); in selected cases, quantitation of T cells (T rosettes, etc.)
      2. Assays for blastoid transformation to mitogens (PHA) for evidence of qualitative lymphocyte deficiency
         In selected cases, additional assays may be needed:
         a. Blastoid response to antigens (e.g., PPD, diphtheria, tetanus toxoid, etc.)
         b. Blastoid response to allogeneic lymphocytes (i.e., MLC)
         c. Spontaneous lymphocyte response
         d. Lymphokine production (e.g., MIF) in response to antigenic stimulation (e.g., PPD)
   C. *In vivo procedures*
      1. Assays for delayed skin hypersensitivity to:
         a. Ubiquitous antigens, e.g., SK-SD, mumps, Candida, trichophyton, PPD, etc.
         b. 2,4-dinitrochlorobenzene
      2. Lymph node biopsy and evaluation of histological state of T areas, especially after antigenic stimulation

Critical levels of IgG. Sufficient amounts of IgG antibodies are crucial for the protection of the individual from pathogenic microorganisms. In spite of relatively low levels of IgG during the 3 to 5 months after birth (see Fig. 4-5, Chap. 4), most infants remain protected from infections. This fact, together with circumstantial evidence derived from adult patients with hypogammaglobulinemia, suggests that the critical, protective threshold level of IgG is approximately 200 to 250 mg per 100 ml. Such levels obtained by RID correspond to approximately 0.3 gm per 100 ml of the total γ-globulin fraction on serum protein electrophoresis [105]. Below these levels, increased susceptibility to infections is usually encountered, and γ-globulin substitution therapy is usually indicated. The normal levels of IgG, approximately 1250 mg per 100 ml, provides a four- to fivefold reserve capacity of protective IgG functions in the normal adult. In this respect, IgG conforms with the general biological rule of a four- to fivefold reserve function of most organ systems, including the heart, liver, bone marrow, and so on. Conversely, the normal abundance of IgG constrains the indications for γ-globulin substitution therapy to patients with critically low IgG levels.

Quantitation of immunoglobulin subclasses. These subclasses can be quantitated by RID or hemagglutination techniques, and their absence can be detected by IEP or Ouchterlony double-diffusion techniques. The routine quantitation of the IgG subclasses IgG_1, IgG_2, IgG_3, and IgG_4, as well as of IgA_1 and IgA_2, however, is presently not feasible, because of the lack of readily available specific antisera.

ASSAY OF FRACTIONAL CATABOLIC RATES OR SYNTHETIC RATES
FOR INDIVIDUAL IMMUNOGLOBULINS

These studies, although desirable for the precise characterization of the immunoglobulin deficiency involved and for the determination of synthetic, catabolic, or loss phenomena, are presently not practical in the general hospital laboratory. Referral of such patients under study to specialized centers may be necessary.

QUANTITATION OF PERIPHERAL BLOOD B-CELLS

Immature and mature B cells in the peripheral blood can be quantitated by the application of surface and intracellular immunofluorescence tests [14] and by the erythrocyte complement-antibody-mediated (ECA) test or B-rosette tests [17, 18].

QUANTITATION OF ANTIBODY CONCENTRATIONS TO ANTIGENS
WIDELY DISTRIBUTED IN NATURE

Such antibodies include isohemagglutinins, antistreptolysin-O antibodies, Schick antibodies, antiviral antibodies, and others. The anti-A, anti-B, anti-AB, and anti-I antibody titers usually reflect IgM antibody activity, and their normal titers in adults (95th percentile) range from 1:8 to 1:2048 [21, 106], with lower titers being found in the elderly (see Fig. 19-6). Antistreptolysin O activity is carried by IgG antibodies. The normal adult person, once having responded to the inevitable exposure to the ubiquitous β-hemolytic streptococci, possesses ASO titers of at least 200 Todd units. The Schick test reflects IgG antibodies to diphtheria toxin. This test is somewhat limited by the fact that not all persons have been exposed to diphtheria antigen. Certain viral antibodies, which are carried by IgG, IgA, and IgM, may also be utilized to evaluate the functional state of the B system. A World Health Organization committee's recommendations for such immunizations have been issued [104].

INTRADERMAL INJECTION OF ANTIGENS

The intradermal injection of killed polio virus vaccine (Pasteur Institute), diphtheria toxoids, and tetanus toxoids provides a valuable test to evoke secondary (or primary) antibody responses in sensitized (or unsensitized) individuals to these antigens. The immunoglobulins responding are predominantly IgG and to a lesser extent IgA or, in response to a primary sensitization, IgM. The elicited antibodies to administered antigens from pneumococcal, meningococcal, and hemophilic polysaccharides evoke mainly an IgM response, both in the unsensitized and presensitized individual. Live vaccines should never be given. Failure to respond to antigenic stimulation can sometimes be demonstrated in patients with normal or increased levels of all serum immunoglobulins. Thus, the presence of normal total immunoglobulin concentrations does not exclude an antibody deficiency, and responses to antigenic stimulation may be essential in the diagnostic evaluation of such patients.

LYMPH NODE BIOPSY

Such biopsy, especially after appropriate antigenic stimulation, allows a correlation with the immunodeficiency state, in particular, with the nature and degree of the deficiency of B cells, T cells, or both.

HYPOGAMMAGLOBULINEMIAS

Since the initial description in 1951 by Löffler of agammaglobulinemia in a patient with chronic lymphocytic leukemia [107] and the subsequent clinical correlation of congenital agammaglobulinemia by Bruton in 1952 [108, 109], patients with a wide variety of immunoglobulin deficiency disorders have been reported. Although the absolute number of patients with primary immunodeficiency disorders is relatively low, the impact of these reports upon the general area of basic, experimental, and clinical immunology has been extraordinary. The study of these "experiments of nature" as Good has called them, has yielded new knowledge that is applicable to areas beyond immunology. These developments have recently been reviewed [110].

Most immunological disorders reflect a deficiency in immune capacity. They may be viewed in the context of the dichotomy of the immune system into T and B systems (see Figs. 19-3 and 19-20). No completely satisfactory classification of primary and secondary hypogammaglobulinemias, agammaglobulinemias, selective immunoglobulin deficiencies, and dysgammaglobulinemias (i.e., imbalanced immunoglobulin levels) is presently available. Recently, a World Health Organization proposal for

Table 19-4. Disorders of Immunoglobulin Synthesis

Primary Immunodeficiencies[a]
    Decreased synthesis of most or all immunoglobulin classes
    1. Immunodeficiency with generalized hematopoietic hypoplasia
    2. Severe combined immunodeficiencies
        (a) Autosomal recessive forms
        (b) Sex-linked forms
        (c) Sporadic forms
    3. Immunodeficiency with short-limb dwarfism
    4. Immunodeficiency with thrombocytopenia and eczema (Wiskott-Aldrich syndrome)
    5. Immunodeficiency with thymoma
    6. Infantile X-linked agammaglobulinemia (Bruton form)
    7. Transient hypogammaglobulinemia of infancy
    8. Variable, common immunodeficiencies

    Decreased synthesis of selected immunoglobulins
    1. Selective IgA deficiency
    2. IgG subclass deficiency
    3. Selective IgM deficiency
    4. Selective kappa-chain deficiency
    5. Sex-linked immunodeficiency with IgM elevation
    6. Immunodeficiency with ataxia-telangiectasia
    7. Agammaglobulinemia with B-lymphocytes, associated with defective plasma-cell differentiation

Secondary Immunoglobulin Deficiencies
    Variable, common immunodeficiencies (unclassified)
    Immunoglobulin deficiency induced by immunosuppressive therapy
    Malignant monoclonal B-cell disorders
    1. Chronic lymphocytic leukemia, lymphosarcoma
    2. Nonsecretory monoclonal gammopathies
    3. "Secretory" monoclonal gammopathies
        (a) Symptomatic monoclonal gammopathies
            (1) Multiple myeloma (IgG-, IgA-, IgD-, IgE-myeloma and light-chain disease)
            (2) Waldenström's macroglobulinemia (IgM)
            (3) Heavy-chain disease (γ, α, μ)
        (b) Asymptomatic monoclonal gammopathies (IgG, IgA, IgM, IgD)

[a] Adapted from Fudenberg, H. H., et al. *Bull. W.H.O.* 45:125, 1971.

the categorization of primary immunodeficiency disorders [17, 111, 112], including T-cell, B-cell, and stem-cell abnormalities, has been adopted (see Table 19-4). The immunodeficiency disorders affecting the immunoglobulins either are genetically determined (primary immunoglobulin deficiencies or primary B-cell deficiencies) or may arise as acquired disorders in association with certain diseases (secondary immunoglobulin deficiencies or secondary B-cell deficiencies). The former are encountered mainly in children, whereas the latter are seen predominantly in adults. The differentiation into primary-congenital and secondary-acquired immune disorders is, however, somewhat arbitrary, because some acquired forms may develop later in life in patients having the conducive genetic background.

DECREASED SYNTHESIS OF IMMUNOGLOBULINS

Primary immunoglobulin deficiencies. Primary immunodeficiencies during childhood that affect the immunoglobulins include those caused by a failure to produce the effectors of the B-cell system, thus leading to decreased synthesis of immunoglobulins (see Table 19-4). A brief characterization of the various categories of primary immunodeficiency disorders is presented.

1. *Immunodeficiency with generalized hematopoietic hypoplasia.* This term refers to a presumed hematopoietic stem-cell deficiency in its purest sense, in which no myeloid elements fully mature in adequate numbers. This rapidly fatal disorder includes a profound hypogammaglobulinemia due to the impaired B-cell development. However, this may be clinically less threatening than the erythrocyte, megakaryocyte, and granulocyte types of hypoplasia.

2. *Severe combined immunodeficiencies.* Three distinct forms of combined immunodeficiencies are recognized: the autosomal-recessive, the sex-linked, and the sporadic forms. The congenital, severe combined immunodeficiency (the Swiss type of agammaglobulinemia) is transmitted as a single autosomal recessive trait. Death occurs in afflicted patients before the age of 2 years. Smallpox vaccination leads to progressive vaccinia in these infants. The immunological defect consists of a combined deficiency of both the humoral and cellular defenses (i.e., a combined B-cell and T-cell deficiency, with lymphoid stem cells involved). The humoral aspect of this defect is clinically reflected by a deficiency of all classes of immunoglobulins and the absence of plasma cells with the predictable predisposition to numerous infections. Cellular deficiency is expressed as a deficiency of peripheral blood lymphocytes (lymphocytopenia), an underdeveloped thymus, decreased phytohemagglutinin (PHA) response and mixed leukocyte culture (MLC) reactions, the absence of delayed hypersensitivity, the inability to reject skin allografts, and a resulting susceptibility to viral, fungal, and other infections. One hypothetical explanation for this constellation of immunodeficiencies is that the stem cells may be defective in this disorder. According to Good [1], this disease resembles the defect produced experimentally in chickens by total body irradiation and complete extirpation of both the bursa of Fabricius and the thymus, which provides the model of the absence of B- and T-functions. The only available treatment modalities reside in the highly experimental and, at present, extremely limited attempts at allotransplantation of bone marrow, thymic tissue, or both [19, 112–116].

3. *Immunodeficiency with short-limb dwarfism.* Lymphocytopenia, impaired in vitro responsiveness to PHA and specific antigens, and disseminated viral infections have been associated with hair-cartilage hypoplasia, a variant of short-limbed dwarfism [116]. From these observations, this particular immunodeficiency would appear to also affect the T-cell system.

4. *Immunodeficiency with thrombocytopenia and eczema (Wiskott-Aldrich syndrome)*. This sex-linked recessive disease [17] is characterized by thrombocytopenia, eczema, recurrent infections, and deficient delayed hypersensitivity but normal lymphocyte response to PHA stimulation. The existence of a defect in the afferent limb of immunity has been suggested, which may lead to a defect of recognition or processing of antigens or a defect of information transfer. Correction by bone-marrow transplantation and administration of transfer factor has been attempted.

5. *Immunodeficiency with thymoma*. Patients with thymoma have a high association of agammaglobulinemia or varying degrees of hypo-gammaglobulinemia. T-cell impairment may also occur in a progressive fashion in association with this neoplasm [116].

6. *Infantile sex-linked agammaglobulinemia (Bruton's disease)*. In 1952, Bruton [108, 109] reported an 8-year-old boy who had suffered from 19 bouts of life-threatening episodes of sepsis during a four-year period. Most of these were due to pneumococci. Each episode responded to the administration of penicillin. The family history did not reveal an abnormality, nor did physical and laboratory examinations. Eventually, Tiselius moving-boundary electrophoresis [22] was employed, and absence of the γ-globulin fraction was demonstrated. This finding prompted the administration of 20 ml of concentrated human γ-globulin which kept the patient symptom-free for approximately one month. There was a dramatic improvement in the patient's lack of susceptibility to infections, and serum γ-globulin levels could be detected. Since that time, this patient has been treated by monthly injections of γ-globulins, albeit in higher doses. He has grown normally, has never experienced another attack of severe sepsis, and has been able to lead a normal life. It has been suggested that this patient did not suffer from the congenital sex-linked recessive disorder, but rather from an acquired form of agammaglobulinemia, possibly secondary to a rubella infection. This argument, however, is irrelevant, since clear-cut and well-characterized cases of congenital sex-linked agammaglobulinemia have been described subsequently that exhibited clinical manifestations identical with those described by Bruton.

Infections in males with sex-linked congenital B-cell deficiency do not become a major problem until 6 to 9 months of age, when an increasing number of acute episodes of infections begin to occur. This early period of protection is due to remaining maternal IgG antibodies. In addition to septicemia, cases of meningitis and skin infections are frequently encountered. The predominant sites for such infections are those that are unprotected because of the absence of secretory IgA in these patients; the most common infections are otitis media, sinusitis, conjunctivitis, and pulmonary disease. Such patients show deficiencies in the humoral defense mechanism, as reflected by a deficiency of plasma cells and blood lymphocytes with surface immunoglobulins, a deficiency of circulating and secretory immunoglobulins, and the inability to form antibodies upon antigenic challenge. Plasma cells and germinal centers are absent in lymphoid tissues, whereas the T-cell areas are intact. Delayed skin hypersensitivity and skin allograft rejection reactions are usually normal, as are the thymic structure and the functions of the lymphocytes. In some patients with agammaglobulinemia, normal numbers of B lymphocytes bearing surface IgM, IgG, and IgA are demonstrable. Such patients may not complete the final stage of plasma cell differentiation, and they therefore may not produce and secrete specific antibodies [117]. This sex-linked recessive form of agammaglobulinemia may be considered conceptually as an isolated deficiency of the B system in which the T system remains intact. Experimentally, such deficiencies can be produced by irradiation and bursectomy in the chicken, leaving the thymus intact. This disorder may represent an efferent-limb defect of the humoral immune system. Treatment of this disorder consists of γ-globulin substitution [118].

7. *Autosomal recessive congenital hypogammaglobulinemia.* In this immunodeficiency, immunoglobulin levels are decreased but not to the degree that is seen in X-linked congenital agammaglobulinemia. The germinal centers are present, and immunoglobulins are detectable on the surface of blood lymphocytes. The prevalent infections are similar to those encountered in Bruton's disease—otitis media, sinusitis, conjunctivitis, and pulmonary disease.

8. *Variable, common immunodeficiencies.* These disorders are discussed under secondary immunoglobulin deficiencies (see Case Report 1 and Fig. 19-21).

9. *Transient hypogammaglobulinemia of infancy.* This type of transient hypogammaglobulinemia of infancy is characterized by the slow development of immunoglobulin production (i.e., "late starters"). The prognosis is good in that the serum immunoglobulin concentrations become normal by 18 to 24 months of age.

10. *Selective IgA deficiency.* Selective IgA deficiency [17] is usually due to the deficient synthesis of serum and secretory IgA [119]. It is the most common form of selective immunoglobulin deficiencies, occurring in 1 of 700 persons [120]. Occasionally, there is synthesis but no release of IgA from the B cells. In other cases, there is synthesis and release, but rapid elimination is brought about by circulating antibodies to IgA [119]. Such antibodies may be directed against genetic determinants not found on the patient's own IgA [121]. In patients with isolated IgA deficiency, anaphylactoid reactions may be experienced following the transfusion of blood that contains even trace amounts of IgA [119]. Such patients should always be studied for the presence of antibodies against IgA, which are found in a significant number of these patients [111]. The majority of patients with selective IgA deficiency are asymptomatic, but the remainder suffer from repeated respiratory infections or steatorrhea because of the lack of secretory IgA antibodies. Also, the incidence of autoimmune diseases in such patients is significantly increased [122]. IgA-producing cells in the respiratory and GI tracts are sharply reduced, but levels of blood lymphocytes with surface IgA molecules often remain normal. The numbers of IgM-producing cells are often increased vi-

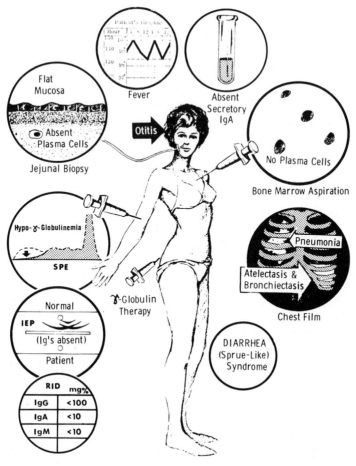

Figure 19-21

Clinical features of hypogammaglobulinemia: common variable form of late onset (see Case Report 1). (Reproduced by permission. From Ritzmann, S. E., and Daniels, J. C. In G. J. Race (Ed.), *Tice's Practice of Medicine,* Vol. 2. New York: Harper & Row, 1974.)

cariously in the respiratory and GI tract, and consequently IgM antibodies are high in the external secretions of such individuals.

11. *Selective IgG subclass deficiency.* In general, patients with IgG subclass deficiencies [17] show great susceptibility to pneumococcal and other high-grade extracellular pyogenic pathogens, which leads to pyogenic infections, progressive pulmonary disease, and so on, just as in patients with generalized B-cell immune deficiency [104]. Selective deficiency of IgG subclasses may affect one subclass [123] or two or three subclasses [124]. Replacement therapy with γ-globulin prevents the recurrence of infections [124].

12. *Selective IgM deficiency.* Selective deficiency of IgM [17, 123] is due to decreased numbers of IgM-producing cells. Affected patients display increased susceptibility to respiratory bacterial infections and sudden, unexpected bouts of septicemia. This susceptibility correlates with decreased levels of neutralizing and opsonizing antibodies and limited complement activation.

13. *Selective deficiency of IgD.* This deficiency has been reported, but its clinical significance is unknown. Afflicted individuals are apparently asymptomatic.

14. *Selective deficiency of IgE.* This has also been recognized, but its clinical implication remains to be established [17].

15. *Selective κ chain deficiency.* A young girl with repeated respiratory infections and diarrhea has been described. Her serum and secretory immunoglobulins were found to have a selective deficiency of κ-type molecules as a result of selective suppression of κ-chain synthesis [125].

16. *Sex-linked immunodeficiency with IgM elevation.* This type of immunoglobulin deficiency is the most frequent form of dysgammaglobulinemia. It is associated with decreased IgG and IgA and increased IgM levels [116]. Other forms of dysgammaglobulinemia include those with decreased IgG and IgM and increased IgA concentrations; normal IgG and decreased IgA and IgM concentrations; and normal IgG, decreased IgM, and increased IgA levels (e.g., Wiskott-Aldrich syndrome). Alterations of the differentiation of the plasma cell lines, which produce results that are similar to several forms of human dysgammaglobulinemias, can be induced experimentally in the chicken by surgically removing the bursa of Fabricius at hatching or by suppressing its development by hormones.

17. *Immunodeficiency with ataxia-telangiectasia.* The ataxia-telangiectasia syndrome [17], which is inherited as an autosomal recessive trait, is characterized by progressive cerebellar ataxia, conjunctival and cutaneous telangiectasias, frequent respiratory infections, often isolated IgA deficiency, and deficient cellular immunity.

The mechanisms leading to immunoglobulin deficiency are varied and incompletely understood. Defective B-cell differentiation appears to exist in most patients. They may have either no detectable B lymphocytes (e.g., patients with X-linked agammaglobulinemia and certain patients with variable immunodeficiencies) or normal to increased numbers of B lymphocytes but no mature plasma cells (e.g., some variable immunodeficiencies, especially those with follicular lymph node hyperplasia, as well as certain forms of selective IgA deficiency and ataxia-telangiectasia syndrome). The latter condition suggests the presence of a block of maturation from immature B cells [15]. Most patients with X-linked infantile agammaglobulinemia have been shown to be deficient in all B lymphocytes and immunoglobulins in the peripheral blood, whereas others have B cells in the blood but no immunoglobulins. There are also others who lack IgG-, IgA-, and IgM-bearing B cells and the corresponding immunoglobulins, but who have normal levels of serum IgE and IgE-bearing B cells in the peripheral blood. This observation suggests that various sites of maturation blocks exist (see Fig. 19-20) within the developmental sequence of immature, nonsynthesizing B cells to nonsecretory B cells and, finally, to mature secretory plasma cells. This observation also suggests the independence of the differentiation of IgE B-cells [126].

There is a high risk of lymphoid and nonlymphoid malignancies [19, 112] (the estimated incidence is 5 to 10 percent [17]) and collagen-like diseases [105] in patients with B-cell defects, especially in those patients with selective IgA deficiency [122] and Wiskott-Aldrich syndrome [111].

Secondary immunoglobulin deficiencies. Secondary immunodeficiencies are primarily encountered in adult patients. They include those due to decreased immunoglobulin synthesis, such as chronic lymphocytic leukemia [107] and lymphosarcoma [127], the various forms of monoclonal gammopathies complicated by decreased residual normal immunoglobulins, and the largely unclassified group of variable, common, or late-onset immunodeficiencies. Most of these immunodeficiencies may be viewed in the context of the dichotomy of the immune system, and their mechanisms can now be relegated to certain "immunological blocks" (see Fig. 19-20).

1. *Variable, common immunoglobulin deficiencies.* The majority of patients with immunodeficiencies cannot yet be unequivocally classified, and such disorders are therefore grouped under the heading of "variable, common immunodeficiency" [111, 112]. This form of immunoglobulin deficiency occurs both in children and adults (i.e., late-onset hypogammaglobulinemia), and it is characterized by the same deficiencies as the sex-linked congenital forms of agammaglobulinemia (see Case Report 1 and Fig. 19-21). In general, however, the B-cell deficiency is severe but not complete, i.e., the major immunoglobulins are usually detectable in amounts that are approximately 10 percent of normal. The clinical complications are usually otitis, bronchitis, and colitis, which reflect the deficiency of secretory IgA. Therapy is restricted to γ-globulin substitution [118] and symptomatic relief measures. Presently, there is no practical approach to the reconstitution of the B-cell system, including the cells that produce secretory IgA. An example of the variable late-onset form of agammaglobulinemia in an adult patient follows:

Case Report 1
N. R., a 26-year-old school teacher, had a history of frequent upper respiratory infections and a progressive cough productive of greenish sputum, which had been prominent since her mid-teenage years. As a child, she had suffered tonsillitis and several bouts of pneumonia. Her family history did not indicate a predisposition to infection. At the time of referral, she was having minimal symptoms of cough, sinusitis, and diarrhea. Physical examination was seemingly normal except for boggy nasal mucosa and scarred tympanic membranes. The patient was afebrile. The chest roentgenogram revealed multiple infiltrates and lingular atalectasis. Because of a gram stain of the sputum showing a dense mixed flora, administration of tetracycline was begun. Bilateral bronchography demonstrated bronchiectasis limited to the left lower lobe. Bronchodilators, expectorants, and postural drainage were

initiated. A jejunal biopsy revealed a sparsity of submucosal plasma cells and a flattened mucosa. A complete blood count was unremarkable, but bone-marrow aspiration showed a severely decreased number of plasma cells. Serum protein electrophoresis revealed a drastically diminished γ-globulin fraction (0.3 gm per 100 ml). IgG, IgA, and IgM were virtually undetectable on IEP. RID demonstrated the IgG concentration to be less than 100 mg per 100 ml, both IgA and IgM to be less than 10 mg per 100 ml, and the IgD to be less than 1 mg per 100 ml. RIA revealed IgE levels of less than 5 ng per milliliter. Salivary secretory IgA was absent. The α_1-antitrypsin levels and C3 and C4 concentrations were normal, and other studies were unrevealing. The lymphocytes responded normally in culture with PHA and MLC. The patient underwent a left lower lobe lobectomy without complications, and she has been maintained relatively free of symptoms on monthly intramuscular injections of 20 ml of γ-globulin (Fig. 19-21).

Final Diagnosis: Hypogammaglobulinemia of late onset, complicated by recurrent infections, sprue-like syndrome, and bronchiectasis requiring surgical treatment.

2. *Immunoglobulin deficiency induced by immunosuppressive therapy.* Corticosteroids are the principal class of immunosuppressants that are effective during the primary and secondary (anamnestic) immune responses. Their efficacy rests mainly on their effects upon the factors of the amplification system, i.e., the inhibition of phagocytosis and the suppression of inflammation. Corticosteroids depress both the circulating B and T lymphocytes numerically as well as functionally. Depressed functions of B lymphocytes are reflected by a fall in serum immunoglobulin levels [128].

3. *Malignant monoclonal B-cell disorders.* These disorders [17, 112, 129] may be classified as follows:

A. *Chronic lymphocytic leukemia.* Patients with chronic lymphocytic leukemia (CLL) [17] possess a defective ability to produce and secrete normal amounts of antibodies and to express humoral hypersensitivity; consequently, their serum immunoglobulin levels are often decreased, particularly during the terminal phase of the disease [127]. Among 104 patients with CLL, low γ-globulin levels were encountered in 37 patients (35.6 percent), normal levels in 50 (48.1 percent), and high levels in 17 (16.3 percent) [127]. This lymphocyte deficiency, involving mainly humoral immunity, may be due to blocked cell maturation of the bone-marrow lymphoid stem cell or the general hematopoietic stem cell itself into functional secretory plasma cells (see Fig. 19-20), thus resulting in hypogammaglobulinemia [130]. Recent analyses using surface immunoglobulin markers indicate that in most patients with CLL, the abnormal lymphocytes are of the B-cell variety. In these, the abnormal cells may reflect a proliferation of B-cell populations with monoclonal immunoglobulin surface markers, but usually without secretion of monoclonal immunoglobulins [16, 130–132]. Lymphocytes from patients with CLL usually display small amounts of surface membrane immunoglobulins but larger amounts internally (usually IgM of either κ or λ type). Different types of lymphocytic leukemias may represent neoplastic counterparts of different stages of B-cell differentiation [133].

B. *"Nonsecretory" monoclonal gammopathies.* An increasing number of patients are being recognized with malignant monoclonal B-cell disorders in whom the B cells produce but do not secrete monoclonal immunoglobulins. Such cells may reflect a state of B-cell differentiation somewhat more mature than those associated with CLL, lymphosarcoma, and Burkitt's lymphoma [134], but which is less mature than those B cells associated with the classic "secretory" monoclonal gammopathies. This cytological state may be reflected clinically by symptoms of multiple myeloma [135–137] or macroglobulinemia [138], but without the accompanying serum M proteins.

C. *"Secretory" monoclonal gammopathies.* These disorders include classic multiple myeloma (i.e., IgG, IgA, IgD, or IgE myeloma or L-chain disease), macroglobulinemia (i.e., IgM-macroglobulinemia), and H-chain diseases (γ-, α-, and μ-chains), as well as the asymptomatic varieties. In these monoclonal gammopathies, it is the plasma cell system that is primarily affected. One clone of plasma cells proliferates, and consequently one homogeneous immunoglobulin is produced in excessive amounts. The remainder of the plasma cell lines and their "normal" immunoglobulin products are either normal or decreased, and the ability of such patients to produce antibodies is often significantly impaired. Not infrequently, clinical complications arise from this antibody deficiency. Such patients possess essentially normal cellular immunity. Delayed hypersensitivity develops, and the rejection of skin allografts proceeds in a normal fashion. In monoclonal gammopathy, the functions of the B-cell system are deficient, whereas the normal functions of the T-cell system are retained, at least at the clinical level. Whether subtle T-cell abnormalities may underlie the loss of normal control mechanisms, thereby playing a "permissive" role in the monoclonal expansion, remains to be elucidated. Since the main feature of these disorders is, however, due to an overproduction and secretion of monoclonal immunoglobulins, they will be described later (see pp. 419–466).

INCREASED LOSS OF IMMUNOGLOBULINS
Excessive loss of immunoglobulins (Table 19-5) may occur from the kidneys (e.g., nephrotic syndrome), the GI tract (i.e., protein-losing gastroenteropathies), the skin (e.g., early stages of thermal burns, eczema, or severe trauma), and into the peritoneal cavity (e.g., ascites with frequent removal). In general, the disorders leading to the loss of immunoglobulins are identical to those associated with the loss of albumin (see Chap. 13).

Urinary loss of immunoglobulins. The nephrotic syndrome is complicated by the loss of small molecular weight proteins, including albumin and often IgG, as well as the hypercatabolism of these proteins [87, 119]. The increase of the endogeneous fractional catabolic rate in such patients may be due to increased exposure of these proteins to the catabolic mechanisms in the renal tubule. Strober et al. [87, 119] have elucidated the principal mechanisms of protein catabolism in renal disease (see Fig. 19-23). In pure glomerular diseases that are associated with large "membrane pores" but little or no tubular dysfunction, there are both increased

Table 19-5.   Disorders Associated with Pathological Loss of
Immunoglobulins[a]

Kidneys—Nephrotic Syndrome
   Chronic glomerulonephritis
   Diabetes mellitus
   Lupus erythematosus
   Others (allergy, syphilis, etc.)

Gastrointestinal Tract—Protein-losing Gastroenteropathies
   Primary disorders
     Whipple's disease
     Ulcerative colitis
     Ménétrier's disease
     Congenital, primary lymphangiectasia

   Secondary disorders
     Tricuspid insufficiency
     Secondary lymphangiectasia associated with
       lymphoma, filariasis, etc.

Skin
   Acute thermal burns
   Eczematous lesions

Peritoneal Cavity
   Ascites with frequent tapping

---

[a] See also Chapter 13, "Albumin Abnormalities."

loss of intact immunoglobulin molecules into the urine and increased endogenous catabolism. In tubular diseases, there is no change in the catabolism of large proteins, which are normally retained by the glomerular basement membrane. The significant proteinuria in such patients is due to the decreased uptake and decreased endogenous catabolism of low molecular weight proteins by the renal tubule. Since the total metabolism is unchanged, serum protein levels of these proteins remain normal.

In chronic renal disease with uremia and nephron loss, there is normal endogenous catabolism and only slight proteinuria of large proteins. However, small proteins that pass into the glomerular filtrate are lost into the urine in normal amounts, and the endogenous catabolism is reduced because of fewer glomeruli and tubules to filter and catabolize these proteins. In these cases, the survival of low molecular weight proteins is prolonged, and the serum levels may be increased. This fact is of considerable clinical importance. For instance, patients with lupus erythematosus complicated by severe renal disease excrete increased amounts of free polyclonal L chains [139]. Similarly, these mechanisms may affect the urinary excretion rates and the serum levels of free monoclonal L chains, i.e., Bence Jones proteins (see Chap. 20), as well as other low molecular weight proteins, such as lysozymes [140].

Protein loss into the gastrointestinal tract.   Protein-losing gastroenteropathies may complicate more than 70 GI diseases (e.g., Whipple's disease and intestinal lymphangiectasia) or other disorders, including cardiac diseases (e.g., constrictive pericarditis and tricuspid insufficiency) and lymphoma [87, 119] (see Chap. 13). In the prototype of protein-losing gastroenteropathies, which is exemplified by intestinal lymphangiectasia, there are dilated lymphatic channels of the small bowel due to either primary abnormal development of central lymphatic channels or secondary blockage of these channels by unrelated pathological processes. In the other group of protein-losing gastroenteropathies, which is exemplified by cardiac disease, there is a high elevation of the central venous pressure that leads to a functional blockage of the lymph channels and a reversal of the lymph flow into the gut. In these disorders, the protein loss occurs throughout the electrophoretic range, regardless of the molecular weight of the protein ("bulk loss" [119]); this loss is associated with hypoproteinemia (see Chap. 1). Additionally, lymphocytes are lost into the gut, resulting in significant lymphocytopenia (see Chap. 13), which has been compared with a "functional thoracic duct fistula" [87, 119]. Surgical or medical correction of the underlying cardiac disease results in the termination of the hypoproteinemic and lymphocytopenic state [87, 119].

Loss from skin. Among the accidents, thermal burns are a leading cause of death in children as well as in older persons [141]. In the United States, there are more than 12,000 deaths per year resulting from burns, and more than 70,000 burn patients are hospitalized each year [141]. The alterations in immunoglobulins as a consequence of acute thermal burn injury are of considerable clinical importance.

The typical serum immunoglobulin profiles [105, 142–144] in burned patients are depicted in Figure 19-22. The mean serum γ-globulin levels and the immunoglobulins IgG, IgA, and IgM decrease to a nadir between the third and fifth days after the burn and then return to the control range at 10 to 12 days. In individual patients, the total γ-globulin and IgG concentrations fall below the "critical" levels of about 0.3 gm per 100 ml and 200 mg per 100 ml, respectively. In deceased patients, the level of γ-globulin is usually significantly lower than in the surviving patients.

The changes in serum immunoglobulin levels in children after burn injury [105, 142] are similar to those in adults [143, 144], except for minor age-group differences. The striking initial decrease of serum immunoglobulin levels is mainly related to exudative loss of proteins from the burn wounds; it is probably also related to a shift of proteins into the extravascular space, to increased protein catabolism, and to decreased protein synthesis during the first week after the burn. The decreased immunoglobulin levels are notably limited to the initial burn period. Serum IgM returns to normal or increased values during the first week, and IgA and IgG return to normal or increased levels during the second and third weeks, respectively ("square root" pattern) (see 19-22). The extent of subsequent increases of immunoglobulins after the initial decreases seems to be age-dependent. For IgG and IgA, there is a significant elevation in the older group of children, but a lesser elevation is observed in the youngest age group. On electrophoresis, however, the "rebound" hypergammaglobulinemia found in the older group does not approach the polyclonal gammopathy pattern that is often encountered in adult burned patients.

The significant decrease of immunoglobulins during the first week after burn injury is of clinical importance [145, 146], especially for those patients whose γ-globulin fractions fall below the "critical" levels. Since the decrease of the electrophoretic γ-globulin fraction reflects mainly the decrease of IgG, serum protein electrophoresis or electroimmunodiffusion appear to be the preferred methods for monitoring burn patients for critical immunoglobulin decreases, especially during the first week following the injury. Since the lowest immunoglobulin levels have been demonstrated to occur in the youngest age group, the frequency of monitoring should be increased for these particularly vulnerable patients [105]. Although some studies suggest that substitution therapy with γ-globulin preparations may not be fully effective in adult patients [147], such treatment in burn patients with severe degrees of hypogammaglobulinemia appears nonetheless indicated, especially in burned children. When purified γ-globulin fractions (which contain almost exclusively IgG) are unavailable in cases of critically depressed γ-globulin levels of burned patients, the emergency use of fresh human serum or plasma appears warranted because of the high incidence of fatality that occurs with such critically low levels in children [148].

Loss of immunoglobulins into peritoneal cavity—ascites with frequent tapping. Of the numerous causes of ascites (see Chap. 13), portal obstructive hepatic disease is the most common. Prior to the development of the more potent diuretic agents now available, mechanical removal of ascitic fluid by repeated peritoneal taps was advocated as a therapeutic modality in cases resistant to sodium restriction, water restriction, bed rest, and the available diuretics. Although peritoneal taps are seldom indicated for nondiagnostic purposes, occasionally one encounters situations where serial drainage of ascitic fluid is mandatory to relieve the pressure effects of severe and rapidly reaccumulating ascites. As would be expected from the mechanical removal without replacement of any body fluid, depletion of the constituents of that fluid may occur. Since ascitic fluid may contain significant amounts of immunoglobulins (usually IgG and IgA but less often IgM), secondary hypogammaglobulinemia may result from aggressive peritoneal drainage.

INCREASED CATABOLISM OF IMMUNOGLOBULINS

Hypermetabolism occurs in association with several disorders (Table 19-6), which results in decreased serum levels of one or more immunoglobulins [87, 119, 149].

Familial (hypercatabolic) idiopathic hypoproteinemia. This condition was observed in two siblings who had hypoalbuminemia and hypogammaglobulinemia with a significant reduction of IgA. The low levels of serum IgG and albumin were due to short survival of the proteins. This condition appears to represent a new disease syndrome.

Thyrotoxicosis and hypercorticism. These conditions may cause a

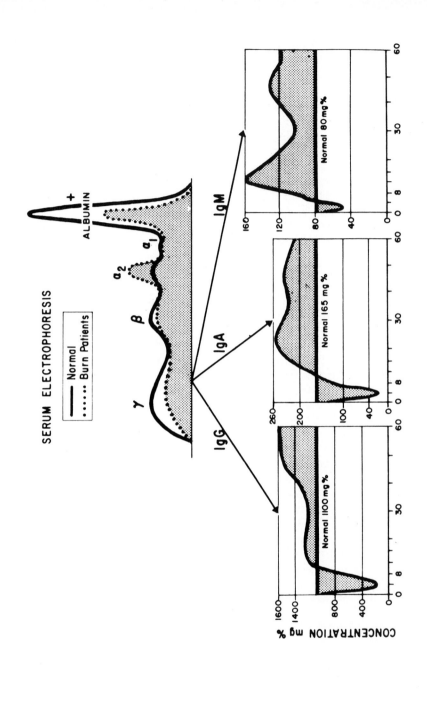

Figure 19-22

Profiles of serum immunoglobulins IgG, IgA, and IgM during 60-day period after thermal burn injury: summary of immunoglobulin profiles for all age groups, related to serum protein electrophoresis. The top panel depicts the profile of the γ-globulin fraction, represented as the mean value of 121 acutely burned patients. The lower left panel depicts the IgG profile for all age groups of the acutely burned patients. Serum IgG falls significantly to low levels during the first 3 to 5 days following the burn injury, but returns to normal by the third week after the burn. Thereafter, the serum IgG levels rise gradually above the normal mean, especially in adult patients, and remain significantly elevated (polyclonal gammopathy). The lower center panel reflects the IgA profiles. The initial decrease is significant on the second and third days after the injury in adults and older children, but is insignificant in children under 5 years of age. After returning to the normal levels, the values remain above this level after the second week. The lower right panel illustrates the IgM profiles. The serum IgM levels decrease somewhat shortly after thermal injury, with a nadir occurring between 2 and 4 days after the burn. A significant increase of IgM occurs during the 5- to 10-day period following the burn, especially in children. The serum IgD levels follow the general pattern of the other major immunoglobulins. They decrease sharply initially. The serum IgE levels also follow the general profiles of the major immunoglobulins. (Reproduced by permission. From Daniels, J. C., et al. *J. Trauma* 12:137, © 1974, The Williams & Wilkins Co., Baltimore.)

Table 19-6.   Disorders Associated with Altered Metabolism of
Immunoglobulins

Hypercatabolism of Immunoglobulins
  Affecting two or more immunoglobulins and other serum proteins:
    Familial hypercatabolic hypoproteinemia
    Hypermetabolic states
    Immunodeficiency with thrombocytopenia and Eczema
      (Wiskott-Aldrich syndrome)
    Nephrotic syndrome

  Affecting one immunoglobulin class:
    Myotonic dystrophy (IgG)
    Anti-immunoglobulin antibodies

Hypocatabolism of Immunoglobulins
  Nephron-loss diseases (L chains and other low molecular
    weight serum proteins)

---

generalized state of hypercatabolism that also affects the levels of immunoglobulins.

Immunodeficiency with Thrombocytopenia and Eczema (Wiskott-Aldrich Syndrome).   This rare immunological disorder appears to be associated with an abnormality of the afferent limb of immunity that affects the humoral and cellular immune responses (see Figs. 19-4 and 19-20) or the antigen processing in the immunodynamic sequence. Patients with this disorder usually have normal immunoglobulin levels but a suppressed capacity for antibody response to antigenic challenge. In these patients, the synthetic rates of all classes of immunoglobulins appear to be elevated, but the fractional catabolic rates of all immunoglobulins (as well as albumin) are increased. The hyperplastic state of the reticuloendothelial system in these patients has led to speculation that this system is involved in the accelerated catabolism of immunoglobulins and albumin.

Myotonic dystrophy.   This autosomal dominant disorder is associated with low levels of serum IgG due to hypercatabolism. The survival time of IgG in patients with this disorder is approximately 50 percent of that of normal persons (i.e., 11.4 days versus 23 days). The serum levels of albumin, IgA, IgM, IgD, and IgE appear normal. Since the catabolism of free L chains is normal, it has been postulated that the catabolic defect is associated with the Fc fragment of the IgG molecule. Furthermore, since isolated IgG from myotonic patients behaves normally in control persons whereas normal IgG displays shortened survival in myotonic dystrophy patients, unknown host factors must be responsible for this metabolic defect.

Immunodeficiency with ataxia-telangiectasia.   Patients with this disorder display thymic hypoplasia, impaired delayed hypersensitivity, and often isolated IgA deficiency. The IgA deficiency in most of these patients is usually due to decreased synthesis, but in others, it is due to circulating anti-IgA antibodies.

Antibodies to immunoglobulins.   Hypercatabolism of immunoglobulins may result from antibodies to these immunoglobulins. For instance, hypercatabolism of IgG may be observed as a result of mixed cryoglobulins that are associated with monoclonal anti-IgG-IgM antibodies, which either complex or form cryoglobulins with IgG. These immune complexes are rapidly catabolized. Shortened IgG survival due to this mechanism has been observed in Sjögren's syndrome, rheumatoid arthritis, and other collagen diseases.

HYPOCATABOLISM ASSOCIATED WITH NEPHRON-LOSS DISEASES

Waldmann, Strober, and associates [87, 119] have elucidated the renal catabolic pathways of serum proteins, which clarifies many hitherto puzzling events. Increased serum concentrations of immunoglobulin L-chain fragments may occur as a result of decreased catabolism in patients with certain renal diseases. The renal tubules have been shown to be the major site of catabolism of small serum proteins (13,000 to 45,000 MW), including free L chains (polyclonal κ or λ L chains, monoclonal κ or λ L chains, or Bence Jones proteins), H chains, lysozyme, and β-microglobulin. This relationship is depicted in Figure 19-23. Normally, approximately 90 percent of such L chains are reabsorbed and catabolized by the tubules, thus effectively catabolizing approximately 20 percent of the circulating L chain pool per day.

In tubular proteinuria, which may be due to either acquired or hereditary disorders of the renal tubules, large amounts of small molecular weight proteins, but only small amounts of larger proteins such as intact immunoglobulins, are excreted into the urine. For example, in tubular proteinuria, 15 to 80 mg per day of free λ light chains may be found, which is 10 to 60 times greater than the 1 to 4 mg per day in the urine of control persons [87]. In these patients, the synthetic and survival rates of serum L chains are normal; thus, in tubular proteinuria, there exists a failure of the proximal renal tubules to reabsorb and catabolize small serum proteins, including L chains, which are filtered normally through the glomerulus. In patients with severe tubular proteinuria (e.g., systemic lupus erythematosus), the urinary L chain concentrations reach values that yield false-positive heat tests. Such a finding may be misinterpreted as reflecting Bence Jones proteins; therefore, confirmatory tests for the distinction between polyclonal free (κ and λ) L chains, which are the result of catabolism of immunoglobulins, and monoclonal free (κ or λ) L chains, which are the result of abnormal synthesis of immunoglobulins, must be employed (see Chap. 20).

In uremia associated with the loss of entire nephrons, there is usually a striking increase in the serum concentrations of low molecular weight proteins; L chains may be elevated tenfold. In these patients, the survival time of L chains may be prolonged 10 times normal and the catabolic rate may be significantly reduced as a result of the loss of entire nephrons, which are the physiological catabolic sites for these microglobulins.

TREATMENT OF IMMUNOGLOBULIN DEFICIENCIES

The management of patients with severe immunoglobulin deficiencies includes appropriate prophylactic measures, administration of antibiotics

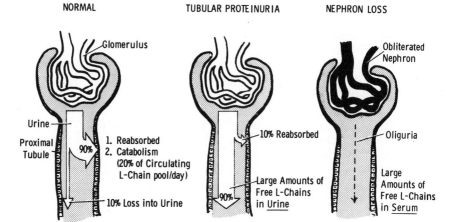

NORMAL   **TUBULAR PROTEINURIA**   **NEPHRON LOSS**

Figure 19-23
Quantitative relationship among glomerular filtration, tubular reabsorption and
catabolism, and excretion of L chains in normal persons, in patients with
tubular proteinuria, and in those with nephron loss in uremia.

when indicated, γ-globulin substitution, and, rarely, the use of transfer
factor and allotransplantation of bone marrow, the thymus, and so on
[17, 111, 113, 150, 151].

γ-Globulin replacement therapy. Intramuscular injections of commercial γ-globulin preparations, at a minimum dose of 0.1 gm per kilogram per month or 0.025 gm per kilogram per week, have been used
with benefit [17]. On this regimen, patients with X-linked hypogammaglobulinemia have reached adult life [109, 111]. Some patients with severe hypogammaglobulinemia (less than 200 mg per 100 ml of IgG),
however, may require twice as much γ-globulin. In these, a loading dose
of 250 mg per kilogram, given intramuscularly over 5 days, followed by
a maintenance dose of 25 mg per kilogram of body weight per week, has
been recommended [118]. About 20 percent of patients on regular replacement therapy may experience side-effects, including dyspnea, faint-
ness, hypotension, flushing, facial swelling, and anxiety [118]. Since
most commercial γ-globulin preparations contain only about 16 percent
IgG, the above dosages are determined by multiplying the gram-per-
kilogram dose by a factor of 6 to obtain the appropriate milliliter per
kilogram dose. Preparations intended for intramuscular use should not
be given intravenously, because of the danger of anaphylactic reactions
due to the IgG aggregates that are commonly formed.

Plasma infusions. Intravenous infusions of plasma [17, 148] may
provide some advantage over intramuscular γ-globulin preparations. Infusion permits the quick replacement of all immunoglobulin classes, it is
less painful, and the prophylactic levels of IgG are maintained somewhat
longer. It has been recommended that the plasma be frozen and thawed

prior to infusion in order to destroy any incompatible T cells as a potential cause of graft-versus-host reactions. Patients with selective IgA deficiency and anti-IgA antibodies, however, should not receive plasma, because of the danger of anaphylactic reactions.

HYPERGAMMAGLOBULINEMIA–POLYCLONAL GAMMOPATHIES
Hypergammaglobulinemia consists essentially of two different varieties, which are usually distinguishable by serum protein electrophoresis (SPE) (see Chap. 1): the polyclonal and monoclonal gammopathies.

DEFINITION AND DIAGNOSTIC ASPECTS
Polyclonal gammopathies (PG) are characterized by a broad, diffuse, and heterogeneous increase of mainly the γ-globulin fraction due to increased proliferation of numerous plasma cell clones (Fig. 19-24). Usually, all three major immunoglobulins are increased, with variable relative concentrations (Table 19-7) [152]. *PG is the second most frequent electrophoretic serum protein abnormality after hypoalbuminemia.* PG is not a primary disease entity, but an expression of an underlying disease, and, as such, it is a nonspecific and objective reflection of an underlying disorder. Monitoring of the PG pattern provides some prognostic information. Clinical improvement of hepatitis, for instance, is associated with a gradual decrease of the polyclonally increased γ-globulin fraction, and, conversely, a progressive increase in γ-globulins may herald an ominous clinical course [153].

DISEASES ASSOCIATED WITH PG
Polyclonal gammopathy is also referred to as *secondary hypergammaglobulinemia,* and it may accompany a wide range of clinical disorders. Some of these are listed in Table 19-7 [152], and they include:

1. *Chronic liver diseases:* Laennec's cirrhosis, infectious hepatitis, chronic active hepatitis (lupoid hepatitis), biliary cirrhosis, hepatoma, and others.
2. *Collagen disorders:* Rheumatoid arthritis, Sjögren's syndrome, Felty's syndrome, lupus erythematosus, and others.
3. *Chronic infections:* Tuberculosis, syphilis, deep fungus diseases, lymphogranuloma venereum, osteomyelitis, chronic bronchitis with bronchiectasis, scarlet fever, chronic pyelonephritis, leprosy, malaria, toxoplasmosis, kala-azar, toxocara infections, trypanosomiasis, trichinosis, and others.
4. *Miscellaneous disorders:* Metastatic carcinoma, sarcoidosis, recovery stages of thermal burns, cystic fibrosis, hyperglobulinemic purpura, diabetes mellitus, acquired hemolytic anemia, and others.

PG patterns are not diagnostic for any disease entity, but they may aid in the differential diagnosis and the evaluation of the clinical course of certain disorders [152–166]. Diagnostic overinterpretations of such patterns, however, must be avoided.

Figure 19-24

Relationship between B-cell proliferation and immunoglobulin concentrations as reflected by serum protein electrophoresis. *A*. B-cell precursors give rise to mature B cells (i.e., plasma cells), which synthesize and secrete five different classes of immunoglobulins (IgG, IgA, IgM, IgD, and IgE). Their electrophoretic migration ranges in relative normal concentrations are indicated. *B*. The normal, agammaglobulinemic, polyclonal gammopathy, and monoclonal gammopathy patterns are exemplified by the IgG class and its cellular sources (IgG plasma cells). (*1*) The normal IgG class contains numerous individual antibodies, each with specific antibody activity. These are elaborated by individual, separate IgG plasma cell clones. (*a*) Agammaglobulinemia, resulting from deficient or blocked B-cell proliferation and consequent lack of immunoglobulin secretion, is reflected by the absence of IgG and specific antibodies. Less complete forms of B-cell deficiency result in various degrees of hypogammaglobulinemia. Depending upon the type of agammaglobulinemia, either the entire IgG class or one, two, or three IgG subclasses may be deficient. (*b*) Polyclonal gammopathy is the result of the proliferation of a wide spectrum of B-cell clones, leading to increased levels of antibody classes and of specific antibodies contained therein. (*c*) Monoclonal gammopathy results from the proliferation of a selective B-cell clone, leading to the production of homogeneous M protein. Such a constellation is often associated with decreased proliferation of the uninvolved B-cell clones, leading to decreased levels of the normal background immunoglobulins.

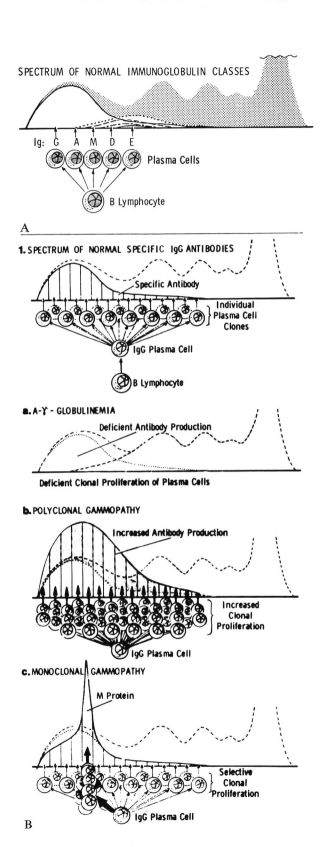

SPECTRUM OF NORMAL IMMUNOGLOBULIN CLASSES

Ig: G A M D E

Plasma Cells

B Lymphocyte

A

1. SPECTRUM OF NORMAL SPECIFIC IgG ANTIBODIES

Specific Antibody

Individual
Plasma Cell
Clones

IgG Plasma Cell

B Lymphocyte

a. A-γ - GLOBULINEMIA

Deficient Antibody Production

Deficient Clonal Proliferation of Plasma Cells

b. POLYCLONAL GAMMOPATHY

Increased Antibody Production

Increased
Clonal
Proliferation

IgG Plasma Cell

c. MONOCLONAL GAMMOPATHY

M Protein

Selective
Clonal
Proliferation

IgG Plasma Cell

B

Table 19-7. Disorders Associated with Polyclonal Gammopathies

Diseases	Serum Immunoglobulin Levels		
	IgG	IgA	IgM
Liver diseases			
Infectious hepatitis	↑↔↑↑	N↔↑	N↔↑↑
Laennec's cirrhosis	↑↔↑↑↑	↑↔↑↑↑	N↔↑↑
Biliary cirrhosis	N	N	↑↔↑↑
Lupoid hepatitis	↑↑↑	↑	N↔↑↑
Collagen disorders			
Lupus erythematosus	↑↔↑↑	N↔↑	N↔↑↑
Rhematoid arthritis	N↔↑	↑↔↑↑↑	N↔↑
Sjögren's syndrome	N↔↑	N↔↑	↓↔↑
Scleroderma	N↔↑	N	↑
Infections			
Tuberculosis	↑↔↑↑	N↔↑↑↑	↓↔N
Subacute bacterial endocarditis	↑↔↑↑	↓↔N	↑↔↑↑
Leprosy	↑↔↑↑	N	↑
Trypanosomiasis	N↔↑	N↔↑	↑↑↔↑↑↑
Malaria	↓↔↑	N	↑↔↑↑
Kala-azar	↑↑	N	N
Infectious mononucleosis	↑↔↑↑	N↔↑	↑↔↑↑
Fungus diseases	N	N↔↑	N
Bartonellosis	↑	↓↔N	↑↑↔↑↑↑
Lymphogranuloma venereum	↑↑	N	N
Actinomycosis	↑↑↑	↑↑	↑↑↑
Sarcoidosis	N↔↑↑	N↔↑↑	N↔↑
Miscellaneous			
Hodgkin's disease	↓↔↑↑	↓↔↑	↓↔↑↑
Monocytic leukemia	↑	↑	↑↑
Cystic fibrosis	↑↔↑↑	↑↔↑↑	N↔↑↑

Note: N = Essentially normal serum immunoglobulin levels. ↓ = Decreased immunoglobulin concentrations.   ↑, ↑↑, ↑↑↑ = Slight, moderate or marked increases in serum immunoglobulin concentrations. ↔ = Range of immunoglobulin levels.

Reproduced by permission. From Ritzmann, S. E., and Levin, W. C. In H. Dettelbach and S. E. Ritzmann (Eds.), *Lab Synopsis,* Vol. 2 (2nd ed.). Somerville, N.J.: Behring Diagnostics, 1969.

Liver diseases. Advanced hepatic parenchymal diseases are generally associated with a significant decrease of albumin and an increase of γ-globulin regardless of the cause. Acute viral hepatitis is often accompanied by hypoalbuminemia and slight to moderate degrees of PG. These changes occur early in the course of disease, frequently before the onset of icterus, but revert to normal within 2 to 3 months. Persistence or increase of PG may be indicative of subacute or chronic hepatitis. Subacute hepatic necrosis may be associated with pronounced hypoalbuminemia and extreme hypergammaglobulinemia. Chronic active hepatitis (lupoid hepatitis), a syndrome of chronic hepatopathy affecting mainly young females, is frequently associated with hypoalbuminemia and a greatly increased γ-globulin fraction, often of the oligoclonal type ("compact γ-globulin band" [161]), which may be mistaken for an M protein, i.e., a pseudo-M protein (see Case Report 2 and Fig. 19-26B).

Laennec's cirrhosis is usually associated with significant hypoalbuminemia and PG. The electrophoretic changes that are observed are usually correlated with the severity of the disease, and serial electrophoretic observations may be of prognostic value. In the majority of such patients, there is "β-γ-bridging" (see Fig. 19-26A). Postnecrotic cirrhosis is characterized by significant hypoalbuminemia and PG. The γ-globulin fraction may be elevated 5 to 7 times above normal levels. Portal cirrhosis is usually associated with significant hypoalbuminemia and a moderate to marked degree of polyclonal gammopathy. When liver tissue is largely replaced by primary or metastatic tumors of the liver, the protein pattern of hepatoparenchymal disease may be noted.

Collagen disorders. In rheumatoid arthritis, a significant degree of hypoalbuminemia and PG is often encountered. For example, among 150 such patients, the albumin fraction was reduced in 55 percent, the γ-globulin fraction was elevated in 37 percent, and in 25 percent of these patients, the protein pattern remained normal [163]. The highest γ-globulin levels occur with severe and continued activity of the disease process. Steroid treatment tends to decrease the γ-globulin concentrations. Sjögren's syndrome is often characterized by a pronounced degree of PG [165]. Lupus erythematosus (SLE) shows a protein pattern similar to that of rheumatoid arthritis. In 36 patients with acute systemic lupus erythematosus, the albumin was reduced in 47 percent, the γ-globulin fraction was increased in 58 percent, and a normal serum protein pattern was found in 14 percent [163]. Corticosteroid treatment often results in an increase of albumin and a decrease of γ-globulin. The nephrotic syndrome that complicates SLE is often characterized by the occurrence of PG (rather than the expected normal or decreased γ-globulin fraction) in addition to hypoalbuminemia and hyperalpha-2-globulinemia. In polyarteritis nodosa, the γ-globulin concentration usually remains within normal limits, although PG may occur. In diffuse scleroderma, the γ-globulin concentration is highly variable. Of 20 patients with scleroderma, a moderate elevation of γ-globulin was demonstrated in nine patients, and there was a slight decrease of albumin in four patients [163]. Patients with dermatomyositis may develop PG.

Infections. The γ-globulin concentrations in acute, subacute, and chronic infections demonstrate a wide spectrum, ranging from normal to dramatically increased levels, depending mainly upon the type and duration of the infection (see Fig. 19-25). A significant degree of transitory PG may be observed in children with scarlet fever [167].

Sarcoidosis. PG may be observed in sarcoidosis, especially in patients with progressive disease and liver involvement. There is no definite diagnostic significance attributable to certain electrophoretic patterns, such as a "stepwise" increase in α_2-, β-, and γ-globulin fractions.

Miscellaneous disorders. In numerous additional diseases, PG may be encountered, although usually not as often or as severe as in liver diseases, collagen disorders, and chronic infections. Among 221 patients with diabetes mellitus, PG was found in 40 percent and hypogammaglobulinemia in 10 percent [164]. PG may be encountered in patients with hypothyroidism, mongolism, adenocarcinoma, acquired hemolytic anemia, idiopathic thrombocytopenic purpura, nonthrombocytopenic purpura, allergic or hyperimmune reactions, drug allergy and other hypersensitivity reactions, hyperglobulinemic purpura (Waldenström) [168], extreme starvation and kwashiorkor, Hodgkin's disease, and others. In other patients with PG, no associated disease is detectable (i.e., idiopathic PG).

SPECIAL PATTERNS OF PG

In additon to the usual pattern of PG, there are special patterns that are of some diagnostic significance (Figs. 19-24B and 19-25).

"β-γ Bridging." Such a pattern is characterized by an increased γ-globulin fraction that fuses with the increased β-globulin fraction (Fig. 19-26A). Such β-γ bridging [160] is due to a significant increase in the anodally migrating portion of IgG, and the IgA and IgM classes, which are mainly located in the β-globulin fraction. Such a combined increase of the immunoglobulins may lead to an increased β-globulin fraction with fusion with the increased γ-globulin fraction. This phenomenon is also known as β/γ *linking* [161] or *beta-gamma fusion* [169]. Such a PG pattern was observed in 63 of 73 cases of cirrhosis that were confirmed by autopsy [161].

Oligoclonal gammopathy. Not infrequently, the increased γ-globulin fraction is of a more restricted heterogeneity than the usual PG; such a pattern is referred to as *oligoclonal gammopathy,* which is manifested as a "compact γ-globulin band" [161] on the electrophoretic separation pattern (see Fig. 19-26B). It is due to a significant increase of only a small portion of the γ-globulin fraction (e.g., part of the IgG class or a subclass), which is nevertheless polyclonal in that both κ and λ light-chain constituents are increased [153]. Oligoclonal gammopathy patterns are often encountered in patients with chronic active hepatitis (lupoid hepatitis or progressive hypergammaglobulinemic hepatitis [162]), as well as in those with disorders associated with high concentrations of circulating immune complexes (e.g., high rheumatoid factor activity [152]). Such oligoclonal patterns may be mistaken for M proteins, but appropri-

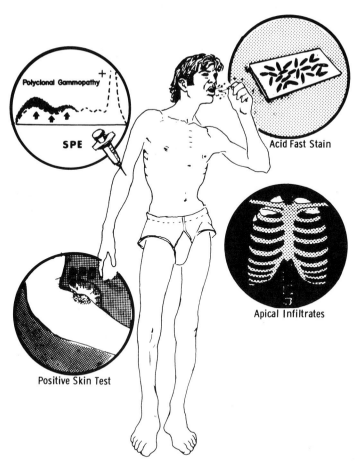

Figure 19-25
Clinical features of polyclonal gammopathy, in this case secondary to pulmonary tuberculosis.

ate studies ordinarily establish the true nature of such proteins [153] (see pp. 43–47).

Case Report 2
A 20-year-old black female was admitted with a maculopapular rash over the dorsum of the arms and legs. Review of systems was essentially negative other than the present illness, except for increasing episodes of bleeding gums. On physical examination, the gums were swollen and red. The neck revealed small nontender lymph nodes on the left. The breasts contained multiple small masses bilaterally in the lateral aspect of each breast; these were nontender, small, and cystic in consistency. Examination of the heart revealed a grade I/VI systolic ejection murmur at the left sternal border. The liver was felt at the right costal margin on inspiration. The spleen was not

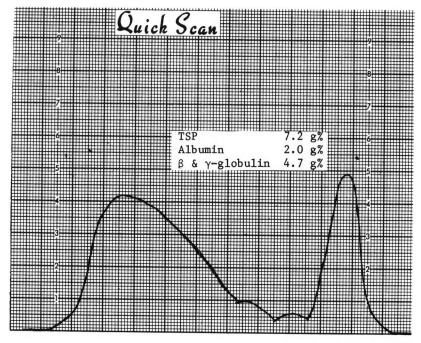

TSP	7.2 g%
Albumin	2.0 g%
β & γ-globulin	4.7 g%

A

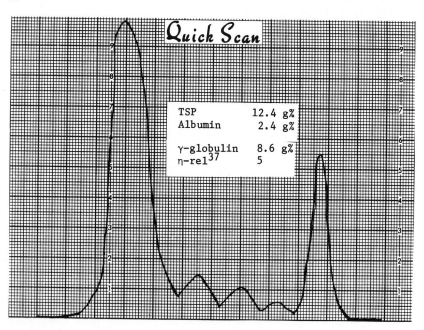

TSP	12.4 g%
Albumin	2.4 g%
γ-globulin	8.6 g%
η-rel^{37}	5

B

Figure 19-26

A. Polyclonal gammopathy with β-γ-bridging in a patient with severe hepatic cirrhosis. *B*. Oligoclonal gammopathy, characterized by a tall and narrow peak that mimicks M protein in a patient with chronic active hepatitis (see Case Report 2).

416

palpable. Examination of the skin revealed maculopapular erythematous lesions on the face, arms, and legs, especially the forearms and lower legs, as well as hypopigmentated macules on the front, hyper- and hypopigmentated areas on the arms and legs, and punctate red lesions on the tips of the toes. There were small vesicles on the inner aspects of the soles of the feet. Skin biopsy tests were consistent with pleomorphic light eruption, and liver biopsy specimens showed chronic active hepatitis. Serum albumin was 2.4 gm per 100 ml and γ-globulin was 8.6 gm per 100 ml (see Fig. 19-26B). There were increased plasma cells on bone-marrow examination (10 percent of total nucleated cells). Serum IgG was 10,763 mg per 100 ml, IgA was 242 mg per 100 ml, and IgM was 285 mg per 100 ml. Hemoglobin was 7 gm per 100 ml. The hematocrit was 23 percent, with a mean corpuscular volume of 67 and a mean corpuscular hemoglobin concentration of 34. The reticulocyte count was 2.1 percent, and the leukocyte count was 10,500 per cubic millimeter with normal differential. The relative serum viscosity was 5 (37°C). There were no cryoglobulins, the rheumatorial arthritis (RA) latex test was negative, and the antinuclear antibody (ANA) test was negative. Both the direct and indirect Coombs' tests were positive. The serum iron was 50 μg per 100 ml.

Final Diagnosis: Chronic lupoid hepatitis, possible systemic lupus erythematosus, hyperviscosity syndrome, and fibrocystic breast disease.

Disposition: The patient was discharged for further evaluation and possible treatment with steroids and plasmapheresis.

Transformation of PG to MG.   Rarely, a PG pattern transforms into MG pattern (see Case Report 3 and Fig. 19-27). Such an event has been described in patients with hepatoma [152, 170], Hodgkin's disease [157], and others. The transition from PG to MG is reminiscent of the events following long-term stimulation of the reticuloendothelial system in BALB/c mice and in Aleutian mink disease (see pp. 457–458).

Case Report 3
A 48-year-old black female blood-bank technologist was under observation for viral hepatitis. Serum protein electrophoresis (SPE) revealed a polyclonal gammopathy pattern (Fig. 19-27), which gradually transformed into an oligoclonal pattern. Fifteen months later, the pattern showed the characteristics of an IgG M protein. There were no osteolytic lesions, and the plasma cells in the bone marrow were only slightly increased. Approximately 8 months later, the patient succumbed to a metastasizing hepatic carcinoma [152].

ETIOPATHOGENIC CONSIDERATIONS
The subject of the etiopathogenesis of PG will be presented in conjunction with that of the MG. Several aspects pertaining specifically to PG, however, will be discussed.

PG in animals.   PG may be found in animals [152], such as BALB/c mice, following intraperitoneal injection of mineral oil, plastics, or other materials. In aged mice, it occurs spontaneously [171], as it does in mink suffering from the virus-induced Aleutian mink disease. In these, the PG pattern may be transformed into a MG pattern, even with the occurrence of Bence Jones proteins [172]. In approximately 10 percent of the affected animals, an M protein evolves in about 3 to 12 months. Aleutian mink disease may also affect man [173].

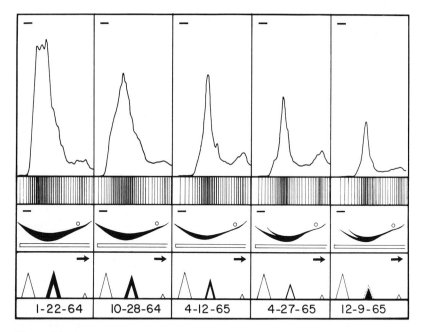

| 1-22-64 | 10-28-64 | 4-12-65 | 4-27-65 | 12-9-65 |

Figure 19-27

Transformation of oligoclonal gammopathy into monoclonal gammopathy. *Top:* Serum electrophoresis reveals (*left to right*) gradual transition from large oligoclonal γ-globulin fraction into a monoclonal configuration with M protein of moderate concentration. *Center:* Immunoelectrophoresis—*left,* increased but qualitatively normal IgG globulin precipitin line; *right,* scooping and abnormal bending of IgG globulin precipitin line and presence of second precipitin line at concave aspect. *Bottom:* Ultracentrifugation reveals slightly increased 7S component with gradual "sharpening" of configuration on follow-up (see Case Report 3). (Reproduced by permission. From Ritzmann, S. E., and Levin, W. C. In H. Dettelbach and S. E. Ritzmann (Eds.), *Lab Synopsis,* Vol. 2 (2nd ed.). Somerville, N.J.: Behring Diagnostics, 1969.)

Familial PG.   A familial form of PG has been described in symptomatic and asymptomatic family members of patients with lupus erythematosus and other diseases [152, 174–179]. In these, a genetically determined tendency for hypergammaglobulinemia may exist.

Antigens and PG.   Infectious agents provide some of the most powerful antigenic stimuli leading to PG. This subject is discussed in conjunction with MG. PG associated with liver disorders is a frequent occurrence [156]. The liver is ordinarily not involved in immunoglobulin production; the polyclonal immune response in such patients has been attributed to defective sequestration of a wide variety of antigens by the von Kupffer cells of the liver or their abnormal release. Results of immunological studies performed on patients with cirrhosis suggest an immunological response to an as yet unidentified stimuli [158, 159, 180].

Similarly, the PG-producing antigenic stimuli that are associated with autoimmune disorders are poorly defined.

INCREASED IgM LEVELS IN CORD BLOOD

Pathophysiological aspects. Increased levels of immunoglobulins may be produced by the fetus in response to intrauterine infections, which may thus provide diagnostic clues to such infections. The human fetus can form increased amounts of IgG with antibody specificity, but the difficulty in distinguishing between the fetal and maternal origin of the IgG precludes its use as a diagnostic aid for intrauterine infections. Increased levels of cord serum IgA may also occur as a result of certain intrauterine infections. IgM is normally present in trace amounts in almost all cord blood sera; therefore, a threshhold level for abnormally increased IgM must be accepted as the diagnostic criterion. It must be recognized, however, that no absolute threshhold level exists that is predictably associated with intrauterine infections: the lower the threshhold level, the more false-positive cases, and the higher the level, the more false-negative instances. In general, a level of approximately 20 mg per 100 ml offers a practical compromise [151]. Since the IgM levels rise appreciably shortly after birth, it is essential to use a sliding scale of increasing threshhold levels with increasing age [80] (Fig. 19-28).

IgM levels in symptomatic neonates with congenital infections. The IgM levels are increased in almost all such cases, and usually the IgM increase is considerable [80, 151, 181]. The screening of subclinical congenital infections in newborns by assaying cord blood IgM is of increasing clinical significance. The easy and rapid detection of cord blood IgM by RID or EID techniques allows its widespread use. The following diseases are frequently associated with neonatally increased IgM levels: syphilis, cytomegalovirus disease, toxoplasmosis, rubella, bacteremia, aseptic meningitis, and others. Screening for cord blood IgM levels has led to the recognition that most chronic congenital infections are "silent" at delivery and occur much more frequently than previously thought [80], with unknown influences on health in later life.

Sources of error. IgM assay for the detection of intrauterine infections represents only a nonspecific approach, and it must be supplemented by specific diagnostic tests. Contamination of cord blood by maternal blood (e.g., placental leaks) may result in high cord blood IgM levels (false-positive results), and newborns with hypogammaglobulinemia may have low or absent cord serum IgM levels, even in the presence of congenital infections (false-negative results).

MONOCLONAL GAMMOPATHIES

In monoclonal gammopathies (MG), one clone of the plasma cells proliferates, producing one homogeneous immunoglobulin in excessive amounts (see Fig. 19-24; see also Chap. 1). Criteria for MG have been defined by Osserman and Takatsuki [182]. An all-inclusive modified definition of MG encompasses the following triad of pathogenic signs: (1) excessive and often neoplastic proliferation of B-lymphocyte

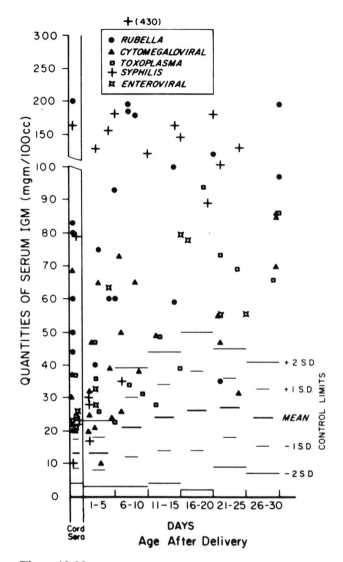

Figure 19-28

Age of neonates in relation to levels of IgM in congenitally infected and control infants. Quantities are shown separately for each type of infection. It is notable that most of the infants with rubella and syphilis had symptomatic types of infections, whereas the others had less severe involvement. (Reproduced by permission. From Alford, C. A. In D. Bergsma and R. A. Good (Eds.), *Immunologic Deficiency Diseases in Man,* Vol. 4. Birth Defects Original Article Series. New York: National Foundation for Birth Defects, 1968. P. 11.)

clones, usually without apparent antigenic stimulus; (2) elaboration of electrophoretically, structurally, and antigenically homogeneous immunoglobulins or comparably homogeneous immunoglobulin subunits, which are usually detectable in serum or urine or both; and (3) frequently, deficiency of the normal immunoglobulins.

HISTORICAL BACKGROUND
Multiple myeloma was first reported more than 135 years ago. An account of the first reported case has been presented by Clamp [47]*:

> In an important series of papers published between 1846 and 1850, John Dalrymple,[1] Henry Bence Jones,[2-4] and William MacIntyre[5] described all the essential features of the disease now known as multiple myeloma. These papers covered the clinical aspects of the disease, the properties of Bence Jones protein, the postmortem findings, and the histological appearances, and left no doubt that the authors considered this a hitherto undescribed disease "essentially malignant in nature" affecting the "osseous system".

WILLIAM MACINTYRE
William MacIntyre was perhaps the most remarkable member of this outstanding trio. He was, at the time he saw the patient in 1845, 53 years of age and physician to the Metropolitan Convalescent Institution and to the Western General Dispensary, St. Marylebone. On Friday, Oct. 30, 1845, he was called from his rooms at 84 Harley Street, to see a patient who had been under the care of Dr. Thomas Watson for several months. From the history and examination, MacIntyre noted many important clinical features of the disease, including the severe bone pains and could later assess the significance of the pathological fractures. Equally remarkable was the care with which he observed the effect of heat on the urine. In view of the history of œdema, one of his first acts when he saw the patient had been to carry out this examination. He thereby noted and later described all the important characteristics of the protein that subsequently and with little justice became known as Bence Jones protein. The ability of the precipitated protein to redissolve with a rise in temperature of the urine, only to reprecipitate as the urine cooled, was clearly described. MacIntyre was also aware of the other property of this protein—namely, its tendency to precipitate at temperatures considerably lower than those of other proteins. Thus, he noticed that the protein redissolved at the "coagulating point" of albumin, namely, 160–170°F (71–77°C) —the inference being that the protein had precipitated at a temperature well below this.

Dr. Watson had evidently not examined the urine during the time that the patient had been under his care. But he appears to have been present during the discovery of this unusual protein or else MacIntyre discussed his perplexing findings with him, since both physicians quite independently sent a specimen of urine to Bence Jones. It was customary then for the specialist services to be provided by practising physicians and surgeons, and Bence Jones had already established a reputation as a chemical pathologist.

BENCE JONES
Henry Bence Jones, of 50 Lower Grosvenor Street, was at this time only 31 years of age and was physician to St. George's Hospital. He was able to

* Reprinted with permission by J. R. Clamp, M.B., Ph.D., University Department of Medicine, Bristol, England, and the publishers of *Lancet*.

confirm MacIntyre's findings and then proceeded to examine the urinary protein in some detail. His papers were therefore concerned with the properties, analysis, and significance of this protein, whereas the paper by MacIntyre dealt mainly with the clinical features of the disease. For this reason, Bence Jones became credited with the discovery of the protein. Further confusion arose over the part played by Dr. Thomas Watson, since Bence Jones quotes the letter from Dr. Watson which accompanied the urine: "The tube contains urine of very high specific gravity. When boiled it becomes highly opaque. On the addition of nitric acid it effervesces, assumes a reddish hue and becomes quite clear; but as it cools assumes the consistence and appearance which you see. Heat reliquefies it. What is it?" Nevertheless, the fact that the urine specimens were sent on Saturday, Nov. 1, 1845—that is, the day after Dr. MacIntyre had been called in for consultation—supports MacIntyre's claim to the discovery, and this is established by the statements made by Bence Jones in his papers. In the first[2] he writes: "On the last day of October, a peculiar state of urine was discovered, through the carefulness of Dr. MacIntyre", and in the second,[4] "He [Dr. MacIntyre] being in attendance on the case with Dr. Watson, had two days previously first observed the peculiar reactions of the urine."

DALRYMPLE

MacIntyre[5] also described the postmortem examination carried out by Mr. Alexander Shaw, surgeon to the Middlesex Hospital. The significant findings were in the bones, particularly the ribs and sternum, and the cervical, thoracic, and lumbar vertebræ. The affected bones were softened, fragile, and easily cut, with the interior replaced with a soft, "gelatiniform", blood-red substance. Some of this material taken from two of the lumbar vertebræ and a rib was referred for histological examination to John Dalrymple, surgeon to the Royal Ophthalmic Hospital, Moorfields, and a member of the Microscopical Society. He described the nucleated cells which were present in great numbers and which formed the bulk of this gelatiniform mass. These cells were said to vary in size and shape but the majority were round or oval with the smaller cells "one and a half to twice larger than the average blood cell or blood disc" (red blood-cells). Dalrymple also noted that the larger and more irregular cells frequently contained two and often three nuclei. These descriptions would be consistent with malignant plasma cells with some multinucleated forms. Dalrymple's paper was illustrated by two woodcuts which were credible drawings of these cells. Both Dalrymple and MacIntyre believed that this disorder was principally a malignant disease of bone. They were puzzled because the tumour had not extended outside the bone, and this they explained by the limited duration of life of the nucleated cells and therefore limited production of bulk by the tumour.

THE PATIENT

The identity of the patient has so far been unknown. It would also be interesting to know the cause of death that appeared on the death certificate of this first recorded case of multiple myeloma. In order to trace this case therefore, the personal details of the patient were taken from the various papers (Table I). Unfortunately, the index of deaths for the first quarter of 1846 gives only the names in alphabetical order, the district of registration, and the volume and page number of the entry in the Register of Deaths. The initial step in the search was therefore to extract from the index the names beginning with M, of all males who died in the London area. In the first quarter

Table I. Details of Patient with Multiple Myeloma Described by William MacIntyre and Henry Bence Jones

	MacIntyre[5]	Bence Jones[2, 4]
Name	Mr. M——	No details
Address	London	London.
Age at death	45	45[2]
		47[4]
Date of death	Jan. 1, 1846	Jan. 2, 1846.
Occupation	Tradesman	Tradesman[2]
		Grocer[4]
Social details	Married early	Wealthy.
	Numerous offspring	
	"Holiday in Scotland"	

of 1846, of the 45,941 males who died in England and Wales, 7259 had names beginning with M, and of these 437 died in the London area. These names were then arranged according to volume and page number to facilitate the search of the Register of Deaths by officers of the General Register Office. The search instructions were to note all names of men aged 45, 46, or 47 years, who died on Jan. 1 or 2, 1846. The expected number of such men can be calculated. Thus, 437 names will represent all deaths from birth onwards, and from the figures in the Annual Report of the Registrar General for that year about 20 of these would be aged 45 to 49 years. Assuming that the death-rate is equal over this age-span, then only about 12 of these men would be aged 45, 46, or 47. These 12 men would have died over the period from Jan. 1 to March 31, and therefore no more than one of these can be expected to have died on Jan. 1 or Jan. 2.

The search agreed with this prediction, since only one man was found who fulfilled all the particulars and this person must therefore be the patient seen by Watson, MacIntyre, and Bence Jones (Table II). It is gratifying to find that the death certificate is consistent with the known personal details, including the holiday in Scotland! Not unexpectedly, the details of the patient given in MacIntyre's paper are correct, in contrast to some of the details given by Bence Jones. The cause of death is given as "atrophy from albuminuria". This was a reasonable diagnosis, since the term albuminuria was used in those days quite non-specifically to mean proteinuria. Alternatively, the cause of death might have been given as "McBean's disease with MacIntyre's proteinuria".

I should like to thank the officers of the General Register Office for their kind cooperation.

1. Dalrymple, J. *Dublin J. Med. Sci.* 1846, ii, 85.
2. Bence Jones, H. *Lancet,* 1847, ii, 88.
3. Bence Jones, H. *Proc. R. Soc.* 1847, *5,* 673.
4. Bence Jones, H. *Phil. Trans. R. Soc.* 1848, p. 55.
5. MacIntyre, W. *Med. Chir. Trans.* 1850, *33,* 211.

In 1889, Kahler [183] described four cardinal features of multiple myeloma: bone pain, fragility and deformity (osteolytic punched-out le-

Table II. Details of Death Certificate

When and where died	Name and surname	Sex	Age	Occupation
First of January 1846 at No. 37 Devonshire Street	Thomas Alexander McBean	Male	45 years	Grocer

Cause of death	Signature, description and residence of informant	When registered	Signature of registrar
Atrophy from Albuminuria Certified	Mary Davidson present at death No. 22 Devonshire Street	Eighth of January 1846	William Clapp Registrar

sions) of the bones, the presence of Bence Jones proteins, and cachexia. The now well-established association of plasma cell proliferation within the bone marrow in this disease was reported by Wright [29] in 1900. In 1944, Waldenström [38] recognized another entity within the group of "malignant" plasma cell disorders, which was characterized by discrete lymphadenopathy and splenomegaly, absence of bone pain and osteolytic lesions, proliferation of plasma cells in the bone marrow, and large amounts of IgM macroglobulins in the serum. Hence, the term *macroglobulinemia of Waldenström* was coined. About 20 years later, Franklin et al. [48] described yet a further malignant plasma-cell disorder, the H-chain diseases. All of these disorders are characterized by the elaboration of "abnormal" immunoglobulins or their subunits.

IMMUNOGLOBULINS ASSOCIATED WITH MG
Plasma cells, or mature B cells, are known to produce at least five classes of normal immunoglobulins: IgG, IgA, IgM, IgD, and IgE. Normally, L and H chains are produced within single plasma cells and are assembled intracellularly into a complete immunoglobulin molecule (see Fig. 19-7). In pathological states, however, L chains may be produced in excess (Fig. 19-29). These free L chains are identical with Bence Jones proteins. Under extreme conditions, myeloma cells may produce only free L chains or Bence Jones proteins. This situation is referred to as *light-chain disease* or *Bence Jones monoclonal gammopathy*. Pathologically,

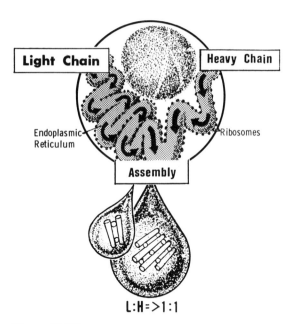

Figure 19-29

In pathological conditions, light and heavy chains may be produced in an asynchronous fashion, i.e., light chain excess (light chains:heavy chains greater than 1:1) or heavy chain excess (light chains:heavy chains less than 1:1). Free monoclonal light chains (i.e., κ or λ chains) are identical with Bence Jones proteins and denote the presence of monoclonal gammopathy. In certain renal diseases associated with nephron loss (e.g., SLE nephropathy), there occur free polyclonal light chains (i.e., κ and λ chains), which must be distinguished from Bence Jones proteins. Free monoclonal light chains are products of altered synthesis or assembly of immunoglobulins, whereas free polyclonal light chains are usually the result of altered catabolic pathways of immunoglobulins.

H chains may also be produced in excess, i.e., the "mirror image" of asynchronous L-chain overproduction. These free H chains are found in what are termed *heavy-chain diseases*.

The term paraprotein was introduced by Apitz in 1940 [184] to denote foreign proteins in the blood, urine, or tissues that are produced by myeloma cells. Gutman [185] coined the term *M protein* for the discrete proteins that are demonstrable by electrophoresis in the sera of patients suffering from myeloma. Riva [154] applied this term to the narrow bands seen by serum electrophoresis that were also associated with macroglobuiinemia.

The clonal concept—that myeloma may be considered the result of unlimited autonomous proliferation of one specific plasma cell clone—is based upon Burnet's hypothesis [100]. Waldenström [174, 186] extended this hypothesis and included all categories of electrophoretically narrowbanded hypergammaglobulinemic conditions as instances of this disorder. He suggested the term *monoclonal gammopathy* (or *gammapathy* [187]) as a comprehensive term for such "abnormal" immunoglobulins and their associated clinical conditions. (This type of hypergammaglobulinemia is in contrast to the electrophoretically broad-based, diffuse hypergammaglobulinemia that is regarded to be polyclonal in nature.) Alternative terms in use include *plasma cell dyscrasias* [182, 188], *paraimmunoglobulinopathies* [189], *immunocytomas* [190], and others.

DIAGNOSIS OF MG

The diagnosis of MG is a matter of practical importance. Although classic MG may be suspected clinically, the diagnosis is supported by evidence of proliferating plasma cells in bone-marrow preparations (Fig. 19-30) or by biopsy of lymphoid organs [191]. The asymptomatic and incipient forms of MG are not suspected clinically. The marrow reveals prominent proliferation of plasma cells, which often display considerable heterogeneity. These cells may be classic plasma cells, "flamed" plasma cells [192], or plasmablasts. In other cases, lymphoid plasma cells predominate. The latter cell type is prominent in Waldenström's macroglobulinemia [193]. The peripheral blood and marrow picture may suggest chronic lymphocytic leukemia in some patients with IgG multiple myeloma, and, conversely, it may suggest the presence of multiple myeloma in patients with IgM macroglobulinemia. Several points are now apparent: First, in most instances, a diagnosis of multiple myeloma or any form of MG cannot be made on cytopathological grounds alone, since Waldenström's macroglobulinemia and other MGs may display similar or identical plasma cells. Second, the cherished concept of the "myeloma plasma cell" [194] must be abandoned. The so-called myeloma cell cannot always be distinguished with certainty from reactive plasma cells or even from lymphocytes. Third, numerous instances of asymptomatic MG, with small numbers of plasma cells in the marrow, often are not detected by the hematologist or surgical pathologist unless serum and urine immunoglobulins are routinely examined. Histopathological criteria likewise may be inconclusive. In most MGs, but particularly in Waldenström's macroglobulinemia and H-chain diseases, the lymphoid organs often are infiltrated by immunoglobulin-producing plasma cells. Biopsy specimens of spleen or lymph nodes may exhibit a lymphosarcoma-like picture. Indeed, most instances of Waldenström's macroglobulinemia are diagnosed histologically as lymphosarcoma. This reflects the necessity of including SPE in the diagnostic screening of patients.

Immunochemical analysis is now the method of choice, and IEP analysis is the sine qua non for the diagnosis of MG [23, 39, 49, 152, 169, 195] (see Chaps. 1 and 2). Specifically, the diagnostic approach to MG requires the examination of serum and urine by electrophoresis and IEP, and, in special instances, by ultracentrifugation analysis and quantitative and qualitative immunological assays of the immunoglobulins. Older diagnostic procedures for MG, which are now obsolete, include the Sia test [196], the formolgel test [155], the acid gel test [197], and others [193]. These tests are insensitive and nonspecific. However, notable rouleaux formation and accelerated erythrocyte sedimentation rates may be diagnostic clues of MG, although they are not pathognomonic [193, 198].

CLINICAL IMPLICATIONS

Classification of MG

1. *Immunochemical classification.* The immunochemical classification of MG is based upon the recognition and characterization of the monoclonal immunoglobulin classes or their elaborated subunits (Table 19-8) (see Chap. 2). At present, the recognized immunochemical varieties of MG include the IgG, IgA, IgM, IgD, and IgE types, which may or may not be associated with free L (κ or λ) or H (γ, α, or μ) chains or other subunits (e.g., low molecular weight IgM or half molecules). *The IgG class of MG accounts for approximately two-thirds of all MG cases* (see Table 19-8), *and the combined IgG, IgA, IgM, and Bence Jones forms of MG constitute more than 95 percent of all cases of MG.* The rare variations of MG (including IgD classes, IgE classes, H-chain diseases, half molecules, low molecular weight IgM, and others) and biclonal and triclonal gammopathies account for less than 5 percent of all gammopathies. (It should be noted that this immunochemical classification of MG includes only the secretory forms of MG as diagnosed by electrophoresis and IEP of serum and other body fluids, but it excludes the nonsecretory forms of MG, such as chronic lymphocytic leukemia, which are recognizable by immunofluorescence assays for intracellular and surface immunoglobulins on B cells.)

2. *Clinical classification.* A correlation between these immunochemical forms of MG and their clinical counterparts has been established:

A. *Symptomatic MG.* Approximately two-thirds of all patients with immunochemical evidence of M proteins are symptomatic in that they may exhibit the classic clinical manifestations of either multiple myeloma (see Case Report 4 and Fig. 19-31), Waldenström's macroglobulinemia (see Case Report 1 in Chap. 20), or a malignant lymphoma-like condition (see Table 19-8). Specifically, approximately two-thirds of these symptomatic patients who exhibit either the IgG, IgA, IgD, IgE, or Bence Jones forms of monoclonal gammopathy experience the classic clinical manifestations of myeloma [41, 45, 169, 187, 199]. Only about two-thirds of the patients with IgM-type of MG are symptomatic and suffer from the classic clinical manifestations of macroglobulinemia [193, 200, 201].

Most patients with H-chain disease present with unique, malignant lymphoma-like pictures. Heavy-chain diseases include γ H-chain disease, α H-chain disease (abdominal lymphoma, found predominantly in patients living in the Near East), and μ H-chain disease (chronic lymphocytic leukemia-like features or splenomegaly) [48–51, 200, 202]. Patients with symptomatic MG displaying these clinical manifestations have what might be termed *classic monoclonal gammopathy* [203] (Tables 19-8 and 19-9). They usually display large amounts of M proteins in their sera (more than 3.0 gm per 100 ml), Bence Jones proteins in their urine, and significant bone-marrow plasmacytosis (more than 10 to 15

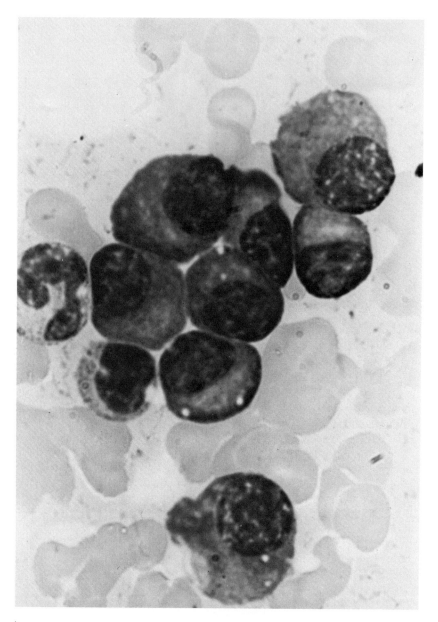

A

Figure 19-30
Bone-marrow smear from patient with symptomatic IgG monoclonal gammopathy, i.e., IgG(κ) multiple myeloma, exhibiting classic plasma cells. *A*. Light microscopy, ×1000. Plasma cells of 8 to 10 μ cellular diameter are characterized by eccentric, dense nuclei and perinuclear clear zones (Golgi

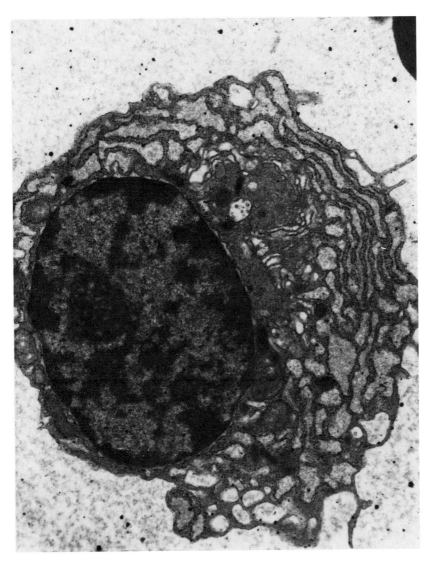

B

apparatus). *B.* Electronmicroscopy, ×5000. Plasma cells are characterized by lamellar endoplasmic reticulum, which is the site of light and heavy chain synthesis. Subsequently, these are assembled to form complete immunoglobulin molecules. (Reproduced by permission. From Ritzmann, S. E., Daniels, J. C., Beathard, G. A., and Levin, W. C. *Tex. Med.* 68:91, 1972.)

Table 19-8. Classification of Monoclonal Gammopathies

I. *Immunochemical Classification* (diagnostic techniques: electrophoresis + immunoelectrophoresis)
  A. IgG MG, with or without Bence Jones proteins: ~60%
  B. IgA MG, with or without Bence Jones proteins: ~15%
  C. IgM MG, with or without Bence Jones proteins, ~10–15%
  D. IgD MG, with or without Bence Jones proteins: ~1%
  E. IgE MG, with or without Bence Jones proteins: <0.1%
  F. Light chain MG, only Bence Jones proteins present: ~15%
  G. Heavy chain MG, either γ, α, or μ chains present: <1%

II. *Clinical Classification*
  A. Symptomatic MG, i.e., "malignant," classic MG; represents <⅔ of all MG
    Criteria: M proteins: >3.0 g%; bone marrow: >10% plasma cells. Hemoglobin, albumin decreased. Progressive course requiring therapy.
    1. Multiple myeloma (MM)
      a. IgG MM: ⅔ of all MM
      b. IgA MM
      c. IgD MM: Rare
      d. IgE MM: Very rare
      e. Light-chain disease (Bence Jones MM)
    2. Waldenström's macroglobulinemia MW)
      a. IgM MW
    3. Malignant lymphoma-like heavy-chain disease
      a. γ H-chain disease
      b. α H-chain disease
      c. μ H-chain disease
  B. Asymptomatic MG,[a] i.e., "benign" MG; represents <⅓ of all MG
    Criteria: M proteins: <3.0 g%; bone marrow: <10% plasma cells. Hemoglobin, albumin normal. Stationary course not requiring treatment.
      a. IgG MG: ⅔ of all asymptomatic MG
      b. IgA MG
      c. IgM MG
      d. IgD MG: rare

---

[a] Asymptomatic MG is that found in healthy persons or in association with non-B-cell disorders (e.g., carcinoma, lipid disorders, chronic infections).

---

percent plasma cells). In approximately 1.6 percent of myeloma patients, plasma-cell leukemia is observed, i.e., more than 20 percent plasma cells in peripheral blood and an absolute plasma cell count of at least 2000 per cubic millimeter are found [204]. The disease progresses relentlessly, although chemotherapy may provide impressive palliation (see Fig. 19-37).

The remaining one-third of the patients with immunochemical evidence of MG are asymptomatic with regard to the clinical expression of the "malignant" B-cell disorders, and either they are apparently healthy or they present with disorders not directly related to B-cell diseases (see Tables 19-8 and 19-9). Such patients with asymptomatic or

Table 19-9.   Monoclonal Gammopathies—Clinical Classification and
Definition

Symptomatic (malignant, classic) MG
   Associated with clinically manifest and progressive B-cell disorders, including myeloma, macroglobulinemia, heavy-chain diseases.

Asymptomatic (benign, idiopathic) MG
   Absence of clinically overt "malignant" B-cell disorders for more than 5
   years. Frequently associated with non-B-cell disorders, including cancer,
   lipid disorders, etc.

Reproduced by permission. From Ritzmann, S. E., et al. *Arch. Intern. Med.*
135:95, 1975.

benign MG usually exhibit low M-protein concentrations (see Fig.
19-36) and slight bone-marrow plasmacytosis, but they usually do not
require specific treatment [203, 205] (see Tables 19-8 and 19-9).

Case Report 4
A 72-year-old man was admitted with a 4-month history of lower back
pain, a 40-pound weight loss over 6 months, and progressive lethargy and
diffuse weakness for several weeks. Three days prior to admission, the back
pain became considerably more intense, with pain in the right gluteal region
radiating down the right leg. He came to the emergency room for this
pain, and, on questioning, he was found to have frequent nausea and vomiting of food contents, a significant dyspnea that was greatly exacerbated by
exercise, a two-pillow orthopnea, occasional transient bilateral ankle edema,
intermittent dull nonpleuritic chest pain unrelated to exercise, and a severe
pleuritic pain of recent origin localized in the region of the anterior segment
of the fourth rib on the right. He denied having had previous severe illnesses
other than pneumonia requiring antibiotic therapy about one year prior to
admission.
   On physical examination, his blood pressure was 170/94, his pulse 110
and regular, his respiration 18 breaths per minute and regular, and his temperature was 99.6°F (orally). Generally, he was a severely emaciated, chronically ill, elderly male in moderately severe pain. He was oriented but with
senile mentation. Other findings were noted as follows. *Eyes:* pupils equal,
round, reactive to light and accommodation; bilateral arcus senilis; sclerae
clear; conjunctivae unremarkable. *Fundi:* normal other than bilateral mild
arteriolar narrowing. *Ears, Nose, & Throat:* edentulous, neck supple, moderate venous distention bilaterally, no bruits, no significant lymphadenopathy,
no thyromegaly. *Lungs:* moderate basilar rales bilaterally, no dullness to percussion. *Heart:* point of maximal impulse, 2 cm lateral to the midclavicular
line in the 6th intercostal space, crisp S_1, S_2 in rapid regular ryhthm with a
loud S_3 gallop, grade II/VI systolic ejection murmur over the lower left
sternal border without radiation, no rubs. *Abdomen:* scaphoid and soft, liver
decreased 4 cm below the right costal margin (14 cm span by percussion)
and tender, spleen and kidneys were not palpable, no other tenderness, bowel
sounds normal. *Back:* no costovertebral angle tenderness; exquisite localized
tenderness at the dorsal aspect of the 4th lumbar vertebra with paravertebral
muscle spasm; impaired range of motion for flexion, extension, and lateral

motion of the spine at this level. *Genitalia:* normal adult male. *Extremities:* 2+ pitting pretibial edema bilaterally to the midcalf level of the lower extremities; decreased range of motion of right hip; no arthritis, clubbing, or cyanosis; pulses palpable and symmetrical. *Neurological:* cranial nerves intact, deep tendon reflexes diffusely decreased and absent knee jerk and Achilles' reflex in right lower extremity, flaccid paralysis of right leg with positive straight-leg raising sign (Lasègue's sign) on the right, sensory loss in right lower extremity, absent Babinski's and Hoffmann's signs. *Skin:* decreased skin turgor, no lesions.

On roentgenological survey, posteroanterior and lateral chest films revealed a cardiomegaly with mild bilateral pulmonary edema. A rib fracture was seen anteriorily on the right in the 4th rib. Rib detail films indicated several scattered osteolytic lesions throughout the thoracic cage. A skull series revealed prominent "punched-out" lesions of the skull. Lumbar spine films revealed a compression fraction at the 4th lumbar vertebra. The remainder of a bone survey was unremarkable except for several osteolytic lesions of the pelvis.

Laboratory examination included electrocardiography, which revealed low voltage with an interventricular conduction defect. A complete blood count revealed hemoglobin of 8 gm per 100 ml, hematocrit 19 percent, with white blood cell count of 8400 and a normal differential. The red blood cell indices indicated a hypochromic microcytic type of anemia. The serum iron and the serum iron-binding capacity were both decreased. The calcium was 12.6 mg per 100 ml and the phosphorus, 2.8 mg per 100 ml. The serum sodium was 134 mEq per liter, the chloride, 96 mEq per liter, the potassium, 2.8 mEq per liter, and the CO_2-combining power, 21 mEq per liter. Serum protein electrophoresis revealed a large M protein in the γ-globulin region of 3.1 gm per 100 ml, which on immunoelectrophoresis proved to be an abnormal IgG. The serum viscosity was normal. The alkaline phosphatase was elevated to 4.6 Bodansky units, with a total serum bilirubin of 1.4 mg per 100 ml with a 1.0 mg per 100 ml direct component. The SGOT was 72 units, the SGPT 49 units, and the LDH 200 units. The serum uric acid was 5.3 mg per 100 ml. Urinalysis showed a specific gravity of 1.012, a negative glucose oxidase test, a negative test for ketones and for occult blood, and a 2+ proteinuria. Examination of the urinary sediment was unremarkable except for the presence of tubular casts. The 24-hour urine protein was 2.6 gm. The BUN was 26 mg per 100 ml, the creatinine, 2.1 mg per 100 ml, and the creatinine clearance, 48.6 ml per minute. A heat test for Bence Jones proteins was positive, and subsequent immunodiffusion tests confirmed the presence of a Bence Jones proteinuria. A bone-marrow aspiration revealed diffuse sheets of plasma cells. A gingival biopsy specimen stained with Congo red and when examined by polarized light, revealed the presence of amyloid. A renal biopsy specimen revealed dilation of tubules containing amorphous material, compatible with the tubular damage of multiple myeloma (Fig. 19-31).

The patient was begun on digoxin, furosemide, and potassium chloride. His congestive heart failure was refractory to these measures and could be controlled only by strict bed rest, salt and fluid restriction, and curtailment of exercise. Open reduction of the compression fracture was successfully performed under spinal anesthesia. During a 3½-week hospitalization, the patient developed two episodes of pneumonia and one acute urinary tract infection; all of which responded to appropriate antibiotics. The patient continued to require heavy analgesia for bone pain. He was discharged to the outpatient clinic, and was followed up on melphalan.

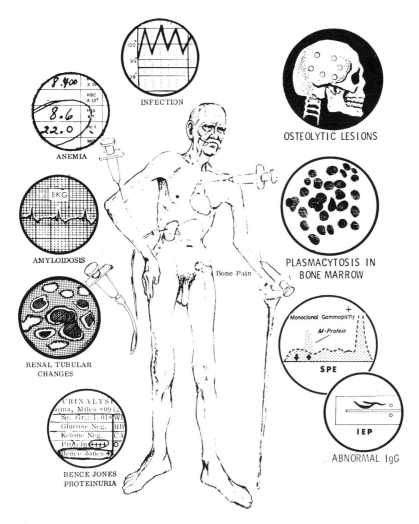

Figure 19-31
Clinical features of IgG multiple myeloma (see Case Report 4).

Final Diagnosis: IgG-multiple myeloma with Bence Jones proteinuria, complicated by (1) pathological and compression fractures secondary to osteolytic lesions, (2) hypercalcemia, (3) renal tubular disease, with mild renal insufficiency, (4) amyloidosis, with intractable heart failure, (5) anemia, and (6) frequent infections, secondary to compromise of normal immunoglobulins.

Prognosis: Fair.

Disposition: Continued treatment with chemotherapy and supportive measures with frequent follow-up.

B. *Asymptomatic MG* [203]. The refinement of diagnostic approaches beyond bone-marrow and histopathological examinations and the reliance upon protein electrophoresis and immunoelectrophoresis have added a new dimension to the study of MG: an increasing number of cases, in both adults and children, have been recognized that show the immunochemical abnormalities of multiple myeloma [206] and macroglobulinemia but lack the corresponding clinical counterparts. In 1952, Waldenström [207] suggested that this "essential hyperglobulinemia" may represent a distinct entity within the spectrum of MG. Subsequently, numerous reports have amplified this concept, and a plethora of synonymous terms has resulted that has led to some obfuscation of this subject (Table 19-10). At present, the terms *asymptomatic, benign,* and *idiopathic* monoclonal gammopathies are most widely used, but none of them is entirely satisfactory. For instance, the causes of multiple myeloma and macroglobulinemia are unknown, and these disorders must therefore be considered to be idiopathic. Furthermore, the meaning of *benign* is not necessarily identical clinically with *asymptomatic.* A more satisfactory terminology and classification of MG must await further clarification of the etiopathogenesis of the syndrome of MG. Since MG overtly represents abnormalities of the B-lymphocyte system, a simplified classification and the corresponding criteria of MG are presented in Table 19-8.

Some individuals with asymptomatic MG appear healthy, whereas others display non-B-cell disorders. Patients with such asymptomatic forms of MG usually have a long life-span, which is considerably in excess of those with symptomatic MG. In general, patients with this form of MG do not progress into the symptomatic forms and do not require specific treatment; however, some exceptions do occur.

C. *Differential diagnostic considerations.* No reliable parameters are available that allow an "instant" differential diagnosis of asymptomatic, benign MG from the symptomatic, malignant forms of MG early in the course of the disease. Long-term follow-up studies of these patients are at present necessary to ascertain their benign nature. A variety of differential diagnostic criteria have been advocated [203, 208]:

Hemoglobin levels: Decreased hemoglobin levels are frequently observed in patients with symptomatic MG, whereas normal hemoglobin levels are usually present in association with asymptomatic MG. Exceptions, however, do occur.

Erythrocyte sedimentation rates (ESR): The ESR is often normal or near normal in both asymptomatic patients and incipient cases of symptomatic MG, but it is increased in patients with fully developed forms of symptomatic MG. Exceptions do occur; for instance, patients with symptomatic MG and cryoglobulinemia may exhibit a decreased ESR.

Bone-marrow examination: A plasma-cell concentration of more than 20 percent of nucleated bone-marrow cells (exclusive of erythroid elements) is generally accepted as a criterion of neoplastic plasmacytic proliferation. Fewer bone-marrow plasma cells (usually less than 10 percent) are seen in patients with asymptomatic MG, but such levels may also be found in patients with early stages of myeloma and macroglobulinemia. There is, however, a wide variation in the amounts of bone-marrow

Table 19-10.   Synonyms for Asymptomatic Monoclonal Gammopathies[a]

Synonym	Author(s)	Year
Essential hyperglobulinemia	Waldenström	1952
Benign paraproteinemia	Olhagen-Liljestrand	1955
Nonmyelomatous paraproteinemia	Smith	1957
γ_1-Syndrome	Knedel	1958
Dysgammaglobulinemic syndrome	Hammack et al.	1959
Atypical dysproteinemias	Creyssel et al.	1959
Symptomless myelomatosis	Baker-Martin	1959
Essential, monoclonal, benign hypergammaglobulinemia	Waldenström	1961
Cryptogenetic and transitory paraproteinemias	Schobel-Wewalke	1961
Essential hyperdysglobulinemia	Olmer et al.	1961
Facultative paraproteinemias	Spengler et al.	1961
Monoclonal gammopathy of unknown etiology	Osserman-Takatsuki	1963
Rudimentary paraproteinemia	Märki-Wuhrmann	1963
Benign, essential, monoclonal nonmacromolecular hyperglobulinemia	Waldenström	1964
Secondary paraproteinemia	Videback-Drivsholm	1964
Idiopathic paraproteinemia	Rádl-Masopust	1964
Companion paraproteinemia	Riva	1964
Symptom-poor paraproteinemia	Huhnstock et al.	1964
Pseudo-myelomatous dysproteinemia	Laroche et al.	1964
Essential or isolated paraproteinemia	Brittinger-König	1965
Essential or atypical dysglobulinemia	Derycke et al.	1965
Atypical paraproteinemia	Klemm et al.	1965
Discrete gammaglobulin (M-) components	Hällen	1966
Asymptomatic monoclonal hypergammaglobulinemia	Allensmith-Chandor	1966
Lanthanic dysimmunoglobulinemia	Zawadzki-Edwards	1967
Nonmyelomatous plasmocytosis with dysproteinemia	Azar	1968
Secondary and primary benign monoclonal immunoglobulin disorders	Michaux-Heremans	1969
Asymptomatic paraimmunoglobulinemia	Engle-Wallis	1969
Asymptomatic paraproteinemia	Meijers et al.	1972
Nonmyelomatous monoclonal immunoglobulinemia	Zawadzki-Edwards	1972
Accompanying paraproteinemia	Siebner	1972
Asymptomatic or occult plasma-cell dyscrasias	Isobe-Osserman	1972

Data from Ritzmann, S. E., et al. *Arch. Intern. Med.* 135:95, 1975.

plasma cells in patients with MG in general, and a reliable differential diagnosis cannot be based upon bone-marrow criteria alone. On electron microscopy, plasma-cell asynchrony (i.e., a disparity between cytoplasmic and nuclear maturation, as reflected by nonaggregated nuclear chromatin, prominent nucleoli, and dilated rough endoplasmic reticulum) has been described as a specific ultrastructural defect in bone-marrow cells from patients with symptomatic MG (myeloma and macroglobulinemia) but not in those from patients with benign MG [209].

Serum albumin levels: Serum albumin levels in symptomatic MG are often decreased, but they remain generally normal in asymptomatic MG. Hypoalbuminemia, however, may occur in the latter disorder because of associated disorders and complications.

Serum viscosity: The finding of hyperviscosity is presumptive evidence of symptomatic MG, and the clinical manifestations of the serum hyperviscosity syndrome are most frequently associated with macroglobulinemia or, less commonly, with IgG (especially IgG$_3$ subclass) or IgA myeloma. Exceptions occur, however, and patients with asymptomatic MG or PG (see Case Report 2) may experience serum hyperviscosity (see Chap. 20). Since only a minority of patients with symptomatic MG develop this complication, this criterion does not offer a reliable differential diagnostic aid.

Anticomplementary activity: Anticomplementary activity is found both in symptomatic and asymptomatic forms of MG, in approximately 15 percent of myeloma patients, and in 11 percent of nonmyelomatous patients.

Serum concentrations of M proteins: In general, patients with symptomatic MG show a relentless increase of the M protein concentration as a reflection of the unabated progression of the malignant B-cell proliferation. Subsequently, plateau levels, following a Gompertzian curve of tumor growth, are attained [210]. In the asymptomatic form of MG, however, the M proteins remain essentially at their low levels throughout the disease process, even when these patients have been followed for many years. Exceptions, however, have occurred after 15 years [211] or 18 years of observation [212]. It is generally accepted that, at present, periodic clinical evaluation and determination of the concentrations of serum M proteins over a period of months is the most reliable differential criterion of asymptomatic *versus* symptomatic MG. Various threshhold levels of M-protein concentrations for distinguishing the asymptomatic from the symptomatic forms have been suggested: less than 1.0 gm per 100 ml for IgA and IgM, less than 2 gm per 100 ml for IgG, and either less than 2.0 gm per 100 ml or less than 3.0 gm per 100 ml for any immunoglobulin class. These values provide only a general rule of thumb at best. In our experience, a threshhold level of less than 3.0 gm per 100 ml for IgG-, IgA-, or IgM-class M proteins appears to be a realistic value for most patients with asymptomatic MG, provided the M-protein level is determined by SPE and not by immunodiffusion techniques (see Chap. 4).

L-chain types of M proteins: The normal 2:1 ratio of κ- to λ-type

L-chain constituents of serum IgG molecules is preserved in M proteins from patients with symptomatic MG as a group. A reversal of this ratio has been found in patients with asymptomatic MG. Even if it is confirmed, such a reversal of the $\kappa:\lambda$ ratio could not provide a reliable differential diagnostic aid, because of its nonexclusive nature.

Concentrations of residual, normal serum immunoglobulins: The symptomatic forms of MG are frequently associated with decreased levels of the "residual," normal immunoglobulins, whereas the asymptomatic forms are usually characterized by essentially normal, slightly decreased, or even increased levels. In one series, the residual immunoglobulins were suppressed in 98 percent of patients with symptomatic MG, but in only 10 percent of those with the benign form [213]. Incipient cases of symptomatic MG, however, usually do not show this inverse relationship yet. Thus, this criterion is not a reliable differential diagnostic aid.

Presence of Bence Jones proteins: The conventional heat test for Bence Jones proteins is rather insensitive (levels of less than 1200 mg per day cannot be detected), whereas the application of newer, extremely sensitive immunological techniques allows the detection of approximately 1 mg of either κ- or λ-type Bence Jones proteins in concentrated urine (see Chap. 5), which corresponds to only a few grams of protein-producing tumor tissue. Using these techniques, a new appreciation of the etiopathogenic role of Bence Jones proteins has been gained. Bence Jones proteinemia, proteinuria, or both is generally regarded as an ominous clinical sign. The incidence of Bence Jones proteinuria or proteinemia and the amounts of Bence Jones proteins excreted (less than 6 mg per 100 ml of urine) are appreciably lower in patients with the asymptomatic forms of MG than in the symptomatic cases [214]. McLaughlin and Hobbs [215] found Bence Jones proteins in a high percentage of patients with myeloma (70 percent among 708 patients), with macroglobulinemia (78 percent among 33 patients), and with chronic lymphocytic leukemia (15 percent among 104 patients). However, among patients with lichen myxedematosus and MG (6 patients), with transient paraproteinemia (5 patients), and with benign MG (40 patients) who were followed for at least 5 years, there was not a single instance of Bence Jones proteinuria.

These newer studies support the earlier contention that the presence of Bence Jones proteins is virtually pathognomonic for symptomatic MG [216], although well-defined exceptions to this rule are being recognized [217]. For instance, we have under observation an individual with IgA and Bence Jones MG who has had a seemingly benign course for more than 6 years. This 60-year-old patient was incidentally found to have a serum M protein in March 1968. At that time, he underwent extensive evaluation with the following findings: normal physical examination; normal electrocardiogram; roentgenologically normal skull, spine, pelvis, and long bones; essentially normal bone-marrow aspirate; the presence of IgA(λ) M protein; a significant degree of λ-type Bence Jones proteinemia and proteinuria, and low normal serum IgG and IgM concentrations. These parameters have remained essentially unchanged during the interim period, but the IgA M-protein levels have fluctuated between 1.5 and 2.5 gm per 100 ml, and the Bence Jones proteins have decreased gradually to intermittently undetectable levels. At present, this individual remains in excellent health with no evidence of progression of the asymptomatic MG.

The occurrence of Bence Jones proteins must be considered to be an important differential diagnostic aid between symptomatic and asymptomatic forms of MG; its usefulness is, however, not absolute, since not all patients with symptomatic MG elaborate Bence Jones proteins. Nevertheless, the combination of high or rising M-protein levels and the presence of Bence Jones proteins is an almost certain indicator of the symptomatic forms of MG; the reverse, however, is not necessarily true for asymptomatic forms of MG.

Low molecular weight 7S IgM: The presence of appreciable amounts of 7S IgM in patients with IgM-type MG usually indicates symptomatic MG, i.e., Waldenström's macroglobulinemia [218].

Chromosomal aberrations: Chromosomal aberrations have been reported in patients with various forms of MG [219–222]. These consist of large extra chromosomes in the AB size range, and additional abnormalities are found in variable percentages of patients with the IgG, IgA, IgM, and IgD types of MG, of either the symptomatic or asymptomatic variety, before and after treatment (see Fig. 19-42). These abnormal chromosomes are probably acquired rather than congenital in nature, since a patient with macroglobulinemia was found to possess the chromosomal abnormalities, whereas his healthy uniovular twin did not [223]. At present, chromosomal analysis does not have differential diagnostic value for the various forms of MG.

ABO blood groups: A preponderance of A-blood groups in patients with MG suggested a possible correlation with these genetic markers [224]. In our patients, however, there was no significant correlation of the ABO profiles in either group of patients with MG.

HL-A and W antigens: An increased frequency of the W-18 [225] and 4C histocompatibility antigens [226] was reported in patients with multiple myeloma. In other studies [203], no increase of W-18 and 4C was found in the asymptomatic IgG-type MG, but there was an absence of W-22, HL-A 7, HL-A 9, and W-15 antigens in symptomatic IgG-type MG. There was also an increased frequency of 4C in the symptomatic group. These parameters, however, are not of definite differential diagnostic significance at the present time.

Lymphocyte response patterns: Salmon and Fudenberg [227] demonstrated a significantly deficient lymphocyte in vitro response to phytohemagglutinin (PHA) in patients with multiple myeloma and macroglobulinemia. In other studies [203], the PHA response and mixed lymphocyte culture reactions were deficient to an equal degree both in patients with symptomatic and asymptomatic IgG-type MG, as well as in patients with IgA- and IgM-type MG. Thus, no differential diagnostic pattern has emerged for symptomatic and asymptomatic forms of MG using such techniques.

Surface immunoglobulins of lymphocytes: In certain patients with chronic lymphocytic leukemia, monoclonal B-cell proliferation is suggested by the demonstration of monoclonal immunoglobulin determinants on the cellular surfaces [14, 15, 17, 132], which may reflect a blocked cell maturation into functional, secretory plasma cells. A redistribution of B cells and T cells as well as altered ratios in the peripheral blood have been described with the reduction of B cells and normal surface immunoglobulins in myeloma patients [132, 228], but preservation of the normal proportion of B cells has been observed in patients with benign MG [228].

Delayed skin hypersensitivity: Based upon earlier studies by Fahey et al. [229], tests for delayed skin hypersensitivity appeared to offer a differential diagnostic aid. Studies with a battery of antigens (including tuberculin PPD, coccidioidin, histoplasmin, and mumps), however, did not yield any useful differential diagnostic parameters [203].

Complications of MG and associated disorders

1. *Complications:* Clinical complications arising in patients with MG may be due directly to the proliferating disease process itself (e.g., myeloma with osteolytic lesions, pathological fractures with attendant pain, and so on); indirectly to the disease process (e.g., hypercalcemia or kidney damage resulting in myeloma kidney); to the suppressive effects upon the physiological immunological functions (e.g., hypogammaglobulinemia and the increased susceptibility to infections); to altered physicochemical properties of the M proteins (e.g., cryoglobulins and hyperviscosity); or to the result of antibody activity of the M proteins (e.g., cold agglutinins). Patients suffering from symptomatic MG often display a bewildering array of clinical manifestations, which may obfuscate the appropriate diagnosis. A few examples of such complications are listed:

   a. *Bacterial infections:* An unusually high incidence of bacterial infections occurs, presumably due to the considerable suppression of "normal" immunoglobulins. Patients with IgG-type MG are particularly susceptible to gram-positive microorganisms, whereas patients with IgM-type MG are particularly prone to gram-negative bacterial infections [193]. The administration of appropriate antibiotics and, in selected cases, γ-globulin substitution are indicated [229].

   b. *Epithelial malignancies:* A high percentage of patients with MG develops epithelial malignancies [152] (Table 19-11). For example, in 25 percent of our patients with Waldenström's macroglobulinemia, carcinoma developed. In some instances, multiple malignancies emerged, such as multiple basal cell and squamous cell carcinomas. Although it is tempting to suggest that the emergence of malignancies in these patients is due to the deficiency of normal immunoglobulins and impaired immunosurveillance for oncogenesis by B cells, the reverse situation—the development of MG in response to epithelial malignancies—cannot be excluded, nor can one exclude the possibility that the same unknown defect that allows neoplastic emergence may also allow the proliferation of an abnormal plasma cell clone.

   c. *Serum hyperviscosity syndrome:* The abnormal immunoglobulins may precipitate or gel upon cooling. Such cryoglobulins often lead to the

Table 19-11.   Cancer in Association with Monoclonal Gammopathy Compared with a Random Series

Type of Cancer	MG with Cancer (75 cases)		Random Series (912 cases)		Ratio (percent MG with cancer to percent random series)
	Number of Cases	Percent	Number of Cases	Percent	
Large bowel	26	34.7	182	19.8	1.8
Rectosigmoid	25	33.4	108	11.9	3.1
Other	1	1.3	74	7.9	0.2
Prostate	23	30.7	176	19.3	1.6
Breast	14	18.7	352	38.6	0.5
Lung	8	10.7	179	19.6	0.5
Adenocarcinoma	5	6.7	18	2.0	3.3
Bronchogenic	3	4.0	161	17.6	0.25
Gall bladder	3	4.0	4	0.4	10.0
Liver	1	1.3	19	2.1	0.6

Adapted from Isobe, T., and Osserman, E. F.   *Ann. N.Y. Acad. Sci.* 190:507, 1971.

serum hyperviscosity syndrome [230, 231] (see Chap. 20). Its manifestations, which are aggravated by cold, include dizziness, mucous membrane bleeding, Menière's syndrome, seizures, and coma. Plasmapheresis, the immediate treatment of choice for this condition, is aimed at reducing and maintaining the serum viscosity below critical levels [232]. The M proteins in some of the patients with hyperviscosity, cryoglobulinemia, or both possess rheumatoid factor activity, i.e., anti-IgG antibody function [193]. The "abnormal" IgM in such patients possessing rheumatoid factor activity is the product of specific B-cell clones that produce IgM with rheumatoid-factor specificity. Therefore, such patients with IgM-type MG may represent a unique clonal form of macroglobulinemia, namely, the *rheumatoid-factor clonal form* [193, 198].

d. *Amyloidosis:* This is another frequent complication of MG, especially in patients with Bence Jones proteins. Amyloid is often related to tissue deposition of fragments of immunoglobulin light chains [195] (see pp. 445–448).

e. *Cold-agglutinin disease:* In certain patients with IgM-type MG, the chief clinical manifestations may be the result of the cold-antibody activity of the "abnormal" IgM [190, 193, 216]. These cold-agglutinin antibodies are usually of the anti-I variety, with extremely high activities that range up to 1:2,000,000 titers [106, 193, 233]. These "abnormal" IgM fractions harboring the high cold-agglutinin activity may be considered to be products of unique IgM cell clones that specialize in the formation of such antibodies. Consequently, such patients may be considered to represent a unique clonal form of macroglobulinemia, namely the "cold-agglutinin clonal form" [106, 193, 198]. In such patients, agglutination of erythrocytes and hemolysis may occur on exposure to cold temperatures (see pp. 489–490, Chap. 20). Cold-agglutinin disease is usually progressive and malignant, but it may occasionally be stationary and benign [234].

Case Report 5
A 65-year-old male had experienced cyanosis, numbness, pain, and coldness of the fingers upon exposure to cold for several years; these manifestations were relieved by warming. Intermittently, he had experienced hemoglobinuria. Upon admission, he was anemic (8 gm per 100 ml), and the cold-agglutinin titer was 1:2 million with a temperature amplitude up to 32°C. The total serum proteins were 5.3 gm per 100 ml, and the γ-globulin fraction on electrophoresis revealed an M protein concentration of 1.5 gm per 100 ml. Using immunoelectrophoresis, this was diagnosed as an IgM(κ) monoclonal gammopathy. There was hepatosplenomegaly. The bone marrow examination revealed erythroid hyperplasia and a moderate increase of lymphoid plasma cells. During the following several years, the patient required multiple blood transfusions and symptomatic treatment for hemolytic crises precipitated by chilling. Three years after the initial admission, a basal-cell carcinoma of the left arm and an epidermoid carcinoma of the periauricular area were removed. One year later, a bilateral herniorrhaphy was performed, which was followed by chilling and a hemolytic crisis requiring multiple blood transfusions. During the ensuing years, he experienced numerous episodes of hemoglobinuria and required numerous blood transfusions. Two years after the herniorrhaphy, he was readmitted. The hemoglobin level was 5.7 gm per 100 ml, the direct Coombs' test was positive, and the red blood cell half-life was 13 days (normal is 28 days) with considerable erythrocyte sequestration in both the liver and spleen. There were prominent hepatosplenomegaly and cholelithiasis. Splenectomy and cholecystectomy were performed. On the sixth postoperative day, the patient's blood pressure became unobtainable, and he died presumably from gram-negative bacterial septicemia. No autopsy was performed [193].

Cold agglutinins are blood-group antibodies usually directed against the I antigens that are ubiquitously distributed on most nucleated cells; others are directed against H, O, Pr, or i antigens [233, 235]. I antigens are present on the erythrocytes of almost all adult persons in low titers (comparable to anti-A and anti-B isoagglutinin titers), whereas erythrocytes in children during the first months of life show the i phenotype, which is gradually replaced by I antigens. Most cold agglutinins are 19S IgM antibodies [236]. A transient polyclonal increase to moderately increased titers (see Fig. 19-32) is observed in certain patients with viral diseases (e.g., infectious mononucleosis) as well as with *Mycoplasma pneumoniae* infections [106, 233, 237]. In contrast, the considerable increase of cold agglutinins in cold-agglutinin disease is usually associated with monoclonal IgM (κ) [106, 233, 237], but occasionally it is also associated with IgM (λ) [238], IgA (κ) [233], IgA (λ) [239], or even IgG (κ) [233].

The serological properties of cold agglutinins are characterized by a temperature-titer relationship. Cold agglutinins reveal their highest erythrocyte agglutination activity at 0°C (Fig. 19-32). Normally, the low-titered cold agglutinins lose their agglutinating activity above 10°C. The transiently increased cold agglutinins following *Mycoplasma pneumoniae* infections usually do not agglutinate erythrocytes above 15° to 25°C, but they may lead to complement-mediated hemolysis if chilling occurs at exposed sites, such as the skin. The excessively increased monoclonal cold agglutinins in patients with cold-agglutinin disease may display erythrocyte agglutination and hemolysis up to 30° to 32°C [106, 193]. Such an event is usually associated with continuous hemolytic anemia and exacerbations leading to paroxysmal cold hemoglobinuria. In such patients, there is severe cold hypersensitivity or cryopathy [240], which is reflected by pallor or acrocyanosis or both, often with numbness of the ear lobes, nose, and lips. Seasonably fluctuating hemolytic anemia, jaundice, and hemoglobinuria occur, which are most pronounced during the winter months. This disease must be considered in the differential diagnosis of Raynaud's phenomenon and cryopathies (see Chap. 20).

2. *Disorders frequently associated with MG:* Both the symptomatic and asymptomatic forms of MG are frequently associated with disorders that are seemingly unrelated to the monoclonal B-cell proliferative process. The association of such disorders with MG is encountered more frequently than would be expected by coincidence [152, 170, 199, 208, 241]. These disorders include cancer or neoplasms of non-B-cell origin; lipid disorders [169, 188, 207, 242–248], such as Gaucher's disease, xanthomatosis, Schüller-Christian-Hand disease, diabetes mellitus, and others; myeloproliferative disorders; and chronic infections, such as syphilis, chronic pyelonephritis, diverticulosis, diverticulitis, and others [199]. In a retrospective study of 128 cases of MG [152], chronic cholecystitis was found in 6 percent, syphilis in 7 percent, and pulmonary tuberculosis in 7 percent of patients with IgG, IgA, or IgM monoclonal gammopathy. Diverticulosis was documented in 25 percent and gastric and duodenal ulcers in 17 percent of all patients with IgM-type MG. The frequency of such mesenchymal abnormalities in association with MG is probably statistically significant [248].

Isobe and Osserman [199] have recently reviewed the clinical and pathological records of 806 cases of MG studied over a 19-year time span, and they have provided the most complete and thorough attempt to define the types of pathological conditions associated with various forms of MG. These authors classified the patients with MG into various categories including: (1) *monoclonal gammopathies of unknown significance*—239 cases in which an M protein was demonstrated in the absence of myeloma, macroglobulinemia, amyloidosis, or an associated nonreticular neoplasm (i.e., asymptomatic, benign MG); (2) *MG with carcinoma*—128 cases in which an M protein was associated with nonreticular neoplasms; (3) *myeloma*—303 cases with evidence of overt plasma-cell myeloma and documented skeletal lesions; (4) *macroglobulinemia*—66 cases with clinically overt evidence of symptomatic macroglobulinemia, i.e., anemia, lymphadenopathy, hepatosplenomegaly, and so on; and (5) *amyloidosis with MG*—70 cases with symptomatic and histologically documented amyloidosis, generally of the so-called primary distribution. The results of this analysis (Table 19-12) indicate that 90 to 95 percent

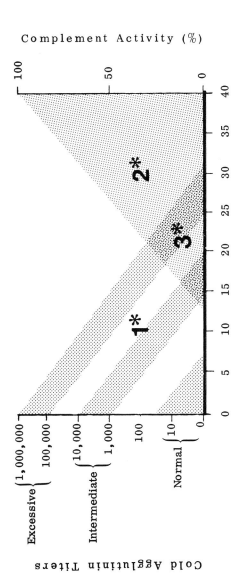

Figure 19-32

Three ranges of cold-agglutinin titers and their respective temperature ranges of activity. (*1*) *Normal range:* Titers of approximately 1:1 to 1:64 and temperature ranges of activity between 0° and 8°C. Under these circumstances, there is no deleterious effect resulting from the auto-anti-I antibodies, since they do not react with their corresponding I antigens that are ubiquitously present on most nucleated cells. (*2*) *Transient increases:* Titers of approximately 1:256 to 1:4000 and temperature amplitudes between 0° and 15° to 20°C. Such increases occur in patients with certain viral infections or *Mycoplasma pneumoniae* infections. Occasionally, significant erythrocyte agglutination and hemolysis may be observed. (*3*) *Excessive increases:* Titers up to 1:2 million and temperature amplitudes between 0° and 32°C. Such increases of cold-agglutinin activity are usually associated with lymphoproliferative disorders, specifically IgM monoclonal gammopathies, i.e., cold-agglutinin disease that is characterized by the triad of jaundice, hemolytic anemia, and paroxysmal cold hemoglobinuria. *: ranges of (*1*) antibody fixation, (*2*) complement activity, (*3*) hemolysis. (Adapted from Schubothe, H. *Semin. Hematol.* 3:27, 1966.)

Table 19-12. Percentage Incidence of Associated Conditions in Monoclonal Gammopathies (MG)

Disorder	MG of Unknown Significance (239)[a]	MG with Carcinoma (128)[a]	Myeloma (303)[a]	Macroglobulinemia (66)[a]	Amyloidosis with MG (70)[a]
Cholecystitis/cholelithiasis	8.8	11.7	11.2	13.6	11.4
Pulmonary emphysema/fibrosis/ chronic bronchitis	7.5	7.0	5.0	7.6	7.1
Peptic ulcer	7.5	10.8	4.3	3.0	7.1
Chronic urinary tract infection {upper	7.1	6.2	3.6	6.1	10.0
Chronic urinary tract infection {lower	7.1	7.8	5.3	3.0	5.6
Liver cirrhosis/chronic hepatitis	7.1	3.9	2.0	3.0	7.1
Syphilis	7.1	4.7	0.7	4.5	4.3
Diverticulitis of the colon	5.4	7.8	3.3	1.5	4.3
Myocardial infarction	5.4	6.2	3.0	3.0	0.2
Peripheral neuropathy/ myopathy	5.4	0.8	1.3	3.0	0.3
Central nervous system disorders	5.0	2.3	1.6	1.5	0.2
(apparently healthy)	4.6	4.7	9.9	9.1	8.6
Rheumatoid arthritis/spondylitis	4.6	3.9	5.0	6.1	5.6
Thyroid/parathyroid	4.6	6.2	5.6	6.1	7.1
Myeloid metaplasia/myelofibrosis/polycythemia vera	4.6	0	0.7	0	0
Lipoma/lipidosis	4.2	3.1	1.6	4.5	4.3
Chronic dermatitis/chronic eczema	2.9	0.8	2.0	4.5	7.1
Peripheral vasculitis/thrombophlebitis	2.5	3.1	2.3	0	0.2
Gaucher's disease	2.1	0	0	1.5	0
Soft tissue calcification	2.1	3.1	2.3	1.5	4.3
Pulmonary tuberculosis	2.1	4.7	3.0	1.5	7.1
Rheumatic heart disease/SBE	2.1	1.6	1.3	3.0	0.3
Diabetes mellitus	2.1	3.9	2.6	3.0	0.2
Drug allergy	1.7	3.1	1.6	3.0	0
SLE/scleroderma/dermatomyositis	1.7	0	1.6	3.0	4.3
Atopy/bronchial asthma/hay fever	1.7	0.8	0.7	6.1	4.3
Ovary, uterus/cyst, polyp, myoma	1.3	4.7	4.0	0	0.2
Paget's disease	1.3	1.6	0.3	1.5	0.2
Malaria	1.3	0	0	0	0
Chronic leg ulcer	0.8	0.8	0.7	0	0
Osteomyelitis	0.8	0	1.3	0	0.3
Sarcoidosis	0.8	0.8	0	3.0	0
Gout	0.8	1.6	0	3.0	0.2
Coombs' positive hemolytic anemia	0.8	0.8	0	3.0	0.2

[a] Number of cases in parentheses.

444

Table 19-12 (*continued*)

Disorder	MG of Unknown Significance (239)[a]	MG with Carcinoma (128)[a]	Myeloma (303)[a]	Macroglobulinemia (66)[a]	Amyloidosis with MG (70)[a]
Idiopathic myocardial hypertrophy	0.8	0	0	0	0.2
Sprue, nontropical	0.8	0	0	0	0
Adrenal gland/adenoma	0.4	0	0.7	0	0.2
Mammary/cyst, fibroma, adenoma	0.4	0	1.3	3.0	0.2
Chronic sinustitis	0.4	0.8	1.3	3.0	0.2
Chronic pancreatitis/cyst	0.4	0	1.3	0	0.2

Adapted from Isobe, T., and Osserman, E. F. *Ann. N.Y. Acad. Sci.* 190:507, 1971.

of all cases in all categories had some significant prior medical illness. Chronic biliary tract disease (i.e., chronic cholecystitis and cholelithiasis) was the most frequently associated background illness in all groups of cases (between 8.8 and 13.6 percent in the various groups). The incidence of peptic ulcer was also remarkably high, especially in the category of MG with carcinoma (10.8 percent).

Table 19-11 depicts the frequency of six types of neoplasms associated with MG. Neoplasms of the rectosigmoid colon (adenocarcinoma, 19.6 percent, and adenomatous polyps, 18.8 percent) represented the most frequent tumors found in association with this group of cases with asymptomatic MG. This high proportion of rectosigmoid lesions in such patients is significantly greater than that in a random series of patients with large bowel tumors. Additionally, in this group of patients, there was a high incidence of neoplasms of the tongue (3.9 percent), biliary tract (2.3 percent), and urinary bladder (2.3 percent). An unknown percentage of cases with benign monoclonal gammopathies are seemingly healthy. Indeed, some of these individuals have served as blood donors prior to diagnosis [224, 249].

Amyloidosis. Amyloid, which was first described in 1842 by Rokitansky [250] and said by Virchow to be starch-like [251], was demonstrated in 1859 to consist primarily of protein [252]. In the century following, there gradually emerged a firm clinical association between the presence of amyloid infiltrates and paraproteinemias [184]. This line of research culminated with a report by Osserman et al. [195] on the identification of monoclonal immunoglobulins or Bence Jones proteins in the sera of the majority of patients with amyloidosis, whether of the primary type (unassociated with other disease) or the secondary type (associated with diseases leading to reticuloendothelial stimulation). Although Osserman implicated the involvement of immunoglobulins in the pathogenesis of amyloidosis, the subsequent decade yielded a vast literature of conflicting data, and there was difficulty in proving this implication [253, 254]. These investigations were based on the available immunological techniques, which were then primarily immunofluorescence and precipitin reactions.

Due to the insoluble nature of amyloid, purification of this substance was not accomplished until recently. Purification of amyloid was performed in 1969 by using ultracentrifugal concentration and solubility techniques developed in the field of membrane chemistry [255]. Electron microscopy established a characteristic fibrillar pattern [256–258] for the substance that had been operationally termed *amyloid* by virtue of its birefringence under polarized light after staining with Congo red [259]. Further x-ray diffraction studies characterized a β-pleated sheet conformation of amyloid [260]. The existence of a purified antigen allowed the preparation of highly specific antisera, which have shown unequivocally that the major protein constituents of the amyloid fibrils are fragments of immunoglobulin polypeptide chains [261]. Certain immunochemical similarities between purified amyloid and immunoglobulin light chains were noted. Two types of amino terminal groups on amyloid correspond to (1) aspartic acid, which is characteristic of κ light chains, and (2) pyrrolidone carboxylic acid (PCA), which is characteristic of λ light chains [262–264].

Thus, purified amyloid has been referred to as κ or λ types, based on the amino terminal grouping and corresponding to the immunoglobulin L chains of the same designation. Specific antisera to κ amyloid reacted with other such κ-amyloid proteins and with 23 of 26 κ-type Bence Jones proteins [265]. There were similar cross-reactivities among λ-type amyloid and λ-type Bence Jones proteins. As with Bence Jones proteins, certain idiotypic reactions were encountered with amyloid fibrils. The similarity between amyloid and Bence Jones proteins was carried further when amino-acid sequence analysis demonstrated a remarkable homology between two purified κ fibrillar amyloid proteins (one from a case of "primary" amyloidosis and the other from a case of "secondary" amyloidosis) and a purified κ-type Bence Jones protein [266]. The amino-acid differences were no greater than those between two different κ-type Bence Jones proteins. The homology resided in the amino terminal portion of the polypeptide chains, thus representing the variable portion of the L chain (Fig. 19-33).

These studies proved that the major protein components of amyloid fibrils are immunochemically and biochemically indistinguishable from monoclonal immunoglobulin L chains, specifically the variable portions. Since the molecular weight of amyloid has been determined to be slightly less than that of Bence Jones protein [262], only a fragment of the L chain must be identical, which is compatible with the localization of homology to the variable portion. However, the molecular weight of amyloid is slightly greater than purified variable portions of L chains alone [262], which implies the presence of nonprotein constituents, most likely

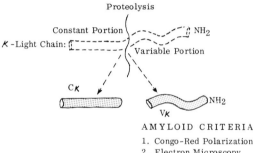

Figure 19-33
Enzymatic degradation of a κ light chain at physiological conditions to a variable portion indistinguishable from amyloid.

AMYLOID CRITERIA
1. Congo-Red Polarization
2. Electron Microscopy
3. X-Ray Diffraction

polysaccharides [262, 267, 268]. The polysaccharide addition to form glycoprotein may be a secondary phenomenon after the initial amyloid deposition.

In recent experiments by Glenner et al. [269], specific enzymatic treatment was employed to separate the variable and constant portions of the polypeptide chain of purified Bence Jones proteins (see Fig. 19-33) in vitro under physiological conditions (37°C, pH 7.42). This resulted in the formation of a β-pleated, fibrillar, Congo-red birefringent material that was indistinguishable from purified amyloid fibril. These studies indicate that variable regions of L chains may become amyloid fibrils under physiological conditions. Preliminary comparisons between the κ and λ light chains suggest that the λ chains of Bence Jones proteins may have a greater tissue affinity and be more "amyloidogenic" than the κ chain [253]. As of present, however, not all monoclonal L chains have been found to conform to these characteristics. Thus, the possibility remains that some cases of amyloidosis may result from the tissue deposition of portions of immunoglobulins other than L chains or of nonimmunoglobulin proteins [17]. Whether the preponderance of L chain involvement is due to the mode of catabolism or to the rate of synthesis of these chains is unknown.

Although the events representing the precursor to amyloid deposition are also unknown, several theories [270] have been advanced: (1) antigen-antibody complexes may be processed by macrophage degradation to amyloid concentrates, which would be distributed into macrophage-rich tissues, such as the spleen and liver; (2) a plasma cell disturbance that results in an asynchrony of L- to H-chain production could lead to excessive L chain formation with consequent deposition due to the insolubility of these chains; (3) a genetic plasma cell disorder could result in a chronic, low-grade, subclinical L-chain disease in which fragments are deposited in tissues, but in which neither urine clearance nor blood accumulation of L chains is attained; and (4) a subtle biochemical perturbation at the plasma-cell level could result in the overproduction of variable portions of L chains, with subsequent tissue fixation. Regardless of any speculations as to the mechanisms involved, it seems firmly established that most, if not all, instances of amyloid deposits that are associated with MG as well as the primary form of amyloidosis represent the tissue deposition of fragments of immunoglobulin L chains, specifically the variable portions of monoclonal L chains [271]. In contrast, the major component of secondary amyloid appears to be a hitherto undescribed protein with a molecular weight of about 8500 daltons, whose amino-acid sequence bears no relationship to any immunoglobulin [271]. It has been postulated that amyloid-related Bence Jones proteins and monoclonal immunoglobulins may be autoantibodies or fragments of autoantibodies directed against normal tissue constituents [272].

Amyloidosis is variously regarded as a disease entity in itself or merely a symptom of the underlying monoclonal gammopathy [216]. The clinical classification of amyloidosis into primary *amyloidosis* (especially in the tongue, heart, GI tract, skeletal and smooth muscles, carpal ligaments, nerves, and skin), secondary *amyloidosis* (especially in the liver, spleen, kidneys, and adrenal glands and found predominantly in patients with chronic infections, rheumatoid arthritis, familial Mediterranean fever, and Hodgkin's disease), and *paramyloidosis* associated with MG is unsatisfactory [258, 272, 273]. In usage, these terms refer either to pathogenic mechanisms or to particular patterns of amyloid distribution. A modified classification of amyloidosis has been proposed that is based on the predominant clinical patterns of amyloid distribution [272]:

Pattern I—principal involvement of organs affected in primary amyloidosis,

Pattern II—principal involvement of organs affected in secondary amyloidosis,

Mixed patterns I and II—representing an admixture of both pathological processes, and

Localized—amyloid deposits exclusively in a single tissue or organ.

These amyloid patterns and the associated immunoglobulin abnormalities in 100 cases are listed in Table 19-13 [272]. M proteins were documented in 88 of the 100 cases. They were found in all 50 (100 percent) pattern I cases, in 26 of 30 (87 percent) mixed pattern I and II cases, but in only 9 of 17 (53 percent) pure pattern II cases. It is particularly noteworthy that 36 of 50 pattern I cases had only Bence Jones proteins and that 10 additional cases had Bence Jones proteins associated with IgG-type (8 cases) or IgA-type (2 cases) M proteins. *Thus, 92 percent of the pattern I cases were associated with the elaboration of Bence Jones proteins.*

Cellular kinetics in MG. In general, the growth of plasma-cell tumors mimicks the pattern of the antibody response following immunization (see Fig. 19-5). The tumor grows initially in an exponential fashion, but it gradually slows its growth rate as it enlarges. Such a growth pattern fits the Gompertzian curve rather than a first-order curve [210] (Fig. 19-34). Repeated measurements of the M-protein levels provide useful information on the rate of growth of the tumor clone [190]. To evaluate this information, it must be considered that the exchangeable pool of the

Table 19-13. Frequency of M Proteins in Different Patterns of Amyloidosis

M Protein	Amyloid Distribution (no. of cases)				
	Pattern I[a]	Mixed (pattern I & II)	Pattern II[b]	Localized	Total
BJκ only	17	3	1		21
BJλ only	19	6			25
IgG only		4	5	1	10
IgG + BJκ	3				3
IgG + BJλ	5	4			9
IgA only	4	2	1		7
IgA + BJκ	1				1
IgA + BJλ	1				1
IgD only		1			1
IgD + BJλ		1			1
IgM only		4	2	1	7
IgM + BJκ		1		1	2
No monoclonal protein detected		4	8		12
Totals	50	30	17	3	100

[a] Involvement of heart, tongue, gastrointestinal tract, etc.
[b] Involvement of liver, spleen, kidneys, etc.
From Isobe, T., and Osserman, E. F. Reprinted by permission from the *New England Journal of Medicine* 290:473, 1974.

M protein (P), and hence its concentration in the serum, is determined by the ratio of its biosynthesis rate (s) and the number of M-protein-synthesizing cells to its fractional rate of catabolism (k) [274]: $P = s/k$. The total body myeloma cell number can be calculated [210] by dividing the total body M-protein synthesis rate by the cellular M-protein synthesis rate.

The techniques for the measurement of M-protein synthesis in vitro and for the study of total body tumor cell numbers have been established [210]. The immunosynthesis rates range from 2.5 pg to 35 pg per myeloma cell per day. Expressed in molecular terms, these rates range from 5200 to 87,500 molecules of immunoglobulin secreted per cell per minute, while the intracellular content of M proteins ranges from 5 to 10 million molecules per cell [210]. There apparently is no correlation between the morphological characteristics of myeloma or macroglobulinemia cells and the immunoglobulin synthesis rates. Since the fractional turnover rate is much higher for IgE (about 0.9 of the plasma pool per day) than for IgA (0.25), IgM (0.11 to 0.19), or IgG (about 0.07) [275], the tumor masses corresponding to a given concentration of these

Figure 19-34
Gompertzian curve of tumor growth for a patient with IgG multiple myeloma. The data points are computer-generated and placed at 1 log intervals up to 10^{12} cells, and are based on retropolation from tumor-cell number determinations in the clinical phase of illness. In this patient, the preclinical phase appears to be less than 1 year in duration. (Reproduced by permission from Grune & Stratton. From Salmon, S. E. Immunoglobulin synthesis and tumor kinetics of multiple myeloma. *Semin. Hematol.* 10:135–147, 1973.)

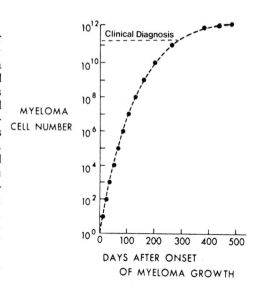

serum M proteins are also much greater in the case of IgE myeloma than in patients with IgA, IgM, or, particularly, IgG. Additionally, the fractional turnover rate of IgG increases with increasing serum concentrations of IgG (IgG_1, IgG_2, and IgG_4, but not IgG_3 [210]) (see Figs. 19-17 and 19-18), which leads to a curvilinear relationship between the tumor mass and the serum IgG concentrations (see Fig. 19-18).

Several general correlations appear to exist between the total body numbers of tumor cells, the tumor weight, its doubling times, the detectability of M proteins, and certain clinical manifestations: (1) The lower limits for the recognition of M proteins by serum protein electrophoresis is about 0.2 gm per 100 ml, which corresponds to a myeloma cell mass of about 2×10^{10} cells or about 20 gm of tumor (10^{12} myeloma cells correspond to approximately 1 kg of tumor mass). (2) Normally, there are approximately 3×10^{11} clones of human antibody-producing cells. With early diagnosis and discernible serum M proteins, myeloma cells may be found in excess of 10 percent in the bone marrow, which corresponds to at least 2×10^{11} myeloma cells present in the body. Patients with less than 1×10^{12} myeloma cells usually do not have significant manifestations of myeloma. Those patients with more than 2×10^{12} myeloma cells usually have evidence of widespread myelomatosis (Fig. 19-35) and a shorter life expectancy; death usually occurs when the tumor load reaches 5 to 7 percent of the body weight. (3) The subclinical period of MG is rather short, averaging only 1 to 2 years from the initial tumor cell doubling to its clinical presentation with 10^{11} to 10^{12} myeloma cells in the body. The initial doubling times of the tumor cells are faster (e.g., 1 to 3 days) than those later in the course (e.g., 4 to 6 months) (see Figs. 19-34 and 19-35).

At the time of clinical diagnosis, the myeloma tumor growth usually has essentially reached a plateau [210]. It is conceivable that asymptomatic, benign forms of MG may differ from symptomatic cases by virtue

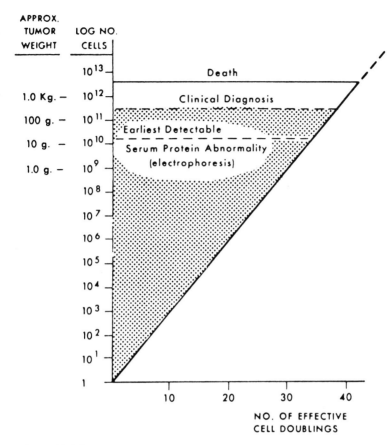

Figure 19-35
Relation of tumor weight and cell number to the number of effective cell doublings from the initiation of a malignant monoclone. It should be emphasized that time is not shown on the abscissa of this graph, because the tumor-cell doubling time is not constant. The illustration is designed to show the "iceberg" of preclinical doublings that go on prior to the potential detection of an M component by serum electrophoresis. Clinical diagnosis is generally about one or more log intervals above that point. (Reproduced by permission from Grune & Stratton. From Salmon, S. E. Immunoglobulin synthesis and tumor kinetics of multiple myeloma. *Semin. Hematol.* 10:135–147, 1973.)

of their earlier plateau formation [210] (Fig. 19-36). The nature of the mechanisms leading to plateau formation of the B-cell growth at different levels is unknown. Feedback promotion and inhibition mechanisms undoubtedly exist, such as those mediated by chalones [276] and possibly B-lymphocytosis factors [277]. These kinetic observations of rapid doubling times early in the course of the disease are in accordance with the observation of transient M proteins expressing themselves within 2 to 4 weeks after antigenic challenge (see Case Report 6 and Fig. 19-39). This recent knowledge of the kinetics involved bears directly on the chemotherapeutic approach to MG [210].

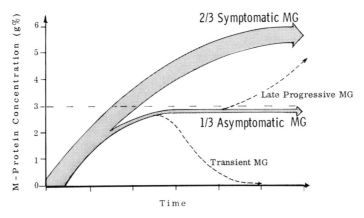

Figure 19-36
Various forms of monoclonal gammopathies. The two principal forms are
symptomatic MG (indicated by the heavy arrow), representing approximately two-thirds of all cases of MG, and asymptomatic MG (indicated by
the thinner arrow). In this latter category, some patients may progress to the
symptomatic form (e.g., a patient with a long-standing asymptomatic IgG-
MG may develop IgG myeloma). Others may regress to normal (i.e., transient MG); rarely, such an event may also be experienced by a patient with
the symptomatic form of MG.

Therapeutic aspects. In general, patients with symptomatic MG require treatment of the underlying B-cell disorder and the associated
complications. In contrast, patients with asymptomatic MG do not usually need treatment except for possible associated disorders. The management of MG is now encouraging [193, 278–284]. Significant improvement in both general management (ambulation with the aid of analgesics
and local irradiation, judicious use of glucocorticoids, adequate hydration, prompt treatment of episodes of hypercalcemia and infections, and
so on) and chemotherapy (melphalan, cyclophosphamides, chlorambucil, and others), as well as the individualized approach to complications
in each case, has resulted in the prolongation of life in the majority of
patients with MG in general and multiple myeloma in particular. Prior
to the use of alkylating agents, the life expectancy of patients with multiple myeloma was 17 months from the onset of symptoms and 7 months
from the beginning of therapy [285]. In contrast, following the introduction of melphalan (Alkeran) and cyclophosphamide (Cytoxan), a three-
to sevenfold increase in the median survival time has occurred [284].

Currently, melphalan and cyclophosphamide may be considered the
drugs of choice for the treatment of multiple myeloma (including the
IgG, IgA, IgD, and Bence Jones types of myeloma) [278, 281, 283,
284], whereas chlorambucil [193, 282] and cyclophosphamide [279]
appear to be the preferred agents for the treatment of macroglobulinemia.
In many instances, the treatment of patients with symptomatic MG may

Figure 19-37
Effect of long-term melphalan treatment upon serum concentration of IgG(κ) M protein (*top*) in a patient with multiple myeloma. After 3 months of melphalan administration, the M protein disappeared on serum protein electrophoresis (*bottom*) and immunoelectrophoresis. It remained undetectable for the remainder of the observation period (5½ years). The patient's general condition was significantly improved.

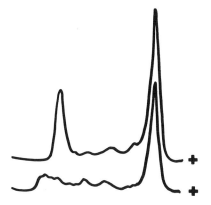

result, over a period of time, in a significant diminution or disappearance of M-protein spikes. Figure 19-37 shows the effect of melphalan therapy in a patient with IgG(κ) myeloma. Symptomatic improvement may become apparent between 2 to 5 days and 2 to 3 weeks after initiating chemotherapy.

Monitoring of the serum M-protein concentrations and urine Bence Jones proteins offers a simple and effective means of objectively assessing the therapeutic response. In view of the more rapid turnover rate of Bence Jones proteins (T½ of about 8 to 12 hours) in comparison to "complete" serum M proteins (e.g., the T½ IgG is about 20 days), a significant decrease in Bence Jones proteinuria after chemotherapy is usually observed sooner than a decrease in the serum M-protein levels. For instance, Bence Jones proteinuria may decrease significantly within one week of chemotherapy, whereas the serum level of IgG M protein may decrease more slowly over a period of several months [284].

Based upon a nine-year experience with intermittent melphalan therapy in 140 patients with multiple myeloma representing various immunochemical categories (IgG, IgA, and κ or λ Bence Jones proteins alone), an objective evaluation was carried out on the patient's response to therapy [278]. A clinical response was registered when the serum myeloma protein level fell by more than 50 percent to less than 4 gm per 100 ml or the daily excretion of Bence Jones proteins fell by more than 90 percent to less than 0.2 gm per 100 ml. Additionally, responders had to satisfy other criteria, such as the maintenance of hematocrit levels above 30 volume percent without transfusions or serum albumin levels above 3.0 gm per 100 ml; the maintenance of serum calcium levels below 12 mg per 100 ml; no progression in the size or number of lytic bone lesions and no decline of any normal immunoglobulin previously in the normal range; the regression of palpable plasmocytomas by more than 50 percent; and, generally, the improvement of bone pain and overall performance. Nonevaluable patients included those who died within four months after treatment or those with inadequate documentation of essential laboratory parameters. These studies demonstrated that (1) 51

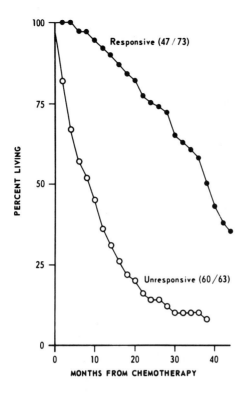

Figure 19-38
Survival of patients responsive to chemotherapy in comparison with unresponsive patients, including those dying early. Figures in parentheses indicate the number dead of the total number of patients. Four patients whose responses were not evaluable because of inadequate data are excluded. (Reproduced by permission. From Alexanian, R. Multiple Myeloma: A Nine-Year Experience with Melphalan Therapy at the M. D. Anderson Hospital. In *Leukemia-Lymphoma.* [A collection of papers presented at the 14th Annual Clinical Conference on Cancer, 1969, at the University of Texas M. D. Anderson Hospital and Tumor Institute, Houston.] Chicago: Year Book, 1970. Pp. 305–316.)

percent of evaluable patients responded to melphalan alone, (2) 75 percent responded to combination chemotherapy with melphalan and prednisone, (3) the survival of responders (median survival of 38 months) was more than two years longer than that of nonresponders (Fig. 19-38), (4) about 20 percent of the responsive patients lived longer than five years, and (5) bone-marrow failure (35 percent) and immunoglobulin failure (32 percent) with severe infections were the most frequent causes of death.

Spontaneous disappearance of M proteins (transient MG). In general, MG proteins do not regress spontaneously. Occasionally, however, M proteins do disappear spontaneously [170, 283, 286–288] coincident

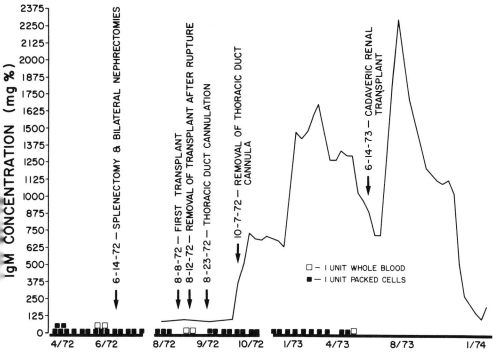

Figure 19-39
Concentrations of IgM during clinical course of transient IgM(κ) monoclonal gammopathy in a 29-year-old male (see Case Report 6).

with the removal of tumors [289, 290], cure of infections [216, 291–294], episodes of hepatitis [182, 188, 295–297], correction of folic acid deficiency [298], cholecystectomy [299], and cessation of blood transfusions [300]. M proteins have also disappeared following prosthetic valve surgery [287] and during the course of primary immune-deficiency disorders [114, 288, 301], as well as under other circumstances.

Case Report 6
A case of transient monoclonal gammopathy [300] is that of a 26-year-old male who developed a transitory IgM(κ) MG shortly after thoracic duct drainage and renal allotransplantation. Three distinct concentration peaks of IgM(κ) (the maximum was 2.3 gm per 100 ml) developed sequentially, which appeared to be related to blood transfusions. After the cessation of transfusions following a second renal allotransplantation 10 months later, the IgM (κ) gradually disappeared within the ensuing 6 months (Fig. 19-39). There were no clinical manifestations of Waldenström's macroglobulinemia, and the patient's clinical condition remained satisfactory. The patient's serum showed a positive test for Wassermann antibodies and several cytotoxic antibodies in low titers, and it inhibited mixed leukocyte culture (MLC) reactions. The purified IgM(κ) was devoid of Wassermann and cytotoxic anti-

Figure 19-40
Age incidence of Waldenström's macroglobulinemia in 46 patients. Cumulative number of cases diagnosed at each decade of life. (Reproduced by permission. From Ritzmann, S. E., Daniels, J. C., and Levin, W. C. Paralymphomatous Disease: The Syndrome of Macroglobulinemia. In *Leukemia-Lymphoma*. [A collection of papers presented at the 14th Annual Clinical Conference on Cancer, 1969, at the University of Texas M. D. Anderson Hospital and Tumor Institute, Houston.] Chicago: Year Book, 1970. Pp. 169–222.)

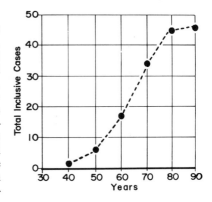

bodies, but it was strongly inhibitory to MLC reactions. These results suggested that the M protein was induced by transfused allogeneic cells and that its antibody activity was directed to MLC-related antigens.

INCIDENCE OF MG

The incidence of MG increases with age; the peak incidence occurs between the seventh and eighth decades of life. The age-related incidence for macroglobulinemia (Fig. 19-40) is similar to that of myeloma. The absolute incidence of MG is difficult to judge. Among 294 Swedish persons over 70 years of age, nine (3 percent) were found to have asymptomatic MG [302]. In screening 6995 serum samples from Swedish residents over 25 years of age (including 3400 males and 3595 females), an overall incidence of MG of 0.9 percent was found (males, 1.1 percent and females, 0.8 percent) [303]. The age prevalence was found to progress from 0.16 percent at 25 to 49 years of age, to 1.61 percent at 50 to 79 years of age, to 9.2 percent at 80 to 89 years of age. The immunochemical variants of M proteins consisted of IgG (61 percent), IgA (27 percent), IgM (8 percent), and biclonal gammopathy (5 percent). Among 446 Czechoslovakian subjects, evidence of MG was obtained in 1.6 percent of 369 individuals age 65 to 79 years, 11.7 percent of 51 octogenarians, and 19 percent of 26 nonagenarians [304]. Fifteen of 500 (about 3 percent) French subjects above the age of 68 exhibited MG [305]. Myeloma was found in two, macroglobulinemia in one, and the remaining persons were asymptomatic.

In a survey [170] of 817 American residents of a hospital for the aged, both SPE and IEP were employed. MG was detected in 3 percent of the 300 males (mean age of 86.2 years) and 1.6 percent of the 517 females (mean age of 86.9 years); the combined incidence was 2.1 percent. Immunochemically, these M proteins were composed of IgG(κ) (5 cases), IgA(κ) (3 cases), IgA(λ) (3 cases), IgM(κ) (1 case), and IgM(λ) (5 cases). It is of interest that only 5 of 17 sera revealed M proteins by electrophoresis, whereas the remainder required IEP for demonstration of M proteins because of their low concentration.

The frequency with which MG occurs has undoubtedly been underestimated in the past. In the 1000 bed hospital facilities of the University of Texas Medical Branch at Galveston, Texas, two to three cases of MG are presently being diagnosed per week (see Chap. 2), which is a frequency exceeding that of chronic lymphocytic leukemia, systemic lupus erythematosus, and Hodgkin's disease combined. *MG is clearly not an uncommon condition.*

The occurrence of MG is infrequent below the age of 30, but recently M proteins have been described even in children and infants, especially those with immune deficiencies [114, 280, 301, 306, 307]. The lowest age groups in which we have encountered MG are as follows: IgG-MG was found in a 2-year-old child with infections, IgA-MG occurred in a 32-year-old patient with myeloma, IgM-MG was observed in a 3-year-old child with congenital rubella syndrome and a 26-year-old renal transplant recipient (see Case Report 6 and Fig. 19-39), and L-chain disease (κ Bence Jones proteins) was present in a 20-year-old patient with nephrotic syndrome secondary to rapidly progressive glomerulonephritis. In children, MG is of the asymptomatic variety, and no convincing cases demonstrating the clinical manifestations of myeloma or macroglobulinemia have been described.

ETIOPATHOGENIC CONSIDERATIONS

The causes and pathogenesis of MG are unknown. Multiple myeloma and macroglobulinemia have been considered to represent autonomous neoplasms of the plasma cells. Increasing circumstantial evidence is being accumulated, however, which suggests that at least some forms of MG may represent reactive and potentially reversible disorders as a result of antigenic stimulation in patients with a conducive genetic background. This etiopathogenetic concept, which was suggested by Waldenström [206] and elaborated by Osserman and co-workers [182, 199], is based upon findings in both animals and humans that encompass a wide variety of factors. Some of these are briefly presented.

MG in animals. MG occurs in animals [152, 241, 308, 309], including the horse, calf, rabbit, dog, cat, hamster, ferret, mouse, parakeet, mink, and others. The demonstration of spontaneously occurring plasma-cell neoplasia, especially in older C_3H strain "breeder" mice [241, 310, 311], provided evidence for the role of genetic factors. The origin of these tumors from the ileocecal region [312] suggested that prolonged and repetitive antigenic stimulation of these tissues may lead eventually to their neoplastic transformation [182] (Fig. 19-41). Subsequently, it was demonstrated that M-protein-secreting plasma-cell tumors could be induced in a high percentage of BALB/c strain mice by the intraperitoneal introduction of a variety of substances, such as plastics, Freund's adjuvants, mineral oil, or branched-chain alkanes [241, 309, 312] (see Fig. 19-41). The common feature of these agents appears to be their ability to act as long-term physical or chemical stimulants to the RES [182]. The initial response to these substances in the peritoneal cavity of BALB/c mice is the occurrence of a diffuse granulomatous peritonitis with the presence of lymphocytes, reticulum cells, and histiocytes. During the ensuing

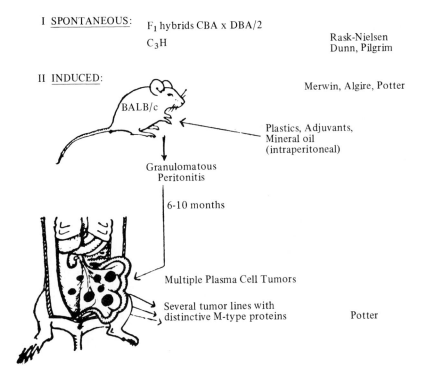

I <u>SPONTANEOUS</u>: F_1 hybrids CBA x DBA/2

C_3H

Rask-Nielsen
Dunn, Pilgrim

II <u>INDUCED</u>:

Merwin, Algire, Potter

BALB/c

Plastics, Adjuvants,
Mineral oil
(intraperitoneal)

Granulomatous
Peritonitis

6-10 months

Multiple Plasma Cell Tumors

Several tumor lines with
distinctive M-type proteins

Potter

Figure 19-41
Principal types of murine plasma-cell tumors. (Reproduced by permission.
From Osserman, E. F., and Takatsuki, K. *Ser. Haematol.* 4:28, 1965.)

weeks, plasma cells emerge in these granulomas, and, after a latent period of several months, multiple plasma-cell tumor nodules develop. Similar plasmocytomas can be induced in NBZ mice [309]. These functionally distinct plasma-cell tumors elaborate their own specific M proteins. Most murine plasmocytomas produce IgA, a fact that may be related to the location of IgA-plasma cells in the lamina propria of the gut and respiratory tracts [309]. There is a reduced incidence of inducible plasmocytomas in germ-free BALB/c mice, which suggests that natural microbial antigens may play a key role in the developmental history of mineral oil-induced plasmocytomas [309].

MG can be induced by immunization in other animal species. For instance, horses hyperimmunized with pneumococcal vaccines [313] and New Zealand rabbits immunized with streptococcal group-specific vaccine [314] elaborate homogeneous immunoglobulins. Aleutian mink disease, which is caused by a known virus [172], is characterized by the early occurrence of polyclonal gammopathy (PG) that progresses in some animals to a MG.

Familial MG. Genetic associations of MG are suggested by its occurrence in relatives of patients with MG. In some families, PG and MG, as well as hypogammaglobulinemia, have been observed [152]. In one family, a female child was found to suffer from systemic lupus erythematosus and her sister from myeloma and reticulum-cell sarcoma [174]. These combinations of immunoglobulin aberrations suggest that they represent different expressions of altered genetic controls of immunoglobulin synthesis [315]. Numerous instances of familial myeloma and macroglobulinemia, as well as familial asymptomatic MG of either the IgG, IgA, or IgM classes, have been reported [152]. Seligmann [316] examined the sera of 216 close relatives of 65 patients with macroglobulinemia. In eight of 216 relatives, an IgM class M protein was identified. Six of these affected individuals were apparently healthy and were more than 50 years old. In a survey of 6995 sera from a normal population, 64 instances of M proteins were found [294, 303]; seven of the persons with M proteins of the IgG, IgA, or IgM class belonged to three families. Williams et al. [317] examined the families of 33 patients with M proteins in comparison with 24 control families. Five of the families of patients with MG had other members with coincidental M proteins; only one family in the control group had a member with MG. Spengler et al. [318] found four families out of 22 with an M-protein propositus to have two members with MG.

These and other reports support the conclusion that familial MG occurs more frequently than expected by chance alone. These findings further suggest the existence of a genetic or environmental predisposition to the development of MG in such families. In an attempt to clarify the possible genetic defects, the M proteins of a mother with multiple myeloma and a son with asymptomatic MG were analyzed [319]. The variable and common regions of the λ light-chain peptides of the two patients were found to be different, which suggested that these polypeptides were encoded by different variable- and common-region structural genes in the plasma-cell clones synthesizing these M proteins. One possible genetic mechanism for the emergence of familial MG may be due to one and the same plasma-cell clone escaping from the control of cell division in relatives, with proliferation of plasma-cell clones accompanied by similar structural genes in such individuals. Such a mode would be expected to yield identical M proteins in the affected relatives. However, in the two patients examined, the M proteins were different, which thus eliminates one possible genetic mechanism for abnormal monoclonal plasma-cell proliferation in familial MG [319]. The occurrence of MG on a familial basis or in spouses [320], however, does not definitively rule out a possible effect of environmental antigens to which the affected family members may have been exposed as a group.

Chromosomal abnormalities. Chromosomal aberrations have been reported in patients with the various forms of MG, including the IgG, IgA, IgM, IgD, and Bence Jones type of MG [193, 219–223, 321, 322]. These consist of large extra chromosomes in the AB size range, as well as additional variable abnormalities that are found in differing percentages of patients with the individual classes of MG (Fig. 19-42). Such abnormal chromosomes do not appear to be pathognomonic of mono-

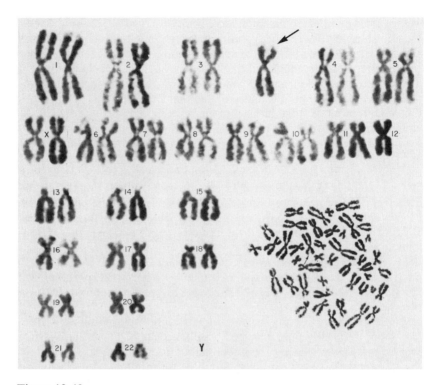

Figure 19-42
Aberrant chromosomal pattern in patient with monoclonal gammopathy, which consists of a supernumerary chromosome in the AB size range and abnormalities in pair 12 chromosomes of group C (e.g., monosomy, trisomy). The morphological appearance of these abnormal chromosomes is similar in patients with IgG, IgA, and IgM monoclonal gammopathies. (Reproduced by permission. From Ritzmann, S. E., Daniels, J. C., Beathard, G. A., and Levin, W. C. *Tex. Med.* 68:91, 1972.)

clonal gammopathies, since indistinguishable chromosomal changes have been observed in patients with acute myeloblastic and acute lymphocytic leukemia [323]. The variety of aberrations in a single patient and the variation in morphological aspects of such aberrant chromosomes from patient to patient are such that a simple causal relationship between any chromosomal abnormality and the etiology of MG appears unlikely. Rather, it has been postulated that some unidentified defect common to all varieties of MG contributes to the formation of MG. Further, these abnormalities may be acquired rather than hereditary in nature, since a patient with macroglobulinemia possessed the described chromosomal abnormalities, whereas his healthy uniovular twin did not [223]. The possibility must also be considered that the abnormal chromosomal patterns may be secondary to the cellular environment, which conceivably could be sufficiently altered by the persistent presence of abnormal immunoglobulins to cause deleterious effects on sensitive chromosomal foci through interference with cellular metabolism [221].

Antibody activity of M proteins. It is presently unknown whether M proteins are abnormal immunoglobulins or simply excessively increased immunoglobulins that are normally present in trace quantities. Increasing circumstantial evidence appears to favor the latter alternative for the majority of M proteins. This is based mainly upon two observations: (1) certain M proteins reflect a monoclonal immune response [324] to certain antigenic stimuli (e.g., infections) and accordingly can recede with the cessation of such stimulation (i.e., transient MG), and (2) M proteins may possess biological (i.e., serological or specific antibody) activity [325].

Harboe [326] has defined criteria for biologically active monoclonal proteins: (1) very high-titered serological activity of serum and a large homogeneous peak on zone electrophoresis, (2) the demonstration of maximal serological activity in the central segments of the peak on preparative electrophoresis, (3) identical electrophoretic mobility of the isolated, serologically active protein and the peak, and (4) the complete disappearance of the peak following immunological absorption. Additional criteria [299] are based on the demonstration of antibody activity residing in the Fab fragment of the immunoglobulin molecule and the lack of activity of the Fc fragment. Human monoclonal immunoglobulins with antibody activity are found in certain patients with either symptomatic or asymptomatic MG [241, 299] (see Case Report 6 and Fig. 19-39).

Human M proteins with antibody activity are directed against a wide spectrum of antigens (Table 19-14). These include erythrocyte antigens, microbial and viral agents, plasma proteins, nitrophenyl ligands, and others. The first M proteins that were shown to possess specific antibody activity were IgM proteins with cold-agglutinin activity to the I, i system from patients with cold-agglutinin disease [327, 328], anti-IgG rheumatoid factor activity [329], and agglutinating activity to aged but not fresh human erythrocytes [330]. Among 47 macroglobulinemic sera, seven instances were found with cold-agglutinin titers ranging from 1:16,000 to 1:2 million, and seven with rheumatoid factor activity having titers varying from 1:5000 to 1:164,000, i.e., a 30 percent incidence [193]. None of the latter patients displayed clinical manifestations of rheumatoid arthritis. It is of interest that 5 of the 7 sera with high rheumatoid factor activity showed positive tests for cryoglobulins, and an additional serum gave a positive test for pyroglobulins. The high incidence of autoantibodies among these patients with IgM-type MG suggests a causal relationship. These "autoantibodies" may be directed against tissue constituents, such as oligosaccharide moieties in blood group substances [331]. Extrinsic stimuli, however, must also be considered as inciting agents, since certain parasites (e.g., ascarides or hydatid-cyst fluid [332]) or microorganisms (e.g., *Mycoplasma pneumoniae* [152, 299]) may evoke anti-I antibodies or rheumatoid factors (e.g., subacute bacterial endocarditis [333]).

In certain murine myeloma proteins, antibody activity against enterobacterial antigens has been demonstrated, and the production of homogeneous antibodies following immunization of rabbits with streptococcal

Table 19-14. Various Antibody Activities Found in Human Monoclonal Immunoglobulins

Antigen	Immuno-globulin Class	Activity in Fab Frag-ment	Quanti-tative Studies
I, i blood group	IgM, IgA		
Sp₁ blood group	IgM		
Aged red blood cells	IgM		
A₁ blood group	IgM		
Streptolysin O	IgG	+	+
Staphylolysin	IgG	+	
Klebsiella	IgM	+	
Brucella	IgG		
Rubella	IgG 1	+	
IgG	IgM, IgG, IgA	+	+
Antigen-antibody complexes	IgM		
Lipoproteins	IgG	+	
Fibrin monomer (?)	IgG	+	
Transferrin	IgG	+	+
Serum albumin	IgM	+	
α_2-macroglobulin	IgG	+	+
DNP	IgM, IgG, IgA	+	+
DNP + aggregated IgG	IgM		
DNP + nucleic acid derivatives	IgG	+	
Cardiolipids	IgM		
Heparin (?)	IgM		
Phosphoryl choline	IgM		

Reproduced by permission from Grune & Stratton. From Seligmann, M., and Brouet, J. C. Antibody activity of human myeloma globulins. *Semin. Hematol.* 10:163–177, 1973.

group-specific vaccines [314] suggests that bacterial antigens elicit certain M proteins in humans. Numerous human IgG M proteins with anti-streptolysin-O (ASO) activity have recently been reported [299, 334]. Other M proteins possess antibody activity against staphylococcal proteins (IgG), *Klebsiella* polysaccharides (IgM), *Brucella* (IgG), *Rubella* (IgG₁[κ]), and others [299]. The antibody activity of M proteins may be directed against human serum proteins such as IgG [299], phospholipids (IgM[κ]) [335], lipoproteins (IgG and IgA), transferrin (IgG₁[κ]), albumin (IgM[κ]), fibrin monomers (IgG and IgA), and α_2-macroglobulin (IgG₁[κ]) [299]. This last myeloma protein was precipitated with horse α_2-M globulin; it was obtained from a patient who had received two injections of horse antitetanus serum 30 years prior to the discovery of the M protein [336]. The most frequently encountered antibody activity is directed against IgG [299]. Most M proteins with such anti-IgG activity are of the IgM class, possess rheumatoid factor activity, and result in mixed cryoglobulins [337] (see Chap.

20), whereas others are of the IgA class (most of which are also cryo-precipitable [299]) or of the IgG class (especially the IgG₃ subclass) which leads frequently to IgG-IgG-cryoglobulins [338].

Murine and human M proteins with antibody activity to nitrophenyl ligands [241, 339, 340] have been demonstrated. They may represent cross-reactions to serum autoantigens, such as nucleic acid components or vitamin K [299]. Other M proteins with antibody activity are directed against cardiolipids (IgM), phosphoryl choline (IgM), and heparin (IgM) [299]. Papular mucinosis (lichen myxedematosus) is frequently associated with M proteins that are extremely basic. For this reason, it has been speculated that such M proteins may be autoantibodies to acidic dermal constituents [341]. The mucopolysaccharides of the dermis are highly acid and consist of repeating polysaccharide units that could elicit homogeneous antibodies.

An increasing number of patients of any age with benign and transient MG are recognized who have either demonstrable or suggestive antibody activity to infectious antigenic stimuli. These include congenital toxoplasmosis [291, 342], malaria [216, 268], congenital syphilis [343], *Pseudomonas* meningitis [344], cytomegalic inclusion disease [345], *Leptospira pomona* [346], subacute sclerosing panencephalitis [347], and possibly the congenital rubella syndrome [306, 348]. The transient nature of some M proteins associated with these infections strongly suggests an essential role of extrinsic antigenic stimulation in the production of these M proteins.

Frequently, M proteins are encountered in primary immunodeficiencies, predominantly in children, which are probably a result of antigenic stimuli, such as infectious agents or incompatible thymic or bone-marrow allografts [114, 347, 349, 350]. Deficiencies associated with M proteins include combined B-T-cell deficiency [315, 351, 352], Aldrich's syndrome [353], hypoglobulinemia [354], ataxia-telangiectasia [301], and others. Two, three, or more separate M proteins may emerge simultaneously in such patients (i.e., biclonal or triclonal gammopathies). To elucidate the mechanisms leading to MG in such immunodeficient subjects, rhesus monkeys were studied after lethal irradiation following bone-marrow transplantation [355]. All irradiated monkeys at first showed a gradual decrease of serum γ-globulins, but in 7 of 18 monkeys, the γ-globulins increased approximately one month after bone-marrow transplantation, reflecting the successful reconstitution of the immune system. In the 6 of 18 monkeys surviving 30 days or longer, one or more serum M proteins emerged (five were IgG; one was IgM), which persisted for several months. In the survivors, the immunoglobulins eventually returned to the normal heterogeneous state. These experimental studies of the causative factors involved in the production of MG should lead to a better understanding of the clinical implications of the disease and, eventually, to the application of this knowledge in humans.

Monoclonal immune response. As previously suggested by Osserman and Takatsuki [182], it is likely that the experimental induction of plasma-cell neoplasia by the introduction of intraperitoneal adjuvants or mineral oil into BALB/c mice and the development of M proteins in rabbits after prolonged immunization with streptococcal C-polysaccharides may be functionally comparable to the pathological processes in humans leading to MG after prolonged antigenic stimulation or adjuvant effects, or both.

At least two general pathogenic mechanisms [332] are recognized, in addition to the possible primary malignant nature of MG. First, repeated antigenic stimulation of specific B-cell clones could lead to monoclonal expansion over a period of years. For instance, repeated infections with streptococci could account for the monoclonal progression of antistreptolysin-O clones: A patient who had suffered three recurrent attacks of rheumatic fever in childhood [356] subsequently developed an IgG M protein that exhibited high antistreptolysin activity. Furthermore, repeated stimulation by a variety of antigens may result in rheumatoid factor activity and immune-complex formation with the host's IgG [356]. In two patients with subacute bacterial endocarditis, a transient excessive increase of rheumatoid factor activity and cryoglobulinemia developed, which receded after successful treatment of the infection [357]. It is conceivable that repeated or prolonged antigenic stimulation may lead to excessive monoclonal stimulation of the rheumatoid factor-producing cell clones.

Second, anomalous adjuvant effects by agents that nonspecifically stimulate the B-cell system may lead to uninhibited monoclonal growth due to the overall across-the-board stimulation of B-cell clones. This mechanism may be exemplified by the plastic and lipid agents that initially produce polyclonal gammopathy and, subsequently, multiple plasma cell tumors and MG in mice [332]. The human analog may be the formation of M proteins that is encountered in a high percentage of patients with various lipid disorders [242–246]. For example, patients with Gaucher's disease [326] initially may show polyclonal gammopathy and later monoclonal gammopathy. Structural lipids may play a major role as possible autoantigens. Similar transitions from polyclonal to monoclonal gammopathies have been observed in nonlipid disorders [152, 170].

Any hypothesis attempting to explain the etiopathogenesis of monoclonal immune responses must account for the various special capabilities of the immune system, including its memory functions, feedback controls, pluripotentiality, and the general aspects of Monod's *"le hasard et la nécessité"* [358].

Heremans [359] has proposed a model for the pathogenesis of MG that is based upon the Darwinian "survival of the fittest" B-cell clone. This model presupposes several assumptions and states that the initial antibody response to an antigen is polyclonal and involves mainly B cells that produce antibodies of moderate affinity. Low affinity cells are not stimulated sufficiently, and there are too few high affinity cells to contribute appreciably to the total amount of antibody. If antigenic stimulation continues, selection occurs in favor of cells that produce high affinity immunoglobulins, presumably because these are more readily stimulated to proliferate and also because high-affinity antibody in the circulation competes with the low-affinity receptors of the cells producing weak antibodies so that these cells are no longer adequately stimulated. Therefore, given sufficient time, a single clone of B cells, the one producing the "fittest" antibody, overcomes its competitors and becomes the sole producer of what is now a monoclonal antibody. In the event of more than one antigenic determinant on the same antigen, the result may be an antibody pattern of restricted heterogeneity rather than a single M protein. The time required to reach this monoclonal limit is shortened if the competition is restricted to a few available B-cell clones. This situation may apply to the restricted heterogeneity patterns (analogous to those of oligoclonal gammopathies) that emerge in patients with immunological deficiency, in immunologically incompetent patients treated with limited numbers of foreign lymphoid cells (e.g., blood transfusions), and in the cerebrospinal fluid of patients with certain infections or autoimmune disorders of the central nervous system (CNS), since the CNS harbors few lymphocytes.

Heremans [359] assumes (1) oncogenesis represents a loss of control mechanisms that govern cell division, (2) the risk of oncogenesis is related to the proliferation activity of the type of cells involved, and (3) the antigen has an affinity for B cells that produce immunoglobulins with potential antibody affinity. He concludes that these factors provide a simple explanation for the observed high incidence of M proteins with antibody affinity to exogenous and endogenous antigens, as well as for the frequent occurrence of lymphomas in immunological deficiency states. This concept may also apply to the case of aged persons and animals [171], who develop senescence of immunity with the implied restriction of antigen-responsive cell clones, thus explaining the increased frequency of MG in the aged.

Rádl et al. [355] attribute the origin of transient M proteins to an unequal development and imbalance of the available B-cell clones. In the normal, immunologically mature subject, the antibody response to most antigens is heterogeneous, and a large number of B-cell clones predictably produce antibodies of different classes, subclasses, types, groups, avidity, and affinity. During the early stages of the maturation process of the immune system, however, only a restricted number of antigen-responsive B cells are available. Such a situation, which may lead to an antibody response with oligoclonal, restricted, or monoclonal immunoglobulins, occurs in several experimental and clinical situations [355]. For example, there is a step-wise establishment of immunological competence toward various antigens during intrauterine maturation in animals; immunization of immunodeficient children who have been reconstituted by thymus or bone-marrow allotransplantation results in a repetition of the normal ontogenesis with the sequential appearance of the various immunoglobulin classes, and it leads to the production of antibodies to some antigens but not to others; and, finally, the M proteins ordinarily regress after the maturation of the immune capability and normalization of the immunoglobulin spectrum.

Thus, the development of polyclonal, oligoclonal, and monoclonal gammopathies must be considered in the context of the various factors governing the host responses and antigenic stimulation that eventually determine the antibody-response pattern in a given patient. This spectrum of antibody responses includes:

1. The normal and usually short-term antigenic stimulation (e.g., acute infections) resulting in heterogeneous antibody response, which is generally not detectable by electrophoretic changes (i.e., "micropolyclonal" gammopathy). This response pattern is by far the most prevalent result of the ordinary antigenic stimulation event.
2. Massive or prolonged antigenic stimulation (e.g., subacute or chronic infections, chronic liver diseases, and so on) leads to antibodies with high affinity and avidity and results in polyclonal gammopathy on electrophoresis.
3. Under specific circumstances of chronic stimulation (e.g., chronic active hepatitis), a restricted immunoglobulin pattern may emerge (i.e., oligoclonal gammopathy), and in others, a transition from polyclonal to monoclonal gammopathy may occur (e.g., in certain autoimmune disorders).
4. Prolonged or repeated stimulation in normal subjects or shorter periods of antigenic stimulation in immunodeficient patients may lead to monoclonal immunoglobulins; these may result either in low M protein levels, i.e., asymptomatic MG, or in high M-protein levels, i.e., symptomatic MG.

The segregation of these two forms of MG is reminiscent of the immunological "nonresponders" and "responders" in the case of some Rh-negative subjects [360] and the HL-A incompatible, polytransfused patients [361] who fail to form anti-Rh or anticytotoxic antibodies to HL-A antigens, respectively, in spite of long, continuous stimulation. Patients with the asymptomatic, benign form of MG probably constitute "partial monoclonal immune responders," whereas those with the symptomatic, malignant form of MG may represent "complete monoclonal immune responders." Thus, two control levels of B-cell proliferation are suggested that are possibly governed by different degrees of expression of the immune-response (Ir) genes due to partial or complete derepression of the latent Ir-gene functions [203]. Recent evidence from studies of experimental animals [324] also emphasizes the importance of genetic factors and the existence of separable categories of low and high, as well as polyclonal and monoclonal, immune responders.

References

1. Good, R. A., and Finstad, J. Adaptive Immunity. In E. D. Frohlich (Ed.), *Pathophysiology—Altered Regulatory Mechanisms in Disease.* Philadelphia: Lippincott, 1972. Pp. 683–710.
2. Pollara, B., Finstad, J., and Good, R. A. The Phylogenetic Development of Immunoglobulins. In R. T. Smith, P. A. Miescher, and R. A.

Good (Eds.), *Phylogeny of Immunity.* Gainesville: University of Florida Press, 1966. Pp. 88–98.

3. Cunningham, B. A., Gottlieb, P. D., Pelumm, M. N., and Edelman, G. M. Immunoglobulin Structure: Diversity, Gene Duplication and Domains. In B. Amos (Ed.), *Progress in Immunology.* New York: Academic, 1971. Pp. 3–24.

4. Cooper, M. D., Kincade, P. W., and Lawton, A. R. Thymus and Bursal Function in Immunologic Development. A New Theoretical Model of Plasma Cell Differentiation. In B. M. Kagan and E. R. Stiehm (Eds.), *Immunologic Incompetence.* Chicago: Year Book, 1971. Pp. 81–104.

5. Fudenberg, H. H., Pink, J. R. L., Stites, D. P., and Wang, A. C. *Basic Immunogenetics.* New York: Oxford University Press, 1972. P. 214.

6. Cohen, S., and Milstein, C. Structure and biological properties of immunoglobulins. *Adv. Immunol.* 7:1, 1967.

7. Mannick, M., and Kunkel, H. G. Two major types of normal 7S γ-globulins. *J. Exp. Med.* 117:213, 1963.

8. Van Loghem, E. Formal genetics of the immunoglobulin system. *Ann. N.Y. Acad. Sci.* 190:136, 1971.

9. Ritzmann, S. E., and Daniels, J. C. Immunology—Summation. In G. J. Race (Ed.), *Laboratory Medicine.* New York: Harper & Row, 1975.

10. Ritzmann, S. E., Daniels, J. C., Sakai, H., and Beathard, G. A. The lymphocyte in immunobiology. *Ann. Allergy* 31:109, 1973.

11. Abdou, N. I., and Abdou, N. L. Bone marrow: The bursa equivalent in man? *Science* 175:446, 1972.

12. Lawton, A. R., Self, K. S., Royal, S. A., and Cooper, M. D. Ontogeny of B-lymphocytes in the human fetus. *Clin. Immunol. Immunopathol.* 1:84, 1972.

13. Somers, H., and Kuhns, W. J. Blood group antibodies in old age. *Proc. Soc. Exp. Biol. Med.* 141:1104, 1972.

14. Grey, H. M., Rabellino, E., and Pirofsky, B. Immunoglobulins on the surface of lymphocytes. IV. Distribution in hypogammaglobulinemia, cellular immune deficiency, and chronic lymphatic leukemia. *J. Clin. Invest.* 50:2368, 1971.

15. Preud'Homme, J. L., Griscelli, C., and Seligmann, M. Immunoglobulins on the surface of lymphocytes in fifty patients with primary immunodeficiency diseases. *Clin. Immunol. Immunopathol.* 1:241, 1973.

16. Unanue, E. R., Grey, H. M., Rabellino, E., Campbell, P., and Schmidt, I. Immunoglobulins on the surface of lymphocytes. II. The bone marrow as the main source of lymphocytes with surface-bound immunoglobulin. *J. Exp. Med.* 133:1188, 1971.

17. Belohradsky, B. H., Finstad, J., Fudenberg, H. H., Good, R. A., Kunkel, H. G., and Rosen, F. Meeting report of the second international workshop on primary immunodeficiency diseases in man. *Clin. Immunol. Immunopathol.* 2:281, 1974.

18. Fudenberg, H. H., and Wybran, J. How clinically useful is T & B cell quantitation? *Ann. Intern. Med.* 80:765, 1974.

19. Good, R. A., Bigger, W. D., and Park, B. H. Immunodeficiency Diseases of Man. In B. Amos (Ed.), *Progress in Immunology.* New York: Academic, 1971. Pp. 699–722.

20. Van Furth, R., Schnit, H. R. E., and Hijmans, W. The immunological development of the human fetus. *J. Exp. Med.* 122:1173, 1965.

21. Mollison, P. *Blood Transfusion in Clinical Medicine* (4th ed.). Philadelphia: Davis, 1968.
22. Tiselius, A. A new apparatus for electrophoresis. Analysis of colloidal mixtures. *Trans. Faraday Soc.* 33:524, 1937.
23. Grabar, P., and Williams, C. A. Méthode immuno-electrophoretique d'analyse de melánges de substances antigéniques. *Biochim. Biophys. Acta* 17:67, 1955.
24. Hitzig, W. H. Die Physiologische Entwicklung der "Immunoglobuline" (Gamma und Beta₂-Globuline). *Helv. Paediatr. Acta* 12:596, 1957.
25. Heremans, J. F. Immunochemical studies on protein pathology. The immunoglobulin concept. *Clin. Chim. Acta* 4:639, 1959.
26. Smith, R. T. Human immunoglobulins. A guide to nomenclature and clinical application. *Pediatrics* 37:822, 1966.
27. World Health Organization. Recommendations for the nomenclature of human immunoglobulins. *J. Immunol.* 108:1733, 1972.
28. Cajal, R. *Mannal de Anatomia Pathologica General.* Barcelona, 1894.
29. Wright, J. H. A case of multiple myeloma. *Trans. Assoc. Am. Physicians* 15:137, 1900.
30. Bing, J., and Plum, P. Serum proteins in leukopenia, contribution on the question about the place of formation of the serum proteins. *Acta Med. Scand.* 92:415, 1937.
31. Kolouch, F. Origin of bone marrow plasma cells associated with allergic and immune states in the rabbit. *Proc. Soc. Exp. Biol. Med.* 34:147, 1939.
32. Bjoerneboe, M., and Gormsen, H. Experimental studies of the role of plasma cells as antibody procedures. *Acta Pathol. Microbiol. Scand.* 20:649, 1943.
33. Fagraeus, A. Antibody production in relation to the development of plasma cells. *Acta Med. Scand.* 130 [Suppl. 204]:1, 1948.
34. Coons, A. H., Leduc, E. H., and Connolly, J. M. Studies on antibody production. I. A method for the histochemical demonstration of specific antibody and its application to a study of the hyperimmune rabbit. *J. Exp. Med.* 102:49, 1955.
35. Good, R. A. Studies on agammaglobulinemia. II. Failure of plasma cell formation in the bone marrow and lymph nodes of patients with agammaglobulinemia. *J. Lab. Clin. Med.* 46:167, 1955.
36. Sherr, C. J., Schenkein, I., and Uhr, J. W. Synthesis and intracellular transport of immunoglobulin in secretory and nonsecretory cells. *Ann. N.Y. Acad. Sci.* 190:250, 1971.
37. McMillan, R., Longmire, R. L., Yelenosky, R., Lang, J. E., Heeth, V., and Craddock, C. G. Immunoglobulin synthesis by human lymphoid tissues: Normal bone marrow as a major site of IgG production. *J. Immunol.* 109:1386, 1972.
38. Waldenström, J. Incipient myelomatosis or "essential" hyperglobulinaemia with fibrinogenopenia—new syndrome? *Acta Med. Scand.* 117:261, 1944.
39. Burtin, P., Hartmann, L., Heremans, J., Scheidegger, J. J., Westendorp-Boerma, F., Wieme, R., Wunderly, C. H., Fauvert, R., and Grabar, P. Études immunochimiques et immuno-électrophoretiques des macroglobulinémies. *Rev. Fr. Étud. Clin. Biol.* 2:161, 1957.
40. Heremans, J. F., Heremans, M. T., and Schultze, H. E. Isolation and description of a few properties of the β₂A-globulin of human serum. *Clin. Chim. Acta* 4:96, 1959.

41. Rowe, D. S., and Fahey, J. L. A new class of human immunoglobulins. I. A unique myeloma protein. *J. Exp. Med.* 121:171, 1965.
42. Rowe, D. S., and Fahey, J. L. A new class of human immunoglobulins. II. Normal serum IgD. *J. Exp. Med.* 121:185, 1965.
43. Ishizaka, K., Ishizaka, T., and Hornbrook, M. M. Physico-chemical properties of human reaginic antibody. IV. Presence of a unique immunoglobulin as a carrier of reaginic activity. *J. Immunol.* 97:75, 1966.
44. Immunoglobulin E. A new class of human immunoglobulin. *Bull. W.H.O.* 38:151, 1968.
45. Johansson, S. G. O., and Bennich, H. Immunological studies of an atypical (myeloma) immunoglobulin. *Immunology* 13:381, 1967.
46. Bence Jones, H. Papers on chemical pathology. *Lancet* 2:88, 1847.
47. Clamp, J. R. Some aspects of the first recorded case of multiple myeloma. *Lancet* 2:1354, 1967.
48. Franklin, E. C., Lowenstein, J., Bigelow, B., and Meltzer, M. Heavy chain disease: A new disorder of serum γ-globulins. Report of a first case. *Am. J. Med.* 37:332, 1964.
49. Osserman, E. F., and Takatsuki, K. Clinical and immunochemical studies of four cases of heavy (Hγ^2) chain disease. *Am. J. Med.* 37: 351, 1964.
50. Seligmann, M., Danon, F., Hurez, D., Mihaesco, F., and Preud'Homme, J. L. Alpha chain disease: A new immunoglobulin abnormality. *Science* 162:1396, 1968.
51. Forte, F. A., Prelli, F., Yount, W. J., Jerry, L. M., Kochwa, S., Franklin, E. C., and Kunkel, H. G. Heavy chain disease of the μ (γM) type: Report of the first case. *Blood* 36:437, 1970.
52. Solomon, A., and Kunkel, H. G. A "monoclonal" type, low molecular weight protein related to γM-macroglobulins. *Am. J. Med.* 42:958, 1967.
53. Hobbs, J. R., and Jacobs, A. A half-molecule GK plasmocytoma. *Clin. Exp. Immunol.* 5:199, 1969.
54. Isobe, T., and Osserman, E. F. Plasma cell dyscrasia associated with the production of incomplete (? deleted) IgGλ molecules, γ-heavy chains and free λ-chains containing carbohydrate: Description of the first case. *Blood* 43:505, 1974.
55. Eisen, H. N. *Immunology: An Introduction to Molecular and Cellular Principles of the Immune Response.* New York: Harper & Row, 1974.
56. Parkhouse, R. M. E., Askonas, B. A., and Dourmashkin, R. R. Electron microscopic studies of mouse immunoglobulin M; Structure and reconstitution following reduction. *Immunology* 18:575, 1970.
57. Edelman, G. M., Cunningham, B. A., Gall, W. E., Gottlieb, P. D., Rutishauser, U., and Waxdal, M. J. The covalent structure of an entire gamma G immunoglobulin molecule. *Proc. Natl. Acad. Sci. U.S.A.* 63:78, 1969.
58. McKelvey, E. M., and Fahey, J. L. Immunoglobulin changes in disease: Quantitation on the basis of heavy polypeptide chains, IgG (γG), IgA (γA) and IgM (γM) and of light polypeptide chains, type K(I) and type L(II). *J. Clin. Invest.* 44:1778, 1965.
59. Putnam, F. W., and Easley, L. Structural studies of the immunoglobulins. I. The tryptic peptides of Bence Jones proteins. *J. Biol. Chem.* 240:1626, 1965.
60. Solomon, A., and McLaughlin, C. L. Immunoglobulin structure de-

termined from products of plasma cell neoplasms. *Semin. Hematol.* 10:3, 1973.

61. Terry, W. D., Tischendorf, F. W., and Osserman, E. F. Subgroup-specific antigenic marker on immunoglobulin λ-chains: Identification of three subtypes of the variable region. *J. Immunol.* 105:1033, 1970.

62. Putnam, F. W., Shimizu, A., Paul, C., and Shinoda, T. Tentative Structure of Human IgM Immunoglobulin. In B. Amos (Ed.), *Progress in Immunology*. New York: Academic, 1971. P. 291.

63. Binghi, R. A. Biological Activities of IgG in Mammals. In B. Amos (Ed.), *Progress in Immunology*. New York: Academic, 1971. Pp. 849–858.

64. Grey, H. M., and Kunkel, H. G. H-chain subgroups of myeloma proteins and normal 7S γ-globulin. *J. Exp. Med.* 120:253, 1964.

65. Terry, W. D., and Fahey, J. L. Subclasses of human γ$_2$-globulin based on differences in heavy polypeptide chains. *Science* 146:400, 1964.

66. Heremans, J. F. Biochemical Features and Biologic Significance of Immunoglobulin A. In E. Merler (Ed.), *Immunoglobulins, Biologic Aspects and Clinical Uses*. Washington, D.C.: National Academy of Sciences, 1970. Pp. 52–73.

67. Tomasi, T. B., Jr. The Gamma A Globulins: First Line of Defense. In R. A. Good and D. W. Fischer (Eds.), *Immunobiology, Current Knowledge of Basic Concepts in Immunology and their Clinical Applications*. Stamford, Conn.: Sinauer Assoc., 1971. Pp. 76–83.

68. Heremans, J. F., and Vaerman, J. P. Biological Significance of IgA Antibodies in Serum and Secretions. In B. Amos (Ed.), *Progress in Immunology*. New York: Academic, 1971. Pp. 875–890.

69. Tomasi, T. B. Secretory immunoglobulins. *N. Engl. J. Med.* 287:500, 1972.

70. Comoglio, P. M., and Guglielmone, R. Immunohistochemical study of IgA transepithelial transfer into digestive tract secretions in the mouse. *Immunology* 25:71, 1973.

71. Franklin, E. C., and Frangione, B. Two serologically distinguishable subclasses of μ-chains of human macroglobulins. *J. Immunol.* 99:810, 1967.

72. Deutsch, H. F., and Morton, J. I. Human serum macroglobulins and dissociation units. I. Physicochemical properties. *J. Biol. Chem.* 231: 1107, 1958.

73. Glenchur, H., Zinneman, H. H., and Briggs, D. R. Macroglobulinemia; Report of two cases. *Ann. Intern. Med.* 48:1055, 1958.

74. Ritzmann, S. E., Coleman, S. L., and Levin, W. C. Effect of some mercaptanes upon a macrocryogelglobulin; Modifications caused by cysteamine, penicillamine and penicillin. *J. Clin. Invest.* 39:1320, 1960.

75. Ishizaka, K. Immunoglobulin E. In E. Merler (Ed.), *Immunoglobulins, Biologic Aspects and Clinical Uses*. Washington, D.C.: National Academy of Sciences, 1970. Pp. 122–136.

76. Ishizaka, K., and Ishizaka, T. Immunoglobulin E and Homocytotropic Properties. In B. Amos (Ed.), *Progress in Immunology*. New York: Academic, 1971. Pp. 859–874.

77. Nisonoff, A. Molecules of Immunity. In R. A. Good and D. W. Fischer (Eds.), *Immunobiology, Current Knowledge of Basic Concepts in Immunology and their Clinical Applications*. Stamford, Conn.: Sinauer Assoc., 1971. Pp. 65–74.

78. Porter, R. R. The hydrolysis of rabbit γ-globulin and antibodies with crystalline papain. *Biochem. J.* 73:119, 1959.

79. Fahey, J. L. Developments in Fundamental Research Related to Clinical Uses of Immunoglobulins. In E. Merler (Ed.), *Immunoglobulins, Biologic Aspects and Clinical Uses.* Washington, D.C.: National Academy of Sciences, 1970. Pp. 15–30.

80. Alford, C. A., Jr. Immunoglobulin determinations in the diagnosis of fetal infection. *Pediatr. Clin. North Am.* 18:99, 1971.

81. Gitlin, D., and Biasucci, A. Development of γG, γA, γM, β_1C/β_1A, C1-esterase inhibitor, ceruloplasmin, transferrin, hemopexin, haptoglobin, fibrinogen, plasminogen, α_1-antitrypsin, orosomucoid, β-lipoprotein, α_2-macroglobulin and prealbumin in the human conceptus. *J. Clin. Invest.* 48:1433, 1969.

82. Hay, F. C., Hull, M. G. R., and Torrigiani, G. The transfer of human IgG subclasses from mother to foetus. *Clin. Exp. Immunol.* 9:355, 1971.

83. Morell, A., Skvaril, F., Steinberg, A. G., Von Loghem, E., and Terry, W. D. Correlations between the concentrations of the four subclasses of IgG and Gm allotypes in normal human sera. *J. Immunol.* 108:195, 1972.

84. Yeager, A. S. Variation of cord IgM level with birth weight. *Pediatrics* 51:616, 1973.

85. Bazaral, M., Orgel, H. A., and Hamburger, R. N. IgE levels in normal infants and mothers and an inheritance hypothesis. *J. Immunol.* 107: 794, 1971.

86. Johansson, S. G. O., Bennich, H. H., and Berg, T. The Clinical Significance of IgE. In R. S. Schwartz (Ed.), *Progress in Clinical Immunology,* Vol. 1. New York: Grune & Stratton, 1972. Pp. 157–181.

87. Waldmann, T. A., Strober, W., and Blaese, R. M. Metabolism of Immunoglobulins. In B. Amos (Ed.), *Progress in Immunology.* New York: Academic, 1971. Pp. 891–903.

88. Waldmann, T. A., Blaese, R. M., and Strober, W. Physiologic Factors Controlling Immunoglobulin Metabolism. In M. A. Rothschild and T. A. Waldmann (Eds.), *Plasma Protein Metabolism. Regulation of Synthesis, Distribution and Degradation.* New York: Academic, 1970. Pp. 269–286.

89. Franklin, E. C. Genetic Regulation of Immunoglobulin Levels in Man. In M. A. Rothschild and T. A. Waldmann (Eds.), *Plasma Protein Metabolism. Regulation of Synthesis, Distribution and Degradation.* New York: Academic, 1970. Pp. 259–268.

90. Waldmann, T. A., Strober, W., and Blaese, R. M. Variations in the Metabolism of Immunoglobulins Measured by Turnover Rates. In E. Merler (Ed.), *Immunoglobulins, Biologic Aspects and Clinical Uses.* Washington, D.C.: National Academy of Sciences, 1970. Pp. 33–51.

91. Fudenberg, H. H. The Immune Globulins. In C. E. Clifton, S. Raffel, and M. P. Starr (Eds.), *Annual Review of Microbiology,* Vol. 19. Palo Alto, Calif.: Annual Reviews, 1965. Pp. 301–338.

92. Solomon, A., Waldmann, T. A., and Fahey, J. L. Metabolism of normal 6.6S γ-globulin in normal subjects and in patients with macroglobulinemia and multiple myeloma. *J. Lab. Clin. Med.* 62:1, 1963.

93. Spiegelberg, H. L. The Submolecular Site Related to the Rate of Catabolism of IgG Immunoglobulins. In M. A. Rothschild and T. A. Waldmann (Eds.), *Plasma Protein Metabolism. Regulation of Synthesis, Distribution and Degradation.* New York: Academic, 1970. Pp. 307–319.

94. Brambell, F. W., Hemmings, W. A., and Morris, I. G. A theoretical model of γ-globulin catabolism. *Nature* 203:1352, 1964.

95. Gitlin, D.   Current Aspects of the Structure, Function and Genetics of the Immunoglobulins. In A. C. deGraff and W. P. Creger (Eds.), *Annual Review of Medicine,* Vol. 17. Palo Alto, Calif.: Annual Reviews, 1966. Pp. 1–22.

96. Barth, W. F., Wochner, R. D., Waldmann, T. A., and Fahey, J. L. Metabolism of human gamma macroglobulins. *J. Clin. Invest.* 42:1036, 1964.

97. Rogentine, G. N., Jr., Rowe, D. S., Bradley, J., Waldmann, T. A., and Fahey, J. L.   Metabolism of human immunoglobulin D (IgD). *J. Clin. Invest.* 45:1467, 1966.

98. Ishizaka, K., and Ishizaka, T.   IgE and reaginic hypersensitivity. *Ann. N.Y. Acad. Sci.* 190:443, 1971.

99. Kunkel, H. G., and Yount, W. J.   Heavy-Chain Subgroups of γG and γA Globulins. In E. Merler (Ed.), *Immunoglobulins, Biologic Aspects and Clinical Uses.* Washington, D.C.: National Academy of Sciences, 1970. Pp. 137–145.

100. Burnet, F. M.   *The Clonal Selection Theory of Acquired Immunity.* Nashville, Tenn.: Vanderbilt University Press, 1959. Pp. 83–86.

101. Kantor, G. L., Van Herle, A. J., and Barnett, E. V.   Auto-antibodies of the IgD class. *Clin. Exp. Immunol.* 6:951, 1970.

102. Rowe, D. S., Hug, K., Forni, L., and Pernis, B.   Immunoglobulin D as a lymphocyte receptor. *J. Exp. Med.* 138:965, 1973.

103. Knapp, W., Bolhuis, R. L. H., Rádl, J., and Hijmans, W.   Independent movement of IgD and IgM molecules on the surface of individual lymphocytes. *J. Immunol.* 111:1295, 1973.

104. Fudenberg, H. H., Good, R. A., Goodman, H. C., Hitzig, W., Kunkel, H. G., Roitt, I. M., Rosen, F. S., Rowe, D. S., Seligmann, M., and Soothill, J. R.   Primary immunodeficiencies; Report of the W.H.O. Committee. *Pediatrics* 47:927, 1971.

105. Daniels, J. C., Larson, D. L., Abston, S., and Ritzmann, S. E.   Serum protein profiles in thermal burns.   I. Serum electrophoretic patterns, immunoglobulins and transport proteins. *J. Trauma* 14:137, 1974.

106. Schubothe, H.   The cold hemagglutinin disease. *Semin. Hematol.* 3:27, 1966.

107. Löffler, H.   Skoda im Wendepunkt der Medizin. *Wien. Med. Wochenschr.* 63:771, 1951.

108. Bruton, O. C.   Agammaglobulinemia. *Pediatrics* 9:722, 1952.

109. Bruton, O. C.   The Discovery of Agammaglobulinemia. In D. Bergsma and R. A. Good (Eds.), *Immunologic Deficiency Disease in Man,* Vol. 4. (Birth Defects Original Article Series.) New York: National Foundation for Birth Defects, 1968. Pp. 2–6.

110. Good, R. A.   Historical Aspects of Immunologic Deficiency Diseases. In B. M. Kagan and E. R. Smith (Eds.), *Immunologic Incompetence.* Chicago: Year Book, 1971. Pp. 149–174.

111. Fudenberg, H. H., Good, R. A., Goodman, H. C., Hitzig, W., Kunkel, H. G., Roitt, I. M., Rosen, F. S., Rowe, D. S., Seligmann, M., and Soothill, J. R.   Primary immunodeficiencies. *Bull. W.H.O.* 45:125, 1971.

112. Rodey, G. E., and Good, R. A.   Immunologic Deficiency Syndromes. In H. A. Azar and M. Potter (Eds.), *Multiple Myeloma and Related Disorders,* Vol. 1. New York: Harper & Row, 1973. Pp. 287–327.

113. Biggers, H. D., Park, B. H., and Good, R. A.   Immunologic reconstitutions. *Annu. Rev. Med.* 24:135, 1973.

114. Rádl, J., and Van den Berg, P. Transitory Appearance of Homogeneous Immunoglobulins—"Paraproteins"—in Children with Severe Combined Immunodeficiency before and after Transplantation Treatment. In H. Peeters (Ed.), *Proteins and Related Subjects. Protides of the Biological Fluids,* Vol. 20. Amsterdam: Elsevier, 1972. Pp. 263–266.

115. Harboe, M., Panda, H., Brandzaeg, P., Tveter, K. T., and Hjort, R. F. Synthesis of donor type γG-globulin following thymus transplantation in hypo-γ-globulinemia with severe lymphocytopenia. *Scand. J. Haematol.* 3:351, 1966.

116. Rosen, F. S. Immunological Deficiency Disease. In F. H. Bach and R. A. Good (Eds.), *Clinical Immunobiology,* Vol. 1. New York: Academic, 1972. Pp. 271–289.

117. Cooper, M. D., Lawton, A. R., and Bockman, D. E. Agammaglobulinaemia with B-lymphocytes. Specific defects of plasma cell differentiation. *Lancet* 2:791, 1971.

118. Management of hypogammaglobulinaemia (Notes and News section). *Lancet* 2:619, 1970.

119. Strober, W., Blaese, R. M., and Waldmann, T. A. Abnormalities of Immunoglobulin Metabolism. In M. A. Rothschild and T. A. Waldmann (Eds.), *Plasma Protein Metabolism. Regulation of Synthesis, Distribution and Degradation.* New York: Academic, 1970. Pp. 287–309.

120. Bachmann, R. Studies on serum γA-globulin level. III. Frequency of a-γA-globulinemia. *Scand. J. Clin. Lab. Invest.* 17:316, 1965.

121. Vyas, G. N., Perkins, H. A., and Fudenberg, H. H. Anaphylactoid transfusion reactions associated with anti-IgA. *Lancet* 2:312, 1968.

122. Ammann, A. J., and Hong, R. Selective IgA deficiency in autoimmunity. *Clin. Exp. Immunol.* 7:833, 1970.

123. Hobbs, J. R., Milner, R. D., and Watt, P. J. Gamma M deficiency predisposing to meningococcal septicaemia. *Br. Med. J.* 4:583, 1967.

124. Schur, P. H., Borel, H., Gelfand, E. W., Alper, C. A., and Rosen, F. S. Selective gamma-G globulin deficiencies in patients with recurrent pyogenic infections. *N. Engl. J. Med.* 283:631, 1970.

125. Bernier, G. M., Gunderman, J. R., and Ruymann, F. B. Kappa-chain deficiency. *Blood* 40:795, 1972.

126. Gajl-Peczalska, K. J., Ballow, M., Hansen, J. A., and Good, R. A. IgE-bearing lymphocytes and atopy in a patient with X-linked infantile agammaglobulinaemia. *Lancet* 1:1254, 1973.

127. Miller, D. G. Immunological Disturbances in Lymphoma and Leukemia. In M. Samter (Ed.), *Immunological Diseases* (2nd ed.). Boston: Little, Brown, 1971. Pp. 548–570.

128. Vaughan, J. H., Blomgren, S. E., and Edgington, T. S. Treatment for rheumatoid arthritis. *Mod. Med.* 5:32, 1973.

129. Alper, C. A. B-lymphocyte malignancy. *N. Engl. J. Med.* 289:154, 1973.

130. Huber, H., Michlmeyr, G., Asamer, H., Huber, C. H., and Braunsteiner, H. Die Differenzierung menschlicher Lymphozyten mit immunologischen und autoradiographischen Methoden. I. Ergebnisse bei Normalpersonen und bei Patienten mit chronischer Lymphadenose. *Klin. Wochenschr.* 51:504, 1972.

131. Hurez, D., Flandrin, G., Preud'Homme, J. L., and Seligmann, M. Unreleased intracellular monoclonal macroglobulin in chronic lymphocytic leukaemia. *Clin. Exp. Immunol.* 10:223, 1972.

132. Knapp, W., Schnit, H. R. E., Bolhuis, R. L. H., and Hijmans, W. Surface immunoglobulins in chronic lymphatic leukaemia, macroglobulinaemia and myelomatosis. *Clin. Exp. Immunol.* 16:541, 1974.
133. Cooper, A. G., Brown, M. C., Derby, H. A., and Wortis, H. H. Quantitation of surface-membrane and intracellular gamma, mu, and kappa chains of normal and neoplastic human lymphocytes. *Clin. Exp. Immunol.* 13:487, 1973.
134. Klein, E., Klein, G., Nadkerni, J. S., Nadkerni, J. J., Wigzell, H., and Clifford, P. Surface IgM-kappa specificity on a Burkitt lymphoma cell in vivo and in derived culture lines. *Cancer Res.* 28:1300, 1968.
135. Kim, I., Harley, J. B., and Weksler, B. Multiple myeloma without initial paraproteins. *Am. J. Med. Sci.* 264:267, 1972.
136. River, G. L., Tewksburg, D. A., and Fudenberg, H. H. "Nonsecretory" multiple myeloma. *Blood* 40:204, 1972.
137. Löffler, H., Knopp, A., and Krecke, H. J. Cases of multiple myeloma (plasmacytoma) "without paraprotein." *Ger. Med. Mon.* 12:226, 1967.
138. Hurez, D., Flandrin, G., Preud'Homme, J. L., and Seligmann, M. Unreleased intracellular monoclonal macroglobulin in chronic lymphocytic leukaemia. *Clin. Exp. Immunol.* 10:223, 1972.
139. Epstein, W. V., and Tan, W. Increase of L-chain proteins in sera of patients with systemic lupus erythematosus and the synovial fluids of patients with peripheral rheumatoid arthritis. *Arthritis Rheum.* 9:713, 1966.
140. Daniels, J. C., Fukushima, M., Fish, J. C., Lindley, J. D., Remmers, A. R., Jr., Sarles, H. E., and Ritzmann, S. E. Studies on lysozyme (muramidase): II. Serum and urine muramidase patterns in chronic uremia, chronic hemodialysis, and renal allotransplantation. *Tex. Rep. Biol. Med.* 30:9, 1972.
141. Lewis, S. R. Magnitude of the Burn Problem. In J. B. Lynch and S. R. Lewis (Eds.), *Symposium on the Treatment of Burns,* Vol. 5. St. Louis: Mosby, 1973. Pp. 5–8.
142. Ritzmann, S. E., and Daniels, J. C. Serum Protein Abnormalities in Thermal Burns. In J. B. Lynch and S. R. Lewis (Eds.), *Symposium on the Treatment of Burns,* Vol. 5. St. Louis: Mosby, 1973. Pp. 31–41.
143. Arturson, G. Serum Immunoglobulin Levels in Severe Burns. In P. Matter, T. L. Barclay, and Z. Konickova (Eds.), *Research in Burns.* Bern: Huber, 1971. Pp. 489–495.
144. Munster, A. M., Hoagland, C., and Pruitt, B. A., Jr. The effect of thermal injury on serum immunoglobulins. *Ann. Surg.* 172:965, 1970.
145. Kefalides, N. A., et al. Role of infection in mortality from severe burns. *N. Engl. J. Med.* 267:317, 1962.
146. Kefalides, N. A., et al. Evaluation of antibiotic prophylaxis and gamma globulin, plasma, albumin and saline-solution therapy in severe burns. *Ann. Surg.* 159:496, 1957.
147. Stone, H. H., et al. Evaluation of gamma globulin prophylaxis against burn sepsis. *Surgery* 58:810, 1965.
148. Stiehm, E. R., Vaerman, J. P., and Fudenberg, H. H. Plasma infusions in immunologic deficiency states: Metabolic and therapeutic studies. *Blood* 28:918, 1966.
149. Blaese, R. M., Strober, W., Levy, A. L., and Waldmann, T. A. Hypercatabolism of IgG, IgA, IgM and albumin in the Wiskott-Aldrich syndrome. A unique disorder of serum protein metabolism. *J. Clin. Invest.* 50:2331, 1971.

150. Schless, A. P., and Harrel, G. S. Human gamma globulin in the treatment of bacterial infections. (Editorial.) *Am. J. Med.* 44:325, 1968.

151. Sever, J. L. (Ed.) Immunological responses to perinatal infections. (Selected papers.) *J. Pediatr.* 75:1111, 1969.

152. Ritzmann, S. E., and Levin, W. C. Polyclonal and monoclonal gammopathies. In H. Dettelbach and S. E. Ritzmann (Eds.), *Lab Synopsis,* Vol. 2 (2nd ed.). Somerville, N.J.: Behring Diagnostics, 1969. Pp. 9–54.

153. Fenoglio, C., Ferenczy, A., Isobe, T., and Osserman, E. F. Hepatoma associated with marked plasmocytosis and polyclonal hyper-γ-globulinemia. *Am. J. Med.* 55:111, 1973.

154. Riva, G. *Das Serumeiweissbild Lehrbuch der Untersuchungsmethoden und der Klinischen Semeiologie der Serum- und Plasmaeiweissveränderungen mit besonderer Berücksichtigung der Elektrophorese.* Bern: Huber, 1957.

155. Wuhrmann, F., and Märki, H. H. *Dysproteinämien und Paraproteinämien. Grundlagen, Klinik und Therpie* (4th ed.). Basel: Schwabe, 1963.

156. Triger, D. R., and Wright, R. Hyperglobulinaemia in liver disease. *Lancet* 2:1494, 1973.

157. Kawai, T. *Clinical Aspects of the Plasma Proteins.* Tokyo: Shoin, and Philadelphia: Lippincott, 1973.

158. Feizi, R. Immunoglobulins in chronic liver disease. *Gut* 9:193, 1968.

159. Paronetto, F., Rubin, E., and Popper, H. Local formation of gammaglobulin in the diseased liver and its relation to hepatic necrosis. *Lab. Invest.* 11:50, 1962.

160. Sunderman, F. W., Jr. Studies of the serum proteins. VI. Recent advances in the clinical interpretation of electrophoretic fractionations. *Am. J. Clin. Pathol.* 42:1, 1964.

161. Demenlenaere, L., and Wieme, R. J. Special electrophoretic anomalies in the serum of liver patients: A report of 1145 cases. *Am. J. Dig. Dis.* 6:661, 1961.

162. Miescher, P. A., Braverman, A., and Amarosi, E. Progressive hypergammaglobulinaemic hepatitis. *Ger. Med. Mon.* 12:162, 1967.

163. Ogryzlo, M. A., Machlachlan, M., Dauphinee, J. A., and Fletcher, A. A. The serum proteins in health and disease. Filter paper electrophoresis. *Am. J. Med.* 26:596, 1959.

164. Wall, R. L. The use of serum protein electrophoresis in clinical medicine. *Arch. Intern. Med.* 102:618, 1958.

165. Bloch, K. J., Buchanan, W. W., Wohl, M. J., and Bunim, J. J. Sjögren's syndrome. A clinical, pathological and serological study of 62 cases. *Medicine* (Baltimore) 44:187, 1965.

166. Sunderman, F. W., Jr. Recent Advances in Clinical Interpretation of Electrophoretic Fractionations of the Serum Proteins. In F. W. Sunderman and F. W. Sunderman, Jr. (Eds.), *Serum Proteins and the Dysproteinemias.* Philadelphia: Lippincott, 1964. Pp. 323–345.

167. Huth, E. Plasmazellendyskrasie mit transitorischer Hypergammaglobulinämie im Kindesalter. *Fortschr. Med.* 87:1116, 1969.

168. Baughan, M. A., Daniels, J. C., Levin, W. C., and Ritzmann, S. E. Hyperglobulinemic purpura (Waldenström). A report of 4 cases and review of literature. *Tex. Rep. Biol. Med.* 29:149, 1971.

169. Heremans, J. *Les globulines sériques du système gamma. Leur nature et leur pathologie.* Brussels: Arscia, and Paris: Masson, 1960.

170. Zawadzki, Z. A., and Edwards, G. A. Nonmyelomatous Monoclonal Immunoglobulinemia. In R. S. Schwartz (Ed.), *Progress in Clinical Immunology,* Vol. 1. New York: Grune & Stratton, 1972. Pp. 105–156.

171. Rádl, J., and Hollander, C. F. Homogeneous immunoglobulins in sera of mice during aging. *J. Immunol.* 112:2271, 1974.

172. Porter, D. D., Dixon, F. J., and Larsen, A. E. The development of a myeloma-like condition in mink with Aleutian disease. *Blood* 25:736, 1965.

173. Chapman, I., and Jiminez, F. A. Aleutian mink disease in man. *N. Engl. J. Med.* 269:1171, 1963.

174. Waldenström, J. Studies on conditions associated with disturbed gamma globulin formation (gammopathies). *Harvey Lect.* 56:211, 1961.

175. Larsson, O., and Leonhardt, T. Hereditary hyper-γ-globulinaemia and systemic lupus erythematosus. I. Clinical and electrophoretic studies. *Acta Med. Scand.* 165:371, 1959.

176. Leonard, T. Hereditable hyper-γ-globulinaemia and systemic lupus erythematosus. II. Serological studies. *Acta Med. Scand.* 165:395, 1959.

177. Lenhardt, T. Familial hyper-γ-globulinaemia and systemic lupus erythematosus. *Lancet* 2:1200, 1957.

178. Gallo, R. C., and Lorde, D. L. Familial chronic discoid lupus erythematosus and hypergammaglobulinemia. *Arch. Intern. Med.* 117:627, 1966.

179. Brunjes, S., Zike, K., and Julian, R. Familial systemic lupus erythematosus. A review of the literature, with a report of ten additional cases in four families. *Am. J. Med.* 30:529, 1961.

180. Hadziyamis, S., Feizi, T., Scheuer, P. J., and Sherlock, S. Immunoglobulin-containing cells in the liver. *Clin. Exp. Immunol.* 5:499, 1969.

181. Stiehm, E. R., Ammann, A. J., and Cherry, J. D. Elevated cord macroglobulins in the diagnosis of intrauterine infections. *N. Engl. J. Med.* 275:971, 1966.

182. Osserman, E. F., and Takatsuki, K. Considerations regarding the pathogenesis of the plasmacytic dyscrasias. *Ser. Haematol.* 4:28, 1965.

183. Kahler, O. Zur Symptomatologie des Multiplen Myeloms: Beobachtung von Albumosurie. *Prag. Med. Wochenschr.* 14:33, 1889.

184. Apitz, K. Die Paraproteinosen (Über die Störung des Eiweissstoffwechsels bei Plasmocytom). *Virchow's Arch. Pathol. Anat.* 306:631, 1940.

185. Gutman, A. B. The plasma proteins in disease. *Adv. Protein Chem.* 4:155, 1948.

186. Waldenström, J. Monoclonal and Polyclonal Gammopathies and the Biologic System of Gamma Globulins. In P. Kallos and B. H. Waksman (Eds.), *Progress in Allergy,* Vol. 6. Basel: Karger, 1962. Pp. 320–348.

187. Waldenström, J. *Diagnosis and Treatment of Multiple Myeloma.* New York: Grune & Stratton, 1970.

188. Osserman, E. F., and Fahey, J. L. Plasma cell dyscrasias: Current clinical and biochemical concepts. *Am. J. Med.* 44:256, 1968.

189. Engle, R. L., Jr., and Wallis, L. A. *Immunoglobulinopathies—Immunoglobulins, Immune Deficiency Syndromes, Multiple Myeloma and Related Disorders.* Springfield, Ill.: Thomas, 1969.

190. Hobbs, J. R. Immunocytoma o'mice an' man. *Br. Med. J.* 2:67, 1971.

191. Azar, H. A. Pathology of Multiple Myeloma and Related Growths,

and The Myeloma Cell. In H. A. Azar and M. Potter (Eds.), *Multiple Myeloma and Related Disorders*, Vol. 1. New York: Harper & Row, 1973. Pp. 1–152.

192. Levin, W. C., and Ritzmann, S. E.   Relation of abnormal proteins to formed elements of blood: Cellular sources. *Annu. Rev. Med.* 16:187, 1965.

193. Ritzmann, S. E., Daniels, J. C., and Levin, W. C.   Paralymphomatous Disease: The Syndrome of Macroglobulinemia. In *Leukemia-Lymphoma*. (A collection of papers presented at the 14th Annual Clinical Conference on Cancer, 1969, at the University of Texas M. D. Anderson Hospital and Tumor Institute, Houston.) Chicago: Year Book, 1970. Pp. 169–222.

194. Zucker-Franklin, D., and Mullaney, V.   Structural features of cells associated with the paraproteinemias. *Semin. Hematol.* 1:165, 1964.

195. Osserman, E. F., Takatsuki, K., and Talal, N.   The Pathogenesis of "Amyloidosis." Studies of the Role of Abnormal Gamma Globulins and Gamma Globulin Fragments on the Bence Jones (L-Polypeptide) Type in the Pathogenesis of "Primary" and "Secondary Amyloidosis," and the "Amyloidosis" associated with Plasma Cell Myeloma. *Semin. Hematol.* 1:3, 1964.

196. Ritzmann, S. E., Wolf, R. E., Lawrence, M. C., Hart, J. S., and Levin, W. C.   The Sia euglobulin test: A re-evaluation. *J. Lab. Clin. Med.* 73:698, 1969.

197. Daniels, J. C., Cobb, E. K., Levin, W. C., and Ritzmann, S. E.   Detection and differentiation of M-proteins by the acid-gel reaction. A re-evaluation. *Tex. Rep. Biol. Med.* 28:541, 1971.

198. Levin, W. C., and Ritzmann, S. E.   Relation of abnormal proteins to formed elements of blood: Effects upon erythrocytes, leukocytes, and platelets. *Annu. Rev. Med.* 17:323, 1966.

199. Isobe, T., and Osserman, E. F.   Pathologic conditions associated with plasma cell dyscrasias: A study of 806 cases. *Ann. N.Y. Acad. Sci.* 190:507, 1971.

200. Bloch, K. J., Lee, L., Mills, J. A., and Haber, E.   Gamma heavy chain disease—An expanding clinical and laboratory spectrum. *Am. J. Med.* 55:61, 1973.

201. Waldenström, J.   Macroglobulinemia. In R. Levin and R. Luft (Eds.), *Advances in Metabolic Disorders*, Vol. 2. New York: Academic, 1965. Pp. 115–158.

202. Bonhomme, J., Seligmann, M., Mihaesco, C., Chauvel, J. P., Danon, F., Brouet, J. C., Bouvry, P., Martine, J., and Clerc, M.   Mu chain disease in an African patient. *Blood* 43:485, 1974.

203. Ritzmann, S. E., Loukas, D., Sakai, H., Daniels, J. C., and Levin, W. C.   Idiopathic (asymptomatic) monoclonal gammopathies. *Arch. Intern. Med.* 135:95, 1975.

204. Kyle, R. A., Maldonado, J. E., and Bayrd, E. D.   Plasma cell leukemia, report on 17 cases. *Arch. Intern. Med.* 133:813, 1974.

205. Waldenström, J.   The occurrence of benign, essential monoclonal (M type) non-macromolecular hyperglobulinemia and its differential diagnosis. IV. Studies in the gammopathies. *Acta Med. Scand.* 176:345, 1964.

206. Waldenström, J.   Die Frühdiagnose der Myelomatose. *Acta Chir. Scand.* 87:365, 1942.

207. Waldenström, J.   Abnormal Proteins in Myeloma. In W. Dock and

I. Snapper (Eds.), *Advances in Internal Medicine,* Vol. 5. Chicago: Year Book, 1952. Pp. 398–440.

208. Waldenström, J. Benign Monoclonal Gammopathies. In H. A. Azar and M. Potter (Eds.), *Multiple Myeloma and Related Disorders,* Vol. 1. New York: Harper & Row, 1973. Pp. 247–286.

209. Bernier, G. M., and Graham, R. C., Jr. Plasma Cell Asynchrony in Myeloma. In *Proceedings of the American Society of Hematology, 16th Annual Meeting,* 1973. P. 38.

210. Salmon, S. E. Immunoglobulin synthesis and tumor kinetics of multiple myeloma. *Semin. Hematol.* 10:135, 1973.

211. Wildhack, R. Verlaufsbeobachtungen bei Paraproteinämien. *Dtsch. Med. Wochenschr.* 94:157, 1969.

212. Kyle, R. A., and Baird, E. D. "Benign" monoclonal gammopathy: A potentially malignant condition? *Am. J. Med.* 40:426, 1966.

213. Hobbs, J. P. Paraproteins, benign or malignant? *Br. Med. J.* 3:699, 1967.

214. Dammacco, F., and Waldenström, J. Serum and urine light chain levels in benign monoclonal gammopathies, multiple myeloma and Waldenström-macroglobulinemia. *Clin. Exp. Immunol.* 3:911, 1968.

215. McLaughlin, H., and Hobbs, J. R. Clinical Significance of Bence Jones Proteinuria. In H. Peeters (Ed.), *Proteins and Related Subjects. Protides of the Biological Fluids,* Vol. 20. Amsterdam: Elsevier, 1972. Pp. 251–254.

216. Michaux, J. L., and Heremans, J. F. Thirty cases of monoclonal immunoglobulin disorders other than myeloma or macroglobulinemia. A classification of diseases associated with the production of monoclonal-type immunoglobulins. *Am. J. Med.* 46:568, 1969.

217. Kyle, R. A., Maldonado, J. E., and Bayrd, E. D. Idiopathic Bence Jones proteinuria—A distinct entity? *Am. J. Med.* 55:222, 1973.

218. Carter, P. M., and Hobbs, J. R. Clinical significance of 7S IgM in monoclonal IgM diseases. *Br. Med. J.* 2:260, 1971.

219. Bottura, C., Farrari, J., and Beige, A. A. Chromosomal abnormalities in Waldenström's macroglobulinaemia. *Lancet* 1:1170, 1961.

220. Gamon, J. L., Biro, C. E., and Bearn, A. G. Chromosomal abnormalities in Waldenström's macroglobulinaemia. *Lancet* 2:48, 1961.

221. Houston, E. W., Ritzmann, S. E., and Levin, W. C. Chromosomal aberrations common to three types of monoclonal gammopathies. *Blood* 29:214, 1967.

222. Dartnell, J. A., Mundy, G. R., and Baikie, A. G. Cytogenetic studies in myeloma. *Blood* 42:229, 1973.

223. Spengler, G. A., Siebner, H., and Riva, G. Chromosomal abnormalities in macroglobulinemia Waldenström. Discordant findings in uniovular twins. *Acta Med. Scand.* [Suppl.] 445:132, 1966.

224. Kohn, J., and Scrieveslove, P. G. Paraproteinemia in Blood Donors and the Aged: Benign and Malignant. In H. Peeters (Ed.), *Proteins and Related Subjects. Protides of the Biological Fluids,* Vol. 20. Amsterdam: Elsevier, 1972. Pp. 257–261.

225. Bertrams, J., Kuwert, V., Böhme, U., Reis, H. E., Galtmeier, W. M., Wetter, O., and Schmidt, C. G. HL-A antigens in Hodgkin's disease and multiple myeloma. Increased frequency of W-18 in both diseases. *Tissue Antigens* 2:41, 1972.

226. Dausset, J. Correlation between Histocompatibility Antigens and Sus-

ceptibility to Illness. In R. S. Schwartz (Ed.), *Progress in Clinical Immunology*, Vol. 1. New York: Grune & Stratton, 1972. Pp. 183–210.

227. Salmon, S. E., and Fudenberg, H. H. Abnormal nucleic acid metabolism of lymphocytes in plasma cell myeloma and macroglobulinemia. *Blood* 33:300, 1969.

228. Lindström, F. D., Hardy, W. R., Eberle, B. J., and Williams, R. C., Jr. Multiple myeloma and benign monoclonal gammopathy: Differentiation by immunofluorescence of lymphocytes. *Ann. Intern. Med.* 78:837, 1973.

229. Fahey, J. L., Scoggie, R., Utz, J., and Swed, C. F. Infection and antibody response in gamma globulin components in multiple myeloma and macroglobulinemia. *Am. J. Med.* 35:698, 1963.

230. Gray, H. M., and Kohler, P. F. Cryoimmunoglobulins. *Semin. Hematol.* 10:87, 1973.

231. Bloch, K. J., and Maki, D. G. Hyperviscosity syndromes associated with immunoglobulin abnormalities. *Semin. Hematol.* 10:113, 1973.

232. Solomon, A., and Fahey, J. L. Plasmapheresis therapy in macroglobulinemia. *Ann. Intern. Med.* 58:789, 1963.

233. Roelke, D. Cold agglutination. Antibodies and antigens. A review. *Clin. Immunol. Immunopathol.* 2:266, 1974.

234. Evans, R. S., Baxter, E., and Gilliland, B. C. Chronic hemolytic anemia due to cold agglutinins: A 20-year history of benign gammopathy with response to chlorambucil. *Blood* 42:463, 1973.

235. Marsh, W. L. Anti i: A cold antibody defining the I:i relationship in human red cells. *Br. J. Haematol.* 7:200, 1961.

236. Fudenberg, H. H., and Kunkel, H. G. Physical properties of the red cell agglutinins in acquired hemolytic anemia. *J. Exp. Med.* 106:689, 1957.

237. Harboe, M., Van Furth, R., Schubothe, H., Lind, G., and Evans, R. S. Exclusive occurrence of kappa chains in isolated cold haemagglutinins. *Scand. J. Haematol.* 2:259, 1965.

238. Macris, N. T., Capra, J. D., Frankel, G. J., Joachim, H. L., Stax, H., and Bruno, M. S. A lambda chain cold agglutinin-cryomacroglobulin occurring in Waldenström's macroglobulinemia. *Am. J. Med.* 48:524, 1970.

239. Andersen, B. R. Gamma A-cold agglutinin: Importance of disulfide bonds in activity and structure. *Science* 154:281, 1966.

240. Ritzmann, S. E., and Levin, W. C. Cryopathies: A review. Classification, diagnostic and therapeutic considerations. *Arch. Intern. Med.* 107:754, 1961.

241. Potter, M. Experimental Plasma Cell Tumors and Other Immunoglobulin-Producing Lymphoreticulum Neoplasms in Mice, and Antigen-Binding M-Components in Man and Mouse. In H. A. Azar and M. Potter (Eds.), *Multiple Myeloma and Related Disorders*, Vol. 1. New York: Harper & Row, 1973. Pp. 153–246.

242. Pratt, P. W., Estren, S., and Kochwa, S. Immunoglobulin abnormalities in Gaucher's disease: Report of 16 cases. *Blood* 31:633, 1968.

243. Levin, W. C., Aboumrad, M. H., Ritzmann, S. E., and Brantly, C. γ-Type I myeloma and xanthematosis. *Arch. Intern. Med.* 114:688, 1964.

244. Beaumont, J. L., Jacotot, B., Beaumont, V., Warnet, J., and Vilain, C. Myélome, hyperlipidémie et xanthomatose. *Nouv. Rev. Fr. Hematol.* 5:507, 1965.

245. Lennard-Jones, J. E. Myelomatosis with lipaemia and xanthometa. *Br. Med. J.* 1:781, 1960.
246. Klemm, D., Nennhuber, J., and Schoop, W. Paraproteinämie bei Hand-Schüller-Christianscher Erkrankung. *Blut* 9:164, 1965.
247. Brittinger, G., and König, E. Für Klinik der Paraproteinämien. *Schweiz. Med. Wochenschr.* 95:1584, 1965.
248. Rhomberg, W. Beitrag zur Kenntnis der Sogenannten Rudimentären Paraproteinämien. *Schweiz. Med. Wochenschr.* 98:568, 1968.
249. Laurell, C. B., Laurell, H., and Waldenström, J. Glycoprotein in serum from patients with myeloma, macroglobulinemia and related conditions. *Am. J. Med.* 22:24, 1957.
250. Rokitansky, K. *Handbuch der pathologischen Anatomie,* Vol. 3. Vienna: Braumüller and Seidel, 1842.
251. Virchow, R. *Cellular Pathology.* Philadelphia: Lippincott, 1863. P. 409.
252. Friedreich, N., and Kekulé, A. Zur Amyloidfrage. *Virchow's Arch. Pathol. Anat.* 16:50, 1859.
253. Glenner, G., Ein, D., and Terry, W. D. The immunoglobulin origin of amyloid. *Am. J. Med.* 52:141, 1972.
254. Cathcart, E., Ritchie, R., Cohen, A. S., and Brandt, K. Immunoglobulins and amyloidosis. *Am. J. Med.* 52:93, 1972.
255. Glenner, G., Cuatrecasas, P., Isersky, C., Bladen, H. A., and Eanes, E. D. Physical and chemical properties of amyloid fibers. II. Isolation of a unique protein constituting the major component from human splenic amyloid fibril concentrates. *J. Histochem. Cytochem.* 17:769, 1969.
256. Spiro, D. The structural basis of proteinuria in man. Electron microscopic studies of renal biopsy specimens from patients with lipid nephrosis, amyloidosis and subacute chronic glomerulonephritis. *Am. J. Pathol.* 35:47, 1959.
257. Cohen, A. S., and Calkins, E. Electron microscopic observations on a fibrous component in amyloid of diverse origins. *Nature* 183:1202, 1959.
258. Azar, H. A. Amyloidosis and Plasma Cell Disorders. In H. A. Azar and M. Potter (Eds.), *Multiple Myeloma and Related Disorders,* Vol. 1. New York: Harper & Row, 1973. Pp. 328–403.
259. Puchtler, H., Sweat, F., and Levine, M. On the binding of Congo red by amyloid. *J. Histochem. Cytochem.* 10:355, 1962.
260. Eanes, E. D., and Glenner, G. G. X-ray diffraction studies on amyloid filaments. *J. Histochem. Cytochem.* 16:673, 1968.
261. Husby, G., and Natvig, J. B. Immunological characterization of amyloid fibrils in tissue sections. *Clin. Exp. Immunol.* 11:357, 1972.
262. Harada, M., Isersky, C., Cuatrecasas, P., Page, D., Bladen, H. A., Eanes, E. D., Keiser, H. R., and Glenner, G. G. Human amyloid protein: Chemical variability and homogeneity. *J. Histochem. Cytochem.* 19:1, 1971.
263. Glenner, G. G., Harada, M., Isersky, C., Cuatrecasas, P., Page, D., and Keiser, H. R. Human amyloid protein: Diversity and uniformity. *Biochem. Biophys. Res. Commun.* 41:1013, 1970.
264. Kimura, S., Guyer, R., Terry, W. D., and Glenner, G. G. Chemical evidence for λ-type amyloid fibril proteins. *J. Immunol.* 109:891, 1972.
265. Isersky, C., Ein, D., Page, D., Harada, M., and Glenner, G. G. Im-

munochemical cross-reactions of human amyloid proteins with human immunoglobulin light chains. *J. Immunol.* 108:486, 1972.

266. Glenner, G. G., Terry, W., Harada, M., Isersky, C., and Page, D. Amyloid fibril proteins: Proof of homology with immunoglobulin light chains by sequence analysis. *Science* 171:1150, 1971.

267. Sox, H. C., and Hood, L. Attachment of carbohydrate to the variable region of myeloma immunoglobulin light chains. *Proc. Natl. Acad. Sci. U.S.A.* 66:975, 1970.

268. Pras, M., Nevo, Z., Schubert, M., Rotman, J., and Matalon, R. The significance of mucopolysaccharides in amyloid. *J. Histochem. Cytochem.* 19:443, 1971.

269. Glenner, G. G., Ein, D., Eanes, E. D., Bladen, H. A., Terry, W., and Page, D. The creation of "amyloid" fibrils from Bence Jones proteins in vitro. *Science* 714:712, 1971.

270. Moore, C. Amyloidosis (Clinicopathology Conference). *Am. J. Med.* 53:495, 1972.

271. Franklin, E. C. The complexity of amyloid. *N. Engl. J. Med.* 290: 512, 1974.

272. Isobe, T., and Osserman, E. F. Patterns of amyloidosis and their association with plasma cell dyscrasia, monoclonal immunoglobulins and Bence Jones proteins. *N. Engl. J. Med.* 290:473, 1974.

273. Kyle, R. A., and Bayrd, E. D. "Primary" systemic amyloidosis and myeloma: Discussion of relationship and review of 81 cases. *Arch. Intern. Med.* 107:344, 1961.

274. Heremans, J. F., and Masson, P. L. Specific analysis of immunoglobulins. Techniques and clinical value. *Clin. Chem.* 19:294, 1973.

275. Waldmann, T. A., and Strober, W. Metabolism of immunoglobulins. *Prog. Allergy* 13:1, 1969.

276. Maugh, T. H. Chalones: Chemical regulation of cell division. *Science* 176:1407, 1972.

277. Sakai, H., Beathard, G. A., and Ritzmann, S. E. B-Lymphocytosis Factors (BLF) in Plasma from Burned Patients (Abstract). In *Proceedings of the Ninth Leukocyte Culture Conference*, Williamsburg, Va., 1974.

278. Alexanian, R. Multiple Myeloma: A Nine Year Experience with Melphalan Therapy at M. D. Anderson Hospital. In *Leukemia-Lymphoma*. (A collection of papers presented at the 14th Annual Clinical Conference on Cancer, 1969, at the University of Texas M. D. Anderson Hospital and Tumor Institute, Houston.) Chicago: Year Book, 1970. Pp. 305–316.

279. Cass, R. M., Anderson, B. R., and Vaughan, J. H. Waldenström's macroglobulinemia with increased serum IgG levels treated with low doses of cyclophosphamide. *Ann. Intern. Med.* 71:971, 1969.

280. Hoogstraten, B. Steroid therapy of multiple myeloma and macroglobulinemia. *Med. Clin. North Am.* 57:1321, 1973.

281. Waldenström, J. *Diagnosis and Treatment of Multiple Myeloma.* New York: Grune & Stratton, 1970.

282. Olesen, H. Chlorambucil, treatment in cold agglutinin syndrome. *Scand. J. Haematol.* 1:116, 1964.

283. Snapper, I., and Kahn, A. *Myelomatosis. Fundamentals and Clinical Features.* Baltimore: University Park Press, 1971.

284. Farhangi, M., and Osserman, E. F. The treatment of multiple myeloma. *Semin. Hematol.* 10:149, 1973.

285. Osgord, E. E. Survival time of patients with plasmacytic myeloma. *Cancer Chemother. Rep.* 9:1, 1960.

286. Klemm, D., Huhnstein, W., and Harwerth, H. W. Für Klassifizierung atypischer paraproteinämischer Hämoblastosen. *Blut* 11:208, 1965.

287. Young, V. H. Transient paraproteins. *Proc. R. Soc. Med.* 62:778, 1969.

288. Seligmann, M., Danon, F., and Clauvel, J. P. Natural history of monoclonal immunoglobulins (myeloma workshop). *Br. Med. J.* 2:321, 1971.

289. Bohrod, M. G. Plasmocytosis and cryoglobulinemia in cancer. *J.A.M.A.* 164:18, 1957.

290. Clubb, J. S., Posen, S., and Neale, F. C. Disappearance of a serum paraprotein after parathyroidectomy. *Arch. Intern. Med.* 114:616, 1964.

291. Oxelius, V. A. Monoclonal immunoglobulins in congenital toxoplasmosis. *Clin. Exp. Immunol.* 11:367, 1972.

292. Laroche, C., Nenna, A., Seligmann, M., Richet, G., Caquet, R., and Bignon, J. Dysprotéinémie pseudo-myélomateuse au cours de pyonèphrose. *Presse Med.* 72:2833, 1964.

293. Levin, W. C., and Ritzmann, S. E. Relation of abnormal proteins to formed elements of blood. *Annu. Rev. Med.* 17:323, 1966.

294. Hällén, J. Discrete gammaglobulin (M-) components in serum: Clinical study of 150 subjects without myelomatosis. *Acta Med. Scand.* 462[*Suppl.*]:179, 1966.

295. London, R. E. Multiple myeloma: Report of a case showing unusual remission lasting 2 years following severe hepatitis. *Ann. Intern. Med.* 43:191, 1955.

296. Nutter, D. O., and Kramer, N. C. Macrocryogelglobulinemia. Report of a case with unusual spontaneous recovery. *Am. J. Med.* 38:462, 1965.

297. Wolf, R. E., Riedel, L. O., Levin, W. C., and Ritzmann, S. E. Remission of macroglobulinemia coincident with hepatitis. Report of a case and review of literature. *Arch. Intern. Med.* 130:392, 1972.

298. Roman, W., and Coles, M. Paraproteins in folic-acid deficiency. *Lancet* 1:211, 1966.

299. Seligmann, M., and Brouet, J. C. Antibody activity of human myeloma globulins. *Semin. Hematol.* 10:163, 1973.

300. Ritzmann, S. E., Sakai, H., Cottom, D., Sakai, H. K., Vyvial, T. M., Remmers, A. R., Jr., and Sarles, H. E. An MLC-inhibiting monoclonal IgM in a transplant patient (Abstract). In *Proceedings of the Fifth International Congress of the Transplantation Society,* Jerusalem, Israel, 1974.

301. Cawley, L. P., and Schenken, J. R. Monoclonal hypergammaglobulinemia of the gamma-M-type in a nine-year-old girl with ataxia-telangiectasia. *Am. J. Clin. Pathol.* 54:790, 1970.

302. Hällén, J. Frequency of "abnormal" serum globulins (M-components) in the aged. *Acta Med. Scand.* 173:737, 1963.

303. Axelsson, U., Bachmann, R., and Hällén, J. Frequency of pathological proteins (M-components) in 6995 sera from an adult population. *Acta Med. Scand.* 179:235, 1966.

304. Englisová, M., Englis, M., Kyral, V., Kourilek, K., and Dvǒrák, K. Changes of Immunoglobulin synthesis in old people. *Exp. Gerontol.* 3:125, 1968.

305. Fine, J., Derycke, C., and Boffa, G. A. Les dysglobulinémies mono-

clonales "essentielles" chez les sujets âgés. In *Proceedings of the 10th Congress of the European Society of Haematology,* Strasbourg, 1965. P. 872, 1967.

306. Friedman, J., and Ritzmann, S. E.   Personal observation.

307. Mawhinney, H., Allen, I. V., Beare, J. M., Bridges, J. M., Connolly, J. H., Hair, E., Nevin, N. C., Neill, D. W., and Hobbs, J. R.   Dysgammaglobulinaemia complicated by disseminated measles. *Br. Med. J.* 2:380, 1971.

308. Kitchen, H.   Comparative biology: Animal models of human hematologic disease. *Pediatr. Res.* 2:215, 1968.

309. Potter, M.   The developmental history of the neoplastic plasma cell in mice: A brief review of recent developments. *Semin. Hematol.* 10: 19, 1973.

310. Rask-Nielsen, R.   On the occurrence of plasma-cell leukemia in various strains of mice. *J. Natl. Cancer. Inst.* 16:1137, 1956.

311. Potter, M., Fahey, J. L., and Pilgrim, I.   Abnormal serum protein and bone destruction in transmissible mouse plasma cell neoplasm. *Proc. Soc. Exp. Biol. Med.* 94:327, 1957.

312. Merwin, R. M., and Algire, G. H.   Induction of plasma-cell neoplasms and fibrosarcomas in BALB/c mice carrying diffusion chambers. *Proc. Soc. Exp. Biol. Med.* 101:437, 1959.

313. Van den Scheer, J., Wyckoff, R. W. C., and Clarke, F. H.   The electrophoretic analysis of several hyperimmune horse sera. *J. Immunol.* 39: 65, 1940.

314. Osterland, C. K., Miller, E. J., Karakawa, W. W., and Krause, R. M.   Characteristics of streptococcal group specific antibody isolated from hyperimmune rabbits. *J. Exp. Med.* 123:599, 1966.

315. Despont, J. P., Fluckiger, R., Ghaith, A., Hausser, E., Jeannet, M., Monnier, J., Scheidegger, J. J., Siegenthaler, P., Wettstein, P., and Crouchaud, A.   Idiopathic paraproteinemia. *Helv. Med. Acta* 34:401, 1969.

316. Seligmann, M.   A genetic predisposition to Waldenström's macroglobulinaemia. *Acta Med. Scand.* 179 [Suppl. 445]:140, 1966.

317. Williams, R. C., Jr., Erickson, J. L., and Polesky, H. F.   Studies of monoclonal immunoglobulins (M-components) in various kindreds. *Ann. Intern. Med.* 67:309, 1967.

318. Spengler, G. A., Bütler, R., and Fischer, C.   On the question of familial occurrence of paraproteinemia. *Helv. Med. Acta* 33:208, 1966.

319. Grant, J. A., Blumenschein, G. R., and Buckley, E. C., III   Familial paraproteinemia. *Arch. Intern. Med.* 128:427, 1971.

320. Kyle, R. A., Heath, J. W., Jr., and Carbone, P. P.   Multiple myeloma in spouses. *Arch. Intern. Med.* 127:944, 1971.

321. Siebner, H., Aly, F. W., and Brann, H. J.   Chromosomenbefund bei γD-Plasmocytom. *Klin. Wochenschr.* 47:884, 1969.

322. Wurster-Hill, D. H., McIntyre, O. R., Cornwell, G. G., III, and Maurer, L. H.   Marker-chromosome 14 in multiple myeloma and plasma cell leukaemia. *Lancet* 2:1031, 1973.

323. Sandberg, A. A., Ishihara, T., Kikucki, Y., and Crosswhite, L. H.   Chromosomal differences among the acute leukemias. *Ann. N.Y. Acad. Sci.* 113:663, 1964.

324. Braun, D. G.   Die monoklonale Immunantwort. *Blut* 25:57, 1972.

325. Metzger, H.   Myeloma proteins and antibodies. *Am. J. Med.* 47:837, 1969.

326. Harboe, M. Biologically active "monoclonal" γM-globulins. *Ser. Haematol.* 4:65, 1965.

327. Christenson, W. N., Dacie, J. V., Croucher, B. E. E., and Charlwood, P. A. Electrophoretic studies on sera containing high titre cold haemagglutinins: Identification of the antibody as the cause of the abnormal γ-peak. *Br. J. Haematol.* 3:262, 1957.

328. Fudenberg, H. H., and Kunkel, H. G. Physical properties of the red cell agglutinins in acquired hemolytic anemia. *J. Exp. Med.* 106:689, 1957.

329. Kritzmann, J., Kunkel, H. G., McCarthy, J., and Mellors, R. C. Studies of a Waldenström-type macroglobulin with rheumatoid factor properties. *J. Lab. Clin. Med.* 57:905, 1961.

330. Ozer, F. L., and Chaplin, H. Agglutination of stored erythrocytes by a human serum, characterization of the serum factor and erythrocyte changes. *J. Clin. Invest.* 42:1735, 1963.

331. Feizi, T., Kabat, E. A., Vicari, G., Anderson, B., and Marsh, W. L. Immunochemical studies on blood groups. LIV. Classification of anti-I and anti-i sera into groups based on reactivity patterns with various antigens related to the blood group A, B, H, Le^a, Le^b and precursor substances. *J. Exp. Med.* 135:1247, 1972.

332. Potter, M. Myeloma proteins (M-components) with antibody-like activity. *N. Engl. J. Med.* 284:831, 1971.

333. Williams, R. C., Jr. Subacute bacterial endocarditis as an immune disease. *Hosp. Practice* 7:111, 1972.

334. Holm, S. E., and Kaijser, B. Extreme ASO Activity in an IgG Kappa Myeloma Protein. In H. Peeters (Ed.), *Proteins and Related Subjects. Protides of the Biological Fluids,* Vol. 20. Amsterdam: Elsevier, 1972. Pp. 207–210.

335. Cooper, M. R., Cohen, H. J., Huntley, C. C., Waite, B. M., Spees, L., and Spurr, C. L. A monoclonal IgM with antibodylike specificity for phospholipids in a patient with lymphoma. *Blood* 43:493, 1974.

336. Seligmann, M., Sassy, C., and Chevalier, A. A human IgG myeloma protein with anti α₂ macroglobulin antibody activity. *J. Immunol.* 110: 85, 1973.

337. Meltzer, M., and Franklin, E. C. Cryoglobulinemia: A study of twenty nine patients. IgG and IgM cryoglobulins and factors affecting cryoprecipitability. *Am. J. Med.* 40:828, 1966.

338. Grey, H. M., Kohler, P. F., Terry, W. D., and Franklin, E. C. Human monoclonal γG-cryoglobulins with anti-γ-globulin activity. *J. Clin. Invest.* 47:1875, 1968.

339. Eisen, H. N., Little, J. R., Osterland, K., and Simms, E. S. A myeloma G-Protein with antibody (anti-2,4-dinitrophenyl) activity. *Symp. Quant. Biol.* 32:75, 1967.

340. Terry, W. D., Boyd, M. M., Rea, J. S., and Stein, R. Human M-proteins with antibody activity for nitrophenyl ligands. *J. Immunol.* 104: 256, 1970.

341. Lawrence, D. A., Tye, M. J., and Liss, M. Immunochemical analysis of the basic immunoglobulin in papular mucinosis. *Immunochemistry* 9:41, 1972.

342. Griscelli, C., Desmonts, G., and Gny, B. Congenital toxoplasmosis: Fetal synthesis of oligoclonal immunoglobulin G in intrauterine infection. *J. Pediatr.* 83:20, 1973.

343. Ainti, F., Ungari, S., and Serrn, G. B.   Immunologic aspects of congenital syphilis. *Helv. Paediatr. Acta* 21:66, 1968.

344. Hochwald, G. M., and Thorbecke, G. J.   Occurrence of myeloma-like γ-globulin in CSF of a four month old infant with hydrocephalus. *Pediatrics* 33:435, 1964.

345. Weinberg, A. G., McCracken, G. H., LoSpalluto, J., and Luby, J. P.   Monoclonal macroglobulinemia in cytomegalic inclusion disease. *Pediatrics* 51:518, 1973.

346. Bain, B. J., Ribush, N. T., Nicoll, P., Whitsed, H. M., and Morgan, T. O.   Renal failure and transient paraproteinemia due to leptospira pomona. *Arch. Intern. Med.* 131:740, 1973.

347. Danon, F., and Seligmann, M.   Transient human monoclonal immunoglobulin. *Scand. J. Immunol.* 1:323, 1972.

348. Schinke, R. N., Bolano, C., and Kickpatrick, C. H.   Immunologic deficiency in the congenital rubella syndrome. *Am. J. Dis. Child.* 118:626, 1969.

349. Hitzig, W. H., and Jako, J.   Monoclonal Immunoglobulins in Children. In H. Peeters (Ed.), *Protides of the Biological Fluids,* Vol. 18. Amsterdam: Elsevier, 1971. Pp. 139–143.

350. Pruzanski, W., Cowan, D. H., Merrett, R. A., and Freedman, M. H.   IgG-1(κ) M-component after bone marrow transplantation. *Clin. Immunol. Immunopathol.* 1:311, 1973.

351. Hitzig, W. H., Landolt, R., Miller, G., and Bodmer, P.   Heterogeneity of phenotypic expression in a family with Swiss-type gammaglobulinemia: Observation on the acquisition of agammaglobulinemia. *J. Pediatr.* 78:968, 1971.

352. Geha, R. S., Schneeberger, E., Gaticu, J., Rosen, F. S., and Merler, E.   Synthesis of an M-component by circulating B lymphocytes in severe combined immunodeficiency. *N. Engl. J. Med.* 290:726, 1974.

353. Dalloz, J. C., Casteing, N., Nezelof, C., and Seligmann, M.   Paraproteinemie transitoire de type gamma: Observation chez un nourisson atteint du syndrome d'Aldrich. *Presse Med.* 73:1541, 1965.

354. Faux, J. A., Ervin, J. D., Rosen, F. S., and Merler, E.   An alpha heavy chain abnormality in a child with hypogammaglobulinemia. *Clin. Immunol. Immunopathol.* 1:282, 1973.

355. Rádl, J., van den Berg, P., Voormolen, M., Hendriks, W. D. H., and Schaefer, U. W.   Homogeneous immunoglobulins in sera of rhesus monkeys after lethal irradiation and bone marrow transplantation. *Clin. Exp. Immunol.* 16:259, 1974.

356. Seligmann, M., Danon, F., Busch, A., and Bernard, J.   IgG myeloma cryoglobulin with antistreptolysin activity. *Nature* 220:711, 1968.

357. Williams, R. C., Jr., and Kunkel, H. G.   Rheumatoid factor, complement, and conglutinin aberrations in patients with subacute bacterial endocarditis. *J. Clin. Invest.* 41:666, 1962.

358. Monod, J.   *Le hasard et la nécessité.* Paris: Editions du Seuil, 1970.

359. Heremans, J. F.   A model for the development of immunocyte monoclones. *Br. Med. J.* 2:319, 1971.

360. Wiener, A. S.   Further observations on isosensitization to the Rh factor. *Proc. Soc. Exp. Biol. Med.* 70:576, 1949.

361. Opelz, G., and Terasaki, P. I.   Histocompatibility matching utilizing responsiveness as a new dimension. *Transplantation Proc.* 4:433, 1972.

Thermoproteins

Robert E. Wolf, William C. Levin, and Stephan E. Ritzmann

20

The term *thermoproteins* [1] refers to plasma or urinary proteins that exhibit abnormal physicochemical behavior at temperatures above or below 37°C. The types of thermoproteins are *cryoglobulins,* which form reversible or irreversible precipitates, gels, or crystals at temperatures below 37°C; *pyroglobulins,* which form irreversible precipitates or gels at 56°C; and *Bence Jones proteins,* which reversibly precipitate at 40° to 60°C, but redissolve at higher and lower temperatures. Bence Jones proteins may also demonstrate cryoglobulin reactions. The discussion in this chapter will be limited to the thermoreactive "abnormal" immunoglobulins, i.e., cryoglobulins, pyroglobulins, and Bence Jones proteins, although it should be recognized that cryofibrinogen as well as other temperature-reactive serum proteins also exist [2–5].

Thermoproteins are usually found in association with systemic disorders such as multiple myeloma, Waldenström's macroglobulinemia, proliferative lymphoreticular disorders, connective tissue diseases, and chronic infections. However, essential, or primary, thermoproteinemia also exists. Clinically, the spectrum ranges from asymptomatic disorders to life-threatening illness.

Cryoglobulins

CLASSIFICATION

Wintrobe and Buell [6] first described the precipitation of proteins from cooled serum in a patient with multiple myeloma. Extensive in vitro studies of one such protein were reported by Lerner and Watson [7, 8], who found the thermoreactive component to be an immunoglobulin in nature, and thus proposed the term *cryoglobulin.* Cold-reactive proteins have been observed that reversibly or irreversibly precipitate (cryoglobulins), gel (cryogelglobulins), or crystallize (crystaloglobulins) at lowered temperatures; more than one type may coexist.

Cryoglobulins are a heterogeneous group of immunoglobulins that

Table 20-1. Disorders Associated with Cryoglobulinemia

Malignant B-Cell Diseases
  Multiple myeloma
  Waldenström's macroglobulinemia
  Chronic lymphocytic leukemia
  Lymphosarcoma (?)

Collagen Diseases
  Rheumatoid arthritis
  Sjögren's syndrome
  Serum immune complexes
  Systemic lupus erythematosus
  Polyarteritis nodosa

Acute and Chronic Infections
  Syphilis
  Kala-azar
  Leprosy
  Subacute bacterial endocarditis
  Infectious mononucleosis
  Cytomegalovirus disease

Other Disorders
  Sarcoidosis
  Acute poststreptococcal glomerulonephritis
  Cirrhosis
  Hemolytic anemia

Essential (Primary) Cryoglobulinemia

have been reported in association with a wide variety of disorders (Table 20-1). The types of cryoglobulins that have been reported are (1) IgG-cryoglobulins, (2) IgM-cryoglobulins, (3) IgA-cryoglobulins (rare), (4) Bence Jones cryoproteins (rare), and (5) Mixed cryoglobulins, including complexes of IgG + IgM mixed cryoglobulins (frequent), IgG + IgA cryoglobulins, IgG + IgA + IgM cryoglobulins, IgG + IgM + complement component cryoglobulins, IgG + IgM + α_2M-globulin cryoglobulins, and IgM + lipoprotein cryoglobulins (see also Chap. 9).

In the mixed types of cryoglobulins, neither of the two components alone may demonstrate cryoreactivity when isolated. The IgM-IgG complex type is most frequently encountered, with the IgM possessing antiglobulin (rheumatoid factor–like) activity. The IgM may be either monoclonal or polyclonal [2, 9–12]. Recent studies indicate a propensity for the IgM to react with the IgG_3 subclass in the formation of these mixed cryoproteins [13]. Additionally, IgG antiglobulin forms cryoreactive complexes with normal IgG, and some cases of apparent "pure" IgG cryoglobulinemia may represent this type of interaction without demonstrable antibody activity in the isolated proteins. Other serological activities have been demonstrated in cryoglobulins [14, 15], such as: (1) anti-IgG rheumatoid factors, (2) anti-nuclear antibodies, (3) antithyroglobulin antibodies, (4) anti-cytomegalovirus antibodies, (5) anti-complementary activity, and (6) anti-erythrocyte antibodies ("cold agglutinins"). DNA has also been detected as the complexed antigen in some instances [15]. The nonmixed types of cryoglobulins probably possess undetected antibody activity.

PATHOPHYSIOLOGY

Cryogelglobulins and the serum hyperviscosity syndrome, which represent entities related to, but somewhat distinct from, the precipitating cryoglobulins in many respects, will be discussed in the next section. Three pathophysiological mechanisms appear to be related to the manifestations of cryoglobulinemia. First, the unique physicochemical characteristic of reversible precipitation on cooling may lead to vascular occlusion. Such occlusion may result either directly by precipitation of protein or more obliquely by precipitated protein that forms a lattice for trapping erythrocytes, thus producing clot formation. Blockade of major arteries or veins, or both, as well as smaller vessels may occur, and organizing thrombi have been observed. Variable and often bizarre clinical manifestations may result from reversible occlusions.

Second, the circulating immune complexes (e.g., IgM-IgG) in association with complement components may lead to immune-complex nephritis, vasculitis, or both [11, 16, 17]. Cutaneous vasculitis with perivascular infiltration of neutrophils, lymphocytes, and plasma cells has been observed, and immunofluorescence studies have demonstrated complement, immunoglobulins, and fibrinogen in the vessel walls [18]. Diffuse, progressive glomerulonephritis has also been found in patients with the mixed IgM-IgG type of cryoglobulinemia. Electron-dense glomerular deposits containing immunoglobulins and complement components [15, 16] in conjunction with lowered serum complement levels [19] suggest that the deposition of immune complexes is causally and pathologically related to the glomerulonephritis.

Third, the intravascular precipitation of the cryoglobulins may have effects other than stasis of the circulation. Vasoconstriction distal to an occlusion may induce the secondary release of histamine and other vasoactive mediators and thus enhance ischemic symptoms.

CLINICAL MANIFESTATIONS

The clinical manifestations of cryoglobulinemia may be related to ischemia, immune-complex deposition, or both. In many cases, a history of cold sensitivity may be elicited (i.e., cryopathy) [2, 3]. Symptoms related to vascular occlusion are highly variable, depending on the organ systems affected, and they may include hemorrhagic diatheses such as purpura, epistaxis, gingival bleeding, as well as gross hemorrhage, abdominal pain, cyanosis or respiratory distress, deafness, peripheral gangrene or ulceration, Raynaud's phenomenon, myocardial injury, and so on (see Fig. 20-5). Thus, cold hypersensitivity should be excluded at least on the basis of the history of patients with pulmonary infarction, angina pectoris or myocardial infarction, mesenteric artery occlusion, transient deficits in auditory or visual acuity, cerebral ischemia, and hemorrhagic diatheses. The differential diagnosis of cold hypersensitivity disorders or cryopathies [2–5] may be guided by the information presented in Table 20-2. Although retinal vessel distension, occlusion, or hemorrhage or neurological manifestations may be found on physical examination, most of the findings will be related to the symptomatology and will not assist in the diagnosis of cryoglobulinemia unless there is a suggestion of the presence of the disorder. Cryoglobulinemia associated with immune-complex disease may be manifested clinically by arthralgia, glomerulonephritis, or vasculitis in some combination. Again, suspicion is the key to relating these clinical entities to cryoglobulinemia. Clinical data must be correlated with laboratory evaluations, since there is no consistent correlation between the amount of cryoglobulin present and clinical symptoms.

LABORATORY DIAGNOSIS
The laboratory diagnosis of cryoglobulinemia is made by observing the formation of a precipitate in cooled serum (Figs. 20-1 and 20-2). Whole blood is drawn and immediately placed at 37°C in a water bath until the serum can be extracted. The serum is placed in a Wintrobe hematocrit tube at room temperature for 4 to 5 hours, and it is then refrigerated at 4°C for 16 to 20 hours. After refrigeration, the tube is centrifuged for 3 minutes at 3000 rpm at 4°C, and the amount of cryoprecipitate is then expressed as a percentage, the *cryocrit* (see Fig. 20-1). A more accurate determination of the amount of cryoprecipitate protein may be made by quantitating the serum proteins before and after cryoprecipitation. Serum rather than plasma must be used for this assay in order to distinguish cryoglobulins from cryofibrinogen. Initial cooling to room temperature before refrigeration is performed, since the optimal temperature for precipitation may vary. In some sera, precipitates may form rapidly at ambient temperature, but they may require refrigeration for several days before developing. Once the precipitate has formed, however, further cooling does not affect its stability.

THERAPY
The ultimate goal of therapy is to decrease the level of circulating cryoglobulins and thus avoid continued pathophysiological alterations. However, symptomatic relief to the patient is also necessary and often more readily achieved. Some immediate symptomatic relief is obtained by instructing the patient to avoid cold (e.g., cold food or drinks, air conditioning, cold baths, and swimming in unheated water) and to wear warm clothing and gloves if necessary. This is an important aspect of therapy and one which many individuals will have learned by experience before seeing a physician. A variety of therapeutic modalities have been used with variable results [2, 11, 15, 17]. These include the avoidance of exposure to cold, the administration of corticosteroids, penicillamine, or antimetabolites, and the use of plasmapheresis. Splenectomy may also be of some value.

Administration of adrenal corticosteroids may provide symptomatic

Table 20-2. Classification of Cryopathies (Cold Hypersensitivity Disorders)

1. *Raynaud's disease.* Idiopathic, essential disorder, mainly affecting females during 2nd to 4th decades, without recognizable underlying disorders upon long-term follow-up.

2. *Cryoproteinemias.* Occurrence of cold-sensitive plasma proteins.
   A. *Cryoglobulinemias.* Found in association with monoclonal (especially Waldenström's macroglobulinemia) or polyclonal gammopathies (e.g., rheumatoid arthritis).
   B. *Cryofibrinogenemia.* Rare.

3. *Paroxysmal cold hemoglobinurias (PCH).* Antibody-caused hemolysis upon exposure to cold. Triad: Acrocyanosis, hemolytic anemia, PCH.
   A. *Cold agglutinin syndrome.* Due to increased cold agglutinins, usually of anti-I-IgM variety; either acute (e.g., *Mycoplasma pneumoniae* infections) or chronic (related to Waldenström's macroglobulinemia, i.e., cold agglutinin disease).
   B. *Cold hemolysin syndrome.* Due to Donath-Landsteiner (i.e., anti-P + P_1) antibodies; either acute (nonsyphilitic) or chronic (syphilitic).

4. *Connective tissue disorders.* These vascular cryopathies include:
   A. Scleroderma (commonly associated with Raynaud's phenomenon).
   B. Lupus erythematosus.
   C. Dermatomyositis.
   D. Rheumatoid arthritis (including its variants).
   E. Polyarteritis nodosa.

5. *Occlusive arterial disease*
   A. Nonoccupational diseases, such as arteriosclerosis obliterans, thromboangiitis obliterans, and arterial embolism.
   B. Occupational diseases, including vibration tool (e.g., pneumatic hammer) diseases and Raynaud's phenomenon in typists, pianists, cashiers, creamery workers, and so on.

6. *Neurovascular compression syndromes* (i.e., shoulder-girdle compression or thoracic outlet syndromes).
   A. Scalenus anticus syndrome.
   B. Cervical rib syndrome.
   C. Hyperabduction syndrome.
   D. Costoclavicular syndrome.

7. *Miscellaneous disorders*
   A. Cold urticarias.
   B. Intoxications (e.g., ergotism or heavy metals such as lead, arsenic, thallium).
   C. Tumors (e.g., glomus tumors or pituitary tumors).
   D. Angiokeratoma corporis diffusum (Fabry).
   E. Paramyotonia congenita.
   F. Injuries to brain, spinal column, or nerve roots or trunks.
   G. Erythrocyanosis.
   H. Myxedema.
   I. Primary pulmonary hypertension.
   J. Unexplained causes of Raynaud's phenomenon.

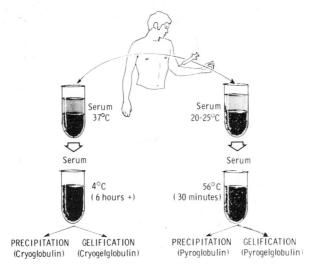

Figure 20-1
Assays for cryoglobulins (*left*) and pyroglobulins (*right*). (For details, see text.)

relief, especially in cases where immune complexes are present, but they do not alter the level of circulating cryoglobulins or the progression of the disease. Penicillamine, which cleaves disulfide linkages and thus depolymerizes macroglobulins in vitro, has been used with some success in lowering serum cryoglobulin concentrations. However, penicillamine probably has some effect on the synthesis of immunoglobulins and, in vivo, acts more like a cytotoxic agent. Concentrations used in vitro are never reached in vivo; suppressed levels of macroglobulins persist for several months after discontinuation of the drug; and diminished levels of all immunoglobulins may result from long-term therapy. Antimetabolite therapy using cyclophosphamide, chlorambucil, urethane, or stilbamidine has also been used successfully to decrease the level of cryoglobulins in some instances. In one case, cyclophosphamide provided symptomatic relief and lowered the concentration of circulating cryoglobulin. However, a precipitous fall in the cryocrit was observed following splenectomy for hypersplenism, and antimetabolite administration was no longer required [17]. A predominance of IgM-forming cells was found in the spleen, which may have been the site of cryoglobulin synthesis. The potential benefits of splenectomy in cryoglobulinemias require further investigation. Finally, plasmapheresis may be beneficial, as will be discussed in the subsequent section on therapy for serum hyperviscosity syndrome. Plasmapheresis has been proved to be useful and practical for long-term therapy of cryogelglobulinemia, and it may be similarly applicable in other cases, especially in IgM-related cryoglobulinemias and life-threatening complications.

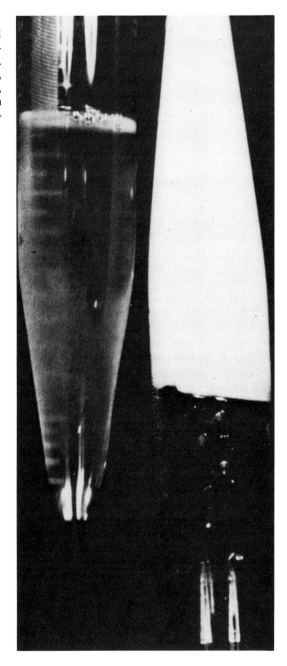

Cryogelglobulins and the Serum Hyperviscosity Syndrome

PHYSIOLOGY

The rate of flow of a liquid—e.g., blood through a capillary tube or the vascular system—is related to the pressure gradient and various factors of resistance according to Poiseuille's equation:

$$\ddot{Q} = \Delta P \times \frac{\pi r^4}{L} \times \frac{1}{\eta}$$

where $\ddot{Q}$ = flow rate, ΔP = pressure gradient, r = radius, L = length, and η = viscosity. If the pressure gradient, radius, and length remain within normal ranges in a physiological system, such as in man, the flow rate is inversely proportional to η, the viscosity. Thus, the elevation of η will decrease the flow rate by affecting increased resistance to flow.

Since a number of factors such as erythrocyte mass in polycythemia vera or leukocyte mass in leukemia may affect whole blood viscosity, and since coexisting cellular phenomena such as rouleaux formation in multiple myeloma may contribute to the symptoms, the determination of serum viscosity is more relevant in serum protein abnormalities [20]. Furthermore, the viscosity is increased in relation as the vessel radius diminishes in the microcirculation. The relationship between the rate of flow and the factors of resistance follows Poiseuille's law in a linear fashion (i.e., Newtonian) for serum or plasma. Relatively small decrements of the vascular lumen result in a disproportionate increment of resistance, however.

In contrast, the viscosity, and therefore the flow rate, of whole blood is non-Newtonian. This difference is due to the suspended particles (erythrocytes and other formed elements) in blood. For particulate suspensions, viscosity may be defined as the ratio of shear stress (blood pressure) to shear rate (the velocity at which the elements move with respect to one another). Assuming the pressure of blood in the microcirculation to be constant, whole blood viscosity and flow rate become directly related to the shear rate [20]. At low shear rates, the viscosity increases exponentially. The dependence of viscosity on the shear rate is further influenced by factors such as plasma proteins (both total and type [21]), erythrocyte protein interaction, erythrocyte aggregation, and red cell charge in hyperviscosity syndromes. Furthermore, the hematocrit (in polycythemia), leukocyte mass (in leukemia), or erythrocyte deformability (in hemoglobinopathies) may be involved in other disorders. The physical characteristics of the plasma proteins affecting viscosity are mentioned later (pp. 495–496). The shear rate of erythrocytes in plasma is much greater than in saline, and only a portion of this difference may be accounted for by the differences in viscosity between plasma and saline. Thus, cell-protein interaction [22] appears to affect the shear rate. When cell aggregation (e.g., rouleaux formation) occurs, a greater proportion of shear stress is employed in shearing the cells,

Figure 20-3
Ostwald viscosimeter. The flow time (in seconds) of serum at 37°C is determined between marks 1 and 2. The viscosimeter is placed in a water bath (37°C) and 5 ml of serum is delivered into reservoir A. After equilibration at 37°C, suction is applied until the upper meniscus of serum is above mark 1. The serum is then allowed to flow freely back into reservoir A. The time required for the upper meniscus of the serum to pass between markers 1 and 2 is measured with a stop watch. (Reproduced by permission. From Ritzmann, S. E., Daniels, J. C., Alami, S. Y., and Lawrence, M. C. In G. J. Race (Ed.), *Laboratory Medicine*. New York: Harper & Row, 1975.)

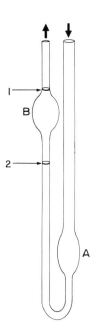

thus causing a decreased flow rate and an increased relative viscosity. Cell charge is related to shear rates in that a decrease in the net negative charge leads to rouleaux formation and cell aggregation. An increase in net negative charge leads to better dispersion of the cell, which results in increased shear rates and blood flow with an effective decrease in viscosity [23]. Although numerous factors may affect whole blood viscosity and flow rates in the microcirculation, the determination of the serum viscosity is most relevant in serum protein abnormalities.

MEASUREMENT OF SERUM VISCOSITY
Serum viscosity measurements are performed using an Ostwald viscosimeter (Fig. 20-3). The measurements are expressed relative to a standard fluid, such as distilled water or saline under constant temperature at atmospheric pressure. The relative viscosity at 37°C is denoted η rel 37°. Initially, the viscosimeter is calibrated by (1) filling the viscosimeter to the upper level of bulb A (see Fig. 20-3) with distilled water, (2) bringing the fluid level to line 1 by suction, thus filling bulb B, and (3) recording the time of gravity flow from line 1 to line 2. Similarly, the timed flow of serum is recorded and converted to η rel by dividing the flow time of serum by the predetermined flow time of distilled water. Thus,

$$\eta \text{ rel} = \frac{\text{flow time of serum}}{\text{flow time of water}}$$

Normal η rel[37] is 1.6 to 2.0. Each viscosimeter must be individually calibrated for each temperature (e.g., 37°, 25°, 13°, and 4°C), since the bulb volume of viscosimeters may vary and since large temperature differences may affect the viscosity of the reference liquid as well as the serum.

PATHOPHYSIOLOGY OF SERUM HYPERVISCOSITY

Serum hyperviscosity may be associated with a variety of clinical disorders and is related to such physical properties of the serum proteins as the total concentration, size, shape, aggregation, and thermoreactivity of the molecules. Although it occurs most frequently in Waldenström's macroglobulinemia [24, 25], hyperviscosity may also be associated with multiple myeloma [26–30] or serum immune-complex disorders [11, 31–35]. The serum hyperviscosity syndrome [26, 36, 37] represents an extremely variable complex of signs, symptoms, and physical abnormalities caused by slowed circulation, decreased cardiac output, diminished oxygenation of tissues, venous engorgement, and other abnormalities (see Figs. 20-4 and 20-5).

Two essential concepts in understanding the hyperviscosity syndrome and its variability are the *symptomatic threshold* [37], which refers to the η rel (relative viscosity) at which a symptom or group of symptoms appear (or disappear with plasmapheresis therapy) (Fig. 20-4) and the *target organs,* which are the organs or organ systems that are affected at various viscosity levels. Although most patients do not exhibit symptoms before an η rel 37° of 6 to 7 is attained, the symptomatic threshold may vary from η rel 37° 4 to η rel 37° 10, and a relatively fixed progression of target organ involvement will occur as the η rel 37° rises above the symptomatic threshold. Both the symptomatic threshold and the target organs are usually constant for a single individual, although both may vary among different patients. Part of the variation in symptomatic thresholds may be due to factors other than serum viscosity that affect shear rates.

SERUM HYPERVISCOSITY SYNDROME

CLINICAL MANIFESTATIONS AND PHYSICAL STIGMATA

The signs, symptoms, and physical aberrations due to the hyperviscosity syndrome are presented in Figures 20-4 and 20-5. Although most symptoms may be directly or indirectly related to aberrations of circulation or oxygenation, other factors may also be operative. Central nervous system involvement may be related to inadequate "flushing" of the pial arteries [38] or precipitation of protein in the Virchow-Robins spaces [39, 40], which may lead to coma paraproteinicum or Bing-Neel syndrome and death. Interference with the countercurrent exchange mechanism or decreased amounts of oxygen available for sodium transport may lead to renal dysfunction, including elevation of the blood urea nitrogen [27, 41]. Vascular endothelial damage, venous distension, coagulopathies possibly due to antithrombin activity, decreased antihemophilic globulin, fibrinolysin, or a defect in the conversion of fibrinogen to fibrin may

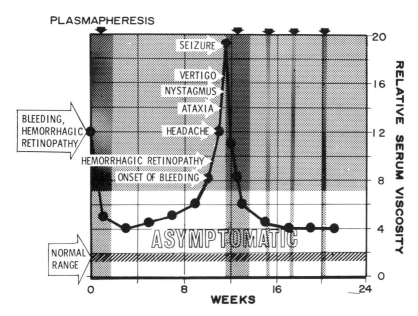

Figure 20-4
Clinical manifestations of the serum hyperviscosity syndrome. These manifestations are aggravated by low temperatures. (For details, see text.) (Modified from Solomon, A., and Fahey, J. L. *Ann. Intern. Med.* 58:789, 1963.)

contribute to hemorrhagic manifestations (gastrointestinal hemorrhage, gingival bleeding, epistaxis, and purpura), but the exact cause or causes are undetermined. Congestive heart failure that is related to decreased cardiac output, increased cardiac work, and, in some cases, an expanded plasma volume [27] may be present, and cardiac arrhythmias and electrocardiographic evidence of myocardial ischemia may also be found.

Although most of the stigmata found on physical examination are related to the symptoms (e.g., hemorrhage, purpura, or deafness), retinal venous engorgement that frequently occurs with segmentation or "boxcarring," retinal hemorrhages, nystagmus, ataxia, peripheral nerve defects, and, less commonly, bizarre neurological findings may also be uncovered. Hemorrhagic diatheses, ocular difficulties, and acousticovestibular dysfunction are the most common manifestations of serum hyperviscosity. In fact, the coexistence of blurred vision and retinal vein segmentation should suggest serum hyperviscosity until proved otherwise.

DIAGNOSIS
The diagnosis of the serum hyperviscosity syndrome is based upon suspicion and a thorough medical history and physical examination. Confirmation is obtained by viscosimetry. The suspicion of the presence of hyperviscosity is extremely important and cannot be overemphasized, since the pertinent symptoms might be overlooked and viscosimetry

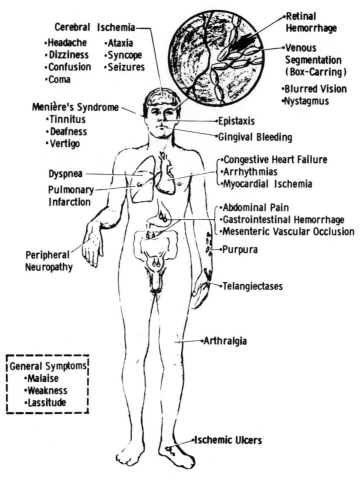

Figure 20-5
Clinical manifestations of serum hyperviscosity.

might never be performed. Since only a few of the many manifestations may be present and since delayed diagnosis may result in a fatal outcome of a treatable disorder, the possibility of serum hyperviscosity syndrome should be considered in any unexplained coma, bizarre neurological disorders, hemorrhagic diatheses, or retinal vein segmentation with any of the other manifestations, as well as in cases with more classic presentations. Naturally, the complete diagnosis of the underlying disease should be undertaken, but in the seriously ill patient, one should not await results of slower diagnostic procedures. Viscosimetry is rapid and simple, and cryogelglobulins may be detected by placing serum in a refrigerator and observing for gel formation. Even a laboratory report that a patient's serum plugged an automatic analyzer device or that the serum was difficult to separate from clotted blood should alert the physician to the possibility of serum hyperviscosity if other suggestive factors are present. Furthermore, viscosimetry and plasma volume determinations may be beneficial preoperative screening tests to be performed on all patients with monoclonal gammopathies in order to avoid potential complications from these problems if either is present.

THERAPY

Approach to treatment. The therapeutic approach should include the treatment of any underlying disorder and its other complications (e.g., transfusion with packed erythrocytes to avoid volume overload if severe anemia coexists and avoidance of cold temperature if cryoproteins are present) which is not aimed directly at correcting serum hyperviscosity. Plasmapheresis [42–45] represents specific therapy for the hyperviscosity syndrome per se. The procedure consists of removal of whole blood followed by replacement of the patient's own packed erythrocytes. It is performed in order to reduce the concentration of the abnormal serum protein and to alleviate the symptoms of hyperviscosity.

Technique of plasmapheresis. This procedure utilizes a two-bag transfer pack system [42]. After phlebotomy, the erythrocytes and other cellular constituents may be separated by either centrifugation or sedimentation at $37°C$. The plasma is then expressed into the transfer bag, and the erythrocytes and buffy layer are reinfused into the patient.

Application of plasmapheresis. Plasmapheresis of 1 to 4 units may be accomplished on the first day. Subsequently, the removal of one to 2 units daily for 1 or 2 weeks may be undertaken. It may be continued as often as two to four times weekly on a long-term basis if serum viscosity measurements or the persistence of symptoms indicate that it is necessary. The response to plasmapheresis is often both rapid and dramatic; cessation of bleeding or the reversal of coma may occur during or within a few hours after the initial plasmapheresis [24, 25, 28, 37, 41, 44, 45]. The requirements of plasmapheresis will vary from one patient to another and therefore must be individualized. The serum viscosity usually may be maintained at near normal levels, and good response to chemotherapy of the underlying disorder may eventually decrease or obviate the necessity of plasmapheresis.

Initially, the effects of plasmapheresis may occur more rapidly and may be longer lasting in Waldenström's macroglobulinemia than in multiple myeloma, since 80 percent of IgM exists intravascularly and therefore is more readily removed by plasmapheresis than IgG, which is evenly distributed between the intravascular and extravascular compartments. Due to the rapid influx of IgG from the tissues, lowering of serum viscosity may be transient or delayed. Once an equilibrium between production and removal is reached, plasmapheresis is equally effective in both disorders.

In the patient with hyperviscosity syndrome, there are no major contraindications to plasmapheresis therapy. Potentially, there are three side-effects of plasmapheresis: hypovolemia, thrombocytopenia, and hypoalbuminemia. By maintaining slow intravenous infusion of normal saline during the withdrawal of blood, hypovolemia may be avoided or easily corrected. Thrombocytopenia may be prevented by reinfusing the buffy coat with the erythrocytes. Since serum albumin levels may be decreased in disorders associated with the serum hyperviscosity syndrome (e.g., Waldenström's macroglobulinemia or multiple myeloma) and since albumin is removed by plasmapheresis, serial determinations of serum albumin should be performed and possible symptoms of hypoalbuminemia should be monitored. Decreasing the frequency or volume of plasmapheresis should be the first step in treating hypoalbuminemia. If this approach is not feasible due to the nature of the symptoms, albumin replacement may be required. However, relatively large quantities of albumin may be required, since continued removal will occur. Thus, a balance between optimal control and the albumin level must be established.

If these precautions are observed, long-term maintenance plasmapheresis therapy for the serum hyperviscosity syndrome is feasible. For example, in one patient with IgM(κ) monoclonal gammopathy and severe clinical manifestations of hyperviscosity, 300 liters (600 units) of blood were exchanged by plasmapheresis during a 6-year period. This resulted in the removal of 180 liters of plasma, 3.5 kg of albumin, and 15 kg of monoclonal IgM. The patient's condition was satisfactory throughout this period, and none of the potential complications mentioned above was encountered. With adequate monitoring, such maintenance plasmapheresis may be performed on an outpatient basis [42].

In addition to severe hyperviscosity states, a trial of plasmapheresis is also indicated in seriously ill patients with monoclonal gammopathies and bizarre symptoms (especially those of hyperviscosity), even in the face of only mildly or modestly elevated serum viscosities in the range of η rel 4 to 6 [28, 29]. Another application of plasmapheresis may be in treating dilutional anemia that is related to an expanded plasma volume and hypervolemia. In such individuals, plasmapheresis rather than transfusion is indicated.

Case Report 1—Waldenström's Macroglobulinemia
A 59-year-old Latin American male was first hospitalized on January 16, 1965 with purpura of the legs that had been precipitated by exposure to cold weather [25]. No cause was established. The patient was readmitted in February 1965 because of pedal edema and persistent purpura. Examination revealed only the presence of purpuric, ulcerated lesions on the lower legs and feet and bilateral pedal edema. The serum protein level was 7.0 gm per 100 ml, and electrophoresis revealed an M-protein concentration of 2.2 gm per 100 ml. Immunoelectrophoresis demonstrated an IgM (κ) monoclonal macroglobulin. Large amounts of 19S components and moderate amounts of 22S components were found on serum ultracentrifugation. Cryogelglobulinemia was detected. The latex test for rheumatoid factors was positive at a 1:40,000 dilution. Bone marrow examination revealed large masses of pleomorphic lymphoid plasma cells, which was consistent with the diagnosis of Waldenström's macroglobulinemia. Additionally, an abnormal chromosomal pattern, i.e., MG chromosome, was demonstrated [46].

Subsequently, the patient required numerous hospitalizations for generalized weakness, malaise, and lassitude. Hemorrhagic diatheses occurred, as well as gingival bleeding, epistaxis, gastrointestinal hemorrhage, purpura, and hematuria. Neurological deficits included numbness of the extremities in a glove-and-stocking distribution, tinnitus, vertigo, partial deafness, syncope, blurred vision, and headache. Clinical evaluation at various times revealed retinal hemorrhages, engorged and segmented retinal veins, nystagmus, neurosensory hearing deficits, mental obtundation and confusion, borderline psychotic behavior patterns, peripheral sensory nerve impairment, purpura, microscopic and gross hematuria, occult or gross blood in the stool, and cardiac arrhythmias (see Fig. 20-5).

The M-protein concentration and serum viscosity increased and the rheumatoid-factor latex test titer rose to 1:160,000. Hemorrhage necessitated transfusions of a total of 9000 ml of whole blood. Throughout this time, manifestations of serum hyperviscosity always necessitated vigorous plasmapheresis. All the signs and symptoms of hyperviscosity syndrome improved rapidly and strikingly with this therapy.

In January 1966, the patient developed Australia-antigen positive hepatitis but became asymptomatic after recovery from the hepatitis. The M-protein concentration, rheumatoid factor activity, and serum viscosity gradually decreased to normal levels. In June 1969, he developed a slight degree of polyclonal gammopathy, but immunoelectrophoresis revealed no evidence of a monoclonal gammopathy. In February 1970, the patient was brought to the hospital after a 6-day illness and died within 6 hours of hospitalization from pneumococcal sepsis. No evidence of macroglobulinemia was found at autopsy.

Pyroglobulins

DIAGNOSTIC CONSIDERATIONS
Heat-reactive thermoproteins were first described by Ellinger [47] in 1898 in a patient with multiple myeloma. The term *pyroglobulins* was applied to these immunoglobulins by Martin and Mathieson in 1953 [48]. In contrast to cryoglobulins and Bence Jones proteins, pyroglobulins irreversibly precipitate or gel when heated to 56°C.

Pyroglobulins are most frequently found in individuals with monoclonal gammopathies, e.g., multiple myeloma, Waldenström's macroglobulinemia, hypervitaminosis D (later developing into macroglobulinemia), but they have been reported in association with lymphosarcoma, carcinoma of the esophagus, lupus erythematosus, "convulsive disorders," chronic infection, or idiopathic hyperglobulinemias [49], as well as in the absence of detectable underlying disease. Usually, pyroglobulins are detected when serum complement is inactivated at 56°C for serological tests ("anticomplementary activity"). In approximately half of these cases, monoclonal gammopathy may be present. The common factor in these disorders is immunoglobulin aberrations [50].

CLINICAL ASPECTS
Clinically, isolated pyroglobulinemia is asymptomatic. Thus, a positive test is of significance only through the association of these proteins with monoclonal gammopathies and other systemic disorders.

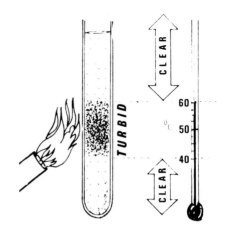

Figure 20-6
Positive heat test for Bence Jone proteins. (Reproduced by per mission. From Ritzmann, S. E. and Daniels, J. C. In G. J Race (Ed.), *Tice's Practice o Medicine,* Vol. 2. New York: Harper & Row, 1974.)

Individuals possessing heat-reactive proteins should undergo thorough screening tests for possible asymptomatic disease. In apparently healthy persons, repeated assays for pyroglobulins and occasional screening tests, especially for monoclonal gammopathies, may be warranted. The assay for pyroglobulinemia is simply performed by extracting the serum from clotted blood and heating the serum at 56°C for 30 minutes (see Fig. 20-1). The formation of an irreversible precipitate or gel constitutes a positive reaction. Since pyroglobulinemia per se is unassociated with symptoms, the only therapy indicated is that for underlying disorders.

Bence Jones Proteins

PHYSIOLOGY AND CHEMISTRY
In 1848 Sir Henry Bence Jones [51, 52] reported on the peculiar thermoreactivity (Fig. 20-6) of the urine from a patient with multiple myeloma. These proteins, which now bear his name, typically form a reversible precipitate when heated at 40° to 60°C but redissolve at higher and lower temperatures (see also Chaps. 5 and 19). Immunochemical analyses have demonstrated that Bence Jones proteins represent free light chains that may occur in monomers, dimers, or tetramers. In fact, isolated "normal" light chains possess similar thermoreactivity [53]. Electrophoretic migration is in the α_2-, β-, or γ-globulin fraction, and ultracentrifugation sedimentation coefficients range from 2.8S to 4.5S or even higher, depending on the degree of polymerization. The usual dimeric form has a molecular weight of approximately 35,000 and a sedimentation coefficient of 3.5S.

Bence Jones proteins may be present in serum as well as urine. Although small amounts of polyclonal free (κ and λ) light chains may be found in highly concentrated, normal urine using sensitive techniques [54], the presence of pathological quantities of Bence Jones proteins (i.e., monoclonal L chains, either κ or λ), as detected by the more commonly applied assays, is usually associated with malignant B-cell diseases such as multiple myeloma, Waldenström's macroglobulinemia, and, rarely, lymphatic leukemias. Most frequently, Bence Jones proteins are associated with monoclonal gammopathies either alone, in conjunction with Bence Jones myeloma or light-chain disease, or coexistent with IgG, IgA, IgM, IgD, IgE or even heavy-chain monoclonal proteins [55–58]. In each case, light-chain production is monoclonal in nature and may be of either type κ or λ. Except for rare cases that represent biclonal gammopathies, Bence Jones proteins are of the same class and amino-acid sequence as the light chains of the monoclonal immunoglobulins.

It has been demonstrated that asynchronous, excessive light-chain synthesis (an exaggeration of the process responsible for light chains in normal urine) rather than hypercatabolism is responsible for the occurrence of Bence Jones proteins [59, 60]. Monomeric light chains are rapidly filtered by the glomeruli due to their small size. These proteins are totally reabsorbed by the tubular cells and catabolized in the kidney. Thus, in the early stages of monoclonal gammopathies associated with Bence Jones proteins, light chains are not detectable in either the serum or the urine. The detection of Bence Jones proteins in the serum or urine, or both, is associated with abnormalities of filtration, reabsorption, or catabolism of the protein [61, 62]. As the disease begins to affect the kidney, excretion and reabsorption continue to be intact, while only partial catabolism occurs. At this time, Bence Jones proteins may be demonstrable in the blood but not in the urine. Progression of renal involvement interferes with reabsorption. With mild to moderate diminution of reabsorption superimposed on decreased catabolism, a stage occurs at which Bence Jones proteins are present both in the serum and urine. Later, the light chains are present only in the urine as total blockade of reabsorption occurs. Terminally, as uremia ensues, renal clearance of Bence Jones proteins may be affected so that the light chains reappear in the serum. It is, therefore, important for both diagnosis and prognosis that Bence Jones proteins be assayed in both serum and urine.

Since λ light chains have a propensity to polymerize in the serum [63], they are not usually found in the urine unless glomerular injury has occurred. In such instances, albumin, transferrin, immunoglobulins, and other serum proteins will also be present, thus making the diagnosis somewhat more difficult. Solomon and Fahey (55) found that 70 percent of cases with Bence Jones proteinemia were λ-type. Instances of Bence Jones myeloma (i.e., light-chain disease) without proteinuria have occurred with tetramers of λ light chains that produce a serum monoclonal spike on electrophoresis [63]. On the other hand, κ light chains may be difficult to demonstrate in serum in spite of heavy Bence Jones proteinuria, because of rapid glomerular clearance. Cases of Bence Jones myeloma have been reported with osteolytic bone lesions, plasma cell infiltration in the bone marrow, and Bence Jones proteinuria, but with normal or low serum γ-globulin levels [64]. Total reabsorption of κ-type Bence Jones proteins by the renal tubules during early stages of the disease is the most likely explanation of the rare cases of myeloma kidney disease without detectable Bence Jones proteinuria.

CLINICAL AND PATHOPHYSIOLOGICAL ASPECTS

Clinically, the presence of Bence Jones proteins is of diagnostic and prognostic importance. Since Bence Jones proteins are highly suggestive of malignant B-cell diseases when present in large amounts, a thorough diagnostic evaluation is required when such proteins are found, and an unrewarding evaluation should be followed up regarding the possibility of subclinical monoclonal gammopathy that may become overt. The quantity of Bence Jones proteins excreted is usually correlated with both the development of monoclonal gammopathy renal disease and the type of underlying disorder. In highly concentrated urine specimens from patients with benign monoclonal gammopathies, low concentrations (0.25 to 6 mg per 100 ml) of light chains may be detectable [57], whereas levels of up to 20 gm per liter have been found in the urine from patients with multiple myeloma [56]. When urine that has been concentrated 300 to 500 times is tested, Bence Jones proteins are detectable in 73 to 87 percent of the specimens from patients with either multiple myeloma or Waldenström's macroglobulinemia [56, 57].

Perhaps more important are the prognostic implications of Bence Jones proteinuria. "Myeloma kidney" changes, which consist of tubules packed with proteinaceous hyaline material, protein within the tubular cells, and giant tubular cells, are closely associated with the excretion of Bence Jones proteins in most cases, and renal failure is the most common cause of death among myeloma patients. The λ chains may polymerize in the serum and may be present in the urine only in association with nonmyelomatous renal dysfunction [63]. In macroglobulinemia, uremia is a rare cause of death. The pathological aberrations seen in the myelomatous kidney appear to be due to the deposition of proteinaceous material in the tubular cells and the tubules [55, 65]. Since tubular precipitation may be related to protein concentration, maintaining a dilute urine is of utmost importance. Thus, a good fluid intake and avoiding tests that require dehydration (e.g., intravenous pyelography) [66, 67] are factors that may slow down renal involvement. In the case of intravenous pyelography, deposition of the contrast medium along with protein in the tubules may be an additive factor. Tubular reabsorption abnormalities in multiple myeloma may lead to a Fanconi-like syndrome [68, 69] with azotemia, hyperchloremic acidosis, hyperphosphatemia, glucosuria, and aminoaciduria. Additionally, hypercalciuria as well as hypercalcemia may coexist. In macroglobulinemia and cases of multiple myeloma without Bence Jones proteins, renal failure can be caused by intense plasma cell infiltrations in the renal parenchyma.

DIAGNOSIS

A variety of assays have been employed for the detection of Bence Jones proteins, including (1) screening tests for proteinuria (Heller's nitric acid ring test and the sulfosalicylic acid test), (2) the heat test, (3) cellulose-acetate electrophoresis, (4) immunoelectrophoresis, and (5) Ouchterlony double diffusion.

SCREENING TESTS

Heller's nitric acid ring test and the sulfosalicylic acid test were initially used for screening. However, since both of these assays detect proteins other than Bence Jones type, they represent only rough screening procedures for proteinuria and are relatively insensitive. It should also be noted that Albustix reagent may fail to detect Bence Jones proteins, even if present in large amounts, and thus it should not be relied upon for screening for Bence Jones proteins [70–72].

HEAT TEST

Snapper and Kahn [65] described a practical heat test in which a small amount of freshly collected and centrifuged urine is tested with 5 percent sulfosalicylic acid. No precipitation suggests the absence of Bence Jones proteins, whereas precipitation is compatible with, but not diagnostic of, their presence. If the sulfosalicylic acid test is positive, the pH of another aliquot of urine is tested with nitrazine paper. If the pH is above 5, it is adjusted with 4 percent acetic acid to pH 5. This urine is slowly heated in a test tube to 60°C in a water bath. If precipitation develops between 40° and 60°C, the presence of Bence Jones proteins is probable. An equal amount of 5 percent sulfosalicylic acid is added, which precipitates all protein in the urine and simultaneously adjusts the urine to pH 3. The urine, which contains a thick, white precipitate, is boiled over a flame; if the precipitate dissolves during boiling and reappears during cooling, the presence of Bence Jones proteins is confirmed (see Fig. 20-6). However, large amounts of other proteins, may obscure the thermoreactivity of Bence Jones proteins. Such proteins can be removed by filtration at temperature ranges near the boiling point or at room temperature, and the heat test is then repeated on such a filtered urine specimen.

Since immunological techniques have become almost universally available in laboratories, these assays have become the primary means of diagnosing Bence Jones proteins and have replaced the heat test for several reasons. Although the heat test is rapid and simple, it is relatively insensitive (it is unreliable at less than 0.5 gm per liter), and some positive urine samples may not show precipitation at temperatures much below the boiling point. False-positive heat tests may be encountered in patients who excrete large amounts of polyclonal (κ and λ) free L chains as a consequence of proximal tubular disease, such as that associated with lupus erythematosus. Furthermore, positive urine samples need to be typed because of the prognostic implications of κ-chain proteinuria, the monoclonal nature of the protein should be confirmed, and negative urine samples require that more sensitive tests be applied before considering them negative for Bence Jones proteins, especially if the clinical data suggest a monoclonal gammopathy.

ELECTROPHORESIS

The demonstration of a monoclonal urinary protein component in the γ- or β-globulin ranges by means of cellulose-acetate electrophoresis

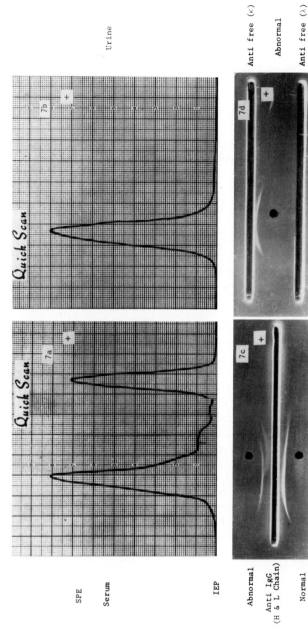

Figure 20-7
Electrophoretic (*top*) and immunoelectrophoretic (*bottom*) assay patterns for Bence Jones proteins.

provides suggestive evidence for the presence of Bence Jones proteins (Fig. 20-7). The frequent need for concentrating the urine prior to electrophoresis renders this test impractical and unreliable, and, in fact, it may be less sensitive than the heat test, which uses unconcentrated urines (see Chaps. 5 and 19).

IMMUNODIAGNOSIS

Bence Jones proteins may be positively identified in serum or urine, even if present in small amounts, by immunoelectrophoresis (IEP) (see Fig. 20-7) or Ouchterlony double diffusion (see Chap. 5) using specific antisera to κ and λ light chains. On IEP, a significant increase of either κ or λ chains is demonstrable, and the electrophoretic position corresponds to the scoop seen on serum IEP using light chain–specific antisera. Usually, the uninvolved light chains are reduced in amount [73–75]. Ouchterlony double diffusion may be performed according to Figure 5-2 (Chap. 5). A precipitin arc between the center (antibody) well and the IgG precipitin line is indicative of the presence of Bence Jones proteins. The availability of rehydratable agarose film has further simplified this immunotest for Bence Jones proteins and has allowed its use in the general clinical laboratory [75]. Using anti-IgG serum containing anti-γ, anti-κ, and anti-λ antibodies, a scooped heavy precipitin line is seen on IEP, with the Bence Jones proteins being indicated by a short precipitin arc at the convex side of the anodic part of the IgG precipitin line and fusing with it (see Chap. 5).

With the Ouchterlony technique, false-positive tests may be obtained when testing sera from patients with IgA monoclonal gammopathy because of the diffusion rate of this immunoglobulin and the immunological cross-reactivity that occurs with the light-chain antibodies. False-negative tests may be encountered occasionally when using serum or urine specimens that have been stored for lengthy periods of time, when using antiserum with low antibody titer to light chains or when dealing with antigen excess. It is therefore imperative to examine serum or urine samples at different concentrations and dilutions, e.g., 100:1 to 1:200.

One of the more difficult diagnostic problems arises in patients who excrete intact immunoglobulin molecules as well as Bence Jones protein in the urine. In these cases, Ouchterlony double-diffusion tests may be diagnostic. IEP may be helpful if only a small precipitin arc is seen with heavy-chain-specific antisera and a heavy scooped arc is demonstrated with κ- or λ-specific antisera. However, when examining urine specimens containing large quantities of intact monoclonal globulin, gel-filtration column chromatography on Sephadex G-200 may be required. With this technique, the low molecular weight Bence Jones proteins are eluted as a shoulder or peak following the albumin fraction [54, 65]. Final confirmation is made by detection of monoclonal light chains in the eluates from this fraction by the employment of IEP with light-chain antisera. Gel-filtration column chromatography may also be used to confirm Bence Jones proteinemia, and it is most beneficial in the unusual cases of Bence Jones myeloma without Bence Jones proteinuria, which may have either an M spike in the α_2- or β-globulin zone on serum electrophoresis or no M protein demonstrable on electrophoresis.

THERAPEUTIC CONSIDERATIONS

Quantitative reduction of Bence Jones proteins is dependent upon successful therapy of the causative disorder (such as myeloma therapy). However, in addition to specific chemotherapy, maintaining good hydration (especially avoiding pyelography) and maintaining an alkaline urine pH are often beneficial in prolonging the onset of renal complications.

References

1. West, E. B.   Identification and Measurement of Thermoproteins (Cryoglobulin, Pyroglobulin, Cryofibrinogen). In F. W. Sunderman and F. W. Sunderman, Jr. (Eds.), *Serum Proteins and the Dysproteinemias.* Philadelphia: Lippincott, 1964. Pp. 217–222.
2. Ritzmann, S. E., and Levin, W. C.   Cryopathies: A review. Classification, diagnostic and therapeutic considerations. *Arch. Intern. Med.* 107: 186, 1961.
3. Kenamore, B. D., Levin, W. C., and Ritzmann, S. E.   Raynaud's phenomenon as leading sign in lupus erythematosus. Report of three cases and classification of cryopathies. *Tex. Rep. Biol. Med.* 26:189, 1968.
4. Moroz, L. A., and Rose, B.   The Cryopathies. In M. Samter (Ed.), *Immunological Diseases* (2nd ed.). Boston: Little, Brown, 1971. Pp. 459–482.
5. Pirofsky, B.   *Autosensitization and the Autoimmune Hemolytic Anemias.* Baltimore: Williams & Wilkins, 1969. Pp. 262–279.
6. Wintrobe, M. M., and Buell, M. V.   Hyperproteinemia associated with multiple myeloma: with report of a case in which an extraordinary hyperproteinemia was associated with thrombosis of the retinal veins and symptoms suggesting Raynaud's disease. *Bull. Johns Hopkins Hosp.* 52:156, 1933.
7. Lerner, A. B., and Watson, C. J.   Unusual purpura associated with the presence of a high concentration of cryoglobulin (cold precipitable serum globulin). *Am. J. Med. Sci.* 214:410, 1947.
8. Lerner, A. B., Barnum, C. P., and Watson, C. J.   Studies of cryoglobulins. II. The spontaneous precipitation of protein from serum at 5°C in various states. *Am. J. Med. Sci.* 214:416, 1947.
9. Lospalluto, J., Dorward, B., Miller, W., and Ziff, M.   Cryoglobulinemia based on interaction between gamma-macroglobulin and 7S gamma-globulin. *Am. J. Med.* 32:142, 1962.
10. Peetoom, F., and Van Loghem-Langereis, E.   IgM-IgG (β_2M-7Sγ) cryoglobulinemia. An autoimmune phenomenon. *Vox Sang.* 10:281, 1965.
11. Meltzer, M., Franklin, E. E., Elias, K., McCluskey, R. T., and Cooper, N.   Cryoglobulinemia. A clinical and laboratory study. *Am. J. Med.* 40:837, 1966.
12. Klein, F., van Rood, J. J., Van Furth, R., and Radema, H.   IgM-IgG cryoglobulinemia with IgM paraprotein component. *Clin. Exp. Immunol.* 3:703, 1968.
13. Cream, J. J., Howard, A., and Virella, G.   IgG heavy chain sub-classes in mixed cryoglobulins. *Immunology* 23:405, 1972.
14. Waldenström, J., Winblad, S., Hällen, J., and Liungman, S.   The occur-

rence of serological "antibody" reagins or similar γ-globulins in conditions with monoclonal hypergammaglobulinemia, such as myeloma, macroglobulinemia, etc. *Acta Med. Scand.* 176:619, 1964.

15. Barnett, E. V., Bluestone, R., Cracchiolo, A., Goldberg, L. S., Kantor, G. L., and McIntosh, R. M. Cryoglobulinemia and disease. *Ann. Intern. Med.* 73:95, 1970.

16. Golde, D., and Epstein, W. Mixed cryoglobulins and glomerulonephritis. *Ann. Intern. Med.* 69:1221, 1968.

17. Mathison, D. A., Condemi, J. J., Leddy, J. P., Callerame, M. L., Panner, B. J., and Vaughan, J. H. Purpura, arthralgia, and IgM-IgG cryoglobulinemia with rheumatoid factor activity. Response to cyclophosphamide and splenectomy. *Ann. Intern. Med.* 74:383, 1971.

18. Miescher, P. A., Paronetto, F., and Koffler, D. Immunofluorescent Studies in Human Vasculitis. In P. A. Miescher and T. Grabar (Eds.), *Proceedings of the Fourth International Symposium on Immunopathology.* New York: Grune & Stratton, 1965. Pp. 446–456.

19. Riethmüller, G., Meltzer, M., Franklin, E. C., and Miescher, P. A. Serum complement levels in patients with mixed (IgM-IgG) cryoglobulins. *Clin. Exp. Immunol.* 1:337, 1966.

20. Wells, R. Syndromes of hyperviscosity. *N. Engl. J. Med.* 283:183, 1970.

21. Wells, A. E., Merrill, E. W., and Gabelnick, H. Shear-rate dependence of viscosity of blood: Interaction of red cells and plasma proteins. *Trans. Soc. Rheology* 6:19, 1962.

22. Wells, R. E. The Effects of Plasma Proteins upon the Rheology of Blood in the Microcirculation. In A. L. Copley (Ed.), *Proceedings of the Fourth International Congress on Rheology,* Part 4. New York: Wiley, 1965. Pp. 431–438.

23. Bernstein, E. F., Castenada, A., Evans, R. L., and Varco, R. L. Alterations in red blood cell charge with extracorporeal circulation. *Surg. Forum* 13:193, 1962.

24. Ritzmann, S. E., Thurm, R. H., Truax, W. E., and Levin, W. C. The syndrome of macroglobulinemia: Review of literature and report of 2 cases of macroglobulinemia. *Arch. Intern. Med.* 105:939, 1960.

25. Wolf, R. E., Riedel, L. O., Levin, W. C., and Ritzmann, S. E. Remission of macroglobulinemia coincident with hepatitis: Report of case and review of literature. *Arch. Intern. Med.* 130:392, 1972.

26. Smith, E., Kochwa, S., and Wasserman, L. R. Aggregation of IgG *in vivo:* I. The hyperviscosity syndrome in multiple myeloma. *Am. J. Med.* 39:35, 1965.

27. Kopp, W. L., Beirne, G. J., and Burns, R. D. Hyperviscosity syndrome in multiple myeloma. *Am. J. Med.* 43:141, 1967.

28. Wolf, R. E., Alperin, J. B., Ritzmann, S. E., and Levin, W. C. IgG-κ-multiple myeloma with hyperviscosity syndrome—Response to plasmapheresis. *Arch. Intern. Med.* 129:114, 1972.

29. Sugai, S. IgA pyroglobulin, hyperviscosity syndrome and coagulation abnormality in a patient with multiple myeloma. *Blood* 39:224, 1972.

30. Pruzanski, W., and Watt, J. G. Serum viscosity and hyperviscosity syndrome in IgG multiple myeloma. *Ann. Intern. Med.* 77:853, 1972.

31. Jasin, H. E., Lospalluto, J., and Ziff, M. Rheumatoid hyperviscosity syndrome. *Am. J. Med.* 49:484, 1970.

32. Wolf, R. E., Ritzmann, S. E., and Levin, W. C. Rheumatoid factors and serum immune complexes. Unpublished data, 1970.

33. Abruzzo, J. L., Heimer, R., and Giuliano, V. The hyperviscosity syn-

drome, polysynovitis, polymyositis, and an unusual 13S serum IgG component. *Am. J. Med.* 49:258, 1970.

34. Blaylock, W. M., Waller, M., and Normansell, D. E. Sjögren's syndrome: Hyperviscosity and intermediate complexes. *Ann. Intern. Med.* 80:27, 1974.

35. Alarcón-Segovia, D., Fishbein, E., Abruzzo, J. L., and Heimer, R. Serum hyperviscosity in Sjögren's syndrome. *Ann. Intern. Med.* 80:35, 1974.

36. Solomon, A., and Fahey, J. L. Plasmapheresis therapy in macroglobulinemia. *Ann. Intern. Med.* 58:789, 1963.

37. Fahey, J. L., Barth, W. F., and Solomon, A. Serum hyperviscosity syndrome. *J.A.M.A.* 192:464, 1965.

38. Rosenblum, W. I., and Asofsky, R. M. Malfunction of cerebral microcirculation in macroglobulinemic mice: Relationship to increased blood viscosity. *Arch. Neurol.* 18:151, 1958.

39. Wanner, J., and Siebenmann, R. Über eine subakut verlaufende osteolytische Form der Makroglobulinämie Waldenström mit Plasmazellenleukämie. *Schweiz. Med. Wochenschr.* 87:1243, 1957.

40. Zollinger, H. V. Die pathologische Anatomie der Makroglobulinämie Waldenström. *Helv. Med. Acta* 25:153, 1958.

41. Williams, R. J., Jr. The hyperviscosity syndromes (Editorial). *Circulation* 38:450, 1968.

42. Ritzmann, S. E., Daniels, J. C., and Levin, W. C. Paralymphomatous Disease. Syndrome of Macroglobulinemia. In *Leukemia-Lymphoma.* (A collection of papers presented at the 14th Annual Clinical Conference on Cancer, 1969, at the University of Texas M. D. Anderson Hospital and Tumor Institute, Houston.) Chicago: Year Book, 1970. Pp. 169–222.

43. Schwab, P. J., and Fahey, J. L. Treatment of Waldenström's macroglobulinemia by plasmapheresis. *N. Engl. J. Med.* 263:574, 1960.

44. Schwab, P. J., Okun, E., and Fahey, J. L. Reversal of retinopathy in Waldenström's macroglobulinemia by plasmapheresis: Report of two cases. *Arch. Ophthalmol.* 64:515, 1960.

45. Skoog, W. A., and Adams, W. S. Plasmapheresis in a case of Waldenström's macroglobulinemia. *Clin. Res.* 7:96, 1959.

46. Houston, E. W., Ritzmann, S. E., and Levin, W. C. Chromosomal aberrations common to three types of monoclonal gammopathies. *Blood* 29:214, 1967.

47. Ellinger, A. Das Vorkommen von Bence Jones' schen Körpern in Harn bei Tumoren des Knochenmarks und seine diagnostische Bedeutung. *Dtsch. Arch. Klin. Med.* 62:255, 1898.

48. Martin, W. J., and Mathieson, D. R. Pyroglobulinemia (heat-coagulable globulin in the blood). *Proc. Mayo Clinic* 28:545, 1953.

49. Martin, W. J., Mathieson, D. R., and Eigler, J. O. C. Pyroglobulinemia: Further observations and review of 23 cases. *Proc. Mayo Clinic* 34:99, 1959.

50. Solomon, J., and Steinfeld, J. L. Pyroglobulinemia. Report of a case, with protein turnover studies. *Am. J. Med.* 28:937, 1965.

51. Bence Jones, H. On a new substance occurring in the urine of a patient with mollities ossium. *Phil. Trans. London* 138:55, 1848.

52. Clamp, J. R. Some aspects of the first recorded case of multiple myeloma. *Lancet* 2:1354, 1969.

53. Schwartz, J. H., and Edelman, G. M. Comparison of Bence Jones pro-

teins and L polypeptide chains of myeloma globulins after hydrolysis with trypsin. *J. Exp. Med.* 118:41, 1963.

54. Berggård, I., and Peterson, P. Immunoglobulin Components in Normal Human Urine. In J. Killander (Ed.), *Nobel Symposium 3, Gamma Globulins, Structure and Control of Biosynthesis.* Stockholm: Almquist and Wiksell, 1967. Pp. 71–78.
55. Solomon, A., and Fahey, J. L. Bence Jones proteinemia. *Am. J. Med.* 37:206, 1964.
56. Dammacco, F., and Waldenström, J. G. Serum and urine light chain levels in benign monoclonal gammopathies, multiple myeloma, and Waldenström's macroglobulinemia. *Clin. Exp. Immunol.* 3:911, 1968.
57. Hobbs, J. R. Paraproteins, benign or malignant? *Br. Med. J.* 3:699, 1967.
58. Williams, R. C., Jr., Brunning, R. D., and Wollheim, F. A. Light chain disease. An abortive variant of multiple myeloma. *Ann. Intern. Med.* 65:471, 1966.
59. Osserman, E. F., Graff, A., Marshall, M., Lawlor, D., and Graff, S. Incorporation of N^{15}-L-aspartic acid into the abnormal serum and urine proteins of multiple myeloma. *J. Clin. Invest.* 36:352, 1957.
60. Putnam, F. W., and Hardy, S. Proteins in multiple myeloma: II. Origin of Bence Jones proteins. *J. Biol. Chem.* 212:361, 1955.
61. Solomon, A., Waldmann, T. A., Fahey, J. L., and MacFarlane, A. S. Metabolism of Bence Jones proteins. *J. Clin. Invest.* 43:103, 1964.
62. Strober, W., Blaese, R. M., and Waldmann, T. A. Abnormalities of Immunoglobulin Metabolism. In M. A. Rothschild and T. A. Waldmann (Eds.), *Plasma Protein Metabolism. Regulation of Synthesis, Distribution and Degradation.* New York: Academic, 1970. Pp. 287–305.
63. Grey, H. M., and Kohler, P. F. A case of tetramer Bence Jones proteinemia. *Clin. Exp. Immunol.* 31:277, 1968.
64. Waldenström, J. G. *Monoclonal and Polyclonal Hypergammaglobulinemia. Clinical and Biological Significance.* Nashville: Vanderbilt University Press, 1968. Pp. 49–64.
65. Snapper, I., and Kahn, A. I. Multiple myeloma. *Semin. Hematol.* 1:87, 1964.
66. Bartels, E. D., Brun, G. C., Gammeltoft, A., and Gjørup, P. A. Acute anuria following intravenous pyelography in patient with myelomatosis. *Acta Med. Scand.* 150:297, 1954.
67. Perille, P. E., and Conn, H. O. Acute renal failure after intravenous pyelography in plasma cell myeloma. *J.A.M.A.* 167:2186, 1968.
68. Sirota, J. H., and Hamerman, D. J. Renal function studies in adults with Fanconi syndrome. *Am. J. Med.* 16:138, 1954.
69. Engle, R. L., and Wallis, L. A. Multiple myeloma and adult Fanconi syndrome. I. Report of case with crystal-like deposits in tumor cells and in epithelial cells of kidney. *Am. J. Med.* 22:5, 1957.
70. Clough, G., and Reah, T. G. A "protein error." *Lancet* 1:1248, 1964.
71. Huhnstock, K. Paraproteinurien mit negativem Ausfall des Albustix-Testes. *Klin. Wochenschr.* 40:1009, 1962.
72. Smith, J. K. The significance of the "protein error" of indicators in the diagnosis of Bence Jones proteinuria. *Acta Haematol.* (Basel) 30:144, 1963.
73. Korngold, L. Abnormal plasma components and their significance in disease. *Ann. N.Y. Acad. Sci.* 94:110, 1961.
74. Tan, M., and Epstein, W. V. A direct immunologic assay of human

sera for Bence Jones proteins (L-chains). *J. Lab. Clin. Med.* 66:344, 1965.

75. Ritzmann, S. E., Lawrence, M. C., and Daniels, J. C. Thermoproteins. In J. B. Fuller (Ed.), *ASCP Workshop Manual, Selected Topics in Clinical Chemistry* (4th ed.). Chicago: American Society of Clinical Pathologists' Commission on Continuing Education, 1973. Pp. 1–155.

Embryonic and Fetal Proteins Associated with Human Neoplasia 21

Robert M. Nakamura and Stephan E. Ritzmann

Tumor-Associated Antigens

When a cell undergoes neoplastic changes, certain antigenic and surface membrane alterations occur. Antigens that are present in tumor cells but absent in normal cells have been termed *tumor-specific antigens*. The antigens that are able to induce an immune response or resistance to tumor growth in the autochthonous host have been called *tumor-specific transplantation antigens* [1]. It has been shown that several of the tumor antigens may be seen in normal tissue, depending upon the age and types of normal cells examined. For example, certain antigens have been found in fetal and tumor tissue and are not found in normal adult tissue. Thus, the term *tumor-associated antigen* is a more appropriate one, since the antigen associated with the tumor can be qualitatively, quantitatively, or temporally different from normal cells [1].

Embryonic or Fetal Protein Antigens

During the events of carcinogenesis, a depressive dedifferentiation [2–4] or retrogenetic expression [5] has been postulated that leads to an increased expression of the genetic information, which is normally repressed in the mature cell. There is a reversion of the cell to the embryonic form, and fetal proteins are formed. The fetal proteins may broadly be separated into two groups:

1. *Macromolecules that can pass from the tumor into biological fluid and are found in the circulation.* These fetal proteins may or may not be observed in normal adult tissue. An unresponsive state exists in normal adults to the majority of these types of fetal proteins, since they do not evoke an immunological reaction.

2. *Macromolecules that have not been shown to pass from the tumor into body fluids.* These fetal proteins may be found in the interior of the cell or associated with plasma membranes, and they may evoke immunological reactions in a tumor-bearing host [6]. There has been increasing

evidence that very small amounts of fetal proteins may be found in adults with diseases other than cancer. However, emphasis will be placed on those fetal proteins that are found in tumors and are released into biological fluids.

The quantitative measurement of fetal proteins in the circulation has become important in the study of human tumors. The presence of a large amount of a fetal antigen in the circulation, such as α_1-fetoprotein, may be diagnostic evidence of a liver embryonal cell carcinoma. However, extremely small amounts of the fetal antigen, may be found in normal individuals and in those with other benign conditions [6, 7].

Clinically Significant Embryonic or Fetal Proteins in Human Cancer

Many of the fetal proteins formed in human tumors are released into biological fluids. Thus, the detection and quantitative measurement of these antigens have become helpful for the diagnosis of malignancy, the monitoring of therapy for cancer, and the evaluation of prognosis.

Lawrence and Munro Neville [7] have outlined four criteria that a specific fetal protein should fulfill before it can be clinically useful. Some of the desired characteristics are: (1) the fetal protein should pass from the tumor into body fluids and ideally persist in circulation; (2) the fetal protein should be associated with certain specific types of tumors (e.g., α_1-fetoprotein is associated with hepatocellular carcinoma and embryonal cell carcinoma)—ideally, the fetal protein should be specific for a particular category of tumor and not seen in other diseases in the absence of cancer; (3) the fetal protein levels should correlate directly with the repression, removal, or recurrence of the tumor; and (4) the fetal protein should be easily quantifiable in the clinical laboratory.

None of the presently known fetal antigens fulfills all of the above criteria. A fetal protein antigen that is specific for a single type of tumor has not been found.

The fetal proteins that are associated with human tumors and found in biological fluids are (1) α_1-fetoprotein antigen, which is produced in the liver and hepatomas [8–10]; α_2-H ferroprotein, which is found in the sera of children and adults with tumors [11, 12]; β-S fetoprotein [13, 14]; Regan alkaline phosphatase (placental alkaline phosphatase) [15–17]; fetal sulfoglycoprotein antigen [18–20]; γ-fetoprotein [21, 22]; and carcinoembryonic antigens (CEA) of the gastrointestinal (GI) tract [23, 24].

α_1-FETOPROTEIN

Normally, the α_1-fetoprotein (AFP) is synthesized in the fetus at 14 to 40 weeks of gestation, and the level of AFP declines rapidly after 2 weeks of age [25, 26]. The AFP is produced by embryonic liver and yolk sac tissues. It has been found in the serum of adults, primarily in association with hepatocellular cancer of the liver and embryonic tumors of the ovary and testes [8, 9, 27–29]. Immunofluorescence studies have shown that fetoprotein is present in human fetal liver and hepatoma tissue [30].

More recently, serum AFP has been detected in cases of gastric carcinoma and prostatic carcinoma [31–33], viral hepatitis [26], and cirrhosis [34]. Thus, it appears that the relative specificity of AFP for hepatomas and embryonal carcinomas is a quantitative phenomenon. Of 380 patients with the diagnosis of hepatoma, 159 (68 percent) had positive tests for serum AFP [35]. Of 355 patients with a neoplasm other than primary hepatoma, only 3.1 percent had positive tests for AFP, and each of these patients had a teratoblastoma [35].

The diagnostic usefulness of AFP detection in serum for the confirmation of a suspected diagnosis of primary liver cancer is well documented [27–29]. Most commonly, agar-gel double-diffusion methods are used, and the sensitivity of the test is approximately 0.1 to 0.3 mg AFP per 100 ml [7, 34, 36] (see Chap. 5). Such levels of AFP are almost always associated with liver or embryonic tumors.

More recently, Abelev [10] has used aggregated hemagglutination and immunoautoradiography to detect AFP levels of 50 ng per milliliter. With the more sensitive radioimmunoassay (RIA) method, levels of AFP down to 0.25 ng per milliliter have been detected [37].

When a sensitive immunoassay procedure is employed, AFP has been detected in apparently normal individuals [34, 36, 37]. Levels in the order of 25 ng per milliliter of AFP have been found in normal persons [38]. AFP levels in the sera of pregnant women at different stages of gestation may range from 100 to 800 ng per milliliter, and are presumed to be of fetal origin [34].

Thus, tests for AFP in serum must be interpreted in light of the method of assay used, and they must also be correlated with the clinical history and physical findings in each particular patient. The quantitative assay of AFP would certainly be of value in the diagnosis and therapeutic monitoring of patients with hepatocellular carcinoma and embryonal cell carcinoma.

Case Report
A 56-year-old, severely jaundiced alcoholic male was admitted with massive ascites. Palmar erythema, testicular atrophy, mild gynecomastia, and numerous spider angiomas were present. The liver was enlarged to the iliac crest. All liver function studies were severely deranged, and a liver scan revealed a 10 cm by 10 cm area of absent radionucleide uptake (i.e., a "cold spot"). Refractory ascites precluded liver biopsy. Examination of the serum was negative for Australia antigen but positive for α_1-fetoprotein. Despite vigorous treatment, the patient went into hepatic coma shortly after admission and died. At autopsy, a large hepatoma was found in the right lobe of the liver (Fig. 21-1).
Final Diagnosis: Hepatoma.

α_2-H FERROPROTEIN
The α_2-H globulin is a protein that is formed in the liver and found in the fetal organs and serum. It is a 17S iron-containing protein [38a], and, with the use of radioimmunodiffusion, one can measure levels of

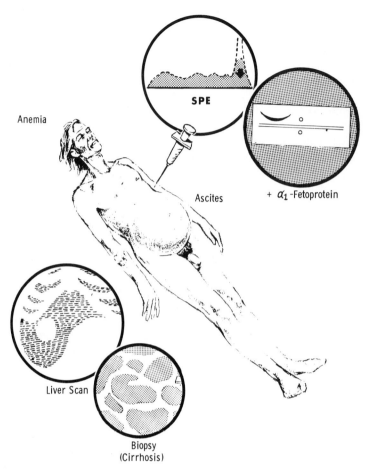

Anemia

SPE

Ascites

+ α_1-Fetoprotein

Liver Scan

Biopsy
(Cirrhosis)

Figure 21-1
Clinical manifestations of AFP-positive hepatoma (see Case Report).

1.5 ng per milliliter of it in the serum [11]. Elevated levels of α_2-H ferroprotein are uncommon in children with noncancerous diseases, but they have been observed in a wide variety of childhood tumors, such as nephroblastoma, neuroblastoma, leukemia, hepatoma, teratoma, lymphomas, osteogenic sarcoma, and brain tumors. There was no correlation between the levels of α_2-H ferroprotein and tumor groups with respect to cell type or location. On the other hand, 8 percent of 122 children with noncancerous diseases had positive results [11, 12, 14].

By conventional serological methods, the protein has not been detected in normal children beyond the age of 2 months. With the use of a radioimmunodiffusion method, the protein was demonstrated in the sera of 81 percent of 334 children with malignant tumors [11].

Elevated serum values of α_2-H ferroprotein were observed in adults with various tumors, including hepatoma, cholangiocarcinoma, and lymphoma. A few adults who have liver disease, without evidence of tumor, may show evidence of elevated α_2-H ferroprotein.

The α_2-H ferroprotein levels are known to rise before or with a recurrence of the tumor [11]; however, further investigation is needed with regard to the correlation between α_2-H ferroprotein levels and successful therapy [7].

β-S FETOPROTEIN

The β-S fetoprotein is a glycoprotein that is found in the cytoplasm of fetal liver cells. This fetoprotein has been detected in the sera of patients with hepatocarcinoma, cholangiocarcinoma, gastric carcinoma, and leukemia and lymphoma [13, 14]. As with other fetal antigens such as α_1-fetoprotein, elevated serum levels were noted in liver diseases without the presence of cancer. The correlation of serum levels of β-S fetoprotein with the removal of tumor remains to be established.

REGAN ALKALINE PHOSPHATASE

An isoenzyme of alkaline phosphatase that is normally absent from adult tissue has been found in the serum of 12 percent of cancer patients [14–16, 39]. The isoenzyme was named for a patient with bronchial carcinoma in whom it was first discovered (Regan), and it is biochemically and immunologically similar to placental alkaline phosphatase. It is identical to placental alkaline phosphatase with respect to L-phenylalanine sensitivity and heat stability at 65°C. The Regan enzyme is probably a product of the tumor, and minute amounts of enzyme may be present in the sera of cancer patients. The Regan isoenzyme is not organ-specific, and it has been observed in many cancer patients with a wide variety of cellular types, including cancers of the lung, ovary, testicle, liver, colon, and uterus, as well as lymphomas [39–42].

Usategui-Gomez and associates [43] have developed an assay to quantitate extremely small amounts of Regan alkaline phosphatase. An antibody is produced to the Regan isoenzyme and is polymerized into a solid immunoadsorbant pellet with ethylchloroformate [44]. The immunoadsorbant allows a tenfold to twentyfold concentration of the Regan isoenzyme by reaction with the antibody. The pellet is then assayed for enzymatic activity, since the antibody complex with the enzyme does not interfere with the enzymatic activity. Using this sensitive assay, the Regan isoenzyme has been noted in normal individuals. The average value obtained in normal sera was 0.29 ± 0.21 international units (IU) per milliliter. Cancer patients with abnormal levels may have 5 to 300 times the average normal value [45]. Thus, Regan alkaline phosphatase may be another fetal antigen that is found in significant amounts in fetal, embryonic, or tumor tissue. Determinations of Regan alkaline phosphatase may provide a reliable means of monitoring the progression or regression of certain tumors during therapy.

FETAL SULFOGLYCOPROTEIN

A sulfoglycoprotein (FSA) present in fetal gut, which has blood group substance A activity, has been found in the gastric juice of patients with

carcinoma of the stomach [18, 19]. FSA is one of three sulfoglycopro-
teins found in the intestinal tract of human fetuses, and it is specifically
located in the superficial epithelial cells of the fetal stomach. FSA is
found in the gastric juice of 0 to 6.67 percent of a normal population between 45 to 65 years of age [18, 19]. However, the antigen is usually
absent in the younger adult. FSA appears to share with carcinoembryonic antigen a common antigenic determinant, which, however, is not
the colon cancer-specific determinant of the carcinoembryonic antigen
molecule [20]. FSA in gastric secretion was found to precede the development of definite cancer cells, and a relationship of FSA to carcinogenesis has been suggested. The detection of FSA in the young adult
population may be helpful in suspected cases of stomach cancer. Upon
removal of gastric carcinoma, however, the FSA levels in the gastric
juice may not disappear [7].

γ-FETOPROTEIN

A fetal protein (γFP), which is distinct from α_1-fetoprotein and carcinoembryonic antigen (CEA), has been found in association with human
neoplasms as well as some tissues of the normal fetus [21, 22]. The
γFP was present in 75 percent of a wide variety of benign and malignant
human tumors, in the sera of 11 percent (23 of 210) of such patients,
and in 2 of 101 specimens of non-neoplastic diseased tissue. The antigen
was not detected by immunodiffusion tests in human tissue or in sera
from normal adults. The γFP does not show species specificity. It has
been reported in the sera of 4 of 6 other mammalian species; however, no tumors of these animals were γFP positive [21, 22]. The
original serum in which γFP was detected had been obtained from a
49-year-old patient with localized medullary carcinoma of the breast.
Antibodies to γFP occur very infrequently, since only 8 of 1030 cancer
patients had evidence of serum antibodies to γFP [21]. The correlation
of serum levels of γFP with therapy is unknown. With the advent of a
more sensitive test than immunodiffusion, one might detect the presence
of γFP in a larger percentage of cancer cases.

CARCINOEMBRYONIC ANTIGEN

IMMUNOCHEMICAL NATURE

The immunochemical properties of carcinoembryonic antigen (CEA)
were discovered by Gold and Freedman in 1965 [23, 24]. CEA was
found to be present in adenocarcinomas of the GI tract as well as in the
embryonic and fetal digestive systems during the first two trimesters of
gestation [3, 23, 34]. The CEA is detected on the surface of the intestinal tumor cells and fetal cells by fluorescence microscopy [46, 47].
CEA was noted to be present in the glycocalices of intestinal cells [47,
48]. Immunofluorescence studies of colonic mucosa in children, ages 1
to 7 years, showed that CEA is a native antigen in the colonic mucosa
[49].

Excellent preparations of CEA have been isolated from tumors of the digestive tract [50, 51], and two molecular sizes (6.8S and 10.1S) have been found. The 6.8S molecule is the one that is usually present in the various tumors [50]. Physicochemical characterization of CEA has indicated it is a glycoprotein that exhibits heterogeneity with immunological identity [52]. Amino-acid sequence studies of CEA preparations from two different tumors suggest that the polypeptide chains are identical [53]. However, the material carrying the CEA activity, may or may not be identical with the protein [53]. A heterosaccharide grouping with a high content of N-acetyl glucosamine may be the major immunological determinant of CEA [54]. The CEA preparations have been found to cross-react with a glycoprotein of normal tissue [55, 56] and the FSA antigen of gastric juice from cancer patients [20].

CONTROVERSY OF POSSIBLE HUMAN ANTI-CEA ANTIBODIES

There has been some controversy as to the existence and nature of CEA antibodies in human patients. In 1967, with the use of a bis-diazotized benzidine hemagglutination technique, Gold [57] demonstrated IgM anti-CEA antibodies in 70 percent of 30 patients with nonmetastatic digestive system cancers and in approximately 70 percent of 18 women in all trimesters of pregnancy. Burtin and co-workers [58, 59] showed that circulating antibodies in patients with colon-rectal cancer could be absorbed by preparations of normal bowel tissue. Other investigators could not demonstrate circulating antibodies to CEA in patients with GI malignancies using a sensitive radioimmunoassay method [58, 60]. Gold and co-workers [61] demonstrated by the use of a radioimmunoelectrophoresis method that anti-CEA antibodies were present in patients with digestive and nondigestive system cancers and in pregnant women. Further, there was some degree of cross-reactivity between CEA and blood group A substance, with anti-A antibodies combined with CEA [61]. The addition of blood group A substance fails to alter the binding of anti-CEA antisera to ^{125}I CEA. This differentiates the A-like site of the CEA from the major antigenic site. The human CEA antibodies do not appear to play any significant role in the protection of the host against the tumor.

There is some evidence that the immune response to CEA in the adult host is not significant. The in vitro tests of lymphocyte functions from patients with CEA-positive GI cancer failed to demonstrate transformation and altered tritiated thymidine incorporation [62]. With the use of the colony inhibition assay, Hellström et al. [63] have demonstrated cellular sensitivity of the lymphocytes of patients with GI cancer against human colonic carcinoma.

Skin reactions of the delayed hypersensitivity type were observed in 17 of 19 patients with carcinoma of the colon and rectum when soluble membrane fractions of autochthonous tumor cells were used as antigens [64]. Further studies of the soluble fractions of human intestinal tumors showed that the skin-reactive intestinal cancer antigen was separate and distinct from CEA [65].

LOCALIZATION OF CEA BY IMMUNOFLUORESCENCE IN NORMAL AND TUMOR TISSUE

The CEA antigen was noted to be on the surfaces and glycocalices of intestinal tumors, fetal cells [47], and colonic cells of normal children [49]. Burtin and co-workers [66] studied intestinal polyps of various histological types by immunofluorescence. They detected CEA-reactive antigen in normal intestinal mucosa as well as in all intestinal polyps, independent of their states of differentiation. The CEA appeared more abundant in differentiated polyps than in the undifferentiated polyps. The localization of CEA in normal tissue may be explained by the presence of normal glycoproteins that can cross-react with CEA [55, 56].

ASSAY FOR CIRCULATING CEA IN EVALUATING HUMAN NEOPLASMS

A hemagglutination inhibition test has been reported for CEA [67]. Preliminary results showed that tests of all 33 patients with endodermally derived carcinoma gave positive results. Also, positive results were seen in some control patients and in 60 percent of patients with rectal polyps, chronic ulcerative colitis, and cirrhosis.

Thompson and co-workers [68] developed a radioimmunoassay (RIA) for CEA. Briefly, the method involves perchloric acid extraction of glycoproteins from the serum. The material is then dialyzed, lyophilized, and converted to a powdered extract. The powdered extract is added to a known anti-CEA antibody and radiolabeled CEA system. The unknown CEA in the perchloric acid extract is quantitated by the inhibition RIA procedure, and the bound and unbound CEA are separated by the coprecipitation of antibody-bound CEA with 50 percent ammonium sulfate.

This method can detect a level of 2.5 ng CEA per milliliter. Circulating CEA up to 320 ng per milliliter may be observed in patients with adenocarcinoma of the colon and rectum [68, 69]. Preoperative levels of serum CEA in cases of colon or rectal cancer may range from 5 to 160 ng per milliliter.

Several investigators [70, 71] used a CEA radioimmunoassay that detects an antigenic site on CEA which is exposed at low ionic strength. Since CEA was found in the serum of patients with either endodermal or ectodermal tumors, they postulated an antigenic site on CEA that was common to several types of tumors [71]. This assay requires perchloric acid extraction of plasma and zirconyl phosphate, which is used to separate antibody-bound CEA from unbound CEA in the RIA procedure.

RIA that can be used directly on serum, which is more adaptable for screening procedures in the clinical laboratory, has been developed by Egan et al. [72, 73] and MacSween et al. [74]. The RIA described by Egan et al. [72, 73] utilizes a double-antibody method for the separation of the bound and unbound CEA, and it may be performed within one day with a 0.2 ml of serum sample. The assay described by MacSween et al. [74] utilized a 25 μ serum sample and requires at least two days; it also utilizes a double-antibody technique. In both of the procedures, one avoids the time-consuming perchloric acid extraction, dialysis, and concentration of the CEA.

Lawrence et al. [75, 76] used a modification of the procedure described by Egan et al. [72, 73] and compared it to the procedure of LoGerfo et al. [71]. Lawrence et al. [75] noted that the upper limit of the normal range, which was 2.5 ng CEA per milliliter by the method of LoGerfo et al. [71], was 12.5 ng CEA per milliliter of plasma [75], and the values of 9 and 24 ng per milliliter of LoGerfo's method corresponded to values of 20 and 40 ng per milliliter.

By the use of a sensitive RIA procedure, Chu et al. [77] demonstrated CEA in normal human plasma. The level of plasma CEA in so-called normal individuals is believed to be 2.5 ng per milliliter [71, 78]. In an extensive study by Reynoso et al. [78], elevated CEA levels were noted in 39 of 48 patients with GI cancers and 90 of 281 with nonentodermally derived tumors.

Other investigators have reported elevated serum CEA levels in a wide variety of diseases other than malignancy, such as severe alcoholic cirrhosis, uremia, and benign inflammatory conditions of the bowel [75, 79, 80]. Low values of CEA have been found in the urine [76], feces [81], and plasma [77] of apparently healthy control subjects. CEA has also been reported in meconium [82] and in the sputum of patients with cystic fibrosis and asthma [83].

CURRENT CLINICAL USEFULNESS OF CEA ASSAYS

It is obvious that much work remains to be done regarding the exact nature and chemical structure of CEA in normal and tumor tissue, the properties of CEA bound in tissue and released into the circulation in different diseases, and the correlation of CEA with the extent of diseases. The CEA assay procedure is, at present, limited as a diagnostic tool; however, it is of value as a presumptive diagnostic test. The CEA assay procedure will not screen out all patients with cancer; a positive result is seen in many non-neoplastic diseases.

In its present form, the major value of CEA assay is that it may be used to monitor cancer patients on therapy. The test can be used to detect recurrences of tumors, since the reappearance of CEA may indicate renewed tumor activity. Serial assays of CEA along with the quantitative levels of CEA may be helpful in the differentiation of cancer of the bowel from benign inflammatory conditions. Patients with inflammatory disease of the bowel may have a transient CEA elevation that disappears with remission [84–86].

REFERENCES

1. Herberman, R. B. Immunological Reactions of Experimental Animals to Tumor Associated Cell Surface Antigens. In H. L. Ioachim (Ed.), *Pathobiology Annals*. New York: Appleton-Century-Crofts, 1973.
2. Anderson, N. G., and Coggins, J. H., Jr. *Proceedings of the First Conference and Workshop on Embryonic and Fetal Antigens in Cancer*. Springfield, Va.: National Technical Information Service, 1971.
3. Gold, P. Antigenic reversion in human cancer. *Annu. Rev. Med.* 22: 85, 1971.

4. Ting, C. C., Lavrin, D. H., Shiu, G., and Herberman, R. B. Expression of fetal antigen in tumor cells. *Proc. Natl. Acad. Sci. U.S.A.* 69:1664, 1972.
5. Stonehill, E. H., and Bendich, A. Retrogenetic expression: The reappearance of embryonal antigens in cancer cells. *Nature* 228:370, 1970.
6. Alexander, P. Foetal "antigens" in cancer. *Nature* 235:137, 1972.
7. Lawrence, D. J. R., and Munro Neville, A. Foetal antigens and their role in the diagnosis and clinical management of human neoplasms: A review. *Br. J. Cancer* 26:335, 1972.
8. Abelev, G. I. Production of embryonal serum globulin by hepatomas: Review of experimental and clinical data. *Cancer Res.* 28:1344, 1968.
9. Alpert, M. E., Uriel, J., and De Nechaud, B. Alpha$_1$ fetoglobulin in the diagnosis of human hepatoma. *N. Engl. J. Med.* 278:984, 1968.
10. Abelev, G. I. Alpha foetoprotein in ontogenesis and its association with malignant tumors. *Adv. Cancer Res.* 14:295, 1971.
11. Buffe, D., Rimbaut, C., Lemerle, J., Schweisguth, O., and Burtin, P. Présence d'une ferroproteine d'origine tissulaire l'α_2 H dans le sérum des enfants porteurs de tumeurs. *Int. J. Cancer.* 5:85, 1970.
12. Martin, J. P., Charlionet, R., and Ropartz, C. The presence of α_2 H in sera from patients with malignant haemopathies and cirrhosis. *Rev. Eur. Etud. Clin.* 26:266, 1971.
13. Takahashi, A., Yachi, A., Anzai, T., and Wada, T. Presence of a unique serum protein in sera obtained from patients with neoplastic diseases and in embryonic and neonatal sera. *Clin. Chim. Acta* 17:5, 1967.
14. Wada, T., Anzai, T., Yachi, A., Takahashi, A., and Sakamoto, S. Incidence of three different fetal proteins in sera of patients with primary hepatoma. In H. Peeters (Ed.), *Protides of the Biological Fluids,* Vol. 18. New York: Elsevier, 1971.
15. Fishman, W. H., Inglis, N. R., Green, S., Anstiss, C. L., and Gosh, M. K. Immunology and biochemistry of Regan isoenzyme of alkaline phosphatase in human cancer. *Nature* 219:697, 1968.
16. Fishman, W. H. Immunologic and biochemical approaches to alkaline phosphatase isoenzyme analysis: The Regan isoenzyme. *Ann. N.Y. Acad. Sci.* 166:745, 1969.
17. Fishman, W. H., Inglis, N. R., and Green, S. Regan isoenzyme: A carcinoplacental antigen. *Cancer Res.* 31:1054, 1974.
18. Häkkinen, I. P. T., Korhoren, L. K., and Saxé, L. The time of appearance and distribution of sulphoglycoprotein antigens in the human fetal alimentary canal. *Int. J. Cancer* 3:582, 1968.
19. Häkkinen, I. P. T., and Viikari, S. Occurrence of fetal sulfoglycoprotein antigen in the gastric juice of patients with gastric disease. *Ann. Surg.* 169:277, 1969.
20. Häkkinen, I. P. T. Immunological relationships of the carcinoembryonic antigen and the fetal sulfoglycoprotein antigen. *Immunochemistry* 9:1115, 1972.
21. Edynak, E. M., Old, L. J., Vrana, M., and Lardis, M. P. A fetal antigen in human tumors detected by an antibody in the serum of cancer patients. *Proc. Am. Assoc. Cancer Res.* 11:22, 1970.
22. Edynak, E. M., Old, L. J., Vrana, M., and Lardis, M. P. A fetal antigen associated with human neoplasia. *N. Engl. J. Med.* 286:1178, 1972.
23. Gold, P., and Freedman, S. O. Demonstration of tumor specific antigens in human colonic carcinomata by immunological tolerance and absorption techniques. *J Exp. Med.* 121:439, 1965.

24. Gold, P., and Freedman, S. O.   Specific carcinoembryonic antigens of the human digestive system. *J. Exp. Med.* 122:467, 1965.
25. Kang, K. Y., Higashino, K., Takahashi, Y., Hasinotsume, M., and Yamamura, Y.   α-Fetoprotein in ill infants. *N. Engl. J. Med.* 287:48, 1972.
26. Smith, J. B.   Occurrence of alpha-fetoprotein in acute viral hepatitis. *Int. J. Cancer* 8:421, 1971.
27. Purves, L. R., Bersohn, I., and Geddes, E. W.   Serum alpha-fetoprotein and primary cancer of the liver in man. *Cancer* 25:1261, 1970.
28. Smith, J. B.   Alpha-fetoprotein: Occurrence in certain malignant diseases and review of clinical applications. *Med. Clin. North Am.* 54:797, 1970.
29. Smith, J. B., and O'Neill, R. T.   Alpha-fetoprotein: Occurrence in germinal cell and liver malignancies. *Am. J. Med.* 51:767, 1971.
30. Purtilo, D. T., and Yunis, E. J.   α-Fetoprotein: Its immunofluorescent localization in human fetal liver and hepatoma. *Lab. Invest.* 25:291, 1971.
31. Alpert, E., Pinn, V. W., and Isselbacher, K. J.   Alpha-fetoprotein in a patient with gastric carcinoma metastatic to the liver. *N. Engl. J. Med.* 285:1058, 1971.
32. Kozower, M., Fawaz, K. A., Miller, H. M., and Kaplan, M. M.   Positive alpha-fetoglobulin in a case of gastric carcinoma. *N. Engl. J. Med.* 285:1059, 1971.
33. Mehlman, D. J., Buckley, B. H., and Wiernik, P. H.   Serum alpha$_1$-fetoprotein with gastric and prostatic carcinoma. *N. Engl. J. Med.* 285:1060, 1971.
34. Purves, L. R., and Geddes, E. W.   A more sensitive test for alpha-fetoprotein. *Lancet* 1:47, 1972.
35. Stillman, A., and Zamcheck, M.   Recent advances in immunological diagnosis of digestive tract cancer. *Am. J. Dig. Dis.* 15:1003, 1970.
36. Purves, L. R., MacNab, M., and Bersohn, I.   Serum alpha-fetoprotein. I. Immunodiffusion and immunoassay results in cases of primary cancer of the liver. *S. Afr. Med. J.* 42:1138, 1968.
37. Ruoslahti, E., and Seppala, M.   Studies of carcino-fetal proteins. III. Development of a radioimmunoassay for α-fetoprotein. Demonstration of α-fetoprotein in serum of healthy human adults. *Int. J. Cancer* 8:374, 1971.
38. Ruoslahti, E., and Seppala, M.   Normal and increased alpha-fetoprotein in neoplastic and in non-neoplastic liver disease. *Lancet* 2:278, 1972.
38a. Alpert, E., and Isselbacher, K. J.   Beta-fetoprotein: Identification as normal liver ferritin. *Lancet* 1:43, 1973.
39. Nathanson, L., and Fishman, W. H.   New observations on the Regan isoenzyme of alkaline phosphatase in cancer patients. *Cancer* 27:1388, 1971.
40. Kang, K. Y., Higashino, K., Hashinotsume, M., Takahashi, Y., Aoki, T., Tsubura, E., and Yamamura, Y.   Production of placental type alkaline phosphatase isoenzyme by lung cancer tissue. *Gann* 63:1388, 1971.
41. Stolbach, L. L., Krant, M. J., and Fishman, W. H.   Ectopic production of an alkaline phosphatase isoenzyme in patients with cancer. *N. Engl. J. Med.* 281:757, 1969.
42. Warnock, M. L., and Reisman, R.   Variant alkaline phosphatase in human hepatocellular cancers. *Clin. Chim. Acta* 24:5, 1969.
43. Usategui-Gomez, M., Yeager, F., and Fernandez de Castro, F.   A sensi-

tive immunochemical method for the determination of Regan isoenzyme in serum. *Cancer Res.* 33:1574, 1973.

44. Avrameas, S., and Ternynck, T.   Biologically active water insoluble protein polymers. *J. Biol. Chem.* 242:1651, 1967.
45. Usategui-Gomez, M., Yeager, F., and Fernandez de Castro, F.   Unpublished data, 1972.
46. Gold, P., Gold, M., and Freedman, S. O.   Cellular location of carcinoembryonic antigens of the human digestive system. *Cancer Res.* 28:1331, 1968.
47. Von Kleist, S., and Burtin, P.   Localization cellulaire d'un antigen embryonnaire de tumeurs coliques humaines. *Int. J. Cancer* 4:874, 1969.
48. Gold, P., Krupey, J., and Ansari, H.   Position of the carcinoembryonic antigen on the human digestive system in ultrastructure of the tumor cell surface. *J. Natl. Cancer Inst.* 45:219, 1970.
49. Burtin, P., Sabine, M. C., and Chavanel, G.   Presence of carcinoembryonic antigen in children's colonic mucosa. *Int. J. Cancer* 10:72, 1972.
50. Coligan, J. E., Lautenschleger, J. T., Egan, M. L., and Todd, C. W.   Isolation and characterization of carcinoembryonic antigen. *Immunochemistry* 9:377, 1972.
51. Krupey, J., Wilson, T., Freedman, S. O., and Gold, P.   The preparation of purified carcinoembryonic antigen of the human digestive system from large quantities of tumor tissue. *Immunochemistry* 9:617, 1972.
52. Coligan, J. E., Henkart, P. A., Todd, C. W., and Terry, W. D.   Heterogeneity of the carcinoembryonic antigen. *Immunochemistry* 10:591, 1973.
53. Terry, W. D., Henkart, P. A., Coligan, J. E., and Todd, C. W.   Structural studies of the major glycoprotein in preparations with carcinoembryonic antigen activity. *J. Exp. Med.* 136:200, 1972.
54. Banjo, C., Gold, P., Freedman, S. O., and Krupey, J.   Immunologically active heterosaccharides of carcinoembryonic antigen of human digestive system. *Nature (New Biol.)* 238:183, 1972.
55. Mach, J. P., and Pusztaszeri, G.   Carcinoembryonic antigen (CEA): Demonstration of a partial identity between CEA and a normal glycoprotein. *Immunochemistry* 9:1031, 1972.
56. Von Kleist, S., Chavenel, G., and Burtin, P.   Identification of an antigen from normal human tissue that cross reacts with the carcinoembryonic antigen. *Proc. Natl. Acad. Sci. U.S.A.* 69:2492, 1972.
57. Gold, P.   Circulating antibodies against carcinoembryonic antigens of the human digestive system. *Cancer* 20:1663, 1967.
58. Collatz, E., Von Kleist, S., and Burtin, P.   Further investigations of circulating antibodies in colon cancer patients: On the autoantigenicity of the carcinoembryonic antigen. *Int. J. Cancer* 8:298, 1971.
59. Von Kleist, S., and Burtin, P.   On the specificity of autoantibodies present in colon cancer patients. *Immunology* 10:507, 1966.
60. LoGerfo, P., Herter, F. P., and Bennett, S. J.   Absence of circulating antibodies to carcinoembryonic antigen in patients with gastrointestinal malignancies. *Int. J. Cancer* 9:344, 1972.
61. Gold, J. M., Freedman, S. O., and Gold, P.   Human anti-CEA antibodies detected by radioimmunoelectrophoresis. *Nature (New Biol.)* 239:60, 1972.
62. Lejtenji, M. C., Freedman, S. O., and Gold, P.   Response of lymphocytes from patients with gastrointestinal cancer to the carcinoembryonic antigen of the human digestive system. *Cancer* 28:115, 1971.

63. Hellström, I., Hellström, K. E., and Shepard, T. H. Cell-mediated immunity against antigens common to human colonic carcinomas and fetal gut epithelium. *Int. J. Cancer* 6:346, 1970.

64. Hollingshead, A. C., Glew, D. H., Bunnay, B., Gold, P., and Herberman, R. B. Skin reactive soluble antigen from intestinal cancer cell membranes and relationship to carcinoembryonic antigens. *Lancet* 1:1191, 1970.

65. Hollingshead, A. C., McWright, C. G., Alford, T. C., Glew, D. H., Gold, P., and Herberman, R. B. Separation of skin reactive intestinal cancer antigen from the carcinoembryonic antigen of Gold. *Science* 177:887, 1972.

66. Burtin, P., Martin, E., Sabine, M. C., and Von Kleist, S. Immunological study of polyps of the colon. *J. Natl. Cancer Inst.* 48:25, 1972.

67. Lange, R. D., Chernoff, A., and Collman, R. I. Experience with a Hemagglutination Inhibition Test for Carcinoembryonic Antigen. In M. G. Anderson and J. H. Coggin (Eds.), *Proceedings of the First Conference and Workshop on Embryonic and Fetal Antigens in Cancer.* Springfield, Va.: National Technical Information Service, 1971.

68. Thompson, D. M. P., Krupey, J., Freedman, S. O., and Gold, P. The radioimmunoassay of circulating carcinoembryonic antigen of the human digestive tract. *Proc. Natl. Acad. Sci. U.S.A.* 64:161, 1969.

69. Gold, P. Tumor specific antigen in GI cancer. *Hosp. Prac.* 7:85, 1972.

70. Chu, T. M., and Reynoso, G. Evaluation of a new radioimmunoassay method for carcinoembryonic antigen in plasma with use of zirconyl phosphate gel. *Clin. Chem.* 18:918, 1972.

71. LoGerfo, P., Krupey, J., and Hansen, H. J. Demonstration of an antigen common to several varieties of neoplasia. *N. Engl. J. Med.* 285:138, 1971.

72. Egan, M. L., Lautenschleger, J. T., Coligan, J. E., and Todd, C. W. Radioimmune assay of carcinoembryonic antigen. *Immunochemistry* 9:289, 1972.

73. Egan, M., Coligan, J. E., and Todd, C. W. Radioimmunoassay for the diagnosis of human cancer. *Cancer* 34:1504, 1974.

74. MacSween, J. M., Warner, M. L., Bankhurst, A. D., and MacKay, I. R. Carcinoembryonic antigen in whole serum. *Br. J. Cancer* 26:356, 1972.

75. Lawrence, D. J. R., Stevens, V., Bettelheim, R., Darcy, D., Leese, C., Turberville, C., Alexander, P., Johns, E. W., and Neville, A. M. Role of plasma carcinoembryonic antigen in diagnosis of gastrointestinal, mammary, and bronchial carcinoma. *Br. Med. J.* 2:605, 1972.

76. Hall, R. R., Lawrence, D. J. R., Darcy, D., Stevens, V., James, R., Roberts, S., and Neville, A. M. Carcinoembryonic antigen in the urine of patients with urothelial carcinoma. *Br. Med. J.* 2:609, 1972.

77. Chu, T. M., Hansen, H. J., and Reynoso, G. Demonstration of carcinoembryonic antigen in normal human plasma. *Nature* 238:152, 1972.

78. Reynoso, G., Chu, T. M., Holyoke, D., Cohen, E., Nemoto, T., Wang, J. J., Chuang, J., Guinan, P., and Murphy, G. P. Carcinoembryonic antigen in patients with different cancers. *J.A.M.A.* 220:361, 1972.

79. LeBel, J. S., Deodhar, S. D., and Brown, C. H. Evaluation of a radioimmunoassay for carcinoembryonic antigen of the human digestive system. *Cleve. Clin. Q.* 39:25, 1972.

80. Zamcheck, N., Moore, T. C., Dhar, P., and Kupchick, H. Immunologic diagnosis and prognosis of human digestive tract cancer: Carcinoembryonic antigens. *N. Engl. J. Med.* 286:83, 1972.

81. Freed, D. L. J., and Taylor, G.   Carcinoembryonic antigen in faeces. *Br. Med. J.* 1:85, 1972.
82. Goldenberg, D. M., Tchilinguirian, N. G. D., Hansen, H. J., and Vandernoorde, J. P.   Carcinoembryonic antigen present in meconium: The basis of a possible new diagnostic test of fetal distress. *Am. J. Obstet. Gynecol.* 113:66, 1972.
83. Abeyounis, C. J., and Milgrom, F.   Studies on carcinoembryonic antigen. *Int. Arch. Allergy Appl. Immunol.* 43:30, 1972.
84. Moore, T. L., Kupchick, H. Z., Marcon, N., and Zarncheck, M.   Carcinoembryonic antigen assay in cancer of the colon and pancreas and other digestive tract disorders. *Am. J. Dig. Dis.* 16:1, 1971.
85. Moore, T. L., Kantrowitz, P. A., and Zamcheck, N.   Carcinoembryonic antigen (CEA) in inflammatory bowel disease. *J.A.M.A.* 222:944, 1972.
86. Rule, A. H., Straus, E., Van de Voorde, J., and Janowitz, H. D.   Tumor associated (CEA reacting) antigen in patients with inflammatory bowel disease. *N. Engl. J. Med.* 287:24, 1972.

Appendix

Serum Proteins—Synopsis of Properties and Characteristics

Protein (synonyms)	Molecular Weight	Peptide Content	Normal Adult Concentration (mg/100 ml serum) Mean Value	Range	Biological Functions (inherited variants)	Abnormalities (hereditary deficiency)
1. Prealbumin	50,000	99%	25	10–40	Thyroxin and retinol binding	Reduced in severe liver diseases
2. Albumin	65,000	100%	4400	3500–5500	Osmotic function; transport of ions, pigments, etc., protein reserve (bisalbuminemia)	Reduced in liver disorders, nephrotic syndrome, etc. (analbuminemia)
3. α_1-Acid glycoprotein (orosomucoid, α_1-seromucoid)	44,100	62%	90	55–140	(Electrophoretic polymorphism) *[handwritten: INACTIVATES PROGESTERONE BY BINDING; ↑ in last trimester pregnancy]*	Increased in chronic inflammatory conditions, rheumatoid arthritis, malignant neoplasms, etc.
4. α_1-Lipoprotein (high-density lipoprotein; LP-A)	180,000–350,000	42%–55%	360	290–770	Transport of lipids, hormones, etc.	Reduced in liver diseases (Tangier disease)
5. α_1-Antitrypsin	54,000	86%	290	200–400	Proteinase inhibitor (trypsin, chymotrypsin, kallikrein etc.) (Electrophoretic polymorphism)	Increased in inflammatory conditions (hypoalpha-1-antitrypsinemia in emphysema)

				5–10 (plasma)	Proenzyme of thrombin	Decreased in liver diseases, anticoagulant therapy
6. Prothrombin (coagulation factor II)	~60,000	—	—	5–10 (plasma)	Proenzyme of thrombin	Decreased in liver diseases, anticoagulant therapy
7. α_1-B-Glycoprotein (easily precipitable α_1-glycoprotein)	50,000	89%	22	15–30	—	—
8. Transcortin	55,700	86%	~7	—	Binding and transport of cortisol	(Syndrome with low cortisol-binding capacity)
9. Thyroxin-binding globulin	36,500	85%	1–2	—	Thyroxin binding	(Familial deficiency of TBG)
10. α_1-T-Glycoprotein (tryptophan-poor α_1-glycoprotein)	~60,000	87%	8	5–12	—	—
11. α_1-Antichymotrypsin (α_1X-glycoprotein)	68,000	73%	45	30–60	Chymotrypsin inhibitor	Increased in inflammatory conditions
12. 9,5S-α_1-Glycoprotein (α_1M-glycoprotein)	308,000	—	5.5	3–8	—	—
13. Retinol-binding protein	21,000	100%	4	3–6	Binding and transport of retinol (vitamin A)	—
14. α_1-Fetoprotein	~68,000	96%	<0.001 10[a]	— 1–40[a]	—	Significantly increased in hepatoma and pregnancy
15. Gc-Globulin (group-specific component)	50,800	96%	40	20–55	(Electrophoretic polymorphism)	Decreased in severe liver diseases

[a] Value for newborn infants.

Serum Proteins—Synopsis of Properties and Characteristics (*Continued*)

Protein (synonyms)	Molecular Weight	Peptide Content	Normal Adult Concentration (mg/100 ml serum)		Biological Functions (inherited variants)	Abnormalities (hereditary deficiency)
			Mean Value	Range		
16. Inter-α_1-trypsin inhibitor	~160,000	91%	45	20–70	Proteinase inhibitor (trypsin)	—
17. Antithrombin III	~65,000	85%	23	17–30	Thrombin inhibitor	Decreased in liver diseases and with oral contraceptives
18. Ceruloplasmin	151,000	89%	35	15–60	Copper binding; oxidase	Increased in malignancies and during pregnancy (decreased in Wilson's disease)
19. Zn-α_2-Glycoprotein	41,000	85%	5	2–15	—	—
20. α_2HS-Glycoprotein (Ba-α_2-glycoprotein)	49,000	87%	60	40–85	—	Decreased in malignancies
21. C1s Inactivator (α_2-neuroaminoglycoprotein, C1-esterase inhibitor)	104,000	57%	24	15–35	Inhibitor for C1r, C1s, plasminogen, kallikrein, and coagulation factor XII	(Decreased in angioneurotic edema)
22. C1s-Component (C1-esterase)	80,000	—	3	2–4	Subunit of C1-esterase	—

	Molecular weight				Function	Clinical significance
23. C9-Component	79,000	–	–	0.1–1	Complement factor	–
24. Histidine-rich 3.8S-α_2-glycoprotein	58,500	–	9	5–15	–	–
25. Erythropoietin	30,000	–	–	–	Erythropoiesis	–
26. Haptoglobin 1-1 type 2-1 type 2-2 type	100,000 80,000 120,000 160,000	81%	170 235 190	100–220 160–300 120–260	Hemoglobin-binding peroxidase (Polymorphism; Hp 1-1, 2-1, 2-2)	Decreased in liver diseases and hemolytic anemias. Increased in inflammatory conditions (hypohaptoglobinemia)
27. α_2AP-Glycoprotein (Xh)	~300,000	–	<0.5	–	–	Increased in inflammatory conditions and pregnancy
28. α_2-Macroglobulin	820,000	92%	Male: 240 Female: 290	150–350 175–420	Proteinase (plasmin, etc.) inhibitor Hormone-binding	Significantly increased in nephrotic syndrome; increased in liver diseases and diabetes mellitus
29. Serum cholinesterase (pseudocholinesterase)	348,000	76%	~1	0.5–1.5	(At least 5 phenotypes)	–
30. Plasminogen (profibrinolysin)	81,000	–	~20	10–30	Proenzymes of plasmin (fibrinolysin) Proactivator	Reduced during fibrinolytic treatment
31. 8S-α_3-Glycoprotein	220,000	–	4	3–5	–	–

Serum Proteins—Synopsis of Properties and Characteristics (*Continued*)

Protein (synonyms)	Molecular Weight	Peptide Content	Normal Adult Concentration (mg/100 ml serum)		Biological Functions (inherited variants)	Abnormalities (hereditary deficiency)
			Mean Value	Range		
32. β-Lipoprotein, LP-B (low-density lipoprotein, LD-B)	2,400,000	~22%	Male: 440[b] Female: 400[b]	220–740[b] 190–600[b]	Transport of lipids, cholesterol, hormones, etc. (polymorphism: Ag, Lp, Ld)	Increased in nephrotic syndrome (abeta-lipoproteinemia)
33. Hemopexin (β1B-globulin)	80,000	77%	75	50–115	Heme-binding protein	Decreased in hemolytic anemias
34. C1r-Component	150,000	—	—	—	Complement factor	–
35. C2-Component	117,000	—	—	1–3	Complement factor	(Familial deficiency of C2)
36. C3-Component (β1C-globulin)	185,000	97%	82[c]	55–120[c]	Complement factor (in serum, converted into C3a [anaphylatoxin], C3c [β1A-globulin], C3d [α2D-globulin]) (Electrophoretic polymorphism)	Decreased in active immunological diseases (glomerulonephritis, lupus erythematosus, etc.)
37. C4-Component (β1E-globulin)	230,000	—	30	20–50	Complement factor	Decreased in active immunological disorders

	Mol. wt.		Conc. (mg)	Normal range	Function	Clinical significance
38. C5-Component (β_1F-globulin)	200,000	81%	8	4–15	Complement factor (in serum, converted into C5a [anaphylatoxin], etc.)	—
39. Transferrin (siderophilin)	90,000	95%	295	200–400	Iron-binding and transport (Electrophoretic polymorphism)	Decreased in nephrotic syndrome, malignancies, and inflammatory conditions
40. Fibrinogen (coagulation factor I)	341,000	97%	300 (plasma)	200–450 (plasma)	Clottable protein (in serum degradation products D and E)	Decreased in liver diseases, hyperfibrinolysis (afibrinogenemia)
41. AHG (coagulation factor VIII)-associated antigen	—	—	—	—	Transport of coagulation factor VIII (von Willebrand factor?)	(von Willebrand-Jürgens syndrome)
42. Fibrin-stabilizing factor (coagulation factor XIII)	340,000	95%	—	1–4 (plasma)	Fibrin cross-linking (transamidase) (In serum, only subunit S)	Decreased levels associated with impaired wound healing
43. C-reactive protein (C-RP)	135,000–140,000	100%	<0.8	—	Phagocytosis-promoting activity	Significantly increased in acute inflammatory conditions
44. β_2-Glycoprotein 1	40,000	81%	20	15–30	—	(Familial deficiency of β_2-glycoprotein 1)
45. C3-Proactivator (glycine-rich β-glycoprotein, properdin factor B)	—	89%	25	10–45	Proenzyme of C3 activator (β_2-glycoprotein II)	—

b Value is age-dependent.
c Measured as C3c (β_1A-globulin).

Serum Proteins—Synopsis of Properties and Characteristics (*Continued*)

Protein (synonyms)	Molecular Weight	Peptide Content	Normal Adult Concentration (mg/100 ml serum)		Biological Functions (Inherited Variants)	Abnormalities (Hereditary Deficiency)
			Mean Value	Range		
46. β_2-Glycoprotein III	35,000	90%	10	5–15	—	—
47. β_2-Microglobulin	11,600	—	—	0.1–0.2	Related to Fc fragments and HL-A antigens	—
48. C1q-Component (11S-component)	400,000	90%	19	10–25	Subunit of C1	Decreased in lupus erythematosus
49. C6-Component	95,000	—	—	1–7	Complement factor	—
50. C7-Component	100,000	—	—	—	Complement factor	—
51. C8-Component	153,000	—	—	—	Complement factor	—
52. Properdin	223,000	—	—	—	Complement activation (alternate pathway)	—
53. IgG (γG-globulin; γ_2, 7S-γ-globulin)	150,000	97%	1250 (144 IU/ml)	800–1800[b] (92–207 IU/ml)	Antibodies (structural polymorphism: Gm, Inv)	Polyclonal increase in chronic liver diseases, chronic infections. Monoclonal increases in IgG myeloma. (Decreased in antibody deficiency syndromes; ataxia-telangiectasia)

(handwritten annotation near row 47: ↑ SJÖGRENS in serum & saliva)

54. IgA (γA-globulin; γ_1A-, β_2A-globulin)	160,000 and polymers	92%	210 (125 IU/ml)	90–450[b] (54–268 IU/ml)	Antibodies, especially in secretions. (Structural polymorphism: Inv)	Polyclonal increase in chronic liver disease, chronic infections, etc. Monoclonal increase in IgA myeloma. (Decrease in antibody deficiency syndromes; ataxia-telangiectasia)
55. IgM (γM-globulin; β_2M-, 19S-γ-globulin)	900,000 and polymers	89%	Male: 125 (144 IU/ml) Female: 160 (184 IU/ml)	60–250[b] (69–287 IU/ml) 70–280 (80–322 IU/ml)	Antibodies, e.g., isoagglutinins. (Structural polymorphism: Inv)	Polyclonal increase in chronic infection, liver diseases (trypanosomiasis, etc.). Monoclonal increases in Waldenström's macroglobulinemia. (Decrease in antibody deficiency syndrome)
56. IgD (γD-globulin)	170,000	88%	3	0–15[b]	Antibodies?	Monoclonal increase in IgD myeloma
57. IgE (γE-globulin)	190,000	89%	~300 ng/ml	10–10,000 ng/ml[b] (5–500 IU/ml)	Antibodies (Reagins, Prausnitz-Küstner antibodies)	Polyclonal increase in allergic diseases. Monoclonal increase in IgE myeloma.
58. Lysozyme (muramidase)	~15,000	100%	12 μg/ml	7–20 μg/ml	Bacteriolysis	Marked increase in monocytic leukemia, certain kidney diseases, etc.

b Value is age dependent.
Adapted from Dettelbach, H., and Ritzmann, S. E. (Eds.), *Lab Synopsis*, Vol. 2 (2nd ed.). Somerville, N.J.: Behring Diagnostics, 1969.

Index

537

in immunoglobulin abnormalities, 17–22, 388
indications for, 22–24
microzone, technique of, 3–5
normal values in, 8
procedures in, 4
of protease inhibitors, 244, 245
of serum proteins, 3–24
sources of error in, 6
total serum protein determinations in, 8–11
of urine proteins, 4
zone, 3
Embryonic and fetal proteins, in carcinogenesis, 513–521
Encephalopathies, and immunoglobulins in CSF, 78
Endocarditis, subacute bacterial, rheumatoid factor in, 323
Enteropathies, protein-losing, 197–203
acute transient, 203
hypogammaglobulinemia in, 18, 19
immunoglobulin loss in, 401–402
Enzymes
immunoassays with, 161–168
advantages of, 165
applications of, 165–168
competitive-binding analysis in, 162–163
disadvantages in, 165
homogeneous, 164
for hormones and haptens, 168
for plasma proteins, 166–168
"sandwich" technique in, 161–162
sources of error in, 165
immunoenzymatic histochemical assays, 149–158
lysosomal, and acute-phase response, 337–338
protease inhibitors, abnormalities of, 243–258
Epithelial malignancies, with monoclonal gammopathies, 439
Erythrocyte sedimentation rate, 332–334
in monoclonal gammopathies, 434
Erythropoietin, properties of, 531
Estrogen. *See also* Contraceptives, oral
and ceruloplasmin levels, 336
and α_2-macroglobulin levels, 253, 254

Fab fragments, 373–376
Factor I, properties of, 533
Factor II, properties of, 529
Factor VIII, properties of, 533
Fc fragment, 373–376
Fd fragments, 375, 376
Felty's syndrome
polyclonal gammopathy with, 19

ultracentrifugation in, 117
α_2-H Ferroprotein, 515–517
Fetal proteins, in carcinogenesis, 513–521
α_1-Fetoprotein, 514–515
enzyme immunoassay of, 166–168
Ouchterlony double-diffusion assay of, 90
radial immunodiffusion of, 67
β-S Fetoprotein, 517
γ-Fetoprotein, 518
Fever, 331
Fibrin-stabilizing factor, properties of, 533
Fibrinogen, 331
normal serum values, 533
properties of, 333, 336–337, 533
radial immunodiffusion of, 67
Fluorescent antibody assays, 133–146
application of, 142–146
for autoantibodies, 143
of biopsy material, for immune complexes, 130–132, 145
competitive inhibition method in, 138
complement-staining method in, 138–140
direct method in, 136
equipment for, 140–142
in immune-complex diseases, 130–132, 143–145
indirect method in, 137–138
for antinuclear antibodies, 314–315
in microbiology, 143
sources of error in, 142
Fungus diseases, polyclonal gammopathy with, 19

Gammopathies
monoclonal, 87, 386, 419–466
ABO blood groups in, 438
albumin levels in, 436
amyloidosis with, 440, 422, 445–448
in animals, 457–458
and antibody activity of M proteins, 461–463
antibody response patterns in, 463–466
anticomplementary activity in, 436
asymptomatic, 430, 433–434
bacterial infections with, 439
Bence Jones proteins in, 19, 45, 424, 437–438, 503–504
bone marrow examination in, 434–436
cellular kinetics in, 448–451
chromosomal aberrations in, 438, 459–460
cold agglutinins in, 440–442

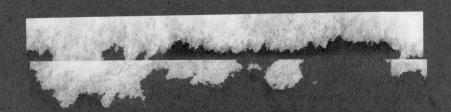